ESSENTIALS OF ORTHOPAEDICS AND APPLIED PHYSIOTHERAPY

Mary Bayonla Banks

ALLIED HEALTH PRESS

Essentials of Orthopaedics and Applied Physiotherapy

Author: **Mary Bayonla Banks**

Allied Health Press
4164 Lakeshore Road
Burlington ON L7L 1A4
Canada
www.alliedhealthpress.com
Email: orders@arclereducation.com

ISBN: 978-1-77956-816-8

ABOUT THE AUTHOR

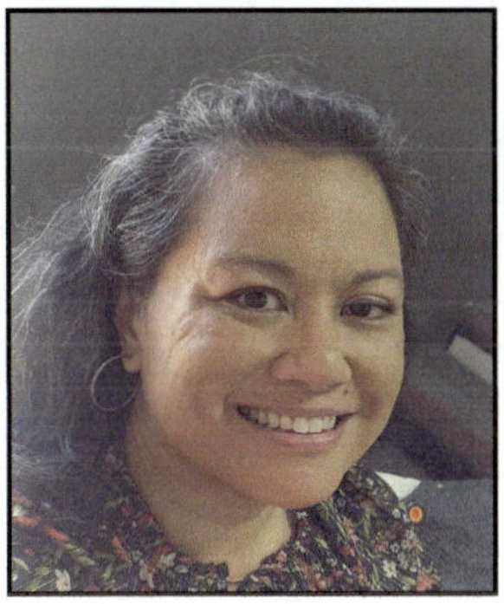

Mary Bayonla Banks is a dedicated physical therapist with a diverse background in pediatrics both school-based and outpatient, geriatrics, and orthopedics. She is also a retired secondary school athletic trainer. She currently works as a staff physical therapist in the Virginia Beach City Public School system where she works with special needs children ranging from ages 2-22 focusing on access to educational program through working on acquisition of gross motor milestones and locomotor skills, as well as attaining and maintaining independent functional mobility. She also works with the geriatric population by providing high quality outpatient orthopedic as well as aquatic physical therapy. Mary attended the Medical Campus of Virginia Commonwealth University in Richmond, VA where she earned her Doctor of Physical Therapy degree in 2004.

Brief Table of Contents

1. Introduction to Orthopedics and Physiotherapy	1
2. Musculoskeletal Injuries and Management	35
3. Fractures and Dislocations	69
4. Soft Tissue Injuries	105
5. Orthopedic Conditions	137
6. Spinal Disorders	169
7. Sports Injury Assessment and Diagnosis	201
8. Pediatric Orthopedics	233
9. Geriatric Orthopedics	267
10. Orthopedic Infections	303
11. Tumors of Bones and Soft Tissues	335
12. Post-Surgical Rehabilitation	369
13. Neurological Disorders with Orthopedic Implications	411
14. Pain Management in Orthopedic Physiotherapy	449
15. Recent Advances in Orthopedics and Physiotherapy	481
Index	515

Detailed Table of Contents

List of Figures xv

Preface xxv

CHAPTER 1

Introduction to Orthopedics and Physiotherapy 1

Introduction 1

1.1. Common Orthopedic Conditions 5

1.1.1. Fractures and Their Classifications 6

1.1.2. Arthritis and Joint Disorders 7

1.1.3. Sports Injuries and Their Management 8

1.2. Principles of Physiotherapy 9

1.2.1. Definition and Role of Physiotherapy 10

1.2.2. Techniques and Modalities Used in Physiotherapy 10

1.2.3. Importance of Physiotherapy in Rehabilitation 11

1.3. The Interdisciplinary Approach 12

1.3.1. Collaboration Between Orthopedic Surgeons and Physiotherapists 13

1.3.2. Role of Other Healthcare Professionals in Orthopedic Care 14

1.3.3. Benefits of an Interdisciplinary Approach for Patient Outcomes 15

1.4. Diagnostic Tools in Orthopedics 16

1.4.1. Imaging Techniques (X-rays, MRIs, CT scans) 17

1.4.2. Physical Examination Methods 18

1.4.3. Importance of Accurate Diagnosis in Treatment Planning 18

1.5. Treatment Options in Orthopedics 19

1.5.1. Surgical Interventions and Procedures 20

1.5.2. Non-Surgical Treatment Options (Medications, Braces) 21

1.5.3. Role of Physiotherapy in Post-Operative Care 22

1.6. Current Trends and Innovations 22

1.6.1. Advances in Surgical Techniques and Technology 23

1.6.2. Emerging Therapies in Physiotherapy 24

1.6.3. Future Directions in Orthopedic Research 25

Summary 27

References 30

CHAPTER 2

Musculoskeletal Injuries and Management 35

Introduction 35

2.1. Types of Musculoskeletal Injuries 38

2.1.1. Acute Injuries 39

2.1.2. Chronic Injuries 40

2.1.3. Common Examples (Sprains, Fractures, Tendonitis) 41

2.2. Causes and Risk Factors 42

2.2.1. Sports-Related Injuries 43

2.2.2. Occupational Hazards 44

2.2.3. Lifestyle Factors (Sedentary Behavior, Obesity) 44

2.3. Symptoms and Diagnosis **45**
2.3.1. Common Symptoms (Pain, Swelling, Limited Mobility) 46
2.3.2. Diagnostic Methods (Physical Examination, Imaging Tests) 47
2.3.3. Importance of Early Diagnosis 48
2.4. Treatment Options **49**
2.4.1. Conservative Management (Rest, Ice, Compression, Elevation) 49
2.4.2. Pharmacological Treatments (Pain Relievers, Anti-Inflammatories) 51
2.4.3. Surgical Interventions (When Necessary) 52
2.5. Rehabilitation and Recovery **52**
2.5.1. Role of Physical Therapy 53
2.5.2. Importance of Gradual Return to Activity 54
2.5.3. Psychological Aspects of Recovery 55
2.6. Prevention Strategies **56**
2.6.1. Importance of Warm-Up and Stretching 57
2.6.2. Use of Protective Gear in Sports 58
2.6.3. Education on Proper Techniques and Ergonomics 59
Summary **61**
References **64**

CHAPTER 3

Fractures and Dislocations 69

Introduction **69**
3.1. Types of Fractures **72**
3.1.1. Closed vs. Open Fractures 74
3.1.2. Complete vs. Incomplete Fractures 74
3.1.3. Common Fracture Types (e.g., Transverse, Spiral) 75
3.2. Types of Dislocations **76**
3.2.1. Shoulder Dislocation 77
3.2.2. Finger Dislocation 78
3.2.3. Hip Dislocation 79
3.3. Causes and Risk Factors **80**
3.3.1. Sports-Related Injuries 81
3.3.2. Falls and Accidents 82
3.3.3. Osteoporosis and Age-Related Factors 83
3.4. Symptoms and Diagnosis **84**
3.4.1. Common Symptoms of Fractures 85
3.4.2. Common Symptoms of Dislocations 86
3.4.3. Diagnostic Imaging Techniques (e.g., X-rays, MRIs) 87
3.5. Treatment Options for Fractures **88**
3.5.1. Non-Surgical Treatments (e.g., Casting, Splinting) 89
3.5.2. Surgical Interventions (e.g., Internal Fixation) 90
3.5.3. Rehabilitation and Recovery 91
3.6. Treatment Options for Dislocations **92**
3.6.1. Reduction Techniques 93
3.6.2. Immobilization Methods 94
3.6.3. Physical Therapy and Rehabilitation 95
Summary **96**
References **99**

CHAPTER 4

Soft Tissue Injuries 105

Introduction **105**
4.1. Types of Soft Tissue Injuries **109**
4.1.1. Sprains 110
4.1.2. Strains 111
4.1.3. Contusions 111
4.2. Causes of Soft Tissue Injuries **112**
4.2.1. Sports-Related Activities 113
4.2.2. Accidents and Falls 114
4.2.3. Repetitive Motion and Overuse 115
4.3. Symptoms of Soft Tissue Injuries **115**
4.3.1. Pain and Tenderness 116
4.3.2. Swelling and Inflammation 117
4.3.3. Limited Range of Motion 118
4.4. Diagnosis of Soft Tissue Injuries **119**
4.4.1. Physical Examination 119
4.4.2. Imaging Techniques (X rays, MRI) 120
4.4.3. Patient history and Symptom Assessment 121
4.5. Treatment Options for Soft Tissue Injuries **122**
4.5.1. Rest, Ice, Compression, Elevation (RICE) 123
4.5.2. Physical Therapy and Rehabilitation 124
4.5.3. Surgical Interventions 125
4.6. Prevention of Soft Tissue Injuries **126**
4.6.1. Proper Warm-Up and Stretching Techniques 126

4.6.2. Use of Appropriate Equipment and Gear 128
4.6.3. Education on Body Mechanics and Ergonomics 129
Summary **130**
References **133**

CHAPTER 5

Orthopedic Conditions 137

Introduction **137**
5.1. Osteoarthritis **140**
5.1.1. Definition and Causes 142
5.1.2. Symptoms and Diagnosis 142
5.1.3. Physiotherapy Treatment Options 143
5.2. Rheumatoid Arthritis **144**
5.2.1. Overview of the Condition 145
5.2.2. Impact on Mobility and Daily Activities 146
5.2.3. Role of Physiotherapy in Management 147
5.3. Fractures **148**
5.3.1. Types of Fractures Commonly Treated 149
5.3.2. Healing Process and Rehabilitation 150
5.3.3. Physiotherapy Interventions Post-Fracture 151
5.4. Tendonitis **152**
5.4.1. Common Types of Tendonitis 153
5.4.2. Symptoms and Risk Factors 154
5.4.3. Physiotherapy Approaches for Treatment 155
5.5. Bursitis **156**
5.5.1. Definition and Common Sites Affected 157
5.5.2. Causes and Symptoms 158
5.5.3. Physiotherapy Strategies for Relief 159
5.6. Sports Injuries **160**
5.6.1. Common Sports-Related Orthopedic Injuries 160
5.6.2. Importance of Early Intervention 161
5.6.3. Rehabilitation Techniques in Physiotherapy 162
Summary **164**
References **167**

CHAPTER 6

Spinal Disorders 169

Introduction **169**
6.1. Anatomy of the Spine **172**
6.1.1. Structure of Vertebrae 173
6.1.2. Intervertebral Discs and Their Function 174
6.1.3. Spinal Cord and Nerve Roots 174
6.2. Common Types of Spinal Disorders **175**
6.2.1. Herniated Discs 176
6.2.2. Spinal Stenosis 177
6.2.3. Scoliosis 178
6.3. Causes of Spinal Disorders **179**
6.3.1. Genetic Factors 180
6.3.2. Lifestyle Choices 181
6.3.3. Age Related Changes 182
6.4. Symptoms of Spinal Disorders **182**
6.4.1. Pain and Discomfort 183
6.4.2. Numbness and Tingling 184
6.4.3. Mobility Issues 185
6.5. Diagnosis of Spinal Disorders **186**
6.5.1. Physical Examination 187
6.5.2. Imaging Techniques 187
6.5.3. Neurological Assessments 188
6.6. Treatment Options for Spinal Disorders **189**
6.6.1. Non-Surgical Treatments 190
6.6.2. Surgical Interventions 191
6.6.3. Rehabilitation and Physical Therapy 192
Summary **194**
References **197**

CHAPTER 7

Sports Injury Assessment and Diagnosis 201

Introduction **201**
7.1. Types of Sports Injuries **204**
7.1.1. Acute Injuries 205
7.1.2. Chronic Injuries 206

7.1.3. Common Examples of Sports Injuries 206
7.2. Mechanisms of Injury **207**
7.2.1. Impact Injuries 208
7.2.2. Overuse Injuries 209
7.2.3. Environmental Factors Contributing to Injuries 210
7.3. Initial Assessment Techniques **211**
7.3.1. Visual Inspection 212
7.3.2. Palpation Methods 212
7.3.3. Functional Testing 213
7.4. Diagnostic Tools and Technologies **214**
7.4.1. Imaging Techniques (X-rays, MRIs) 215
7.4.2. Ultrasound in Injury Assessment 216
7.4.3. Role of Diagnostic Software 217
7.5. Role of Medical Professionals **217**
7.5.1. Sports Physicians 218
7.5.2. Physical Therapists 219
7.5.3. Athletic Trainers 220
7.6. Treatment Protocols **221**
7.6.1. Immediate Care and First Aid 222
7.6.2. Rehabilitation Strategies 222
7.6.3. Return-to-Play Criteria 223
Summary **225**
References **228**

CHAPTER 8

Pediatric Orthopedics 233

Introduction **233**
8.1. Developmental Anatomy and Physiology **237**
8.1.1. Growth Patterns in Children 238
8.1.2. Differences Between Pediatric and Adult Musculoskeletal Systems 239
8.1.3. Impact of Growth on Orthopedic Conditions 240
8.2. Common Pediatric Orthopedic Conditions **241**
8.2.1. Congenital Deformities (e.g., Clubfoot, Hip Dysplasia) 241
8.2.2. Acquired Conditions (e.g., Fractures, Scoliosis) 242
8.2.3. Inflammatory and Infectious Conditions (e.g., Osteomyelitis) 243
8.3. Diagnostic Approaches **244**
8.3.1. Clinical Evaluation and History Taking 245
8.3.2. Imaging Techniques (e.g., X-rays, MRI) 246
8.3.3. Role of Physical Examination in Diagnosis 247
8.4. Treatment Modalities **248**
8.4.1. Non-Surgical Interventions (e.g., Physical Therapy, Bracing) 249
8.4.2. Surgical Options and Considerations 250
8.4.3. Post-Operative Care and Rehabilitation 251
8.5. Challenges in Pediatric Orthopedics **252**
8.5.1. Variability in Growth and Development 253
8.5.2. Psychological Impact of Orthopedic Conditions on Children 254
8.5.3. Access to Specialized Care and Resources 254
8.6. Advances in Pediatric Orthopedic Research **255**
8.6.1. Innovations in Surgical Techniques 256
8.6.2. Development of New Treatment Protocols 257
8.6.3. Future Directions in Pediatric Orthopedic Research 258
Summary **260**
References **263**

CHAPTER 9

Geriatric Orthopedics 267

Introduction to Geriatric Orthopedics **267**
9.1. Common Orthopedic Conditions in the Elderly **271**
9.1.1. Osteoporosis and Its Implications 272
9.1.2. Hip Fractures and Their Management 273
9.1.3 Arthritis and Joint Disorders 274
9.2. Risk Factors for Orthopedic Issues in the Elderly **276**
9.2.1. Age-Related Physiological Changes 276
9.2.2. Lifestyle Factors and Their Impact 277
9.2.3. Comorbidities and Their Influence on Orthopedic Health 278
9.3. Diagnostic Approaches in Geriatric Orthopedics **279**
9.3.1. Imaging Techniques and Their Relevance 280
9.3.2. Clinical Assessments and Evaluations 281
9.3.3. Importance of Patient History in Diagnosis 282

9.4. Treatment Options for Geriatric Orthopedic Patients 283
9.4.1. Surgical Interventions and Considerations 284
9.4.2. Non-Surgical Management Strategies 285
9.4.3. Rehabilitation and Physical Therapy 286
9.5. Challenges in Geriatric Orthopedic Care 287
9.5.1. Polypharmacy and Its Effects on Treatment 288
9.5.2. Communication Barriers with Elderly Patients 288
9.5.3. Ethical Considerations in Treatment Decisions 289
9.6. Innovations and Advances in Geriatric Orthopedics 290
9.6.1. Technological Advancements in Surgical Techniques 291
9.6.2. Research on Age-Specific Treatment Protocols 292
9.6.3. Role of Telemedicine in Geriatric Care 293
Summary 295
References 298

CHAPTER 10

Orthopedic Infections 303

Introduction 303
10.1. Types of Orthopedic Infections 306
10.1.1. Osteomyelitis 307
10.1.2. Septic Arthritis 308
10.1.3. Prosthetic Joint Infections 309
10.2. Causes and Risk Factors 310
10.2.1. Bacterial Pathogens 311
10.2.2. Surgical Procedures and Trauma 312
10.2.3. Patient-Related Factors (e.g., Diabetes, Immunocompromised Status) 313
10.3. Symptoms and Diagnosis 314
10.3.1. Common Clinical Symptoms 315
10.3.2. Diagnostic Imaging Techniques 316
10.3.3. Laboratory Tests and Cultures 316
10.4. Treatment Options 317
10.4.1. Antibiotic Therapy 318
10.4.2. Surgical Intervention 319
10.4.3. Adjunctive Therapies (e.g., Hyperbaric Oxygen Therapy) 320
10.5. Complications of Orthopedic Infections 321
10.5.1. Chronic Pain and Disability 322
10.5.2. Amputation Risks 323
10.5.3. Systemic Infections and Sepsis 323
10.6. Prevention Strategies 324
10.6.1. Preoperative Measures 325
10.6.2. Postoperative Care 326
10.6.3. Patient Education and Awareness 327
Summary 328
References 331

CHAPTER 11

Tumors of Bones and Soft Tissues 335

Introduction 335
11.1. Types of Bone Tumors 338
11.1.1. Primary Bone Tumors 338
11.1.2. Secondary (Metastatic) Bone Tumors 339
11.1.3. Benign vs. Malignant Bone Tumors 340
11.2. Types of Soft Tissue Tumors 341
11.2.1. Classification of Soft Tissue Tumors 342
11.2.2. Common Types of Benign Soft Tissue Tumors 343
11.2.3. Common Types of Malignant Soft Tissue Tumors 344
11.3. Symptoms and Diagnosis 345
11.3.1. Common Symptoms Associated with Bone Tumors 346
11.3.2. Diagnostic Imaging Techniques 346
11.3.3. Biopsy Procedures for Tumor Confirmation 347
11.4. Treatment Options for Bone Tumors 348
11.4.1. Surgical Interventions 349
11.4.2. Radiation Therapy 350
11.4.3. Chemotherapy and Targeted Therapies 351
11.5. Treatment Options for Soft Tissue Tumors 352
11.5.1. Surgical Excision 353
11.5.2. Role of Radiation Therapy 354
11.5.3. Emerging Therapies and Clinical Trials 355
11.6. Prognosis and Outcomes 356
11.6.1. Factors Influencing Prognosis 357
11.6.2. Survival Rates for Different Tumor Types 358

11.6.3. Long-Term Effects of Treatment 359
Summary **361**
References **364**

CHAPTER 12

Post-Surgical Rehabilitation 369

Introduction **369**
12.1. Phases of Post-Surgical Rehabilitation **373**
12.1.1. Immediate Post-Operative Phase 373
12.1.2. Early Rehabilitation Phase 374
12.1.3. Advanced Rehabilitation Phase 376
12.2. Assessment and Evaluation **376**
12.2.1. Pre-Rehabilitation Assessment 377
12.2.2. Ongoing Evaluation Techniques 378
12.2.3. Outcome Measurement Tools 379
12.3. Role of Healthcare Professionals **380**
12.3.1. Physical Therapists 381
12.3.2. Occupational Therapists 382
12.3.3. Physicians and Surgeons 382
12.4. Rehabilitation Techniques and Modalities **383**
12.4.1. Manual Therapy 384
12.4.2. Exercise Prescription 385
12.4.3. Modalities for Pain Management 386
12.5. Patient Education and Engagement **387**
12.5.1. Importance of Patient Involvement 388
12.5.2. Strategies for Effective Communication 388
12.5.3. Resources for Patient Education 389
12.6. Psychological Aspects of Rehabilitation **390**
12.6.1. Coping with Post-Surgical Pain 391
12.6.2. Addressing Anxiety and Depression 392
12.6.3. Building Motivation and Resilience 392
12.7. Challenges in Post-Surgical Rehabilitation **393**
12.7.1. Common Barriers to Recovery 394
12.7.2. Managing Complications 395
12.7.3. Addressing Patient Compliance 396
12.8. Innovations in Rehabilitation Technology **397**
12.8.1. Telehealth and Remote Monitoring 398
12.8.2. Wearable Technology 399
12.8.3. Virtual Reality in Rehabilitation 399
Summary **401**
References **404**

CHAPTER 13

Neurological Disorders with Orthopedic Implications 411

Introduction **411**
13.1. Functional Neuroanatomy Relevant to Physiotherapy **415**
13.1.1. Key Brain Regions and Their Functions 416
13.1.2. Spinal Cord Anatomy and Function 418
13.1.3. Neurotransmitters and Their Role in Movement 418
13.2. Common Neurological Conditions **420**
13.2.1. Stroke: Types and Impact 421
13.2.2. Spinal Cord Injury (SCI): Causes and Consequences 422
13.2.3. Multiple Sclerosis (MS): Symptoms and Management 423
13.3. Other Neurological Disorders **424**
13.3.1. Cerebral Palsy (CP): Overview and Treatment 425
13.3.2. Parkinson's Disease: Pathophysiology and Symptoms 426
13.3.3. Epilepsy: Types and Treatment Options 427
13.4. Signs and Symptoms of Neurological Disorders **428**
13.4.1. Upper Motor Neuron (UMN) Lesions: Characteristics 429
13.4.2. Lower Motor Neuron (LMN) Lesions: Characteristics 429
13.4.3. Diagnostic Approaches for Neurological Symptoms 431
13.5. Principles of Neuroplasticity **432**
13.5.1. Definition and Importance of Neuroplasticity 433
13.5.2. Mechanisms of Neuroplasticity in Recovery 434
13.5.3. Implications for Rehabilitation and Therapy 435
13.6. Assessment and Diagnosis of Neurological Disorders **436**

13.6.1. Clinical Evaluation Techniques 437
13.6.2. Imaging Techniques in Neuroanatomy 438
13.6.3. Neuropsychological Assessments 439
Summary **441**
References **444**

CHAPTER 14

Pain Management in Orthopedic Physiotherapy 449

Introduction **449**
14.1. Understanding Pain **451**
14.1.1. Types of Pain: Acute vs. Chronic 452
14.1.2. Physiological Mechanisms of Pain 453
14.1.3. Psychological Factors Influencing Pain Perception 454
14.2. Assessment of Pain **455**
14.2.1. Tools and Techniques for Pain Assessment 456
14.2.2. Role of Patient History in Pain Evaluation 458
14.2.3. Importance of Objective Measures in Assessment 459
14.3. Treatment Modalities **460**
14.3.1. Physical Therapy Techniques for Pain Relief 461
14.3.2. Pharmacological Interventions in Pain Management 462
14.3.3. Complementary Therapies and Their Effectiveness 462
14.4. Role of Exercise in Pain Management **463**
14.4.1. Benefits of Exercise in Orthopedic Rehabilitation 464
14.4.2. Types of Exercises for Different Orthopedic Conditions 465
14.4.3. Guidelines for Safe Exercise Practices 466
14.5. Patient Education and Self-Management **467**
14.5.1. Importance of Educating Patients About Pain 468
14.5.2. Strategies for Self-Management of Pain 469
14.5.3. Role of Support Systems in Pain Management 469
14.6. Challenges in Pain Management **470**
14.6.1. Barriers to Effective Pain Management in Physiotherapy 471
14.6.2. Ethical Considerations in Pain Treatment 472
14.6.3. Future Directions for Improving Pain Management 473
Summary **474**
References **477**

CHAPTER 15

Recent Advances in Orthopedics and Physiotherapy 481

Introduction **481**
15.1. Technological Innovations in Orthopedics **485**
15.1.1. Robotics in Surgical Procedures 486
15.1.2. 3D Printing for Custom Implants 487
15.1.3. Telemedicine for Pre- and Post-Operative Care 488
15.2. Advances in Physiotherapy Techniques **488**
15.2.1. Use of Virtual Reality in Rehabilitation 489
15.2.2. Evidence-Based Practice in Treatment Protocols 490
15.2.3. Integration of Manual Therapy and Exercise 491
15.3. Regenerative Medicine in Orthopedics **492**
15.3.1. Stem Cell Therapy for Joint Repair 493
15.3.2. Platelet-Rich Plasma (PRP) Injections 494
15.3.3. Tissue Engineering for Cartilage Regeneration 495
15.4. Pain Management Strategies **496**
15.4.1. Multimodal Analgesia Approaches 497
15.4.2. Neuromodulation Techniques 498
15.4.3. Role of Physiotherapy in Pain Management 499
15.5. Evidence-Based Research and Clinical Trials **500**
15.5.1. Importance of Clinical Trials in Orthopedics 501
15.5.2. Recent Studies on Physiotherapy Outcomes 502

15.5.3. Impact of Research on Treatment Guidelines 502
15.6. Interdisciplinary Collaboration **503**
15.6.1. Role of Orthopedic Surgeons and Physiotherapists 504
15.6.2. Benefits of a Team Approach in Patient Care 505
15.6.3. Case Studies Showcasing Successful Collaboration 506
Summary **508**
References **511**
Index **515**

LIST OF FIGURES

Figure 1.1. Orthopedics is a vital branch of medicine that concentrates on the diagnosis
Figure 1.2. The field of orthopedics encompasses the comprehensive study
Figure 1.3. The field of orthopedics plays a pivotal role in healthcare
Figure 1.4. Common orthopedic conditions are vital to the practice of both orthopedics and physiotherapy
Figure 1.5. Arthritis and joint disorders represent a significant concern within the field of orthopedics and physiotherapy
Figure 1.6. Physiotherapy serves as a foundational component in both orthopedic
Figure 1.7. Techniques and modalities used in physiotherapy
Figure 1.8. An interdisciplinary approach to recovery
Figure 1.9. Collaboration between orthopedic surgeons and physiotherapists
Figure 1.10. Role of other healthcare professionals in orthopedic care
Figure 1.11. Diagnostic tools in orthopedics play a pivotal role in the assessment and management of musculoskeletal disorders
Figure 1.12. Imaging techniques play a fundamental role in orthopedics and physiotherapy
Figure 1.13. Accurate diagnosis is a cornerstone of effective treatment planning in orthopedics and physiotherapy
Figure 1.14. Surgical interventions and procedures
Figure 1.15. The role of physiotherapy in post-operative care
Figure 1.16. The evolution of surgical techniques and technology
Figure 1.17. Emerging therapies in physiotherapy
Figure 2.1. Musculoskeletal injury
Figure 2.2. Sprains
Figure 2.3. Ankle instability
Figure 2.4. Tendinitis
Figure 2.5. Sports-related injuries
Figure 2.6. Consequences of a sedentary lifestyle
Figure 2.7. Sign and symptoms of musculoskeletal injuries
Figure 2.8. Musculoskeletal ultrasound
Figure 2.9. RICE method
Figure 2.10. Nonsteroidal anti-inflammatory drugs (NSAIDs)

Figure 2.11. A man with a leg muscle injury receiving orthopedic
Figure 2.12. Gradual return to activity
Figure 2.13. Dynamic warm-up
Figure 2.14. Protective gear
Figure 2.15. Ergonomics
Figure 3.1. The context of musculoskeletal injuries
Figure 3.2. The fractures and dislocations
Figure 3.3. Fractures are classified into various types based on their characteristics and the forces that caused them
Figure 3.4. Fractures are classified primarily into two categories: closed and open fractures
Figure 3.5. Fractures are categorized based on their characteristics and mechanisms of injury
Figure 3.6.
Figure 3.7. Shoulder dislocation represents a significant clinical concern
Figure 3.8. Finger dislocation represents a significant concern within the broader context of fractures and dislocations
Figure 3.9. Hip dislocation
Figure 3.10. The sports-related injuries
Figure 3.11. As individuals age, the risk of developing osteoporosis markedly increases
Figure 3.12. Common symptoms of fractures
Figure 3.13. The diagnosis of fractures and dislocations relies heavily on advanced imaging techniques
Figure 3.14. Non-surgical treatments
Figure 3.15. Surgical interventions have become a cornerstone in the treatment of fractures and dislocations
Figure 3.16. Treatment options for dislocations are largely determined by the type
Figure 3.17. The immobilization of fractures is a fundamental aspect of orthopedic treatment
Figure 4.1. Soft tissue injuries represent a significant category of trauma that affects various structures
Figure 4.2. Soft tissue injuries encompass a range of conditions affecting the connective tissues
Figure 4.3. Soft tissue injuries encompass a variety of damage to connective tissues
Figure 4.4. The various classifications of soft tissue injuries
Figure 4.5. Contusions
Figure 4.6. Engagement in sports-related activities
Figure 4.7. Accidents and falls are prevalent contributors to soft tissue injuries
Figure 4.8. The symptoms of soft tissue injuries are crucial for timely diagnosis and effective treatment
Figure 4.9. Swelling and inflammation are common responses to soft tissue injuries
Figure 4.10. The diagnosis of soft tissue injuries
Figure 4.11. The physical examination serves as a cornerstone for diagnosing soft tissue injuries

Figure 4.12. Imaging techniques (X-rays, MRI)
Figure 4.13. The management of soft tissue injuries
Figure 4.14. Rest, ice, compression, elevation (RICE)
Figure 4.15. Surgical interventions
Figure 4.16. The significance of proper warm-up techniques before physical activity cannot be overstated
Figure 4.17. Education on body mechanics and ergonomics
Figure 5.1. Common Orthopedic Conditions
Figure 5.2. Osteoarthritis (OA)
Figure 5.3. Causes of osteoarthritis (OA)
Figure 5.4. Physiotherapy in the management of osteoarthritis of the knee
Figure 5.5. Rheumatoid arthritis
Figure 5.6. Hand deformity, sometimes called a *swan deformity*, in an elderly person with rheumatoid arthritis
Figure 5.7. Physiotherapy for rheumatoid-arthritis
Figure 5.8. Types of fractures
Figure 5.9. Fracture healing
Figure 5.10. Post fracture physiotherapy
Figure 5.11. Achilles tendonitis
Figure 5.12. Common symptoms of tendonitis
Figure 5.13. Physical therapy exercises for Achilles tendonitis
Figure 5.14. Bursitis
Figure 5.15. Physical therapy for bursitis restores mobility and relieves pain
Figure 5.16. Common sports injuries
Figure 5.17. Sports injury rehabilitation
Figure 6.1. Spinal disorders encompass a broad spectrum of conditions that affect the spinal column
Figure 6.2. The anatomy of the spine is a complex and vital component of the human musculoskeletal system
Figure 6.3. The structure of vertebrae
Figure 6.4. The spinal cord, a critical component of the central nervous system
Figure 6.5. Herniated discs
Figure 6.6. The most common spinal disorders
Figure 6.7. Scoliosis, defined as an abnormal lateral curvature of the spine
Figure 6.8. The multifactorial etiology of spinal disorders encompasses a wide array of biological factors
Figure 6.9. The impact of lifestyle choices on spinal health
Figure 6.10. The symptoms of spinal disorders can manifest in a variety of ways
Figure 6.11. Numbness and tingling
Figure 6.12. The diagnosis of spinal disorders

Figure 6.13. Imaging techniques play a pivotal role in the diagnosis and management of spinal disorders

Figure 6.14. Neurological assessments play a critical role in the comprehensive evaluation of patients with spinal disorders

Figure 6.15. The treatment landscape for spinal disorders encompasses a variety of modalities

Figure 6.16. The landscape of non-surgical treatments for spinal disorders has expanded significantly

Figure 6.17. Surgical interventions play a critical role in the management of various spinal disorders

Figure 7.1. Sports injury evaluation

Figure 7.2. The importance of early treatment of sports injuries

Figure 7.3. ACL injury

Figure 7.4. Whiplash associated disorder (WAD)

Figure 7.5. Optimizing sprint technique to reduce hamstring injury risk

Figure 7.6. Medial tibial stress syndrome

Figure 7.7. Injury assessment and diagnosis Aisling Flynn athletic-therapy

Figure 7.8. Sustentaculum tali palpation

Figure 7.9. Cardiopulmonary exercise test

Figure 7.10. Physician evaluating a student athlete's head injury

Figure 7.11. Integration of point-of-care ultrasound (POCUS) in sports injury assessment

Figure 7.12. Injury assessment and treatment

Figure 7.13. Role of physical therapists in sports injury assessment and diagnosis

Figure 7.14. Management of multifilament knee injuries (MLKIs)

Figure 7.15. Shoulder separations in sports

Figure 7.16. The return-to-play (RTP) criteria represent a crucial aspect of sports

Figure 8.1. Pediatric orthopedics is a specialized branch of medicine focused on the diagnosis

Figure 8.2. Pediatric orthopedics encompasses a specialized branch of medicine focused on the diagnosis

Figure 8.3. The importance of specialized care for children

Figure 8.4. Embryological development is integral to understanding pediatric orthopedics

Figure 8.5. The growth patterns in children

Figure 8.6. The impact of growth on orthopedic conditions

Figure 8.7. Congenital deformities

Figure 8.8. Acquired conditions in pediatric orthopedics

Figure 8.9. The effective diagnostic approaches are pivotal for accurate assessment and treatment intervention

Figure 8.10. In the field of pediatric orthopedics, imaging techniques play a crucial role in the accurate diagnosis

Figure 8.11. The treatment modalities encompass a range of approaches tailored to address the unique musculoskeletal challenges

Figure 8.12. Non-surgical interventions such as physical therapy and bracing
Figure 8.13. Post-operative care and rehabilitation
Figure 8.14. The landscape of pediatric orthopedics
Figure 8.15. The psychological impact of orthopedic conditions on children
Figure 8.16. Recent advancements in pediatric orthopedic research
Figure 8.17. The realm of pediatric orthopedics has witnessed remarkable innovations in surgical techniques
Figure 8.18. Future directions in pediatric orthopedic research
Figure 9.1. The field of geriatric orthopedics
Figure 9.2. Geriatric orthopedics is a specialized branch of orthopedic medicine
Figure 9.3. In geriatric orthopedics, a variety of common conditions are treated
Figure 9.4. The prevalence of orthopedic conditions significantly increases
Figure 9.5. The prevalence of osteoporosis in geriatric populations presents significant implications
Figure 9.6. Hip fractures and their management
Figure 9.7. Arthritis and joint disorders represent a substantial challenge in geriatric orthopedics
Figure 9.8. The aging process brings about significant physiological changes
Figure 9.9. The presence of comorbidities significantly influences the management and outcomes of orthopedic health in geriatric patients
Figure 9.10. Imaging techniques and their relevance
Figure 9.11. The importance of obtaining a comprehensive patient history
Figure 9.12. Treatment options for geriatric orthopedic patients
Figure 9.13. Surgical interventions in geriatric orthopedics are often complex
Figure 9.14. The integration of rehabilitation and physical therapy
Figure 9.15. The challenges inherent in geriatric orthopedic care
Figure 9.16. Communication barriers with elderly patients are critical challenges in the field of geriatric orthopedics
Figure 9.17. Recent advancements in geriatrics have significantly impacted the field of orthopedics
Figure 9.18. The technological advancements in surgical techniques have revolutionized the field of geriatric orthopedics
Figure 9.19. Role of telemedicine in geriatric care
Figure 10.1. The prevalence of orthopedic infections marks a pressing concern in clinical practice
Figure 10.2. The term orthopedic infections
Figure 10.3. Orthopedic infections can be primarily categorized based on their anatomical location and mode of onset
Figure 10.4. Osteomyelitis, an inflammatory condition of the bone caused by infection
Figure 10.5. Septic arthritis represents a significant complication

Figure 10.6. The incidence of prosthetic joint infections (PJIs)
Figure 10.7. The bacterial pathogens emerge as the primary culprits
Figure 10.8. Orthopedic infections are significantly influenced by various patient-related factors
Figure 10.9. Common clinical symptoms
Figure 10.10. Laboratory tests and cultures
Figure 10.11. The role of antibiotic therapy in the management of orthopedic infections
Figure 10.12. The role of surgical intervention in managing orthopedic infections
Figure 10.13. Adjunctive therapies have gained increasing recognition in the management of orthopedic infections
Figure 10.14. The relationship between chronic pain and disability
Figure 10.15. The decision to proceed with amputation as a treatment for orthopedic infections
Figure 10.16. Preoperative measures play a crucial role in mitigating the risk of orthopedic infections
Figure 10.17. The significance of patient education and awareness
Figure 11.1 A tumor is defined as an abnormal mass of tissue
Figure 11.2. A diverse array of classifications exists, each presenting unique characteristics and clinical implications
Figure 11.3. The classification of primary bone tumors
Figure 11.4. The emergence of secondary (metastatic) bone tumors
Figure 11.5. The classification of soft tissue tumors in the body
Figure 11.6. The classification of soft tissue tumors is paramount in facilitating appropriate diagnosis and treatment
Figure 11.7. The spectrum of benign soft tissue tumors encompasses
Figure 11.8. Common symptoms associated with bone tumors
Figure 11.9. Biopsy procedures play a crucial role in the confirmation and characterization of tumors in bones and soft tissues
Figure 11.10. The management of bone tumors often necessitates a multidisciplinary approach
Figure 11.11. Surgical interventions
Figure 11.12. The integration of radiation therapy
Figure 11.13. The treatment landscape for tumors of bones and soft tissues
Figure 11.14. Surgical excision serves as a primary treatment modality for tumors of bones and soft tissues
Figure 11.15. Radiation therapy plays a multifaceted role in the management of tumors of bones and soft tissues
Figure 11.16. The prognosis and outcomes of tumors affecting bones and soft tissues
Figure 11.17. The prognosis of tumors of bones and soft tissues
Figure 11.18. Survival rates for different tumor types vary significantly
Figure 12.1. Post-surgical rehabilitation is defined as a multifaceted approach designed to restore

patients' pre-operative functionality following surgical interventions
Figure 12.2. The spectrum of surgical procedures necessitating rehabilitation is vast, encompassing various orthopedic, gastrointestinal, and cardiovascular interventions
Figure 12.3. The immediate post-operative phase is a critical period wherein the initial recovery and rehabilitation of patients begin
Figure 12.4. Early rehabilitation targets several objectives, including minimizing disuse atrophy, reducing pain, and enhancing the range of motion
Figure 12.5. Understanding a patient's psychological state, social support systems, and adherence to rehabilitation protocols is crucial for successful recovery
Figure 12.6. Ongoing evaluation techniques are fundamental in post-surgical rehabilitation, facilitating a tailored approach to patient recovery
Figure 12.7. Physical therapists play a critical role in the landscape of post-surgical rehabilitation, acting as key facilitators in the recovery process following surgical interventions
Figure 12.8. The role of physicians and surgeons is pivotal in the landscape of healthcare, particularly in relation to post-surgical rehabilitation
Figure 12.9. Manual therapy encompasses hands-on techniques such as mobilization, manipulation, and soft tissue techniques aimed at alleviating pain and restoring function
Figure 12.10. Effective pain management is a crucial component of post-surgical rehabilitation, influencing recovery times and overall patient satisfaction
Figure 12.11. By actively engaging patients in their rehabilitation journey, healthcare professionals can enhance patient adherence to prescribed therapies and establish more meaningful relationships
Figure 12.12. Effective patient education is pivotal in post-surgical rehabilitation, supporting patients understanding of their recovery processes and enabling active participation in their care
Figure 12.13. Coping with post-surgical pain is a multifaceted challenge that significantly impacts the rehabilitation process for patients
Figure 12.14. Patients frequently confront emotional challenges, such as fear of pain or anxiety about their physical capabilities
Figure 12.15. Recovery following surgical procedures can be significantly hindered by various barriers that patients face during the rehabilitation process
Figure 12.16. Educational initiatives aimed at informing patients about the post-operative process can play a pivotal role in enhancing adherence
Figure 12.17. The integration of telehealth and remote monitoring into post-surgical rehabilitation represents a significant advancement in patient care
Figure 12.18. The integration of virtual reality (VR) into post-surgical rehabilitation represents a transformative approach aimed at enhancing patient outcomes and optimizing therapy engagement
Figure 13.1. Central nervous system
Figure 13.2. Peripheral-nervous-system
Figure 13.3. Basics-of-functional-neuroanatomy
Figure 13.4. Regions of the brain and their function

Figure 13.5. Neurotransmitters and their functions
Figure 13.6. Upper-lower-motor-neuron-lesions
Figure 13.7. Lower motor neuron injury
Figure 13.8. The intricate nature of neurological disorders
Figure 13.9. Cerebral palsy
Figure 13.10. Epilepsy – seizure types, symptoms and treatment
Figure 13.11. Common neurological disorders: causes & symptoms
Figure 13.12. Cranial nerves, brainstem, dorsal
Figure 13.13. Principles of neuroplasticity
Figure 13.14. Microbiota and the gut-brain axis
Figure 13.15. Multiple sclerosis
Figure 13.16. Assessment and diagnosis of neurological disorders
Figure 13.17. Imaging techniques in neuroanatomy
Figure 14.1. Illustration of orthopedic pain points
Figure 14.2. Acute vs. chronic pain
Figure 14.3. Pain mechanism
Figure 14.4. Pain scale
Figure 14.5. One-dimensional pain scales depicting examples of pain ratings. Pain is assigned to a range between 0 and 100 mm (VAS), a selection of possible answers (VRS), a numerical value between 0 and 10 (NRS), or a facial expression (SAS). (A) Visual analogue scale (VAS). (B) Numerical rating scale (NRS). (C) Verbal rating scale (VRS). (D) The 'Smiley' analogue scale (SAS)
Figure 14.6. McGill Pain Scale
Figure 14.7. Pain management
Figure 14.8. Expert physiotherapist for pain treatment
Figure 14.9. Pharmacological management of pain
Figure 14.10. Complementary therapy
Figure 14.11. benefits of exercise for pain management
Figure 14.12. Top 10 orthopedic exercises
Figure 14.13. Educating patients about pain
Figure 14.14. Ethical considerations
Figure 15.1. The definition of orthopedics has evolved significantly from its inception
Figure 15.2. Physiotherapy
Figure 15.3. The integration of technological innovations in orthopedics
Figure 15.4. Robotics in surgical procedures
Figure 15.5. The advent of 3D printing technology has significantly transformed the landscape of orthopedics

Figure 15.6. Advances in physiotherapy techniques
Figure 15.7. The integration of manual therapy and exercise
Figure 15.8. The field of regenerative medicine has made significant strides
Figure 15.9. Stem cell therapy for joint repair
Figure 15.10. Platelet-rich plasma (PRP) injections
Figure 15.11. The integration of innovative pain management strategies
Figure 15.12. Multimodal analgesia approaches
Figure 15.13. Neuromodulation techniques
Figure 15.14. The landscape of orthopedics and physiotherapy
Figure 15.15. Importance of clinical trials in orthopedics
Figure 15.16. The concept of interdisciplinary collaboration
Figure 15.17. The implementation of a team approach in patient care

PREFACE

Orthopedics and physiotherapy are an essential synergy in the comprehensive management of musculoskeletal disease. Ranging from trauma-related injuries to degenerative disorders, the combined expertise of orthopedic surgeons and physiotherapists assures not only structural reconstruction but functional rehabilitation as well. The synergy aims at the restoration of mobility, strength, and endurance, all measures of good quality of life. The career is constantly evolving, incorporating innovations in diagnosis, surgical interventions, and modes of treatment, and so students and professionals must maintain a firm foundation of knowledge while adapting to innovations.

Physiotherapy supports the orthopedic management with the resolution of movement dysfunctions through the application of manual therapy, exercise, electrotherapy, and patient education. Physiotherapy contributes to pain relief, avoidance of disability, and maintenance of long-term health following orthopedic treatment or trauma. Integration of physiotherapy into the treatment regimen allows for shorter recovery times and supports sustainable health benefits. Greater understanding of holistic rehabilitation has generated a high emphasis on the interdisciplinarity of knowledge that integrates anatomical correction with functional autonomy.

Essentials of Orthopedics and Applied Physiotherapy is designed to equip readers with a comprehensive understanding of musculoskeletal well-being, causes of injuries, and modes of treatment. The book is designed to provide a balanced understanding that brings together anatomical facts, clinical judgement, and evidence-based practice. It is a handy reference textbook for undergraduate students, interns, and foundation-level professionals wishing to gain competence in both orthopedics and physiotherapy disciplines. Weaving theoretical foundations with practical applications, the text prepares readers to meet patient care head-on with confidence and discernment.

Chapter 1 is an overview of the fundamental tenets of orthopedics and physiotherapy. It introduces general concepts, professional roles for each specialty, and the interdependence required for practice in clinical circumstances.

Chapter 2 is devoted to the explanation of various musculoskeletal injuries, such as common mechanisms, examination protocols, and initial management regimes to minimize long-term damage.

Chapter 3 discusses fractures and dislocations at length, defining types, classification systems, diagnostic methods, and medical or surgical management methods.

Chapter 4 covers soft tissue injuries such as ligament sprain, muscle strain, and tendon rupture with assessment and rehabilitation planning techniques.

Chapter 5 covers orthopedic conditions such as osteoarthritis, rheumatoid arthritis, and bone deformities by highlighting clinical presentation, diagnostic challenge, and physiotherapeutic treatment.

Chapter 6 covers spinal conditions such as scoliosis, herniated disc, and spinal stenosis with an emphasis on assessment techniques and conservative versus surgical plans.

Chapter 7 addresses the diagnosis and assessment of sports injuries. It is focused on functional assessment tools, detection of patterns of injury, and individualized rehabilitation pathways for players.

Chapter 8 addresses pediatric orthopedics, including congenital conditions, developmental conditions, and growth conditions. This chapter outlines age-related assessment and intervention plans.

Chapter 9 shifts focus to geriatric orthopedics and addresses conditions in older persons such as osteoporosis, joint degeneration, and falls injuries, with an emphasis on safety, mobility, and independence during rehabilitation.

Chapter 10 deals with orthopedic infections like osteomyelitis and septic arthritis, a review of symptoms, risk factors, microbiological evaluation, and multi-disciplinary treatment protocols.

Chapter 11 deals with benign and malignant tumors of bone and soft tissues, reviewing diagnostic imaging, biopsy procedures, staging systems, and post-treatment physiotherapeutic interventions.

Chapter 12 deals with rehabilitation after surgery, reviewing total joint replacements, spinal surgery, and fracture fixations with step-by-step protocols for recovery of strength, coordination, and endurance.

Chapter 13 discusses neurological disorders with orthopedic implications, i.e., cerebral palsy, stroke, and spinal cord injury. It addresses musculoskeletal subtleties in neurological disorders and physiotherapy interventions to improve function.

Chapter 14 addresses pain management techniques in orthopedics, i.e., pharmacologic, non-pharmacologic, and physiotherapy-based modalities in the attenuation of acute and chronic pain.

Chapter 15 summarizes the current orthopedic and physiotherapeutic advances, from the least invasive surgery advances to novel physiotherapeutic modalities including dry needling, kinesiology taping, and virtual rehabilitation platforms.

This book is of immense benefit to medical and physiotherapy students, interns, and new clinicians beginning practice in musculoskeletal. The book serves as a reference book for practitioners aiming to establish fundamental knowledge or apply holistic treatment methods. Merging both the orthopedic and physiotherapeutic perspectives, the book presents an even and clinically applicable learning process.

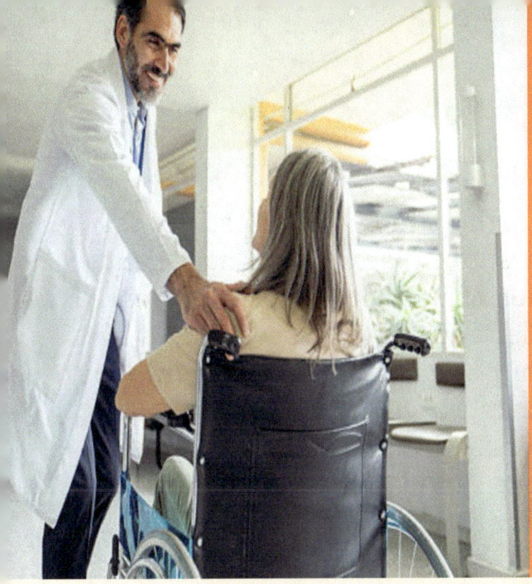

Chapter 1

INTRODUCTION TO ORTHOPEDICS AND PHYSIOTHERAPY

Contents

Introduction 1
1.1. Common Orthopedic Conditions 5
1.2. Principles of Physiotherapy 9
1.3. The Interdisciplinary Approach 12
1.4. Diagnostic Tools in Orthopedics 16
1.5. Treatment Options in Orthopedics 19
1.6. Current Trends and Innovations 22
Summary 27
References 30

Introduction

Orthopedics is an essential branch of medicine that deals with the prevention, treatment, and diagnosis of musculoskeletal diseases. Orthopedics entails interventions for disorders like arthritis, fractures, sports injuries, and congenital deformities. Orthopedic knowledge is important not only in the management of injury but also in improving patients' functional ability and general well-being. Meanwhile, the practitioners are battling to restore mobility and alleviate pain and incorporate a range of therapeutic strategies, including surgical procedures, physical therapy, and rehabilitation programs. These are supplemented by advances in medical technology and evidence-based practice, which expand and improve the technology employed in orthopedic care. Inclusion of physiotherapy as a discipline under the field of orthopedics is particularly significant, since both practice the same aim of enhancing patient outcomes and enabling recovery. Physiotherapists are crucial in the healing process through the utilization of modalities such as manual therapy, exercise prescription, and patient instruction towards enabling healing. This concerted effort is particularly critical, especially following surgery or injury, where attempts are aimed at restoring strength, flexibility, and functional movement. Of interest, studies have identified that the application of audience response systems (ARS) in training has encouraged greater interaction between students and instructors, with the potential to innovate pedagogical methods in physiotherapy education, eventually contributing to the orthopedic field (Bertoni et al., 2023).

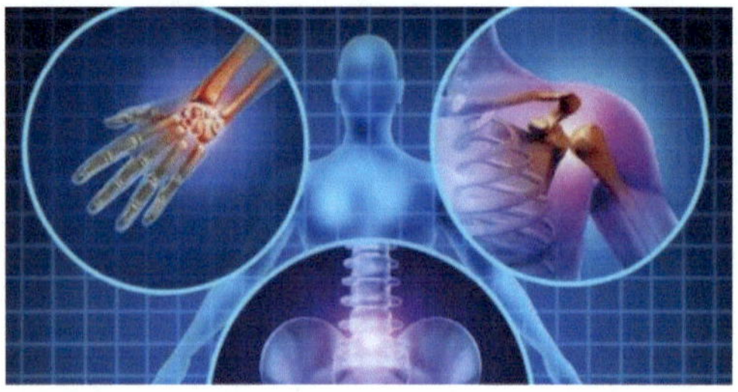

Figure 1.1. Orthopedics is a vital branch of medicine that concentrates on the diagnosis.

Source: https://reliva.in/wp-content/uploads/2023/12/pc-orthopedic-specialization-1.webp.

Hospital-based quality assurance in physiotherapy is crucial to effectiveness and patient satisfaction. A quality framework can provide systematic methods of evaluating and enhancing physiotherapy services, focusing on orthopedics. Existing literature emphasizes mechanisms such as feedback, lifelong learning, and peer observation as essential components of the framework (Steenbruggen et al., 2023). It is through such methods that medical practitioners can build strengths and weaknesses in terms of offering services, hence optimizing treatment outcomes. The long-term vision is to set up an adaptive and responsive physiotherapy setting that not only meets but exceeds patient expectations. Lastly, the integration of orthopedics and physiotherapy is the solution to delivering holistic care that addresses both the physical and emotional healing needs (Figure 1.1).

Definition and Scope of Orthopedics

The field of orthopedics encompasses the comprehensive study, diagnosis, management, and rehabilitation of musculoskeletal conditions. The field handles a variety of issues caused by trauma, congenital abnormalities, degenerative conditions, and injuries involving bones, joints, ligaments, tendons, and muscles. Orthopedics is not just about surgical interventions but is also directed towards conservative treatment modalities, such as physical rehabilitation, that are essential in the recovery of function and improvement of the quality of life of patients. In addition, the emphasis on prevention and patient education regarding musculoskeletal well-being also enhances the breadth of orthopedics and makes it an integral component of modern healthcare systems. Consequently, orthopedic clinicians are progressively needed to embrace interdisciplinary practice with the aid of physiotherapy experts to maximize patient outcomes. An important component of orthopedics is the incorporation of advanced treatment modalities that optimize recovery and improve proper rehabilitation. In the last two decades, there has been a remarkable change in the application of electrophysical agents in physiotherapy practice to support orthopedic care. The availability of various electrotherapy modalities has shown trends of increase as well as decline in various locations, which reflect various gradations of acceptance and utilization in the clinical setting. Specifically, modalities such as ultrasound, pulsed shortwave diathermy, and transcutaneous electrical nerve stimulation have shown trends of increase in utilization in certain nations, whereas others, including microwave diathermy, are showing declining trends of utilization and availability (Shah & Farrow, 2012). These variations can greatly influence the training and practice of the physiotherapists, and therefore, there should be an adaptation to continuously emerging evidence-based protocols of orthopedic treatment. Another very important area of orthopedics is an increased focus on triage protocols within outpatient departments, especially in the case of patients who present with musculoskeletal conditions. As much as outpatient departments are faced with mounting pressures from high and complicated and chronic conditions, the establishment of good triage services is now a priority in orthopedic clinics. Systematic review of triage models revealed large variation in process and definition and a need for standardization in order to further best practices in orthopedic care (Morris et al., 2014). These standardization initiatives will not only serve to simplify the handling of referrals but also improve treatment trajectories for patients with appropriate and timely care. Lastly, establishing explicit and effective triage procedures further reinforces the interdisciplinary aspect of orthopedics, which blends clinical proficiency, patient-centered practice, and evidence-based treatment practices to deal with musculoskeletal health (Figure 1.2).

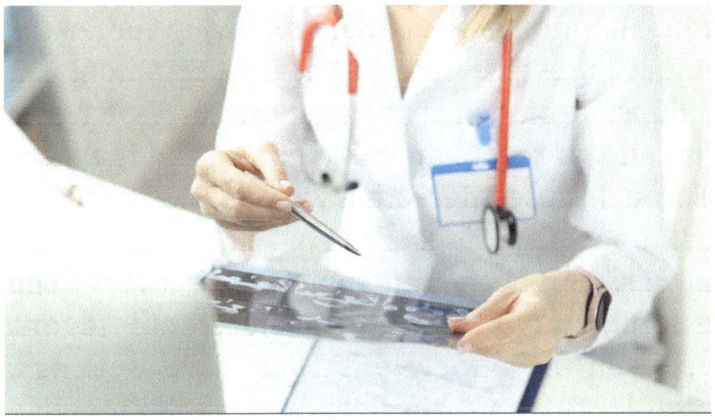

Figure 1.2. The field of orthopedics encompasses a comprehensive study.

Source: https://bonetumorclinic.in/wp-content/uploads/2022/03/scope-of-orthopedic-oncology.jpg.

Historical Development of Orthopedic Medicine

The evolution of orthopedic medicine is inextricably intertwined with advances in the understanding of musculoskeletal diseases as well as the evolution of therapy modalities. Born initially as a specialty for the correction of skeletal abnormalities in children, orthopedics proceeded to expand multiple times larger through the centuries. Ambroise Paré and then later, Joseph Lister were trailblazers who laid basic foundations by integrating surgery techniques with those of hygiene and asepsis. The 19th century was a milestone period because the profession began to adopt scientific principles, away from the exclusive use of mechanical solutions towards a more comprehensive response with both surgical and non-surgical solutions. This transformation, besides focusing on anatomical knowledge, also allowed for the development of specialty instruments and procedures that enhanced the level of patient care. Due to this, orthopedic medicine became recognized as a significant component of healthcare, which catered to a range of disorders and impairments. Due to the greater understanding of musculoskeletal disorders, the 20th century witnessed explosive developments in the specialty field, particularly with the advent of radiology and physical therapy. X-rays revolutionized diagnosis for the good, allowing for more precise identification of fractures, deformities, and bone and joint diseases. Doctors began employing high-technology imaging techniques to not only diagnose but also manage treatment regimens successfully. Furthermore, concurrent innovations in physiotherapy provided patients with the required rehabilitation centers to aid recovery and restore function after injury or surgery. The employment of modalities such as ultrasound, electrical stimulation, and specific exercise programs assisted the three-dimensional management of orthopedics. These developments established the interconnectedness of orthopedic medicine and physiotherapy by highlighting the need for an integrated treatment strategy to enhance patient outcomes and recovery. New developments in orthopedic medicine have continued breaking new ground in the horizon of the effectiveness of treatment, particularly with ailments such as cerebral palsy and

X-linked hypophosphatemia (XLH). Advances in technology, such as the application of botulinum toxin type A (BoNT-A), have been promising in symptom reduction in spastic patients, showing the value of understanding muscle function and morphology (Multani et al., 2019). The use of BoNT-A has contributed to better treatment outcomes, although clinical trials show mixed responses to functional improvement, indicating the challenge in managing neuromuscular disorders. Moreover, multiscalar management of conditions like XLH requires a multidisciplinary management strategy from various healthcare specialists, enhancing diagnosis and treatment results (Haffner et al., 2019). Such advancements best depict how orthopedic medicine never pauses in evolving since it integrates new facts with practice to enhance response to the diverse needs of patients during a lifetime. In view of this, the history of orthopedic medicine in the past reflects significant strides towards complete care and improved patient outcomes.

Importance of Orthopedics in Healthcare

Orthopedics is an essential specialty within the healthcare sector since it deals with the complexities of the musculoskeletal system, which comprises bones, joints, ligaments, tendons, and muscles. Orthopedic illnesses such as fractures, arthritis, and birth deformities take away the mobility and quality of life of a person, necessitating orthopedic treatments. Orthopedic surgeons employ surgical and non-surgical treatments for these conditions and, in some instances, operate in collaboration with other healthcare providers to deliver full care. The growth in the prevalence of musculoskeletal diseases with active lifestyles and aging populations further underscores the necessity of orthopedic care. Therefore, innovation in minimally invasive procedures and regenerative medicine to perform orthopedic procedures highlights the evolving nature of this specialty and its capacity to make significant changes in patient outcomes. In addition to hands-on patient treatment, orthopedics also enhances the health system by impacting policies and procedures that lead to improved overall musculoskeletal health. Evidence-based treatment, drawn from continuous research in orthopedics, informs treatment practices and preventive interventions. Some examples of such studies include issues of informal caregiving, which address the complexities that arise when caring for an individual with chronic musculoskeletal pain (Smith et al., 2021). These findings inform healthcare professionals about the broader social landscape of musculoskeletal disorders so they can craft interventions that not only treat the condition but also address the emotional and practical needs of the family. This evidence-based holistic practice model is a classic demonstration of the worth of using orthopedic knowledge in an extended-range-of-care plan. In addition, orthopedics and physiotherapy need to interact so that the rehabilitation of the patient following surgery or injury is restored. Physiotherapy, commonly an adjunctive branch of orthopedic treatment, treats patients to regain mobility, power, and function. Through close interaction with physiotherapists, orthopedic specialists can provide a continuum of care for better outcomes in recovery. The establishment of multi-professional teams, as seen in effective stroke care settings, highlights the significance of collaborative knowledge and skills on the part of medical professionals (Kilbride et al., 2005). These collaborations foster an organizational culture that is conducive to innovation and patient-focused care, highlighting the critical role that orthopedics plays not only in relation to surgical care but also to optimizing interdisciplinary collaboration in healthcare settings. Therefore, the importance of orthopedics transcends its medical usage, influencing the future horizon of the delivery of healthcare and rehabilitation of patients (Figure 1.3).

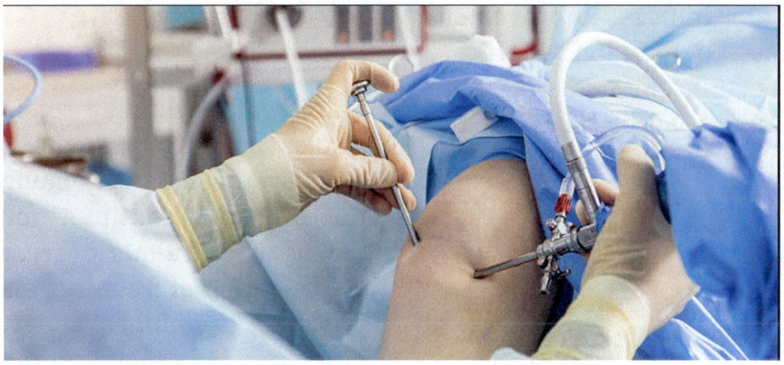

Figure 1.3. The field of orthopedics plays a pivotal role in healthcare.

Source: https://www.muktahealthcare.com/images/department/1613206078COrthopedics-PXsUFugs.jpg.

1.1. Common Orthopedic Conditions

Orthopedic conditions is necessary in order to practice both physiotherapy and orthopedics, since orthopedic conditions have direct impacts on patients' functional ability and quality of life. Among numerous musculoskeletal disorders, frozen shoulder, or adhesive capsulitis, is one such common condition that frequently occurs in middle-aged adults. Painful and stiff by admission, frozen shoulder can potentially severely limit the gliding movements and spinning movements in the shoulder joint and thus influence activities of daily living.

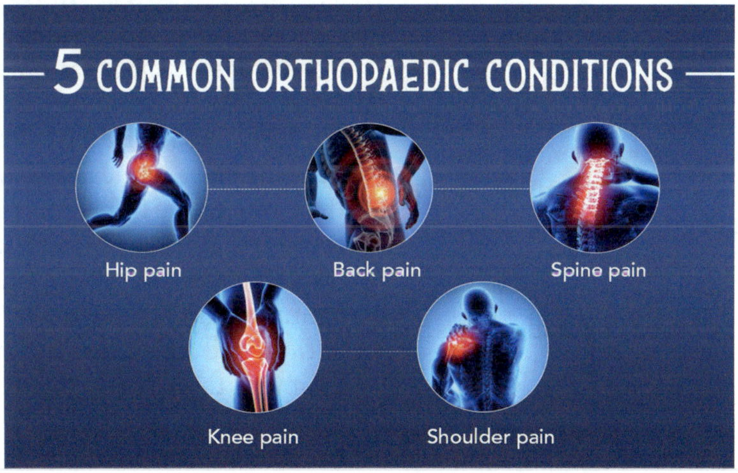

Figure 1.4. Common orthopedic conditions are vital to the practice of both orthopedics and physiotherapy.

Source: https://kdahweb-static.kokilabenhospital.com/kdah-2019/tips/1714655085.jpg.

Proper management calls for an adequate understanding of the etiology of the condition and the application of correct therapeutic procedures. Recent studies suggest that controlled physiotherapy treatment can lead to significant improvement in the function of the shoulder and relief from pain, hence placing significant stress on early and efficient treatment procedures in the management of this common condition. The management strategies for frozen shoulder demonstrate the varying effectiveness of physiotherapy modalities, and the necessity for tailored interventions. More recent evidence indicates that group exercise classes can deliver substantial improvements in shoulder function, being superior to individual physiotherapy sessions and home exercise programs. Specifically, group class members showed considerable improvement in their Constant score, from a baseline mean of 39.8 to 88.1 at one year (Russell et al., 2014). It illustrates the potential benefit of social encouragement and support through group exercises, which may enhance rates of compliance with physiotherapy regimes. In addition, increased levels of anxiety within the subjects also emerged as a significant finding, supporting that physical activity can offer psychological compensation along with physical rehabilitation (Russell et al., 2014). Besides frozen shoulder, other common orthopedic pathologies, such as rotator cuff injuries and osteoarthritis, also require attention according to prevalence and impact on the elderly population. A typical clinical case would involve a patient complaining of shoulder pain in relation to recent activity, e.g., painting, exacerbating pre-existing conditions such as rotator cuff tendinopathy. Appropriate assessment and intervention methods must be employed in these instances, as they enable clinicians to modify rehabilitation protocols that target both functional recovery and pain reduction. By prioritizing the patient-centered model and evidence-based practice, the physiotherapy interventions can become more effective as a whole and help to mitigate the long-term effects of these common orthopedic ailments (Figure 1.4).

1.1.1. Fractures and Their Classifications

Fractures are the key concern of orthopedics, insofar as they can influence short and long-term patient outcomes. Any environment may see a fracture or discontinuity of bone, most often secondary to trauma, overuse, or pathology. The classification of fractures makes the diagnostic process easy, guides the treatment plan, and influences the rehabilitation process. The most common classifications are based on etiology, mechanism of injury, and pattern of the fracture. For instance, fractures are typically classified as closed, when the skin remains intact, or open, when there is an open wound communicating with the fracture point. Such classifications help to determine the probability of developing complications, such as infection, and in structuring ensuing options for management in orthopedic treatment and physiotherapy. Also, fracture classification can be done based on their pattern and nature, such as transverse, oblique, spiral, and comminuted fractures. Transverse fractures, often caused by a direct impact, have a clean break through the bone, whereas oblique fractures result from a diagonal force and lead to a tilted break. Spiral fractures, which commonly occur with twisting injuries, and comminuted fractures, which involve numerous fragments, need distinct clinical management because of their respective implications in healing. Further, there are certain types of fractures, like stress fractures, caused by repetitive stress and are common among sportsmen and individuals with active lifestyles. By understanding these nuances, therapists can design individualized rehabilitation protocols that address not just the mechanical stability required for fracture healing but also the functional recovery required for patient return to play or athletic competition. The consequences of fractures extend well beyond their acute medical management, impacting patients' functional outcomes and general quality of life after injury. Recovery from fracture involves a multi-disciplinary strategy with adequate surgical or conservative treatment and follow-up by an effective regime of physiotherapy to re-establish strength, mobility, and function. The evidence shows that, while younger patients present more rapid and better outcomes depending upon age, gender, and patient factors, complications can arise. For instance, recent findings indicate age-differential trends in pain and function after trauma, and customized rehabilitation is crucial in optimizing recovery outcomes (Sivhugwana, 2022). This highlights the necessity for practitioners to consider not just the nature of injury but also the patient's individual case in providing effective rehabilitation and treatment plans (Sivhugwana, 2022). Knowledge of the complexity encompassed in fracture classification and rehabilitation is paramount in the wide scope of orthopedics and physiotherapy.

1.1.2. Arthritis and Joint Disorders

Arthritis and joint diseases are a serious problem in the field of orthopedics and physiotherapy because of their commonality and impact on the quality of life. They represent an entire spectrum of illnesses, such as osteoarthritis, rheumatoid arthritis, and frozen shoulder, each presenting specific challenges in diagnosis and management. Osteoarthritis, the most common condition, results from wear and tear on the joints, with pain, stiffness, and restriction of function. In contrast, rheumatoid arthritis is a chronic inflammatory autoimmune condition that significantly impairs the function of the joints as well as overall health. The variability in symptoms and variable severity testifies to the necessity for a system of individualized treatment in orthopedic intervention as well as physiotherapy, so that patients are managed with an individualized modality that is suitable, so that they can restore function and relief. Successful arthritis and joint disorders management frequently involves physiotherapy as part of its integral treatment. Evidence highlights the importance of nonoperative intervention in enhancing patient outcomes, particularly for frozen shoulder and other conditions. A study evaluating the effectiveness of different physiotherapy methods showed substantial improvement in formal exercise class-attending patients compared to one-on-one therapy or home-exercise-only patients. The research shows that group settings are capable of enhancing motivation and treatment compliance, resulting in remarkable improvements in range of motion, along with decreased pain scores.

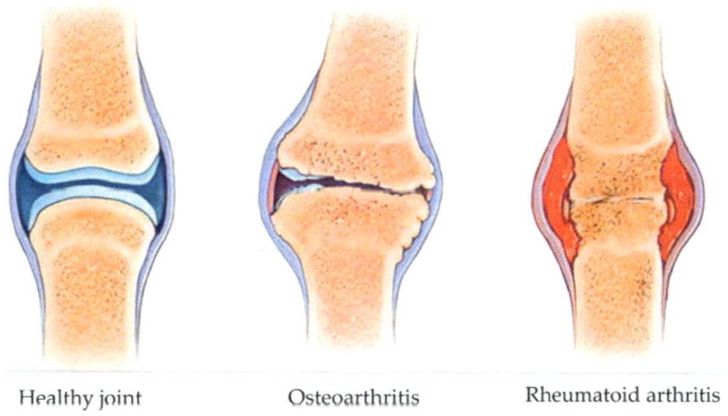

Figure 1.5. Arthritis and joint disorders represent a significant concern within the field of orthopedics and physiotherapy.

Source: https://www.mayoclinic.org/-/media/kcms/gbs/patient-consumer/images/2013/11/15/17/44/ds01122_ds00020_im03689_mcdc7_arthritis_typesthu_jpg.jpg.

Such research is important in evidencing the pivotal role played by physiotherapy as a whole in managing joint diseases, where a judicious combination of rehabilitation techniques can induce remarkable functional gain and increased patient satisfaction (Russell et al., 2014). Furthermore, arthritis and joint disorders research needs to be given a high priority due to the increasing healthcare load posed by these conditions. Among the most problematic soft tissue conditions for physiotherapists, according to a recent study, were frozen shoulder, plantar fasciitis, and tennis elbow. These results support the case for specialized research to determine more about the mechanisms of these conditions as well as their recalcitrance to conventional treatment. Greater diagnostic accuracy and therapeutic intervention can assist medical practitioners in managing such complex diseases more effectively. But the study also points to prevailing unpredictability in treatment outcomes, which is a consequence of inconsistency in clinical practice and triaging procedures among physiotherapists. Hence, it is imperative to create coordination among researchers and clinicians in order to standardize treatment protocols and ultimately enhance patient care in orthopedics and physiotherapy (Poltawski et al., 2008) (Figure 1.5).

1.1.3. Sports Injuries and Their Management

Sports injuries form a major issue in orthopedics as well as in physiotherapy since they can affect any player, from amateur to professional sportspeople. Injuries may range from acute trauma, including fractures and ligament sprains, to chronic injuries like tendinitis and bursitis. Proper management of these injuries is not only essential to heal the disease but also to prevent future complications. The treatment approach for sports injuries is generally multifaceted, comprising immediate management, rehabilitation, and, when indicated, surgical correction. Prompt intervention and proper care can have a major impact on recovery time and the overall performance of the athletes. Further, awareness of the underlying mechanics and risk factors for certain injuries can help in the formulation of directed prevention programs, ultimately reducing the athlete's vulnerability to injuries within their sport. The role of physiotherapy in the rehabilitation of sporting injuries cannot be overstated. The physiotherapist has a central role in rehabilitation, with an arsenal of techniques and modalities used to create function and strength. These may include manual therapy, therapeutic exercises, as well as application of clinical prediction rules (CPRs) to guide treatment. The use of CPRs in practice physiotherapy has been shown to be promising in enhancing clinical reasoning and decision-making skills among practitioners, even though a study has shown that pre-professional students of physiotherapy are not sufficiently familiar with these tools (Knox et al., 2017). The gap in knowledge is indicative of the necessity for training and education in physiotherapy programs to equip future professionals with the necessary expertise to effectively manage sports injuries. Moreover, sports medicine background history informs contemporary practice in the treatment of sports injuries. The profession has a burgeoning past, and over the last few decades, it has evolved from primitive treatments to more evidence-driven procedures with increased focus on long-term performance and athlete health (Reynolds & Tansey, 2009). The emergence of sports medicine as an accepted specialty has also facilitated developments in injury management through multidisciplinary teamwork between physiotherapists, orthopedic surgeons, and sports scientists. This evolution reflects a broader recognition of the concerns related to sports injuries and a necessity for complete rehabilitation programs in line with personal athlete needs. As research advances further, it is of paramount importance that sport managers are aware of new facts and techniques for optimal recovery and safe participation in physical activity.

1.2. Principles of Physiotherapy

Physiotherapy is an integral part of orthopedic rehabilitation as well as the overall health sector. Its foundations are rooted in facilitating mobility, restoring function, and alleviating pain, which are indeed very much in line with the goals of orthopedic care. Fundamental techniques utilized by physiotherapists include manual treatment, exercise prescription, and modalities such as ultrasound or electrical stimulation. Every intervention is personalized to the individual patient's needs, with their specific health status and recovery objectives becoming the primary focus. Through evidence-based practice, physiotherapists are able to make informed decisions regarding treatment planning, which is important in maximizing patient outcomes. This patient-centered mechanism not only facilitates healing of injuries and surgeries but also a better quality of life on an international basis, making physiotherapy the central partner along the journey to physical wellness (Samoy et al., 2016). With the inclusion of cutting-edge technology and traditional physiotherapy therapy, novel techniques are emerging that revolutionize rehabilitation practice. For instance, automated and semi-automated systems are being developed to facilitate physiotherapy and rehabilitation. They use sophisticated technologies, ranging from robots to online communication software, making them more efficient and involving the patient. An example of such is the NeXOS project aimed at lower limb rehabilitation through engineering design integration into physiotherapist practice. By providing ease of access to these sophisticated tools for physiotherapists, treatment effectiveness can be significantly maximized, making rehabilitation environments more flexible. Furthermore, such technological mergers enable physiotherapists to provide tailored care to patients, enabling independent rehabilitation with an emphasis on improving the client experience (Bradley et al., 2009). Central to the ideology of physiotherapy is the emphasis placed on the adaptation and constant reassessment of treatment plans according to patient progress. Such an active response promotes not only accountability but also ensures that the rehabilitation process is made flexible to accommodate changing patient needs. Through ongoing monitoring, physiotherapists can identify the success of interventions and adjust accordingly to promote recovery. By gaining an integrated understanding of each patient's physical strengths and weaknesses, physiotherapists are able to create supportive healing climates. The practice of adaptability is particularly important in orthopedic settings, in which patients can exhibit differential rates of improvement from injury or surgery. Ultimately, physiotherapy tenets emphasize a commitment to continuous learning and responsiveness, maintaining the ethic of personalized patient care within orthopedic rehabilitation frames (Samoy et al., 2016) (Figure 1.6).

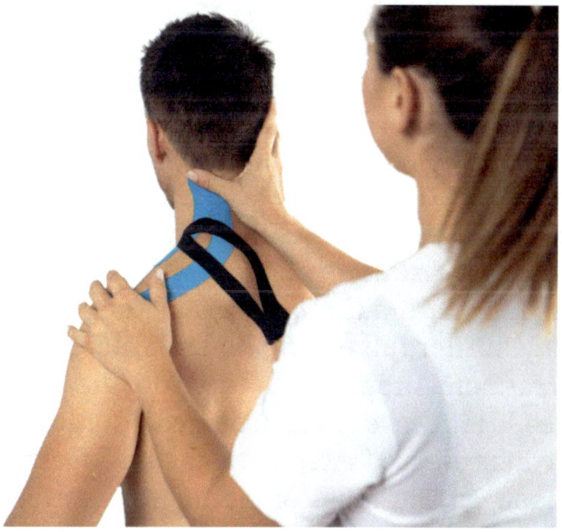

Figure 1.6. Physiotherapy serves as a foundational component in both orthopedic.

Source: https://gmcdhcc.com/wp-content/uploads/2023/10/physiotherapist-applying-elastic-medical-bandage-male-patient-scaled.jpg.

1.2.1. Definition and Role of Physiotherapy

Physiotherapy is a valuable health profession practice dedicated to the prevention, assessment, and treatment of movement disorders. Physiotherapy utilizes an integrated approach combining not only physical rehabilitation but also facilitating optimal health and well-being in various patient groups. Essentially, physiotherapy aims to restore function, encourage mobility, and enhance the quality of life for people recovering from injury, surgery, or disease. By utilizing approaches such as therapeutic exercise, manual therapy, and education, physiotherapists permit patients to take an active role in their recovery process, instilling a sense of self-determination and control that is essential to ensuring maximum outcomes in orthopedic treatment. This multi-dimensional function serves to highlight the central importance of physiotherapy in the continuum of patient care, further emphasizing its integrative role in harmonizing medical, surgical, and rehabilitative therapies. It is where orthopedics is concerned that physiotherapy intervention becomes of critical significance due to the nature of musculoskeletal injury or surgery, which requires comprehensive rehabilitation for a successful return. After procedures such as joint replacement or fracture fixation, patients experience some issues that hinder their rehabilitation process. Physiotherapists implement personalized treatment programs tailored to the patient's needs to recover from orthopedic surgery using evidence-based interventions that address pain management, range of motion restoration, and muscle strengthening. This intervention not only enhances physical recovery but also minimizes the risk of complications such as stiffness or re-injury. Apart from this, physiotherapy is not an after-operation intervention to be adopted promptly; it trains patients in how to recover safely to their pre-injury status, improving general well-being and functional autonomy, which is vital for an efficient, long-term, positive outcome of orthopedic rehabilitation. Literature supports the pivotal role that physiotherapy plays in achieving successful healthcare outcomes in orthopedics. Studies indicate that inter-professional approaches, where physiotherapists are engaged and collaborate with surgeons and other health professionals, enhance overall patient care. Inter-professional working allows for the comprehensive understanding of patients' needs, leading to the use of suitably focused rehabilitation strategies aimed at physical, emotional, and psychological recovery. For instance, the findings of an action research intervention emphasize the importance of team harmony in creating an effective stroke service, demonstrating how collaboration between healthcare professionals results in improved patient outcomes (Kilbride et al., 2005). Similarly, the low abstract-to-publish rate reported in orthopedic literature also shows the need to attach greater importance to the reporting of evidence supporting the effectiveness of physiotherapy during clinical practice, thereby reasserting its vital role in evidence-based orthopedics (Collier et al., 2018).

1.2.2. Techniques and Modalities Used in Physiotherapy

Physiotherapy has a wide range of techniques and modalities that tend to enhance recovery and maximize the outcome for the patient. Manual therapy, therapeutic exercises, and physical modalities are some of the most commonly used techniques. Manual therapy is hands-on treatment encompassing the mobilization and manipulation of soft tissue and joints to minimize pain and maximize mobility. Therapeutic exercises are individualized programs for restoration of strength, flexibility, and functional movement and are the building blocks of the rehabilitation process. Utilization of the techniques tends to result in enhanced health status in musculoskeletal disorder patients, further solidifying the significant position physiotherapists play in the healthcare continuum. In addition to exercise and manual therapy, physiotherapy is frequently blended with physical modalities such as electrotherapy, ultrasound, and heat application. These modalities serve various purposes, including pain relief, anti-inflammatory reduction, and muscle recuperation. Electrotherapy modalities, such as transcutaneous electrical nerve stimulation (TENS), are particularly useful in the management of acute and chronic pain. Similarly, ultrasound can be employed to enhance tissue healing by augmenting blood flow and tissue repair. With current literature, judicious use of these modalities can achieve optimal treatment effectiveness, but evidence-based practice guidelines regarding dosing and combinations remain scarce.

The physiotherapists thus consistently develop and advance their capabilities and further sharpen treatment guidelines according to emerging evidence to ensure optimal practice. Advances in the practice of physiotherapy point towards the importance of evidence-based practice within clinical settings. Addition of such modalities as acupuncture, laser therapy, and mechanical traction has proven to be effective for the management of a variety of conditions, especially chronic neck pain (Samoy et al., 2016). Evidence is moderate supporting acupuncture and laser therapy for pain management, although some modalities are of limited benefit. Pulsed ultrasound and infrared therapy, for instance, have been found to be no more beneficial than a placebo in neck pain in some cases. To cater to practitioners' changing patterns of practice, involving new approaches guarantees a responsive practice that can accommodate different patient needs. Continued exploration and examination of the results are needed, allowing physiotherapists to maintain the integrity of their own practice while providing customized care in line with current scientific understanding (Samoy et al., 2016) (Figure 1.7).

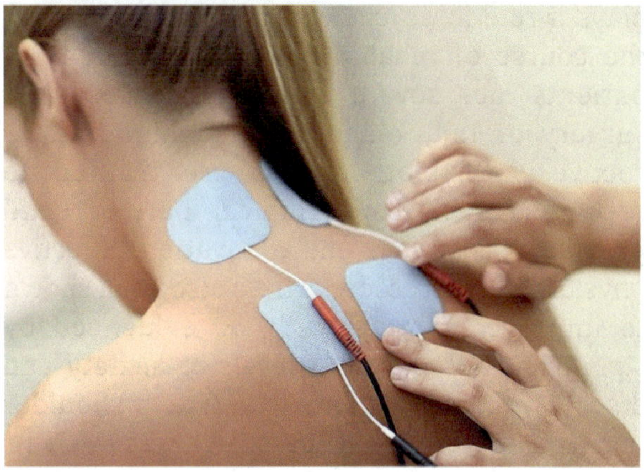

Figure 1.7. Techniques and modalities used in physiotherapy.

Source: https://pillarsofwellness.ca/wp-content/uploads/2024/07/electrical-muscle-stimulation-ems-physiotherapy-burlington-960x675.jpg.

1.2.3. Importance of Physiotherapy in Rehabilitation

The role of physiotherapy in rehabilitation is crucial, particularly following surgery or trauma to the musculoskeletal system. Physiotherapy employs a variety of interventions, including manual therapy, exercise prescription, and patient education, all aimed at restoring function, reducing pain, and enhancing quality of life. For instance, in cases of frozen shoulder, research has established that physiotherapy can lead to significant improvements in function and range of motion. Evidence demonstrated that intensive exercise programs, particularly hospital-based exercise classes, were better than single treatments or home exercises alone, pointing to the strength of group effects and professional supervision during rehabilitation (Russell et al., 2014). Also, the continuous availability of physiotherapists can motivate patients to adhere to exercise therapy, which is a major determinant of long-term rehabilitation. Moreover, physiotherapy not only aims to improve body functions but also plays a role in psychological treatment during the course of rehabilitation. The majority of patients face severe emotional issues after surgery or injury, and this can hinder their recovery. Physiotherapists are trained to recognize such psychological barriers and provide reassurance and motivation. Effective physiotherapy procedures have also been shown to improve mental health, as evidenced by significant reductions in levels of anxiety and disability among patients with frozen shoulder undergoing treatment (Russell et al., 2014). This comprehensive approach reinforces the role of physiotherapy as a comprehensive rehabilitation method, emphasizing the fact that physical recovery goes hand in hand with mental health intervention. In children, for example, in bilateral spastic cerebral palsy, physiotherapy has very important implications not only on the physical development but also on the ultimate result of function. Recent methods in physiotherapy, such as whole-body vibration and resistance training, have proved to be able to enhance muscle force, bone mineral density, and general motor function. Findings from recent studies reveal that targeted physiotherapy contributes significantly towards the improvement of gross motor function in impaired children, demonstrating an overall advantage extending beyond mere physical rehabilitation. Such improvements reinforce the crucial role of physiotherapy in infantile rehabilitation, highlighting its immediate need for maximizing the developmental track of young patients and consequently providing both short- and long-term health advantages.

1.3. The Interdisciplinary Approach

Interdisciplinary practice is one of the defining characteristics of orthopedic and physiotherapeutic practice, enabling integrated patient care through inter-professional collaboration among multi-disciplinary healthcare providers. By combining various fields of expertise, ranging from medicine, physical therapy, and rehabilitation sciences, interdisciplinary practice enables practitioners to address patients' complex needs appropriately. In clinical settings, exercise therapists, for instance, utilize many didactic and methodological strategies for promoting physical activity according to the underlying principle of interprofessional working. These encompass individualized exercise programs and theoretical training integrated with implementation practice, which allow for better patient outcomes and satisfaction (Geidl et al., 2019). Thus, the interdisciplinary model not only enriches the clinical practice but also empowers patients by providing them a sense of personal responsibility towards their health and well-being. A successful interdisciplinary model also relies upon the identification of barriers and facilitators that affect collaboration between the healthcare teams. Structural factors, including the availability of resources and the layout of clinical facilities, can profoundly influence the effectiveness of collaboration in orthopedics and physiotherapy. For example, in clinical environments where staff or equipment is not sufficient, the opportunity for inter-professional practice diminishes, usually compromising patient care (Ernstzen et al., 2015). In addition, patients' experience and expectation as rehabilitants are also a leading factor in determining therapeutic alliance. By involving patients directly in their care, practitioners can form a deeper appreciation of their individual needs, and this raises motivation for rehabilitation. Thus, finding resolutions to these problems is imperative to the continued development and success of interprofessional practice in restoring health and function. Aside from improving patient outcomes, the interprofessional approach in orthopedics and physiotherapy has a vital role in the evolution of professional education and training. As is evidenced by the clinical education of undergraduate physiotherapy students, the choice of training sites plays a vital role in their preparation for the practical world ahead. Convenience of access to schools and the prevalence of multidisciplinary offerings greatly add to learning outcomes (Ernstzen et al., 2015). Second, exposure to diverse clinical settings enhances problem-solving and critical thinking skills, critical thinking in a fast-changing healthcare system. Consequently, the interdisciplinary model enhances not only collaborative practice but also education curricula, empowering future healthcare providers to prepare for orthopedics and physiotherapy patient care complexity (Figure 1.8).

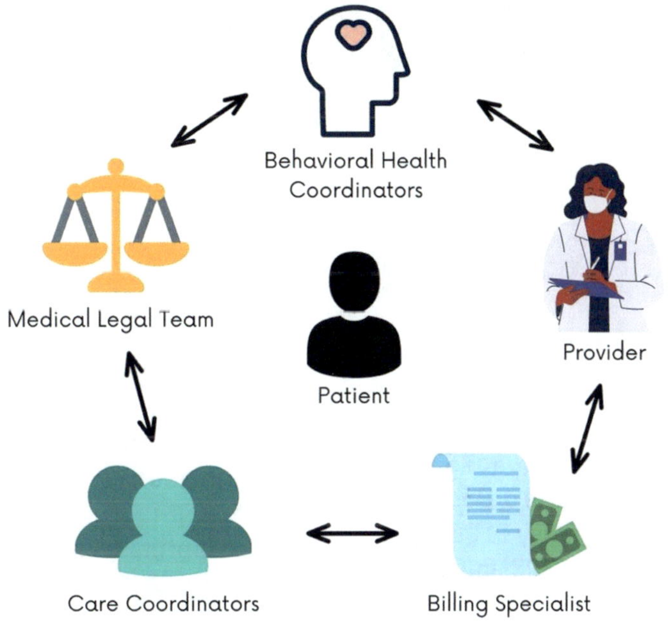

Figure 1.8. An interdisciplinary approach to recovery.

Source: https://www.nationalhealthcorps.org/sites/default/files/uploads/Patient%20-%20NHC%20 Communications.jpg.

1.3.1. Collaboration Between Orthopedic Surgeons and Physiotherapists

Orthopedic surgeon-physiotherapist collaboration is critical for achieving optimal patient outcomes in musculoskeletal well-being. The interdisciplinary collaboration between the two professions ensures a holistic treatment strategy that is integrated from the technical surgical solutions to structural problems and the rehabilitative solutions from physiotherapists who facilitate functional recovery. This collaboration is particularly essential in rotator cuff related shoulder pain (RCRSP) since the outcome of findings reveals that an exercise program, well designed, can be as effective as surgery. The existence of this evidence highlights the significance of combining both surgery and physiotherapeutic methods to treat the complexity of shoulder conditions appropriately, offering patients the most appropriate treatment in relation to their individual needs (Lewis, 2016). The co-operation of these two medical specialties additionally enriches the patient experience. With their cooperative environment, orthopedic surgeons and physiotherapists can communicate better with one another regarding patient assessments, therapeutic management, and patient progress.

Multidisciplinary case meetings and day-to-day discussions allow for better refinement of therapeutic skills and adjustment of treatment plans based on patient response and clinical observations.

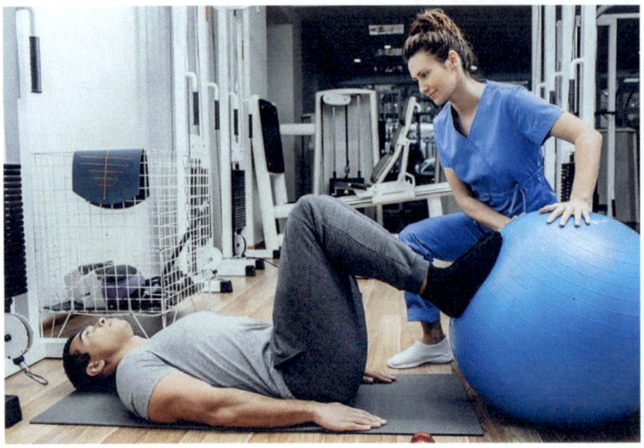

Figure 1.9. Collaboration between orthopedic surgeons and physiotherapists.

Source: https://static.wixstatic.com/media/11062b_134fdd6885f445a194cb61c6b5b75202~mv2.jpeg/v1/fill/w_980,h_647,al_c,q_85,usm_0.66_1.00_0.01,enc_avif,quality_auto/11062b_134fdd6885f445a194cb61c6b5b75202~mv2.jpeg.

For instance, shoulder pain problems concerning causes and origin are better addressed when the two professionals are working together, adding depth to the patient's condition and therefore resulting in more targeted interventions. Such communication ensures that treatment not only addresses immediate needs but also examines long-term functional outcomes, ultimately translating into increased patient satisfaction and recovery rate (Reynolds & Tansey, 2009). Moreover, physiotherapy in combination with orthopedic surgery is indispensable in the management of post-surgical rehabilitation. Physiotherapists play a pivotal role in facilitating recovery following orthopedic procedures and regaining mobility. They apply their expertise to design individualized rehabilitation programs so that patients can transition smoothly from surgical recovery to optimal function. This is particularly evident in populations treated with surgery for conditions like RCRSP, where a combined plan of surgical correction and rehabilitative exercises is used to optimize strength and mobility. Moreover, ongoing feedback from the physiotherapists to the surgeons about patient status enables follow-up therapy to be adjusted and an iterative process of observation and adjustment of treatment protocols. Such a model of collaboration not only improves clinical results but also maintains the importance of team practice in achieving holistic patient well-being (Lewis, 2016) (Figure 1.9).

1.3.2. Role of Other Healthcare Professionals in Orthopedic Care

Within orthopedic practice, coordination among a variety of healthcare providers is key to overall management of the patient. Orthopedic surgeons can work in close collaboration with physiotherapists, occupational therapists, and pain management specialists to develop multidisciplinary treatment strategies. This interdisciplinary model not only maximizes the quality of care but also maximizes patient recovery. For example, physiotherapists play a great role in rehabilitation through the application of personalized exercise regimens in order to develop muscle, increase mobility, and decrease pain following surgical interventions. Through such unity, these specialists ensure to administer patients with round-the-clock care during the healing process. Consequently, the coordination of different health practitioners optimizes results and enables patients to manage their healing process more effectively. Further, orthopedic treatment is also offered by informal caregivers, albeit at times underappreciated in the professional environment. According to Smith et al. (2021), most of these caregivers are the key support for patients with chronic musculoskeletal pain and, as such, have a direct impact on their wellbeing and recovery journey. The dynamics of this patient-caregiver relationship can influence treatment compliance and emotional support, both of which are key to an effective outcome. Informal caregivers typically serve as a liaison between patients and health professionals, communicating patient needs and facilitating adherence to treatment plans. Acknowledging informal caregivers' roles as active members of the healthcare team fortifies the overall care plan for patients.

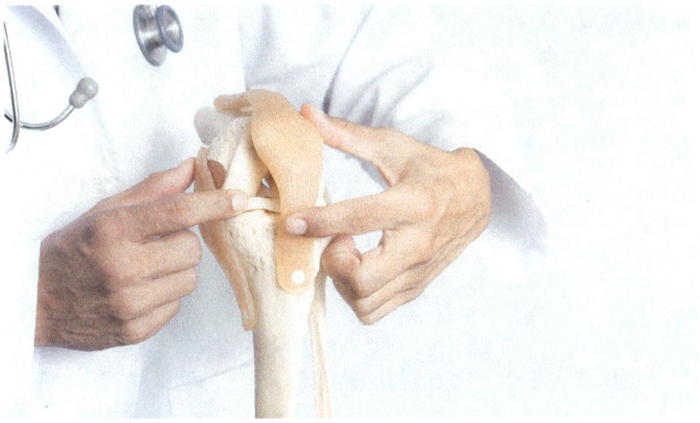

Figure 1.10. Role of other healthcare professionals in orthopedic care.

Source: https://vishwarajhospital.com/wp-content/uploads/2023/08/Ortho.jpg.

The interdependent model emphasizes that caregivers must be included in the process of treatment planning to further empower patients and enhance recovery. Consistency in communication and terms among healthcare professionals is vital in treating musculoskeletal disorders and providing quality care. Inconsistent use of medical terms by Scott et al. (2019) can lead to confusion among providers and patients, potentially affecting the treatment process. It can break down patient trust and stall their recovery process when experts fail to agree on diagnosis or treatment methods. Establishment of consistent language and collaborative channels of communication encourages mutual comprehension of conditions such as tendinopathy, ultimately contributing to an enhanced patient experience. It is, therefore, crucial to develop an open communication and collaborative environment among all healthcare practitioners, such as orthopedic surgeons, physiotherapists, and other specialists, to enhance patient outcomes and holistic care in orthopedics (Figure 1.10).

1.3.3. Benefits of an Interdisciplinary Approach for Patient Outcomes

The use of inter-disciplinary treatment methods in the field of healthcare, particularly in orthopedics and physiotherapy, significantly enhances the quality of treatment given to patients with their improvements. With the integration of the professional skills of various healthcare experts like physiotherapists, orthopedic surgeons, and occupational therapists, the treatment protocols can be more personalized and holistic depending on the unique patient needs. This integration makes it possible to identify and manage complex musculoskeletal disorders that are usually recalcitrant to traditional methods of therapy. For instance, studies have proven that conditions such as frozen shoulder and plantar fasciitis, which are among the most difficult in musculoskeletal care, benefit from an interdisciplinary treatment approach that leverages more than one skill and perspective in diagnosis and treatment interventions (Poltawski et al., 2008). Such coordination, thus, not only promotes clinical outcomes but also patient satisfaction due to the holistic care provided during the process. Further, the interdisciplinary setting encourages a more adaptive and innovative healthcare environment. As different professional backgrounds converge, the team can exchange learning experiences that enrich their clinical practices. This, in turn, can lead to the development of new procedures of treatment that are evidence-based and rooted in practical experience. For instance, action research from one of the London teaching hospitals revealed that from the acknowledgment of joint input of multidisciplinary team members, there were significant improvements in the quality of patient care through enhanced team relationships, practice development, and an overall climate of support within the organization (Kilbride et al., 2005). Such conditions foster innovative problem-solving, which is central to tackling the complex nature of patient management, especially in the settings of orthopedics and physiotherapy. Finally, an interdisciplinary approach maximally facilitates communication and collaboration among medical health providers. Better interprofessional communication allows for easier exchange of important patient information, which is essential to effective treatment planning and implementation. Open communication that facilitates teamwork like this is sure to maintain continuity of care and also prevent the risks of misdiagnosis or treatment in isolated health environments. The study of challenging disorders further highlighted that the lack of coordination could result in less-than-optimal patient outcomes due to inadequate differential diagnosis and no uniform patterns of treatment (Poltawski et al., 2008). In this way, inter-professional cooperation not only optimizes individual therapies but also strengthens the overall healthcare system, which ultimately benefits the delivery of patient care and health outcomes in orthopedics and physiotherapy.

1.4. Diagnostic Tools in Orthopedics

Orthopedic diagnostic equipment is at the forefront of musculoskeletal disease evaluation and management. The equipment ranges from advanced imaging equipment to formal clinical assessment equipment. Ultrasound imaging (USI) and magnetic resonance imaging (MRI) are two of the available technologies that offer soft tissue high-level visualization, enabling accurate diagnosis for conditions like tears in ligaments or injuries to tendons. The application of USI is increasingly recognized within physiotherapy practice, particularly in New Zealand, where its use has been identified as a trend among physiotherapists for both diagnostic and rehabilitative purposes. Notably, understanding the contexts of these diagnostic tools and the barriers to their uptake can enhance clinical education, ensuring that practitioners can leverage these technologies effectively to improve patient outcomes.

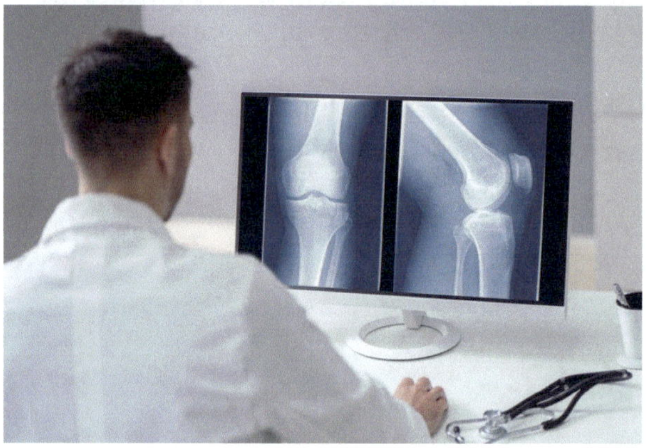

Figure 1.11. Diagnostic tools in orthopedics play a pivotal role in the assessment and management of musculoskeletal disorders.

Source: https://dearbornassoc.com/wp-content/uploads/sites/274/2023/12/shutterstock_1619489473.jpg.optimal.jpg.

Moreover, clinical prediction rules (CPRs) are also significant orthopedic diagnostic tools. CPRs are rational tools to assist clinicians in determining the probability of specific conditions based on clinical findings. Their presence within physiotherapy education, however, creates a concern regarding the unfamiliarity of students. A study established that as much as 60% of final-year physiotherapy students remained unaware of CPRs, although most of those familiar with them found them helpful in enhancing clinical reasoning skills. The gap demonstrates the need for curriculum reforms to incorporate CPR training into the course of study, therefore equipping future physiotherapists with critical diagnosis skills. Through the optimal use of such equipment in learning environments, the quality of assessment of patients can be significantly improved. Challenges of adopting new diagnostic equipment need to be overcome to improve clinical practice for orthopedics and physiotherapy. The findings of the research on USI utilization barriers point to the fact that access issues to machines, finances, and differences in training can significantly hinder the adoption. Thus, steps to improve provision for training and availability of necessary technology can facilitate integration of USI into routine practice. Moreover, consideration of the barriers as a collective can provide insight into systemic reform, promoting more varied use of effective diagnostic practice across the healthcare sector. Thus, enhancement of physiotherapy training and practical application of diagnostic tools can develop an effective and responsive system of orthopedic care (Figure 1.11).

1.4.1. Imaging Techniques (X-rays, MRIs, CT scans)

Imaging modalities play a pivotal role in physiotherapy and orthopedics, providing vital information to support clinicians in the diagnostic process as well as treatment. X-rays, CT scans, and MRIs are the most common of these modalities, each with its own specific advantages in a particular clinical scenario. X-rays are typically the imaging modality of first choice when assessing bone fractures as well as joint alignment due to their speed and high availability. The primary shortcoming of X-rays is that they cannot provide satisfactory images of soft tissues, which are responsible for imaging the specifics of injuries to cartilage, ligaments, and muscles. Hence, newer imaging modalities such as MRI and CT scans are typically employed to complement provisional assessments so that a comprehensive evaluation of musculoskeletal structures in patients with more complex situations or atypical presentations can be made. Magnetic Resonance Imaging (MRI) is particularly valuable in orthopedic settings due to its special ability to image soft tissue anatomy without exposing patients to ionizing radiation. MRI is an imaging technique that utilizes strong magnetic fields and radio waves to produce good-quality images of muscle, tendons, and ligaments, allowing for conditions such as tears, inflammation, and degenerative change to be detected.

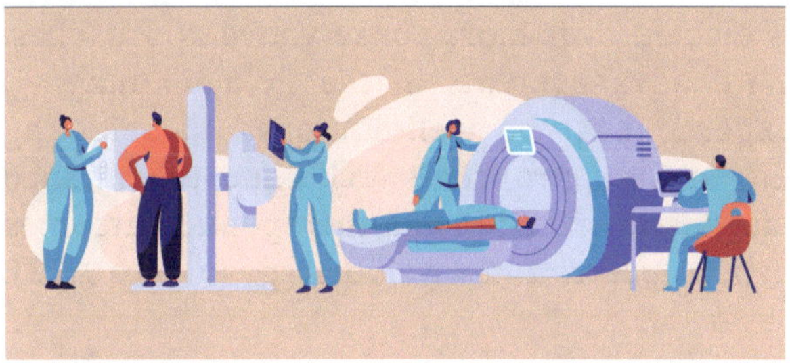

Figure 1.12. Imaging techniques play a fundamental role in orthopedics and physiotherapy.

Source: https://buzzrx.s3.amazonaws.com/bd7421d7-c49e-4b95-9e3c-38cc21be6a21/X-RayvsCTScanvsMRI-UnderstandingtheDifferencesinImaging.png.

Further, MRI has proved particularly useful in the diagnosis of diseases like idiopathic scoliosis, where the evaluation of three-dimensional spinal deformity is important for treatment planning. MRI data can be used to guide the use of orthotic management or surgical intervention in correcting spinal deformities, complementing growing interest in non-surgical means of treatment in orthopedics and physiotherapy. With advancements in imaging modalities, the integration of these techniques into clinical practice becomes increasingly important to achieve maximum patient benefits. Computed Tomography (CT) scans are another powerful imaging modality in orthopedics when it comes to requiring high-resolution images of complex bone anatomy. CT scans take cross-sectional images of bones and joints, which can have fractures not seen on an X-ray, for instance, of the spine or pelvis. Also, pre-surgical planning and post-surgical evaluation are commonly done with CT, so the anatomy and location of implants can be precisely measured. While useful, CT scans do involve a radiation exposure, and practitioners are therefore compelled to balance the diagnostic gains against the dangers present. In benign and malignant bone tumors, subtle visualization by CTs can make a significant difference in whether or not surgery is elected over more conservative approaches. With advancements in the field of imaging, experts must be well-equipped in selecting the most appropriate technique to enhance diagnostic precision and therapeutic outcomes in orthopedics and physiotherapy (Figure 1.12).

1.4.2. Physical Examination Methods

The assessment of musculoskeletal disorders is a cornerstone in orthopedics and physiotherapy, pointing to the importance of physical examination methods. The techniques enable practitioners to gather crucial information regarding the status of a patient, on which further treatment will be based. Initial examinations may include inspection and palpation, where practitioners can check for structural abnormalities and identify areas of inflammation or tenderness. Additionally, range of motion tests quantify the extent of joint movement, which is particularly important in conditions like frozen shoulder. In keeping with current evidence, a careful and systematic assessment with the assistance of physical examination methods significantly enhances the accuracy of diagnoses, in turn changing the treatment course in patients who present with shoulder disorders (Russell et al., 2014). Aside from the core assessments, a more in-depth examination of clinical thinking must be undertaken by physiotherapy students while they learn for practical purposes. The majority of final-year pre-professional physiotherapy students were unaware of CPRs, which are essential in guiding decisions in the context of physical examinations, based on a cross-sectional survey (Knox et al., 2017). Such regulations not only serve to enhance clinical judgment but also improve the overall effectiveness of the process of physical examination. Emphasis on the practical application of CPRs in educational training may serve to narrow the gap between knowledge and practice. Thus, the integration of various physical examination methods with evidence-based guidelines could facilitate improved assessment methods among students, thereby preparing them for their prospective roles within the healthcare system. Also, proper physical examination methods can lead to better patient function and satisfaction. Empirical research confirms that properly designed exercise routines, founded upon thorough examination, yield improved function and range of motion in patients who have conditions like frozen shoulder (Russell et al., 2014). Physiotherapists are tasked with developing individual rehabilitation plans based on findings from such examinations. These individualized approaches not only remove specific barriers but also empower the patients through learning and full engagement in the healing process. Using holistic physical examination methods, practitioners can construct elaborate treatment models, maximizing effectiveness and client coherence throughout the therapeutic process.

1.4.3. Importance of Accurate Diagnosis in Treatment Planning

Accurate diagnosis is the cornerstone of effective treatment planning in orthopedics and physiotherapy, which has a profound effect on patient outcomes. The process of making a correct diagnosis is an art that transcends being a technical process; it is what forms the starting point for developing treatment plans that are tailored to the individualized requirements of particular patients. Poor or inefficient therapy may result from incorrect diagnoses, potentially aggravating existing conditions and causing more problems. As new diagnostic technologies become better, such as artificial intelligence diagnostics, the accuracy of diagnosis will increase. The new diagnostic technologies make it simpler for medical experts to filter through plenty of data efficiently, enhance their ability to identify fractures and tumors and predict the outcomes of patients. Nevertheless, the use of such technology demands that one understand fully how they are to be used and their ability to avert clinical decision-making errors (Lisacek-Kiosoglous et al., 2023). In physiotherapy, proper diagnosis cannot be overemphasized since it determines the rehabilitation goals and interventions employed. Effective intervention relies on adequate assessment of the patients' physical capacity and restrictions. Accurate identification of the musculoskeletal pathology allows for the formulation of evidence-based interventions that target the condition of the individual. Also, constant monitoring of progress by way of newer technologies, such as wearable sensors, can offer information regarding the therapeutic interventions. These allow for recovery milestones to be monitored and provide real-time feedback, which is important in refining treatment plans. In addition, correct diagnosis maximizes patient empowerment and cooperation since patients will more likely be compliant with treatment protocols if they are aware of the specifics of their personal conditions and the reasons for their therapies (Palumbo et al., 2021). Lastly, the importance of accurate diagnosis transcends its application in initial treatment planning; it also involves long-term management and aftercare. Early and correct identification of issues enables the medical team to foretell complications in advance, potentially preventing the need for invasive treatments or prolonged rehabilitation. By bridging a multidisciplinary setting that includes diagnostics from imaging studies, clinical findings, and patient-reported information, medical professionals can enable improved decision-making processes and construct more effective treatment protocols. Moreover, as the healthcare landscape continues to evolve, the inclusion of ongoing learning and education about new diagnostic technologies will be crucial in guaranteeing quality care. Guaranteeing accuracy not only benefits the individual patient but also the overall efficacy of orthopedics and physiotherapy treatments (Lisacek-Kiosoglous et al., 2023) (Figure 1.13).

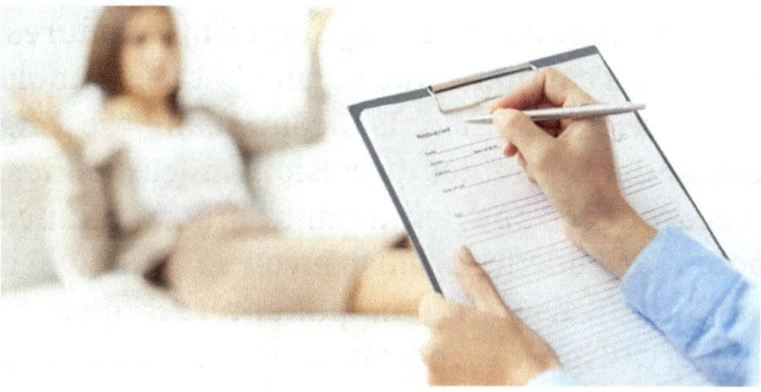

Figure 1.13. Accurate diagnosis is a cornerstone of effective treatment planning in orthopedics and physiotherapy.

Source: https://advantagementalhealthcenter.com/wp-content/uploads/2024/05/The-Importance-of-Accurate-Diagnosis-in-Mental-Health-Treatment.webp.

1.5. Treatment Options in Orthopedics

The orthopedic treatment scene is heterogeneous, a reflection of the heterogeneity of musculoskeletal disorders. Doctors can start with conservative treatment in the form of physical therapy, medication, and lifestyle modifications. They are non-invasive treatments that try to eliminate pain and bring about mobility, a preliminary step prior to more invasive procedures. For certain disorders like osteoarthritis or simple fractures, rehabilitation exercises and analgesics can bring about considerable recovery of function. According to Smith et al. (2015), musculoskeletal disorders, particularly of soft tissues, are quite hard to treat; giving priority to them in treatment planning is critical to optimize patient outcome and utilization of resources. Nevertheless, if conservative management fails, surgery may be inevitable. This is particularly true with recurrent disorders such as patellar dislocation, where it is critical to choose between surgical and non-surgical management. Recent studies, as summarized in Smith et al. (2015), demonstrate impressive reductions in recurrence rates following surgical procedures, but with a caution to the quality of the available evidence. While there is a continually growing demand for greater precision in guidelines, researchers and clinicians must balance potential benefits against involved risks when handling variability in patient response to surgery. The incorporation of physiotherapy with rehabilitation after surgery is essential to achieve the best recovery and to gain long-term functional improvement. An individualized program of physiotherapy, which may include strength training, range-of-motion exercises, and neuromuscular re-education, may help eliminate complications associated with surgery and with non-surgical interventions. The collaborative interaction among orthopedic professionals and physiotherapists is essential in the diagnosis and treatment of the most demanding disorders, as highlighted in Poltawski et al. (2008). Through the maintenance of appropriate rehabilitation procedures, the orthopedic profession will be able to enhance outcomes and allow patients to restore their functional capacity in daily life.

1.5.1. Surgical Interventions and Procedures

Surgery is a dominant methodology employed to treat musculoskeletal diseases, thereby influencing orthopedic practice to a great extent. Surgeries are only prescribed when non-surgical interventions such as drug therapy and physiotherapy fail to meet expectations. For instance, patellar dislocations are one such application. Evidence suggests that surgical interventions can cause a much reduced risk of recurrent dislocations compared to non-surgical options, particularly in the short-term follow-up of patients. The quality of such evidence is associated with considerable restrictions, like high risks of bias in appraising studies evaluating surgical interventions. Therefore, surgical treatment should be decided on after careful weighing of individual patient cases and complications, such as the potential for future surgery, which is indicative of the nuance of surgical decision-making within orthopedic care (Smith et al., 2015). Along with that, evolution in surgical procedures continues to enhance patient care for a variety of orthopedic pathologies. For example, orthopedic treatments for damage control have emerged on the front line in addressing war injuries in war zones, as observed with practices adopted during the Libyan civil war. The priority that such treatments accord is rapid stabilization and appropriate treatment of wounds, addressing the main need of patients who sustain serious spine and limb injuries. The treatments not only focus on sustaining the life of the patient but also accelerating recovery and rehabilitation through multidisciplinary treatment approaches. Depth analysis of trauma cases and application of the newest surgical trends ensure that treatment is tailored to the particular issues brought about by various kinds of injuries, particularly in high-risk cases where normal procedures are given up (Ng et al., 2015). Furthermore, the overall impact of surgical procedures also carries over to rehabilitation and physiotherapy, reiterating a symbiotic integration of these disciplines. After surgical interventions, patients may need to undergo organized rehabilitation programs that enable restoration of function and protection against complications. For example, post-operative physiotherapy after knee surgery is an important aspect in the recovery process, improving the range of motion and alleviating pain. There is a need for joint participation between orthopedic surgeons and physiotherapists to provide patient-specific rehabilitation plans that take into account the specific surgical procedure undertaken. This cooperation brings an integrated system of patient treatment with emphasis on the need for not only correcting the immediate problems of surgery but also maintenance of long-term recovery through effective physiotherapeutic methods. Thus, the intersection of surgical procedures and subsequent physiotherapy is necessary in the optimization of patient outcomes in orthopedic care (Smith et al., 2015) (Figure 1.14).

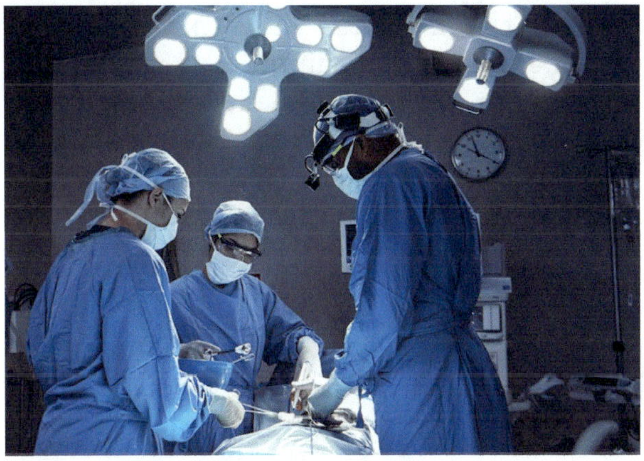

Figure 1.14. Surgical interventions and procedures.

Source: https://www.hopkinsmedicine.org/-/media/images/health/2_-treatment/surgical-care/common-surgical-hero.jpg?h=500&iar=0&mh=500&mw=1300&w=1297&hash=FD277EB2AEE62E1B53537767AEE778CE.

1.5.2. Non-Surgical Treatment Options (Medications, Braces)

In physiotherapy and orthopedics, non-surgical treatments such as medication and braces are now the main tools for treating many musculoskeletal ailments. Medication is typically the first line of treatment, alleviating pain and inflammation through the use of non-steroidal anti-inflammatory drugs (NSAIDs) or other analgesics. It is essential that the role of medication does not negate the need for holistic management techniques. For instance, effective drug management must be accompanied by physical modalities such as specific exercise therapy to address underlying pathology and stimulate long-term recovery. This dual approach is particularly crucial for cases like patellofemoral pain (PFP) and patellar tendinopathy (PT), in which exercise therapy is suggested as the primary treatment modality in order to improve outcomes and diminish reliance on drug interventions (Ophey et al., 2025). Bracing is yet another fundamental non-surgical intervention in the management of spinal deformity and musculoskeletal trauma. In deformities such as adolescent idiopathic scoliosis (AIS) and hyperkyphosis, bracing is applied to correct or reduce deformities and enhance functional capabilities as well as cosmetic acceptance.

Rigid bracing has established effectiveness in the retardation of progression of such conditions, particularly among teenagers. Evidence suggests that bracing not only contributes to the enhancement of spinal alignment but also supports the development of core stability, which is of utmost importance for overall musculoskeletal health (Ophey et al., 2025). In addition, in elderly individuals with spinal deformities, bracing has been established to enhance balance and alleviate pain, reflecting its use across diverse age groups. Though valuable, nonsurgical methods of bracing and medication are not enough, requiring incorporation of these modalities into a comprehensive rehabilitation treatment for optimal benefit. Physiotherapeutic interventions, along with conservative treatment such as bracing, enable functional rehabilitation and enhance the quality of life for patients. Illustrative examples are patients with conditions like AIS for whom physiotherapeutic scoliosis-specific exercise (PSSE), which is used with braces, is beneficial. This multimodal intervention generates greater, more durable improvements. Last but not least, a well-optimized treatment plan must consider the unique patient needs of each, so that pharmacologic as well as mechanical assistance is utilized judiciously to achieve therapeutic effects, as outlined in current literature favoring conservative management (Bettany-Saltikov et al., 2017).

1.5.3. Role of Physiotherapy in Post-Operative Care

The role of physiotherapy in post-operative care is essential to facilitate maximum recovery and rehabilitation after surgical procedures. It incorporates a range of therapeutic interventions for the purpose of restoring the function, alleviating pain, and eradicating complications arising after surgery. Reduced muscle strength and mobility are typically encountered by patients after procedures, and they may be required to undergo long periods of rehabilitation if not attended to early. Physiotherapy treatment, including exercise guidance and manual therapy, can best improve the outcome by improving circulation, increasing flexibility in the joints, and building up the muscles. Most importantly, these treatments not only accelerate the process of physical recovery but also assist in controlling psychological elements of anxiety, ultimately leading to a more integrated approach to post-operative recovery. Moreover, inclusion of evidence-based physiotherapy treatment into the post-operative care leads to improved patient satisfaction and quicker rehabilitation time. A study of various physiotherapy treatments for frozen shoulder conditions showed that subjects treated with organized physiotherapy experienced tremendous improvement in function and pain when compared to home exercise programs (Russell et al., 2014). This implies that the expertise and experience of physiotherapists are of paramount significance in designing the rehabilitation programs to cater to the unique needs of each patient. Successful physiotherapy minimizes post-operative complications like stiffness, reduced range of motion, and even mental issues, hence making it an integral component of comprehensive post-operative management. In the context of trauma cases, say in the form of war-induced cases, for instance, physiotherapy has a fundamental role to play in the management of complex injuries as well as in aiding recovery. For instance, in the assessment of orthopedic trauma casualties arising from the Libyan civil war, application of the multidisciplinary process incorporating physiotherapy was pivotal towards the achievement of speedy recovery and early mobilization of patients (Ng et al., 2015). This emphasizes the versatility and urgency of physiotherapy in various medical environments, particularly in cases where patients have extreme physical disabilities. Through the deployment of custom-made rehabilitation plans, physiotherapy promotes overall quality of care, enabling patients to go back to their routines with recovered functionality and confidence following their operations (Figure 1.15).

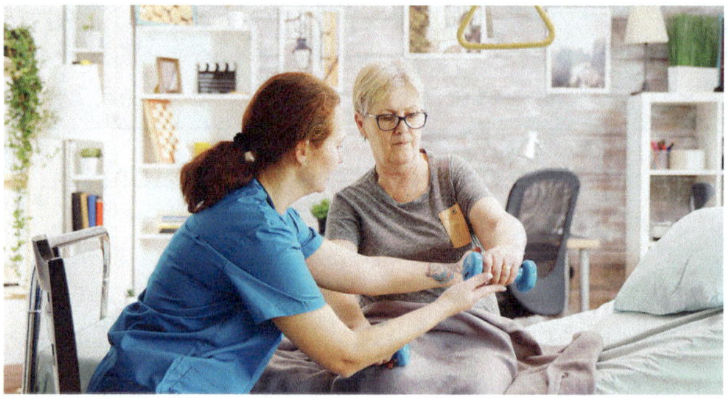

Figure 1.15. The role of physiotherapy in post-operative care.

Source: https://rustingtonconvalescenthome.co.uk/wp-content/uploads/2023/05/TheRoleofPhysiothe rapyinPostOperativeCareandR.jpg.

1.6. Current Trends and Innovations

The orthopedics and physiotherapy environment is more and more affected by current trends and advances that highlight the dynamic nature of healthcare delivery. The most important trend is the integration of advanced information technology, which has revolutionized patient care through telehealth and electronic health records. These advances enable practitioners to monitor patient progress remotely and improve treatment plans, improving patient-centered practice. Furthermore, the use of data analytics in primary care allows for the identification of health trends, which allows providers to respond and address patients' needs beforehand. According to Baldacchino et al. (2014), constant evolution of primary healthcare highlights its central role in improving general health outcomes and closing gaps, so technology becomes an essential ally in dealing with the new challenges facing modern healthcare. Apart from information technology, the design and implementation of novel devices to quantify spasticity are also a typical instance of the interconnection between rehabilitation science and engineering. Recent studies have centered on designing mechatronic devices solely for spasticity measurement of specific joints, such as the ankle, elbow, and knees. The operation principle of such devices is based on the speed-dependent characteristic of tonic stretch reflexes, which provides a true measurement of the degree of spasticity in various patient populations. Further development of these devices is essential, as it provides clinicians with quantitative data to guide treatment planning and assess functional outcomes. Clinical validation of these measurement systems, as recommended in Ferreira et al. (2010), is also vital to determine if the devices will be useful in the clinical setting and ultimately lead to improved rehabilitation protocols for individuals with spasticity. Lastly, interdisciplinary collaboration is an innovative approach in orthopedics and physiotherapy whereby professionals with various expertise collaborate to further the care of patients. The collaboration not only optimizes treatment outcomes but also innovation through idea exchange and skill set compatibility. For instance, physiotherapists, orthopedic surgeons, and occupational therapists can collaborate in developing holistic rehabilitation plans specially tailored to the needs of post-surgical or injured patients. In addition, the trend facilitates shared decision-making and comprehensive care, addressing both physiological and psychological rehabilitation issues. As noted in Baldacchino et al. (2014), the need for equal access to quality healthcare necessitates creative models that enhance collaboration, hence enabling patients to receive the best and best-coordinated care.

1.6.1. Advances in Surgical Techniques and Technology

The evolution of surgical technique and technology has revolutionized the landscape of orthopedics, with improved results and quality of patient experience. The course of history in the evolution of total hip replacements from the late 1930s is also a useful example here. Initial experiences were marred with complications such as infections and failure of implants. However, collaborative efforts of British surgeons and engineers led to the maximization of surgical procedures and prosthetic devices, ultimately resulting in extremely effective solutions. Evolution of material technology and materials, along with the introduction of controlled theatres in operating theatres, was responsible for reducing complications and maximizing the durability of implants. The establishment of national hip registers in the latter part of the twentieth century has also contributed to this field by providing evidence relating to implant performance, thereby determining clinical practice as well as the innovations in orthopedic surgery in the future (Reynolds & Tansey, 2007). In contemporary orthopedic practice, the incorporation of digital technology has changed patient management and surgical precision. Methods such as robot-assisted surgery and deeply sophisticated imaging devices, such as 3D modeling, enable surgeons to plan and conduct complex operations more accurately. Such technology not only enhances safety in surgical outcomes but also minimizes recovery times as well as complications. Telemedicine technologies too have emerged into consideration, especially post-COVID-19 crisis, to aid remote consultations and continuous monitoring of patients through wearable technology. These technological advancements allow health professionals to deliver personalized care more efficiently, addressing each patient's specific needs.

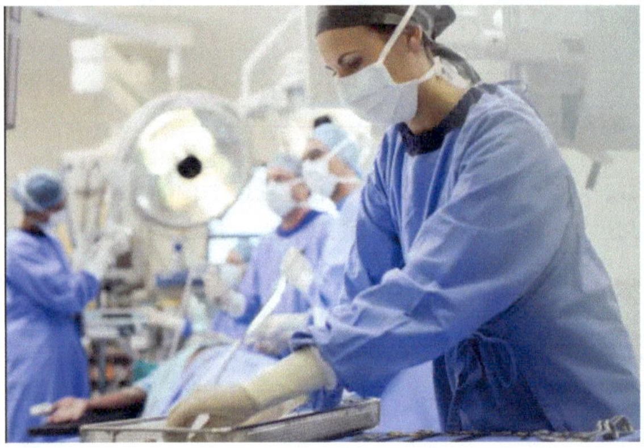

Figure 1.16. The evolution of surgical techniques and technology.

Source: https://b3378418.smushcdn.com/3378418/wp-content/uploads/2023/07/operating-room-surg-tech.jpg?lossy=2&strip=1&webp=1.

As such, traditional physical consultation and rehabilitation models are being reengineered with potential for improved delivery of healthcare in orthopedics (Youssef et al., 2024). Further, the application of immersive technologies in orthopedic procedures is rapidly becoming more prominent. Virtual, mixed, and augmented reality are being increasingly applied in training and patient rehabilitation. Virtual realities enhance the learning process for surgical trainees since they can practice real simulation of surgeries, thus improving their skills without endangering patients. In patient rehabilitation, virtual environments can motivate patients in physical therapy, enabling them to become more participative in the recovery process. This intersection of technology not only results in enhanced educational outcomes for healthcare professionals but also empowers patients with the capability to lend their own energies towards their rehabilitation process. As these technologies advance and become integrated into orthopedic processes, they have the capacity to keep enhancing surgical practices, patient outcomes, and the overall efficiency of care within orthopedics (Youssef et al., 2024) (Figure 1.16).

1.6.2. Emerging Therapies in Physiotherapy

The physiotherapy profession has experienced phenomenal growth over the last several years, driven by advances in new therapies that enhance patient outcomes. Of these newer therapies, the use of technology, specifically virtual reality (VR) and robotic rehabilitation, has revolutionized traditional practices. VR constructs interactive worlds that engage patients and simulate real-world challenges, actually enhancing motor control and functional independence. This technology allows for personalized rehabilitation sessions that are both interactive and responsive to the patient's individual gains, accommodating a more personalized recovery plan. Robotic-assisted devices also provide vital support with the execution of repetitive exercises that strengthen muscles and coordination without endangering injury. With these new therapies integrated into physiotherapy, it is possible to provide more efficient interventions and ultimately enhance the recovery process for patients with various conditions. Apart from innovation in technology, modality-based directed treatments such as neuromuscular electrical stimulation (NMES) are gaining popularity in physiotherapy. NMES is a form of stimulation of muscle contractions through electrical currents, and, therefore, improves rehabilitation in patients with impaired mobility or muscle disuse. It is useful, not only to increase the strength of the muscles but also to prevent muscle atrophy, which is crucial in surgery or injury patients. In addition, the application of NMES in conjunction with other traditional physiotherapy methods can support improved neuromuscular re-education, thus accelerating the process of rehabilitation.

As more physiotherapists become familiar with these techniques, the likelihood of enhancing the outcomes of patient care becomes increasingly apparent, particularly in patients with illnesses such as stroke, where muscle re-education is necessary to regain independence and mobility. Finally, teamwork among healthcare providers plays a crucial role in maximizing therapeutic gains in physiotherapy.

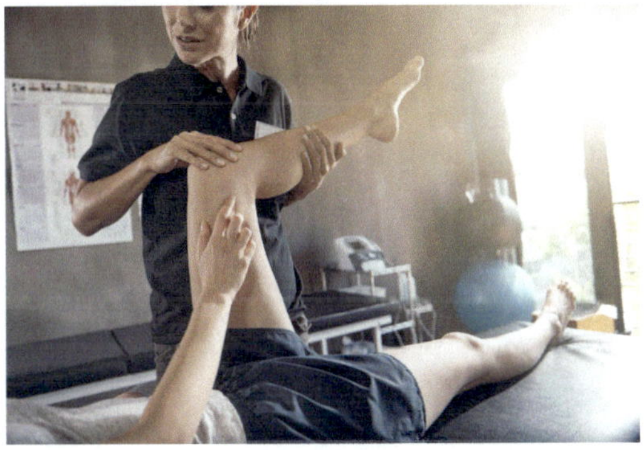

Figure 1.17. Emerging therapies in physiotherapy.

Source: https://www.opencolleges.edu.au/cdn/shop/articles/physio_fil_1.jpg?v=1692607890.

Multidisciplinary care is most clearly evident in the management of fibrous diseases such as hemophilic arthropathy, where comprehensive treatment involves the expertise of hematologists, physiotherapists, and orthopedic specialists. Outcome relies on prompt intervention strategies involving joint protection techniques and reparative physical therapy (Knobe & Berntorp, 2011). In addition, new orthotic devices are being studied to improve mobility and functional capacity in cerebral palsy patients, with physiotherapy playing a central role in their implementation (Morris, 2002). By promoting collaboration and integrating changing therapy, physiotherapy not only improves the quality of care but also ensures that the patients gain the benefit from the cumulative knowledge and experience of different health professionals in their own rehabilitation processes (Figure 1.17).

1.6.3. Future Directions in Orthopedic Research

As we move towards the orthopedic future of research, a lot of focus is on integrating newer technologies for optimizing outcomes of surgery and patient care. The most notable development in this context is the application of robotic-assisted surgical systems. These technologies have the potential to increase precision and uniformity of procedures, thereby reducing complications and recovery times. As robotics evolves further, orthopedics can benefit from the added functionality that will make minimally invasive techniques a standard. Not only do these advancements allow for more successful procedures, but they also set the stage for future studies on their long-term results, with the ultimate goal being to improve patient outcomes and quality of life (Liang et al., 2024). This route will involve extensive study of patient-by-patient response to robotic intervention, depending on their specific anatomical needs and medical histories. Other newer fields, such as regenerative medicine, are also going to change the course of orthopedic research in the coming times. Techniques such as stem cell therapy and platelet-rich plasma (PRP) injection are finding fame for their capability to accelerate healing and facilitate tissue regeneration. Research is currently underway to maximize these uses in order to enhance their effectiveness for the treatment of chronic musculoskeletal conditions. By researching factors such as dosage and when to apply these therapies, researchers aim to make the best practice that can lead to revolutionary improvement in joint function and mobility (Liang et al., 2024). As such methods improve, so too remains the challenge to critically assess their long-term implications and translate research into practice, giving practitioners the information required for informed treatment decisions. The intersection of artificial intelligence (AI) with orthopedic science also holds great promise for future diagnosis and treatment methods. The use of machine learning techniques in the analysis of patient data can lead to more accurate diagnoses and personalized treatment plans that consider the unique characteristics of every patient. This shift towards precision medicine gives the hope of considerable advancement in the treatment of orthopedic disorders, with practitioners more informed about optimal interventions that are tailored to particular needs. In addition, as witnessed in recent research, the integration of AI in clinical operations can also streamline processes and improve decision-making (Liang et al., 2024). The incorporation of these technologies into orthopedic research will not only contribute to better clinical outcomes but also to a holistic understanding of patient experiences, cementing orthopedics as a pioneer in innovative medical interventions.

SUMMARY

It is important to emphasize the profound interdependence of musculoskeletal medicine and orthopedic manual therapy in orthopedic condition management and treatment. The healing application of physiotherapy, illustrated through musculoskeletal conditions like frozen shoulder, highlights the ability of musculoskeletal medicine to wield the therapeutic benefits of certain exercise regimens to deliver astounding improvements in patient health. Empirical evidence supports that patients who went to organized exercise sessions had better recovery rates than with single physiotherapy or even home exercises. These findings highlight the importance of engaging proactively in group therapies because they not only offer physical enhancement but also promote social support among the patients, enhancing holistic recovery (Russell et al., 2014). Moreover, treatment of osteoporotic conditions, particularly in older adults, further highlights the pivotal importance of preventive interventions in orthopedics. The outcomes of more recent studies indicate that the timing of anti-osteoporotic treatment, for instance, bisphosphonates, can significantly impact long-term patient health. The proof of reduction in rates of re-fracture as well as the decline in mortality rates among patients on these medications attests to the extreme importance of an integrated pathway of care post-surgery. This strategic approach not only enhances individual health results but also helps alleviate the broader economic cost to healthcare systems, corresponding to the need for multiplicative treatment paradigms in orthopedic practice (Cuschieri et al., 2016). Lastly, the conclusion of this study calls for the importance of continuous developments and studies in orthopedics and physiotherapy to optimize patient care. It is very important to encourage evidence-based practices that integrate therapeutic exercise with effective pharmacological treatment directed toward the unique circumstances of each patient. The findings of several studies highlight the point that even the best optimized treatment regimens contribute significantly to increased quality of life and healthcare cost savings. As both fields evolve, ongoing communication among medical practitioners will be central to the process of improving treatment and ensuring that patients have complete and effective care for their musculoskeletal conditions and hence closing the gap between rehabilitation and overall well-being. An in-depth understanding of orthopedics and physiotherapy is crucial to the effective management of musculoskeletal disease and the enhancement of patient outcomes. The following essay presents pertinent arguments regarding the interface between the two disciplines, highlighting the role of physiotherapy in rehabilitation following orthopedic intervention. The integrated application of therapeutic modalities alleviates discomfort, promotes mobility, and aids functional restoration. Besides, physiotherapists serve as a focal point for educating patients about self-management skills and prevention measures, reinforcing long-term wellness. By adopting a multidisciplinary ethos, equal emphasis is placed on the physical and psychosocial dimensions of care, thereby ensuring an ideal setting for holistic healing. Technological advancements also significantly contribute to the practice of orthopedics and physiotherapy. The development of automated and semi-automated systems, such as those born out of the NeXOS project, is a quintessential case of engineering and rehabilitation specialists fusion to enhance patient care. This prototype illustrates how novel concepts can structure therapy interventions to change the amount of support offered to patients in recovery. Through enhancing physiotherapist skill levels through technology, these systems can optimize treatment effectiveness and accommodate more personalized provision of care. This intersection of physiotherapy and engineering not only makes rehabilitation processes easier to optimize but also may improve the accessibility of care, such that interventions can be provided in patients' homes. A further prominent aspect discussed in this essay is the complexity of long-term musculoskeletal pain and its implications for informal caregivers and patients. An understanding of caregivers' everyday reality is critical in the creation of an integrated care model. Evidence indicates that informal caregivers often navigate between multiple complicated roles, including those of confidants and middlemen to healthcare workers, and this may result in overwhelming emotional and physical burdens. Considering this complicated relationship between care receivers, caregivers, and healthcare providers, interventions can be designed to cater to the needs of all the involved stakeholders. Lastly, support for the caregiver experience enhances the care recipient's pathway too and develops a more resilient caregiving dyad, leading to better health outcomes for those with chronic pain (Smith et al., 2021).

CLOSER LOOK

ORTHOPEDICS AND PHYSIOTHERAPY

Orthopedics is the branch of medicine dedicated to the care of the musculoskeletal system, which includes bones, joints, muscles, ligaments, tendons, and nerves. It focuses on the prevention, diagnosis, treatment, and rehabilitation of conditions that affect movement and physical function. Orthopedic care is essential for people of all ages, from children with congenital deformities to elderly individuals with degenerative bone and joint diseases. Orthopedic specialists manage a wide range of conditions such as fractures, arthritis, osteoporosis, sports injuries, spinal disorders, and joint problems. Diagnosis typically involves clinical examination supported by imaging technologies like X-rays, MRI, and CT scans. Treatment approaches vary from non-surgical methods, including medication, physiotherapy, braces, and lifestyle modification, to advanced surgical procedures such as joint replacements, arthroscopy, and minimally invasive spine surgery.

Rehabilitation is a core part of orthopedic care, helping patients regain strength, mobility, and independence after injury or surgery. Preventive care is also emphasized through posture training, ergonomics, injury prevention strategies, and physical fitness programs. Overall, orthopedics plays a vital role in improving mobility, reducing pain, and enhancing quality of life. With continuous advancements in medical technology and treatment techniques, orthopedic care continues to evolve, offering safer procedures, faster recovery, and better long-term outcomes for patients.

REFERENCES

1. Bradley, David, Acosta-Marquez, C., Hawley, Mark et al. (3 more authors) (2009) *NeXOS - The design, development and evaluation of a rehabilitation system for the lower limbs.* Mechatronics, 19 (2). pp. 247-257. ISSN 0957-4158(accessed on 26th June 2025).
2. Scott, A., Squier, K., Alfredson, H., Bahr, R., Cook, J. L., Coombes, B., de Vos, R. J., Fu, S. N., Grimaldi, A., Lewis, J. S., Maffulli, N., Magnusson, S. P., Malliaras, P., Mc Auliffe, S., Oei, E. H. G., Purdam, C. R., Rees, J. D., Rio, E. K., Gravare Silbernagel, K., Speed, C., ... Zwerver, J. (2020). ICON 2019: International Scientific Tendinopathy Symposium Consensus: Clinical Terminology. *British journal of sports medicine, 54*(5), 260–262. https://doi.org/10.1136/bjsports-2019-100885(accessed on 26th June 2025).
3. Russell, S., Jariwala, A., Conlon, R., Selfe, J., Richards, J., & Walton, M. (2014). A blinded, randomized, controlled trial assessing conservative management strategies for frozen shoulder. *Journal of shoulder and elbow surgery, 23*(4), 500–507. https://doi.org/10.1016/j.jse.2013.12.026(accessed on 26th June 2025).
4. Smith, T. O., Gaukroger, A., Metcalfe, A., & Hing, C. B. (2023). Surgical versus non-surgical interventions for treating patellar dislocation. *The Cochrane database of systematic reviews, 1*(1), CD008106. https://doi.org/10.1002/14651858.CD008106.pub4(accessed on 26th June 2025).
5. Auckland University of Technology, Forrest, G., Jedrzejczak, M., Leech, S., McKiernan, B., Ministry of Health, New Zealand Medical Radiation Technologists Board, et al. (2018). Exploring the clinical use of ultrasound imaging: A survey of physiotherapists in New Zealand. https://core.ac.uk/download/155776972.pdf (accessed on 26th June 2025).
6. Youssef, Y., De Wet, D., Back, D. A., & Scherer, J. (2024). Digitalization in orthopaedics: a narrative review. *Frontiers in surgery, 10,* 1325423. https://doi.org/10.3389/fsurg.2023.1325423(accessed on 26th June 2025).
7. Baldacchino, M., Bezzina, G., Sammut, M. R., Scerri, A., et al. (2014). A review of certain recent advances in primary healthcare. https://core.ac.uk/download/46603060.pdf (accessed on 26th June 2025).
8. Collier, T., Roadley-Battin, M., Darlow, C., Chant, P., Hing, C. B., & Smith, T. O. (2018). Analysis of conference abstract-to-publication rate in UK orthopaedic research. *BMJ evidence-based medicine, 23*(1), 7–11. https://doi.org/10.1136/ebmed-2017-110831(accessed on 26th June 2025).
9. Knobe K, Berntorp E. Haemophilia and joint disease: pathophysiology, evaluation, and management. *J Comorb.* 2011;1:51-59. Published 2011 Dec 27. doi:10.15256/joc.2011.1.2(accessed on 26th June 2025).
10. Bertoni, G., Marchesini, E., Zanchettin, F. E., Crestini, M., Testa, M., & Battista, S. (2023). Use of audience response systems (ARS) in physiotherapists' training: A qualitative study. *BMJ Open, 13,* e073025–e073025. https://doi.org/10.1136/bmjopen-2023-073025 (accessed on 26th June 2025).
11. Bettany-Saltikov, J., Turnbull, D., Ng, S. Y., & Webb, R. (2017). Management of Spinal Deformities and Evidence of Treatment Effectiveness. *The open orthopaedics journal, 11,* 1521–1547. https://doi.org/10.2174/1874325001711011521(accessed on 26th June 2025).

12. Ophey, M., Koëter, S., van Ooijen, L., van Ark, M., Boots, F., Ilbrink, S., Lankhorst, N. A., Piscaer, T., Vestering, M., den Ouden Vierwind, M., van Linschoten, R., & van Berkel, S. (2025). Dutch multidisciplinary guideline on anterior knee pain: Patellofemoral pain and patellar tendinopathy. *Knee surgery, sports traumatology, arthroscopy : official journal of the ESSKA, 33*(2), 457–469. https://doi.org/10.1002/ksa.12367 (accessed on 26th June 2025).

13. Ng, C., Mifsud, M., Borg, J. N., & Mizzi, C. (2015). The Libyan civil conflict: selected case series of orthopaedic trauma managed in Malta in 2014. *Scandinavian journal of trauma, resuscitation and emergency medicine, 23,* 103. https://doi.org/10.1186/s13049-015-0183-2(accessed on 26th June 2025).

14. Morris C. (2002). A review of the efficacy of lower-limb orthoses used for cerebral palsy. *Developmental medicine and child neurology, 44*(3), 205–211. https://doi.org/10.1017/s0012162201001943(accessed on 26th June 2025).

15. Smith, T., Fletcher, J., & Lister, S. (2021). Lived experiences of informal caregivers of people with chronic musculoskeletal pain: a systematic review and meta-ethnography. *British journal of pain, 15*(2), 187–198. https://doi.org/10.1177/2049463720925110(accessed on 26th June 2025).

16. Poltawski, L., Watson, T. & Byrne, G., (2008). Physiotherapists' perceptions of problematic musculoskeletal soft tissue disorders. International Journal of Therapy and Rehabilitation 2008 15:10, 437-444. https://core.ac.uk/download/1638527.pdf (accessed on 26th June 2025).

17. Carlesso, L., Graham, H., Gross, A., Ho, C., et al. (2013). An ICON overview on physical modalities for neck pain and associated disorders. https://core.ac.uk/download/pdf/56363907.pdf (accessed on 26th June 2025).

18. Choudhary, A., Pisulkar, G., Taywade, S., Awasthi, A., & Salwan, A. (2024). A comprehensive review of total hip arthroplasty outcomes in post-traumatic hip arthritis: Insights and perspectives. *Cureus.* https://doi.org/10.7759/cureus.56350 (accessed on 26th June 2025).

19. Costa, L. (2024). Maturation of the spine and its consequences for conservative treatment of adolescent idiopathic scoliosis. https://core.ac.uk/download/621383344.pdf (accessed on 26th June 2025).

20. Cuschieri, S., Gatt, R., & Grech, S. (2016). Bisphosphonates: A cost benefit analysis patient. https://core.ac.uk/download/46603883.pdf (accessed on 26th June 2025).

21. Morris JH, James RE, Davey R, Waddington G. What is orthopaedic triage? A systematic review. *J Eval Clin Pract.* 2015;21(1):128-136. doi:10.1111/jep.12260(accessed on 26th June 2025).

22. Geidl, W., Wais, J., Fangmann, C., Demisse, E., Pfeifer, K., & Sudeck, G. (2019). Physical activity promotion in daily exercise therapy: the perspectives of exercise therapists in German rehabilitation settings. *BMC sports science, medicine & rehabilitation, 11,* 28. https://doi.org/10.1186/s13102-019-0143-7 (accessed on 26th June 2025).

23. Williams L.G. Ernstzen D.V. Statham S.B. Hanekom S.D. (2015). Evaluation of clinical sites used for training undergraduate physiotherapy students: Factors that may impact on learning. https://core.ac.uk/download/478426891.pdf (accessed on 26th June 2025).

24. Shah, S. G. S., & Farrow, A. (2012). Trends in the availability and usage of electrophysical agents in physiotherapy practices from 1990 to 2010: a review. *Physical Therapy Reviews, 17*(4),

207–226. https://doi.org/10.1179/1743288X12Y.0000000007(accessed on 26th June 2025).

25. Ferreira, J. A. O., Machado, J. M., Rodrigues, P., Soares, D., et al. (2010). An approach for spasticity quantification based on the stretch reflex threshold. International Conference 2nd International Conference on Innovations, Recent Trends and Challenges in Mechatronics, Mechanical Engineering and New High-Tech Products Development MECAHITECH'10 . https://core.ac.uk/download/55616435.pdf (accessed on 26th June 2025).

26. Kilbride, C., Meyer, J., Flatley, M., & Perry, L. (2005). Stroke units: the implementation of a complex intervention. *Educational Action Research*, *13*(4), 479–504. https://doi.org/10.1080/14759390500200301(accessed on 26th June 2025).

27. Haffner, D., Emma, F., Eastwood, D. M., Biosse Duplan, M., Bacchetta, J., Schnabel, D., Wicart, P., et al. (2019). Clinical practice recommendations for the diagnosis and management of X-linked hypophosphatemia. *Nature Reviews Nephrology, 15*, 435–455. https://doi.org/10.1038/s41581-019-0152-5 (accessed on 26th June 2025).

28. Knox, G. M., Snodgrass, S. J., Stanton, T. R., Kelly, D. H., Vicenzino, B., Wand, B. M., & Rivett, D. A. (2017). Physiotherapy students' perceptions and experiences of clinical prediction rules. *Physiotherapy*, *103*(3), 296–303. https://doi.org/10.1016/j.physio.2016.04.001(accessed on 26th June 2025).

29. Lewis, J. (2016). Rotator cuff related shoulder pain: Assessment, management and uncertainties. https://core.ac.uk/download/132614159.pdf (accessed on 26th June 2025).

30. Liang, W., Zhou, C., Bai, J., Zhang, H., Jiang, B., Wang, J., Fu, L., et al. (2024). Current advancements in therapeutic approaches in orthopedic surgery: A review of recent trends. *Frontiers in Bioengineering and Biotechnology, 12*. https://doi.org/10.3389/fbioe.2024.1328997 (accessed on 26th June 2025).

31. Lisacek-Kiosoglous, A., Powling, A. S., Fontalis, A., Gabr, A., Mazomenos, E. B., & Haddad, F. S. (2023). Artificial intelligence in orthopedic surgery. *Bone and Joint Research, 12*, 447–454. https://doi.org/10.1302/2046-3758.127.bjr-2023-0111.r1 (accessed on 26th June 2025).

32. McKeown, M. D. (2009). Back pain episodes of care in family practice: Analysis using electronic medical record data. https://core.ac.uk/download/560854259.pdf (accessed on 26th June 2025).

33. Multani, I., Manji, J., Hastings-Ison, T., Khot, A., & Graham, H. K. (2019). Botulinum toxin in the management of children with cerebral palsy. *Pediatric Drugs, 21*, 261–281. https://doi.org/10.1007/s40272-019-00344-8 (accessed on 26th June 2025).

34. Sivhugwana, Innocentia (2022). Factors related with the functional outcome of patients who sustained tibial plateau fractures. Dissertation (MSc (Physiotherapy))--University of Pretoria, 2022. https://core.ac.uk/download/565849089.pdf (accessed on 26th June 2025).

35. Stark, C., Nikopoulou-Smyrni, P., Stabrey, A., Semler, O., & Schoenau, E. (2010). Effect of a new physiotherapy concept on bone mineral density, muscle force and gross motor function in children with bilateral cerebral palsy. *Journal of musculoskeletal & neuronal interactions, 10*(2), 151–158. (accessed on 26th June 2025).

36. Palumbo, A., Vizza, P., Calabrese, B., & Ielpo, N. (2021). Biopotential signal monitoring systems in rehabilitation: A review. *Sensors, 21*, 7172–7172. https://doi.org/10.3390/s21217172 (accessed on 26th June 2025).

37. Reynolds, L. A., & Tansey, E. M. (2007). Early development of total hip replacement. https://core.ac.uk/download/30696185.pdf (accessed on 26th June 2025).

38. Reynolds, L. A., & Tansey, E. M. (2009). The development of sports medicine in twentieth-century Britain. The transcript of a Witness Seminar held by the Wellcome Trust Centre for the History of Medicine at UCL, London, on 29 June 2007. https://core.ac.uk/download/30696172.pdf (accessed on 26th June 2025).

39. Samoy, Y., Saunders, J., & Van Ryssen, B. (2016). Physiotherapy in small animal medicine. https://core.ac.uk/download/154408470.pdf (accessed on 26th June 2025).

40. Steenbruggen, R. A., Maas, M., Hoogeboom, T. J., Brand, P. L. P., & van der Wees, P. J. (2023). A framework to improve quality of hospital-based physiotherapy: A design-based research study. *BMC Health Services Research, 23.* https://doi.org/10.1186/s12913-023-09062-x (accessed on 26th June 2025).

41. Vassallo, K. (2008). Shoulder pain in general practice. https://core.ac.uk/download/46602184.pdf (accessed on 26th June 2025).

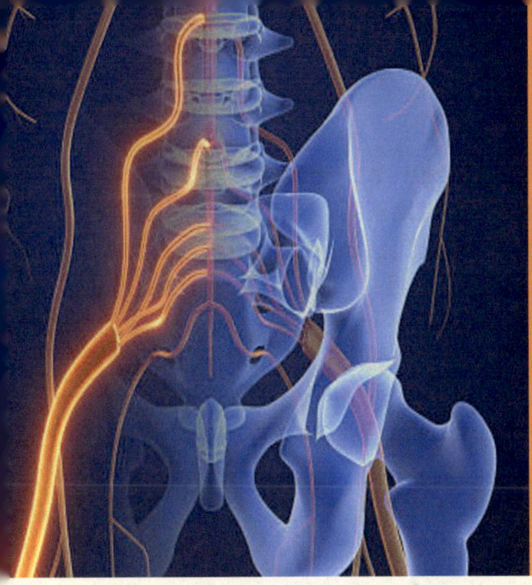

Chapter 2
MUSCULOSKELETAL INJURIES AND MANAGEMENT

Contents

Introduction....35
2.1. Types of Musculoskeletal Injuries....38
2.2. Causes and Risk Factors....42
2.3. Symptoms and Diagnosis....45
2.4. Treatment Options....49
2.5. Rehabilitation and Recovery....52
2.6. Prevention Strategies....56
Summary....61
References....64

Introduction

The diagnosis of musculoskeletal injury is now at the forefront of clinical practice and public health debate, considering that musculoskeletal injuries present significant morbidity. Musculoskeletal injuries are a broad range of tissue damages that include muscle strains, ligament sprains, and fractures, often caused by acute trauma or repetitive strain. These injuries are common among sports teams but also in the general population, largely due to lifestyle. As they are prevalent, knowing the mechanisms behind these injuries is essential to developing effective care practices. There is a demand for improved awareness and knowledge about prevention and care practices for health professionals so that they can offer focused interventions that increase recovery rates and decrease long-term consequences associated with these injuries (Khalek et al., 2024). Management of acute pain is at the core of treating musculoskeletal trauma, particularly in the emergency setting, in which early treatment has a major influence on subsequent patient outcomes. Relieving pain not only to improve current comfort but also to enable early mobilization and rehabilitation is important. With this, challenges still abound in the provision of rapid delivery of analgesics, as seen in the emergency departments, where there are rampant delays. Evidence has shown that optimizing processes of analgesia can have enormous effects on the provision of care. A very recent pilot project, for instance, demonstrated that the employment of formal interventions and protocols can reduce time to first dosing of an analgesic significantly, with commensurate improvement in patient satisfaction and clinical efficacy (Sadasivam et al., 2024). This reinforces the need for an integrated treatment plan that combines pharmacological and non-pharmacological interventions in pain treatment. When treating musculoskeletal trauma, having a holistic model that focuses on both physical rehabilitation and psychological guidance is necessary. The multidimensional nature of recovery benefits patients with a whole-person approach that, besides pain alleviation, provides education in the prevention of the mechanism of injury and lifestyle modification. Awareness of causal factors of musculoskeletal injuries, such as ergonomic behavior and proper methods of exercise, contributes significantly to prevention. Furthermore, integrating multidisciplinary teams into the management process can enhance treatment outcomes by ensuring patients receive treatment in a manner that addresses their unique needs and stages of recovery. Ultimately, musculoskeletal injury management improvement is derived from creating collaboration among medical specialties with emphasis on ongoing research and evidence-based guideline development.

Definition of Musculoskeletal Injuries

Musculoskeletal injury is a broad spectrum of conditions affecting the muscles, bones, joints, tendons, and ligaments and leading to pain, disability, and reduced quality of life. The injuries may arise from various etiologic factors, including acute trauma, overuse, or degenerative changes. Some examples of these include sprains, strains, tendinitis, fractures, and arthritis. Musculoskeletal injuries can be classified by individual diagnoses, where the diagnosis directs the healthcare provider to give appropriate intervention and modify management approaches. As they are leading causes of absence from work and can become chronic conditions if not managed appropriately, awareness of their nature and impact is necessary for effective management both in clinic and occupational settings. The biopsychosocial model of health which is centered on the interaction between biological, psychological, and social elements, is increasingly regarded as indispensable in explaining and managing musculoskeletal injury. By dealing with both the physical presentation of injuries as well as their psychosocial features, this model helps practitioners design a holistic treatment program. The literature indicates that treatment of only the biological aspects of musculoskeletal complaints often will not improve outcomes, particularly in occupational environments. Instead, the incorporation of psychosocial interventions that engage patients and create a nonthreatening environment is essential. This multifaceted approach not only addresses the root musculoskeletal impairment but also lessens the overall impact of injuries on the individual's workplace and overall well-being, as stressed by increasing evidence in the field (Kendall et al., 2015). Incorporating active management of musculoskeletal injury within workplace settings has been shown to considerably reduce its overall impact on work performance and health. The development of tools such as the Health ↔ Work Toolbox illustrates an innovative solution that combines primary prevention and health delivery. The tool offers evidence-based principles and practices to allow employers and workers to address work-related health issues with efficiency. Through the development of a healthy work culture, organizations can lower the incidence rate of musculoskeletal injuries as well as empower workers to maintain productivity. Implementing stringent management strategies and creating a cultural shift that acknowledges the psychosocial nature of injury are both needed. Therefore, the integration of multimodal interventions remains at the forefront in achieving the optimal outcomes for employees whose job is affected by such prevalent conditions in the workplace (Kendall et al., 2015) (Figure 2.1).

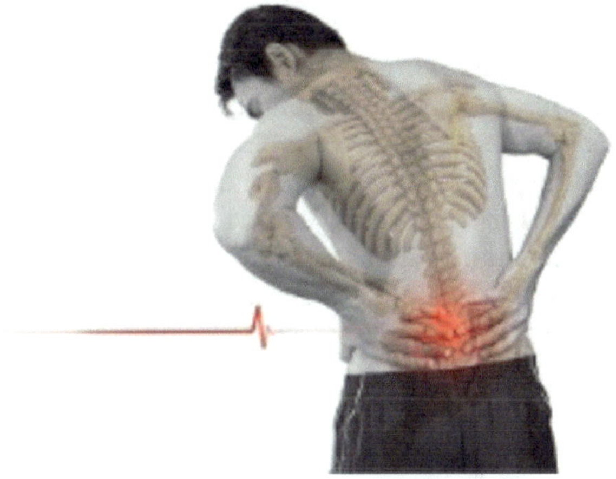

Figure 2.1. Musculoskeletal injury.

Source: https://www.landscapeprofessionals.org/images/LP/Safety/images/BackPainBanner.jpg.

Importance of Understanding These Injuries

A key element in musculoskeletal injuries is the thorough understanding of their etiology and implications for recovery and performance. For equine or human sports horses, an understanding of musculoskeletal injuries enables more targeted rehabilitation as well as training programs. This type of recognition not only guarantees effective injury management but also avoids re-injury, ultimately contributing to the longevity of athletes in their respective sports. This recognition serves as a platform for developing more individualized treatment regimens, making it possible for athletic trainers, coaches, and medical professionals to synchronize their efforts in addressing the complexity of injured athletes. With continued advancements in medical science, the ability to innovate and develop in therapeutic approaches continues to become increasingly feasible, thereby enabling the provision of maximal care to athletes in the recovery process. Additionally, knowledge of various types of musculoskeletal injury—which range from tendonitis to fracture—provides critical information regarding prevention of injury strategies. For instance, the complex presentations of injury, as well as knowledge regarding factors such as biomechanics and load-carrying capacities, can guide training adjustments. In the world of competitive sport, where the stress of performance is so high, an anticipatory strategy drawing on an understanding of probable injuries can make a considerable contribution to injury reduction. Training and exercise preparation adjustments can predispose an athlete towards physiological vigor, reducing the likelihood of incidence of injury in pressure competition. Hence, a knowledge of kinds of injuries and what they imply has a dual advantage: optimizing short-term treatment and enhancing long-term athletic fitness and performance. Moreover, an optimal knowledge of musculoskeletal injuries is necessary in order to facilitate effective communication among healthcare teams, athletes, and coaching staff. Delivery of quality care relies upon an effective strategy where all individuals possess a shared understanding of an athlete's status and development. If trainers and team physicians receive up-to-date information about various therapeutic modalities, both conservative and new advances in regenerative treatments, they can more effectively carry out their responsibilities. In-depth discussions regarding optimal management strategies, as described in the sports medicine team consensus reports, are crucial in optimizing the athlete's recovery and return to competition. Consequently, ongoing education and dialogue on this issue are essential since they lead to informed decision-making that eventually serves players by allowing them to achieve their best performance safely, as quoted by Herring et al. (2024) and Reis et al. (2024)

Overview of Management Strategies

An effective management strategy for musculoskeletal injuries requires a general understanding of injury etiology, diagnosis, and rehabilitation. Most closely examined are the etiology and description of individual injuries, e.g., hamstring strains typical of elite-level athletes. The long head of the biceps femoris muscle has been identified as most susceptible during the terminal swing phase of sprinting, emphasizing the need for specific preventative measures. Evidence-based interventions, like exercise, like the Nordic hamstring curl, have been shown to be effective in reducing the rate of injury by enhancing eccentric strength and flexibility. Further, exercise and load management, like the acute–chronic workload ratio (ACWR), help monitor and adjust training loads to limit the risk of overuse and acute injury among athletes, yielding a more resilient performance with time (Kim & Lee, 2025). Other than preventive care, acute pain control is integral to the management of musculoskeletal injury. The early response to injury is significant in the rehabilitation process since effective pain management abolishes pain and allows for early rehabilitation. Both pharmacologic, e.g., nonsteroidal anti-inflammatory agents (NSAIDs), and non-pharmacologic, e.g., ice pack application and physical modalities, treatments are integral components of acute care protocols. Despite heterogeneity in current protocols, a thorough review of the methods identifies their potential to yield outstanding relief and enable healing (Khalek et al., 2024). It is important that it is performed with an individualized strategy, considering the specific nature and severity of the injury, and patient-specific aspects, to realize maximal recovery outcomes. With progressive rehabilitation, there is a focus on long-term recovery processes, favoring functional recovery and return to sport. This phase is characterized by the combination of progressive exercise in restoring strength, range of motion, as well as general functional capacity. Rehabilitation regimens must be adapted with sport-specific movements to restore required skills in the particular activity. Moreover, psychosocial factors such as motivation and mental readiness must be resolved here for ensuring rehabilitation protocol compliance as well as optimal recovery results. Mechanisms such as feedback through performance appraisals guarantee that rehabilitation approaches are responsive and adaptive as they evolve in accordance with the healing process. Through the combination of these intricate management techniques, the holistic management of musculoskeletal injury is possible, allowing successful recovery and return to sport.

2.1. Types of Musculoskeletal Injuries

Musculoskeletal injuries constitute a wide range of bone, muscle, tendon, ligament, and nerve conditions. Acute and chronic injuries are both present, with each presenting its own difficulties in diagnosis and treatment. Acute injuries, such as fractures and sprains, typically result from an acute traumatic or an acute applied force to the musculoskeletal system. For instance, a fracture results from a blow or fall, but a sprain results from overstretching or tearing ligaments. Chronic injuries, on the contrary, develop gradually over time and are often due to overuse and repetitive stress, such as tendinitis or stress fractures. This difference is essential to utilize correct management principles, guiding therapeutic interventions in addition to prevention measures. Identification of the nuances of these injuries makes for better clinical outcomes and improved efficacy in rehabilitation strategies. Among the most common musculoskeletal injuries are tendinopathies, which greatly impact an individual's quality of life and functional capacity. Tendinopathies are usually caused by repetitive tendon stress, with pain, inflammation, and decreased strength.

Classic examples include Achilles tendinopathy and rotator cuff injury, both with distinct clinical presentations and challenges. Management of these injuries is most often a multifaceted endeavor using physiotherapy, activity modification, and in some cases, surgical intervention. Emerging advances in regenerative medicine, such as adipose-derived stem cell therapy, are also investigated as novel treatments for tendon injuries. These approaches have the potential to enhance tendon healing capacity, reduce recovery time, and prevent chronicity. All these various forms of tendinopathy need to be understood for the development of effective therapy protocols and optimization of outcomes in the management of musculoskeletal injury. One of the most significant groups of musculoskeletal injuries is the spine, commonly presenting as cervical strain or back pain. Spinal injuries can be produced by a variety of mechanisms, ranging from acute trauma to long-standing conditions resulting from bad posture or repetitive strain. Disc herniations, for example, occur when intervertebral discs protrude and compress adjacent nerves, inducing pain and impairment of function. In addition, disorders such as sciatica demonstrate how spinal injuries can refer pain elsewhere, complicating diagnosis and treatment. Spinal injuries are typically treated by an integrated scheme of pain management, physical therapy, and lifestyle modification to prevent recurrence. As more research comes out, the inclusion of newer therapy and rehabilitation techniques remains the key to counteracting the complexities of spinal musculoskeletal injury and enhancing recovery in affected individuals.

2.1.1. Acute Injuries

Acute injuries represent a critical musculoskeletal injury category that is usually caused by acute trauma or overuse while performing physical exercise. Acute injuries can manifest differently, including as fractures, sprains, and strains, all presenting unique diagnostic and management issues. Early evaluation of an acute injury is crucial since interventions made early can substantially affect recovery outcomes. Understanding of the underlying mechanisms—i.e., the extent of tissue destruction and the inflammatory response of the body—provides us with information for optimal treatment planning. Early intervention in the acute injury allows healthcare providers to reduce pain and prevent musculoskeletal trauma's long-term sequelae. The impact of acute injury on the functional capability of an individual provides a strong rationale for the implementation of a unified management approach encompassing not only physical rehabilitation but also psychological counseling in the rehabilitation process. A sophisticated treatment plan addressing both immediate as well as long-term problems of the injured individual is required for optimal management of acute injuries. Part of the key aspects of acute injury care includes pain relief, which may be achieved through several pharmacological and non-pharmacological interventions. The inclusion of pain management protocols is critical to the provision of recovery since uncontrolled pain can readily overwhelm rehabilitation efforts. Furthermore, evidence-based practices guarantee that the care pathways that address the tailored needs of the patient are formulated. Current literature has highlighted the need to evaluate various pain management techniques within the sports and clinical settings, with a focus on the requirement for further research and revised procedures towards maximizing recovery rates from acute injury (Khalek et al., 2024). This holistic method requires all healthcare specialists to work together to attain the best possible recovery patterns for the affected individuals. Outside of pain relief and physical rehabilitation, the treatment of acute injury must also consider the long-term implications of musculature and skeletal integrity.

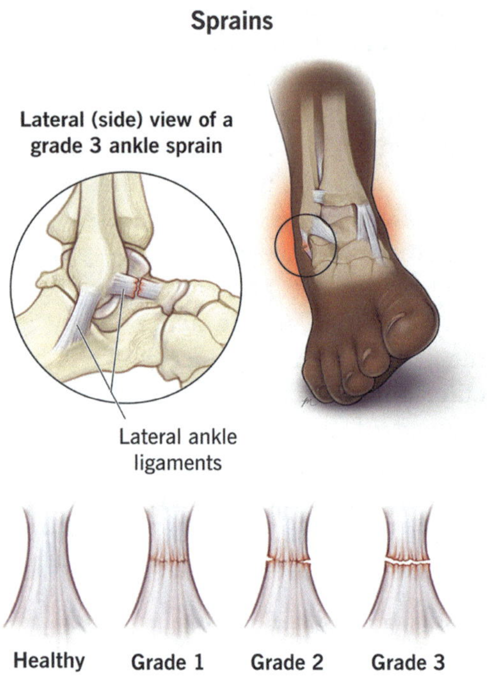

Figure 2.2. Sprains.

Source: https://my.clevelandclinic.org/-/scassets/images/org/health/articles/15461-sprains.

In cases of volumetric muscle loss (VML), obstacles to treatment extend beyond the confines of early healing. VML is likely to require innovative multi-phase treatment protocols for addressing the complexities of healing and tissue regeneration. Research has identified the effectiveness of provisional muscle void fillers, including polyvinyl alcohol (PVA), in stabilizing injury, enabling a two-stage treatment strategy that can offer more promising functional results in the long run (Clark et al., 2024). Research into these new treatments illustrates the importance of adapting protocols of injury treatment to include the current understanding of musculoskeletal pathobiology. In general, appropriate acute injury management not only aims for immediate recovery but also seeks to create a sustainable pathway towards the recovery of long-term health and function (Figure 2.2).

2.1.2. Chronic Injuries

Chronic injury is a very severe musculoskeletal health problem that typically arises from badly treated or rehabilitated acute injuries. Such injuries can lead to constant pain, dysfunction, and decreased quality of life. For instance, ankle conditions such as chronic ankle instability are seen when initial trauma to the lateral ligaments is badly treated. When patients fail to rehabilitate properly following a sprain of the ankle, they can be predisposed to repeated injury and chronic instability.

The identification of these chronic degenerative processes allows physicians to establish an efficient management protocol that will address both acute pain as well as long-term rehabilitation. Preventive measures, early intervention, and rehabilitative protocols become essential in avoiding the transition from an acute injury to a chronic process, improving overall patient outcomes and function. The treatment of chronic injury is generally a mix of conservative and surgical approaches. Contemporary studies indicate the effectiveness of non-invasive procedures such as Kinesio taping and low-level laser therapy in stimulating the healing and pain relief for ankle sprain survivors. A clinical trial also established that both modalities significantly influence Numeric Pain Rating Scale ratings and functional outcome measures like the Foot and Ankle Ability Measure in chronic ankle sprain patients (Yasin et al., 2025). Although both interventions were positive, low-level laser therapy was established to exhibit superior pain reduction and functional enhancement compared to kinesio taping. This evidence attests to the necessity for clinicians to consider patient-specific factors and characteristics of the injury when making decisions regarding the optimal management plan for chronic injuries. Surgical treatment would, on the other hand, be required for those chronic injuries that are resistant to conservative treatment.

For example, in chronic lateral ligament instability with patients failing to exhibit adequate recovery with even six months of conservative management, surgery becomes unavoidable. Research revealed the benefits of internal brace augmentation of open ligament repair with superior functional outcomes and earlier return to pre-injury activity levels than isolated ligament repair (Sethi et al., 2024). Whereas operations are often considered as a final resort, they may be the solution for restoring function in chronic injury and preventing complications. Effective management of chronic musculoskeletal injury thus involves a complete evaluation of both conservative and surgical management, each patient's individual needs being well addressed (Figure 2.3).

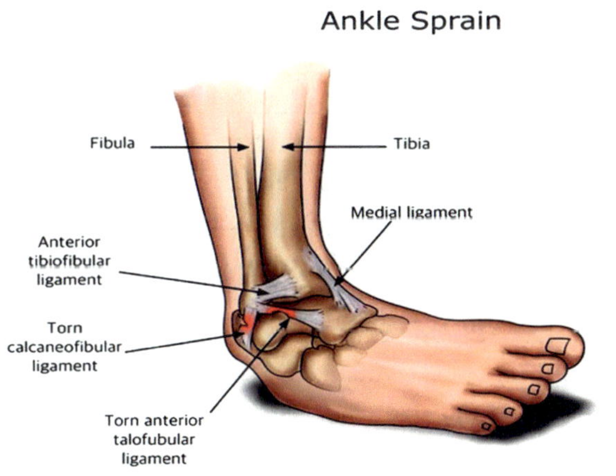

Figure 2.3. Ankle instability.

Source: https://redefinehealthcare.com/wp-content/uploads/2023/03/Ankle-Instability.jpg.

2.1.3. Common Examples (Sprains, Fractures, Tendonitis)

Musculoskeletal injury is prevalent, and sprains, fractures, and tendonitis are among the most common forms that significantly impact one's functionality. A sprain occurs when ligaments, which are fibrous connective tissues that unite bones at joints, are stretched or torn and typically occur due to abrupt movements when one is playing sports or exercising. A sprain can range from mild over-stretching to complete tearing, leading to pain, swelling, and loss of mobility. It is most important to understand the mechanisms of sprains, both prevention and treatment, as rehab attempts to regain the range of motion and to strengthen the surrounding muscles. Furthermore, ergonomic work practices can diminish the threat of such an injury, which most often leads to days lost for recovery (Bureau of Statistics, 2014). Bones can break in a fracture due to trauma, stress, or disease that has weakened the bone. Injuries are not just distinguished based on where they occur—that is, in appendages like wrists or ankles—but also based on type, and simple fractures, in which the bone remains in continuity, exist, as do compound fractures, in which the bone becomes open to the surface of the skin. Fractures need immediate medical evaluation to determine the best intervention, which may involve immobilization, realignment, or surgical intervention. Rehabilitation measures following fractures are crucial, not only to promote physical restoration but also to remove anxiety and fear of re-injury. The wide-ranging process ensures a comprehensive management of fractures so that individuals regain pre-injury activity levels (McArthur et al., 2020). Tendonitis is the result of inflammation of tendons, commonly a consequence of over-stretching or repetitive strain, and occurs in athletes and those who have job-related heavy physical labor. Tendonitis normally occurs at the shoulders, elbows, wrists, and knees and manifests as localized pain and tenderness that intensifies upon movement. Effective cure of tendonitis requires a combination of rest, anti-inflammatory medication, and physical therapy to strengthen and enhance flexibility in the affected area. Additionally, prevention strategies like proper warm-ups and technique adjustment in sports or manual work can lower the risk of tendonitis. Awareness of these common musculoskeletal injuries and modality of care not only benefits subjects in the healing process but also for wider knowledge sharing regarding the prevention of injury across various environments (Bureau of Statistics, 2014) (Figure 2.4).

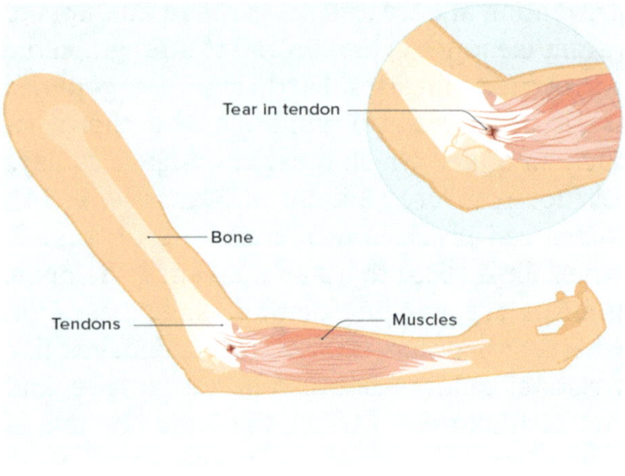

Figure 2.4. Tendinitis.

Source: https://i0.wp.com/post.healthline.com/wp-content/uploads/2021/09/1580068-Visual-intent-What-Is-Tendinitis-1296x728-header-body.png?w=1155&h=1862.

2.2. Causes and Risk Factors

Musculoskeletal injuries, being prevalent in most populations, are largely caused by a combination of intrinsic and extrinsic factors. Intrinsic factors include the individual's age, physical status, and genetics, which all contribute to musculoskeletal health. For instance, older individuals will lose bone and muscle strength from the natural process of aging and thus become more susceptible to injury. Others with a past history of injury or current disease will also be at greater risk. Conversely, extrinsic causes overwhelmingly comprise occupational and environmental factors. Poor ergonomic methods in the workplace, such as improper lifting practices and unsatisfactory seating arrangements, are heavily responsible for the occurrence of musculoskeletal disorders. Specifically, improper ergonomic job design ranks among the most common reasons for occupational disease, accounting for perhaps a third of employers' bills under state workers' compensation plans (Rappaport, 2001). These causative factors with numerous aspects need a complete understanding to offer effective management and prevention strategies. The intrinsic character of the working conditions is what determines the risk factors for musculoskeletal traumas. Occupations involving repetitive movements, sustained awkward positions, or lifting have more instances of these traumas. For instance, healthcare professionals tend to carry out activities that involve lifting or transferring patients and thus put themselves at a high risk of back injuries. Besides, technology introduction has introduced new dangers; a sedentary lifestyle resulting from high levels of computer usage has led to musculoskeletal disorders such as carpal tunnel syndrome and neck pain. The firms not only have to bear the cost of treatment but also suffer from low productivity as their workers are injured. For eliminating these hazards, it is essential to apply ergonomic assessment and workflow process redesign. As claimed in research, federal and state guidelines stress the necessity of preventive interventions and education programs to inform workers about information related to safe practices in their particular settings (Kriebel et al., 2011). Understanding the etiology and risk factors of musculoskeletal injuries also encompasses intervention in lifestyle habits and individual behavior. Typical high-risk groups are those individuals who engage in poor physical exercise, leading to weakening of muscles and reduced flexibility. Further, involvement in recreational or sporting activities without proper technique and training may result in increased risk of injury. Behavioral factors, such as poor posture during everyday activities or not paying attention to warm-up exercises, can also contribute to higher incidence rates for musculoskeletal disorders. Education on proper techniques of exercise, together with protection of physical fitness, plays a key role in ensuring musculoskeletal well-being. A strategy that integrates occupational ergonomics with personal habits will facilitate more effective prevention and management of such injuries, therefore optimizing overall health outcomes and healthcare system burdens.

2.2.1. Sports-Related Injuries

Sport injury is an important concern in the musculoskeletal health field, and it cuts across age and level of skill among athletes. They range from minor sprains and strains to severe ones such as fractures and tearing of ligaments, typically due to physical stresses of activity, overuse, or collision with other participants. Thus, understanding the nature and extent of sport injuries is the cornerstone for developing effective management strategies. Increasing evidence indicates that as participation in sports grows among different groups of the population, so does the incidence of sport-related injuries, hence creating the need for specialized interventions. Not only does the trend highlight preventive intervention, but also the training of practitioners with comprehensive treatment modalities, particularly where pain management and rehabilitation are concerned. Effective management of musculoskeletal sports injuries revolves around pain relief and functional rehabilitation. More recent studies build on the treatment view with an emphasis on the role of non-steroidal anti-inflammatory drugs (NSAIDs) and particularly their topical use as great choices in pain control of low-level injuries. Evidence shows that topical use of NSAIDs can provide pain relief without the systemic side effects associated with oral administration, and therefore is appropriately suited to outpatient therapy. Moreover, their application alongside physical therapy can potentially enhance recovery results through enabling early mobilization and reducing inflammation.

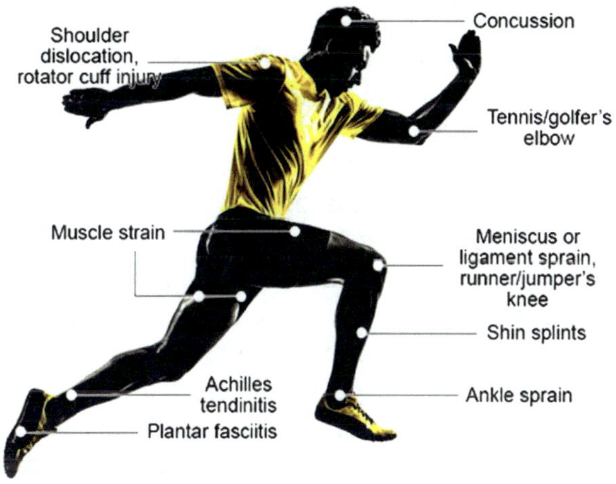

Figure 2.5. Sports-related injuries.

Source: blob:https://cbphysiotherapy.in/1e489205-6a93-4d9d-9f37-58ba58dd105e.

With the focus on these evidence-based techniques, therapists can create an environment that lends itself to faster rehabilitation, allowing athletes to return to activities with reduced lost time and fewer re-injury risks. Outside of the pharmacologic control, an important aspect of controlling sports injury is the implementation of preventive strategies that are sport- and risk-specific. Instruction in proper technique, flexibility exercises, and conditioning is important in minimizing the risk of injury. Furthermore, integrating biomechanics and ergonomics principles into training methodologies can significantly reduce the occurrence of repetitive stress injuries. Regular screening and assessment for possible vulnerability in athletes should also exist before vulnerabilities develop. The multi-faceted system of combining effective pain management with aggressive preventive care is the key to ensuring that long-term musculoskeletal health in athletes is obtained. As studies in sports injury continue to unravel, measures from these results will be crucial to guide our management and comprehension of such injuries among sports persons (Deokar et al., 2007, 2010) (Figure 2.5).

2.2.2. Occupational Hazards

Occupational hazards cover a broad spectrum of risks that could negatively affect workers' health, particularly when it comes to musculoskeletal injuries. The workplace and the physical demands of it are key factors in the prevalence of such injuries. Professions that deal with repetitive motion, weighty lifting, or forced postures could lead to long-term pain and disability, thus contributing significantly to the loss of a person's capacity to perform their work efficiently. Furthermore, the psychosocial aspects of work, like job satisfaction and stress can also exacerbate physical conditions and hinder recovery mechanisms. Recent studies state that fighting against these physical and mental illness problems in workplaces is essential in reducing the incidence of musculoskeletal injuries as well as overall worker well-being (Paladugu et al., 2025). The interaction between various occupational hazards and musculoskeletal injuries reflects the necessity for holistic safety and health practices. Recent research points to the importance of understanding the determinants and impacts of occupational health and safety (OSH) within different sectors. This involves looking at the situation of OSH infrastructure that includes legislation, prevention strategies, and work environment conditions management. Such frameworks play an important role in determining and limiting chemical agents, ergonomic deficiencies, and other physical hazards-related risks leading to injuries (Pouliakas & Theodossiou, 2010). Through interdisciplinary approaches that incorporate both economic and psychological theory, businesses can develop better injury prevention and employee support strategies. Prevention and control measures to be undertaken against musculoskeletal injuries should be multidisciplinary and include both individual and organizational elements. For instance, the implementation of ergonomic interventions would make a significant difference in avoiding the risks associated with physical workplace hazards. Apart from that, developing a work culture of health and safety not only prevents injuries but also increases worker morale and performance. Additionally, frequent training and awareness programs are essential for equipping workers with the knowledge to identify hazards and use protective measures effectively. Lastly, creating a comprehensive strategy towards OSH helps in minimizing the social and economic consequences of occupational hazards, which leads to improved workplace health and improved labor outcomes (Pouliakas & Theodossiou, 2010).

2.2.3. Lifestyle Factors (Sedentary Behavior, Obesity)

The relationship between lifestyle factors such as sedentary behavior and obesity is pivotal in the understanding of the prevalence of musculoskeletal injury. Sedentary behavior, where there are long periods of inactivity, has been found to have a direct impact on levels of obesity. This relationship evolves into a vicious cycle that sees excess body weight placing additional stress on joints, muscles, and ligaments, thus increasing the incidence of musculoskeletal injury. With a large proportion of the adult population failing to meet guideline physical activity levels, intervention on these lifestyle determinants has never been more warranted. Pregnancy, menopause, and retirement are stages of life when the population is most likely to be susceptible to increased sedentary lifestyles and obesity, also raising specifically the risks associated with musculoskeletal health

(Skelton & Mavroeidi, 2018). Furthermore, the effects of obesity are not merely mechanical stress; it also influences inflammatory and metabolic pathways that can compromise musculoskeletal integrity. Pro-inflammatory cytokines secreted by excess fat tissue have been reported to cause damage to tendon and ligament structure in the long term. This inflammation is of particular concern to those who are already physically active and who are likely to increase their risks for injury when their bodies are unable to recover or adapt to stress. Sedentary living is increasingly prevalent in various populations, and risk factors contributing to musculoskeletal injury become increasingly intricate; and hence, prevention and management should be dealt with holistically (Yadav & Choudhary, 2024). Interventions that minimize sedentary behavior and maximize active living can considerably mitigate the risk of obesity-related musculoskeletal injury. Engaging with people at points of change, such as in adulthood or following significant health events, is key to starting long-term adaptations in behavior. Programs that emphasize strengthening and balance training, particularly in high-risk populations, can optimally promote physical function and reduce the rate of injury. In addition, ongoing health promotion interventions must be formulated to address the specific needs of various population groups to motivate increased participation in physical activity (Skelton & Mavroeidi, 2018). Through priorities in lifestyle change, health professionals can contribute significantly to improved musculoskeletal health, resulting in an improved active and healthy population (Figure 2.6).

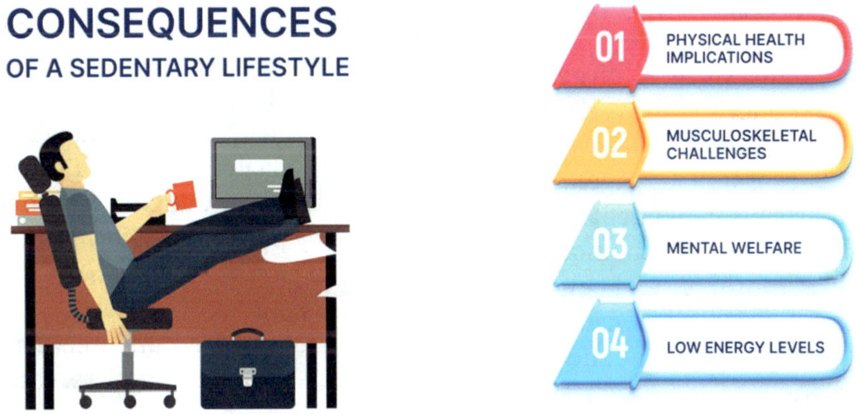

Figure 2.6. Consequences of a sedentary lifestyle.

Source: https://allinjuryrehab.com/wp-content/uploads/2024/03/consequences-of-a-sedentary-lifestyle.jpg.

2.3. Symptoms and Diagnosis

Recognition of symptoms of musculoskeletal injury is important for accurate diagnosis and management. The most frequent signs and symptoms are pain, swelling, stiffness, and limited range of motion. Symptoms typically consist of local pain that is brought on or aggravated by particular movements or activities. For instance, in the case of healthcare workers with lower back pain (LBP), they may exhibit symptoms associated with bad body mechanics, which are exacerbated when the person spends longer hours standing or does repetitive movements, such as healthcare workers (Shashi et al., 2025). Identification of these symptoms is also essential in differentiating between acute injuries, which present suddenly, and chronic conditions resulting from the passage of time due to overuse or poor ergonomics. Diagnoses of musculoskeletal trauma typically involve a comprehensive approach that incorporates clinical testing and imaging studies. Health workers make choices depending on detailed patient histories and physical assessments to identify the area of interest. For example, knee trauma evaluation typically includes evaluation of joint mechanics function and ligament stability, whereas LBP diagnosis can be made dependent upon identifying risk factors such as work-related strains (Aldanyowi & AlOraini, 2024). Imaging modalities such as X-rays or MRIs increase the diagnostic sensitivity by visualizing the structural pathology. Ultimately, accurate diagnosis is paramount since it directs the patient's management plan and thus maximizes recovery while decreasing the potential for recurrent injury. Successful management of musculoskeletal injuries is dependent on early detection and appropriate treatment modalities addressing both symptoms and etiology. Multimodal treatment regimens commonly include both pharmacological and non-pharmacological therapies. Medication, such as nonsteroidal anti-inflammatory drugs (NSAIDs), may provide quick pain relief, while physical therapy rehabilitates the affected area through targeted exercises and ergonomic training (Shashi et al., 2025). In addition, addressing psychological factors through counseling can also enhance patients' compliance with rehabilitation protocols and overall well-being (Aldanyowi & AlOraini, 2024). By combining these methods, medical professionals can create a comprehensive approach that not only addresses pain but also facilitates functional recovery and enhanced quality of life for the victims of musculoskeletal trauma.

2.3.1. Common Symptoms (Pain, Swelling, Limited Mobility)

It is essential to note the common symptoms of musculoskeletal injuries for the right management and treatment. Pain most often proves to be the most immediate and troubling symptom experienced by patients, typically after injury to muscles, tendons, ligaments, or joints. The nociceptive pain response not only serves as a notice of injury but can also lead to chronic conditions when not managed appropriately. Pain may be of different quality and intensity, varying from sharp, burning pain to irritating, aching discomfort. Pain perception, too, is not simple, being influenced by both physiological and psychological factors. Failure to treat it leads to the limitations imposed by pain that interfere with daily living and diminish the overall quality of life of patients, and therefore, its timely and comprehensive control plays an important role in musculoskeletal practice. Other important associated symptoms of musculoskeletal injury include swelling, often a result of tissue damage or mechanical stress-induced inflammation. Swelling occurs when fluid collects in the injured tissue, producing visible distension and frequently palpable tenderness. Inflammation is a normal part of healing; however, pathological or prolonged swelling can exacerbate pain as well as limit joint function. The relationship between mobility and swelling reinforces a cycle of viciousness: swelling may restrict movement, but the lack of movement adds to more challenges, such as joint stiffness and weakening of nearby muscles. As discussed in modern literature, de-swelling through procedures such as corticosteroid joint injection helps alleviate symptoms and promote healing, propelling patients toward better functional outcomes when addressing musculoskeletal challenges (Shoukri, 2025). Restrictive mobility is a serious musculoskeletal injury outcome that compromises the performance of both simple and complex activities of daily living. Swelling and pain complicate a patient's movement of the limbs or weight-bearing function, resulting in a considerably reduced level of physical functioning. This reduced mobility not only obstructs rehabilitation but also manifests as secondary complications of muscle atrophy and joint rigidity, which can further perpetuate the patients' pain. In those patients already battling their baseline conditions, as suggested by Kwan et al. (2023), these limitations can also manifest in deleterious effects on their overall quality of life. Effective management of injury involves handling mobility restriction through the use of rehabilitation methods that enhance progressive motion and strengthening exercises, thus maximizing improvements in function and enhancing the patient's independence (Figure 2.7).

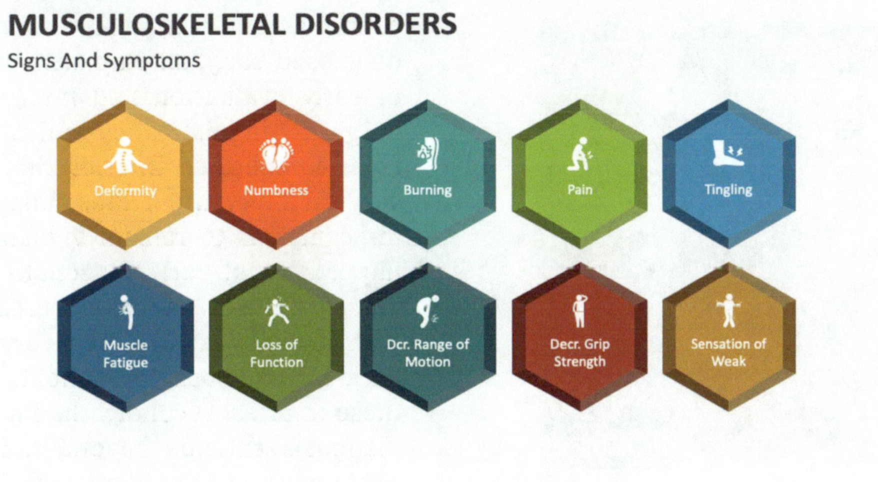

Figure 2.7. Signs and symptoms of musculoskeletal injuries.

Source: https://www.collidu.com/media/catalog/product/img1/7/c/7ca88f16794ea6019c4687b6444268534335384b6b3fe363a3191758573c2f88/musculoskeletal-disorders-slide3.png.

2.3.2. Diagnostic Methods (Physical Examination, Imaging Tests)

Diagnostic methods are pivotal in the management of musculoskeletal trauma, foremost among them being the physical exam and imaging. Physical exam is typically the initial method employed to establish the degree and nature of an injury. A systematic assessment of the affected area is undertaken by clinicians to assess for tenderness, swelling, motion, and muscle strength. This interactive examination is of pivotal importance in the formation of a preliminary diagnosis and the further guidance of testing. Its efficacy rests with the skill and expertise of the clinician, since even minimal positive signs may underlie severe underlying pathology. Therefore, although the physical examination provides valuable data, its constraints necessitate the integration of more advanced diagnostic techniques in the evaluation of musculoskeletal trauma. Imaging tests, particularly magnetic resonance imaging (MRI) and X-rays, complement physical exams with increased visualization of musculoskeletal structures. MRI is particularly useful in identifying soft tissue injuries, such as ligament or cartilage rupture, which are not visible on plain X-rays. The existing literature has pointed towards a high correlation between age and prevalence of imaging-diagnosed conditions, such as superior labral anterior-posterior (SLAP) tears, with older patients having a greater prevalence (Lansdown et al., 2018). Prevalence by age reminds us of the necessity of optimal imaging protocols depending on the patient demographics to achieve improved diagnoses. Later, the combination of physical examination with imaging tests improves overall diagnostic accuracy, directing effective treatment modalities for musculoskeletal injuries. In addition to MRI, ultrasound has been a useful diagnostic tool in the evaluation of musculoskeletal injuries. It allows real-time visualization of activities and enables clinicians to visualize dynamic movements, such as the movement of joints.

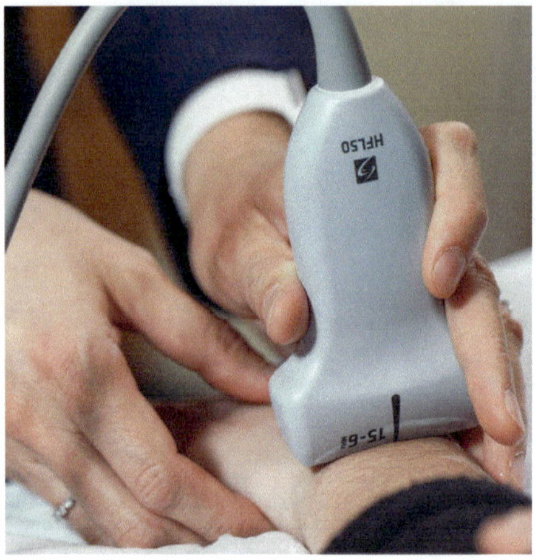

Figure 2.8. Musculoskeletal ultrasound.

Source: https://ysm-res.cloudinary.com/image/upload/ar_1:1,c_fill,dpr_3.0,f_auto,g_faces:auto,q_auto:eco,w_500/v1/yms/prod/a3b05f8e-064f-40e4-a60d-ff74b4130b5d.

This is particularly valuable in the case of repeated evaluation, for example, follow-up of recovery or of recurring injuries. Moreover, ultrasound is cost-effective and non-invasive when compared to other imaging modalities. However, it does require special training and qualification to properly interpret the results. The combination of ultrasound and MRI gives a solid foundation for the diagnosis of complex musculoskeletal disorders, supplementing treatment planning and patient outcomes. With advancing imaging technology, the pattern of diagnosis of musculoskeletal injuries will improve and be more sophisticated, providing clinicians potent tools for effective management (Blyth et al., 2015) (Figure 2.8).

2.3.3. Importance of Early Diagnosis

The need for timely diagnosis of musculoskeletal injuries cannot be stressed enough, as it is instrumental in facilitating maximal treatment and minimizing complications. Timely identification of injuries leads to efficacious management approaches that can directly influence the outcome of patients. Literature indicates that fractures are able to develop complications like avascular necrosis if not diagnosed early, an emphasis on the necessity of early evaluation and intervention. It also helps distinguish uncomplicated contusions from complicated injuries that might require surgical intervention, thus making it imperative for clinicians to remain vigilant. Through the importance of early detection, physicians are able to initiate effective treatment pathways that not only expedite recovery but also yield an ideal prognosis for patients suffering from these injuries. Secondly, the impact of delayed diagnosis extends beyond individual health outcomes and to public health implications on a broader scale. For instance, a failure to provide early recognition of severe musculoskeletal trauma has grave implications for healthcare spending and resource allocation. The prevalence of complications, as in chest trauma where attendant traumas prolong recovery, illustrates the broader implications of failed early diagnostic processes (Lema et al., 2011). Further, the cost of managing complicated injuries can strain healthcare systems, and therefore there is a need to improve the capacity to diagnose and protocols. Investment in early diagnostic equipment can potentially lower both the direct costs of prolonged treatment and recovery times as well as indirect costs, justifying the need for rapid and accurate diagnosis of musculoskeletal injuries. Within the clinical setting, the role of training and education in enabling the diagnostic skills of health professionals is important. Ensuring medical practitioners are well-versed in the detection of signs and symptoms for musculoskeletal trauma allows for the provision of care to patients preemptively. For instance, studies have examined the long-term effects of various fractures and emphasized the fact that surgical timing is associated with success rates (Biz et al., 2019). Well-educated awareness of the consequences of delayed diagnosis not only equips clinicians to act early but also instills confidence in them to handle complex cases. This proactive thinking, grounded in good education and training, ultimately leads to better patient satisfaction and fosters a culture of excellence in the management of musculoskeletal injury. The provision of structured training and sensitization courses can thus bridge gaps in early diagnosis, enhancing the quality of care to patients.

2.4. Treatment Options

In the management of musculoskeletal trauma, a complete understanding of surgical and non-surgical interventions is absolutely necessary. Surgery normally entails arthroscopic repair or reconstructive surgery, most prominently for conditions like rotator cuff tears that drastically impair mobility and function. The selection of surgery is often determined by the nature of the injury, patient age, and lifestyle demands. Surgery will often result in more effective pain reduction and function, yielding long-term benefits that can balance the additional cost of such procedures at inception. But remember that non-surgical intervention, including physical therapy and corticosteroid injections, will likewise yield beneficial outcomes, particularly for minor pathology or in more resilient patients who may be less susceptible to surgical intervention. This delicate strategy highlights the importance of individually targeted treatment protocols consistent with patient profile and injury information (Altamimi et al., 2024). Rehabilitation is a part of non-surgical management for musculoskeletal injuries. Well-organized rehabilitation covers a variety of therapeutic interventions such as physiotherapy, customized exercise routines, and the goal of achieving strength in addition to a range of motion. Apart from this, nutritional interventions have also been reported to be part of the recovery process. The literature shows that a high-protein and carbohydrate-based diet can significantly enhance the healing process in athletes as well as non-athletes. This kind of dietary intervention not only facilitates tissue repair but also enhances the efficiency of recovery in patients undergoing rehabilitation. Additionally, supplement use, like the use of collagen and omega-3 fatty acids, has shown promising potential to speed recovery, but this needs more clinical trials to confirm these findings (Giraldo-Vallejo et al., 2023). Lastly, treatment options need to be selected with a focus on an interdisciplinary approach, considering both physical rehabilitation as well as psychological well-being. Patients also get frustrated and anxious because of mobility limitations from their injuries, and mental care is a necessary component of holistic treatment. Effective communication among healthcare practitioners, including orthopedic surgeons, physical therapists, and dietitians, can guarantee an all-inclusive treatment plan, both physically and psychologically. Emphasis on educating the patient about treatment options available can enable individuals to be actively involved in the recovery process. Sustaining a collaborative work environment among medical practitioners can translate into greater patient success with respect to achieving the best results in the treatment of musculoskeletal injuries (Giraldo-Vallejo et al., 2023; Altamimi et al., 2024).

2.4.1. Conservative Management (Rest, Ice, Compression, Elevation)

In the management of musculoskeletal injury, conservatively, the most popular initial intervention is the RICE method—Rest, Ice, Compression, and Elevation. This broad measure is used to alleviate pain, restrict swelling, and ensure healing. Resting is critical after an injury has occurred because this allows the damaged tissues to recover without additional stress. Concurrently, the application of ice serves to constrict blood vessels, thereby decreasing swelling and numbing pain in the involved area. Research indicates enhanced early focus on conservative care, observing its immediate benefits to patients with conditions such as acute ankle sprain, which is prevalent among active populations (Borg & Pickard, 2008). Elevation and compression maximize the rest, ice, and principles of conservative management, which are highly effective. Compression bandages applied correctly will efficiently decrease swelling by exerting constant pressure on the damaged area and inhibiting the flooding of fluids into the location. Elevation, typically a question of keeping the afflicted limb higher than heart level, decreases blood flow to the location and drops inflammation accordingly. A systematic review is bringing to the fore disparate rates of conservational rehabilitation methods, particularly emphasizing the significance that when initiated early, the techniques will play a role towards enhanced recovery outcomes in clinical conditions like ankle sprain (Puhakka & Koistinen, 2014). Not only for symptom relief, but this integrated approach is also crucial in preventing the onset of complications arising from suboptimal initial management. Then, going on to rehabilitation, the need for conservative treatment is evident because it creates the basis for what comes afterwards in terms of therapy. Once active symptoms have passed and the acute process has resolved, active rehabilitation modalities such as physical therapy, strengthening, and range-of-motion exercises can be applied to regain function. It is worth noting that while RICE is a foundational cornerstone in the acute phase, its integration into an overall recovery plan is essential to maximizing long-term outcomes. By minimizing initial symptoms with effective mitigation and promoting tissue repair through conservative management, practitioners are facilitated in their efforts to make the transition more comfortable to more aggressive treatment and, subsequently, restore patients to baseline levels of function and quality of life (Borg et al., 2008) (Figure 2.9).

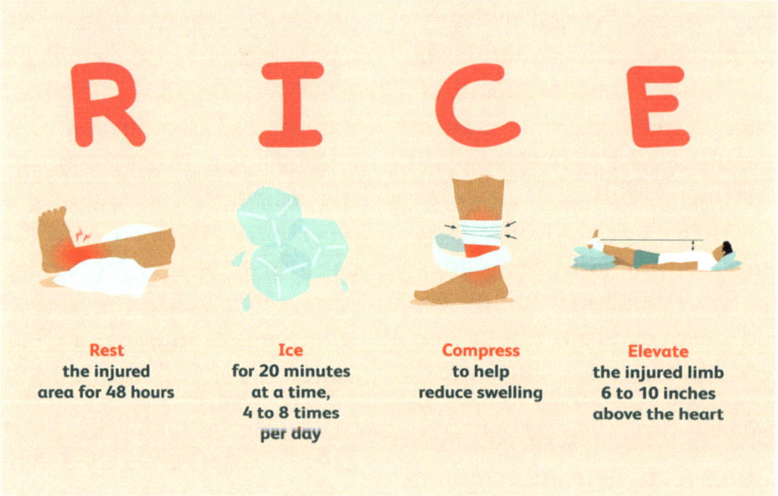

Figure 2.9. RICE method.

Source: https://www.verywellhealth.com/thmb/ML1jw4V5NleI8om7I7Ipo-uKX5Q=/1500x0/filters:no_upscale():max_bytes(150000):strip_icc()/what-is-rice-190446_FINAL-5bc5fcebc9e77c005135258d.png.

2.4.2. Pharmacological Treatments (Pain Relievers, Anti-Inflammatories)

Pharmacological treatments are very crucial in the management of musculoskeletal injuries, predominantly through the administration of painkillers and anti-inflammatory agents. Nonsteroidal anti-inflammatory drugs (NSAIDs) are commonly used to manage pain and inflammation resulting from injuries like sprains, strains, and tendonitis.

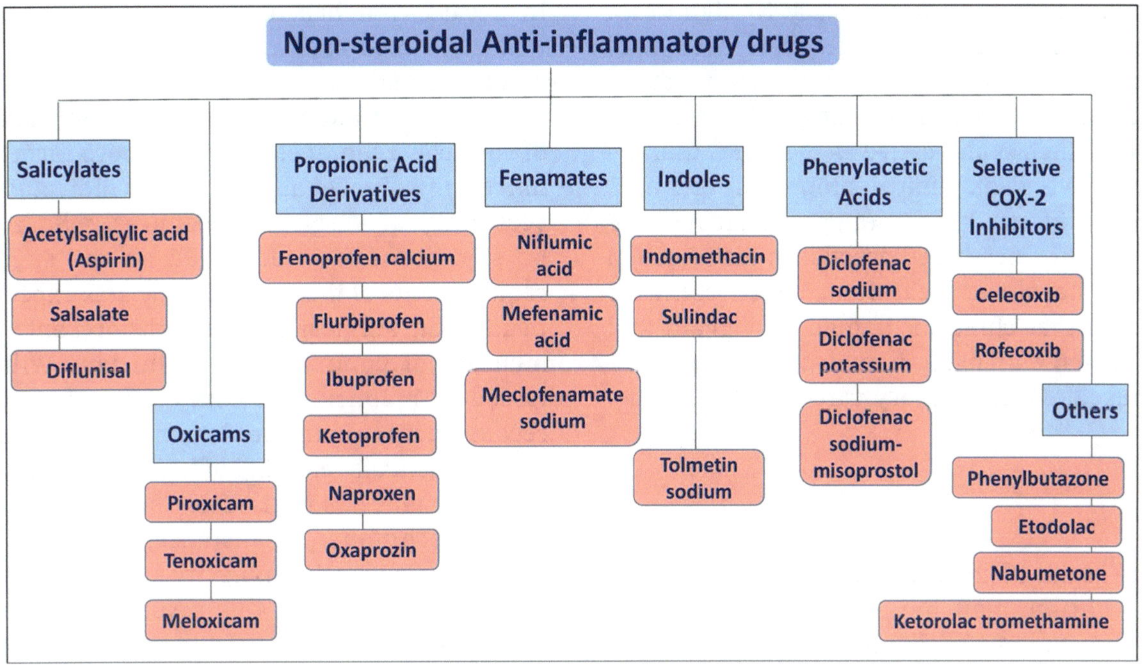

Figure 2.10. Nonsteroidal anti-inflammatory drugs (NSAIDs).

Source: https://media.springernature.com/lw685/springer-static/image/art%3A10.1208%2Fs12249-023-02649-x/MediaObjects/12249_2023_2649_Fig1_HTML.png.

These agents act by inhibiting cyclooxygenase enzymes, which play a very important part in the inflammatory process. The resulting reduction in inflammation and pain can aid in the restoration of mobility and accelerate the rehabilitation process. Caution, however, is required in that prolonged administration of NSAIDs can yield gastrointestinal symptoms and cardiovascular side effects. Thus, effective in the short run, careful observation and consideration of certain patient risk factors are required to ensure maximum safety and efficacy in musculoskeletal injury management. Besides, the scene of pain management has evolved with the introduction of multi-modal therapy employing a variety of pharmacological weapons to optimize outcomes. Opioids, although suitable for acute pain, are employed with caution due to their tendency to cause addiction and rising cases of opioid-related overdoses in the United States. An area of concern witnessed was an unprecedented increase in the prescription of opioids starting in 1999, when pharmaceutical companies promised healthcare professionals that they were not addictive. This has caused a public health crisis, with opioids becoming more and more linked to overdose deaths, now officially categorized as a leading cause of injury-related mortality (Meldrum, 2016). With growing opioid dependence, clinicians are prompted to explore alternative approaches to pain management and, where possible, favor non-opioid medications. Novel interventions, such as intermittent pneumatic compression, have also been explored for effectiveness in the management of musculoskeletal pain, particularly with regard to conditions like delayed onset muscle soreness (DOMS). As much as this method has been employed following exercise with the objective of lessening pain, evidence supports the potential limitation of its efficacy. No significant differences in pain reduction were seen with intermittent pneumatic compression versus placebo therapy between healthy volunteers and DOMS, which is indicative that such a therapy would have weak clinical support in this area (Lindahl, 2016). This finding underscores the value of evidence-based practice in the selection of pharmacologic treatment, which confirms the idea that clinicians should be vigilant and alert when employing new drugs of treatment in musculoskeletal injury care (Figure 2.10).

2.4.3. Surgical Interventions (When Necessary)

In the realm of musculoskeletal injury, surgical intervention may be required for optimal recovery and return to function. If conservative treatments—bracing or physical therapy—are ineffective, then surgery becomes the turning point. The choice of a surgical procedure usually depends on the nature and severity of the injury. For instance, there are some suturing techniques for soft tissue repair that are crucial to attain healing as well as maintain structural support. A systematic review mandated setting these techniques into categories based on the structural principles behind them, elevates clinical guidelines' validity, thereby assisting surgeons in making tactical decisions based on requirements specific to cases (Liu et al., 2024). This underscores the importance of evidence-based practice in surgical treatment, where surgical interventions are individualized to the unique requirements of each musculoskeletal injury. Surgical treatment also encompasses cases of extensive soft tissue damage, where simple suturing might not be sufficient. For example, scalp avulsion wounds resulting from traumatic injuries are likely to need very advanced surgical repair techniques, including free flaps—a method of surgery that can successfully treat extensive tissue loss. Such cases are typical of the sophistication of surgical treatment for musculoskeletal trauma. In a case that has been reported, a patient with near-complete avulsion of the scalp was reconstructed successfully using a latissimus dorsi free flap, indicating the remarkable ability of surgical techniques to restore both form and function (Paudel et al., 2024). This indicates the versatility of surgical procedures, which can be significantly varied based on the specific requirements of the injury and what is expected. In addition, surgical interventions present their own set of complications. Clinicians will be forced to reconcile the complexity of surgical reconstruction with the demands of a durable and aesthetically pleasing outcome, especially in the treatment of soft tissues. The most optimal suture technique, for instance, must balance against procedural complexity and the strength of the repair, making this a very complicated decision-making process for surgeons (Liu et al., 2024). Refining techniques and surgical methods is required to enhance the safety and efficacy of procedures aimed at minimizing musculoskeletal injuries. Ultimately, the process of combining surgical innovation and evidence-based practice has a strong influence on determining recovery patterns, improving long-term patient outcomes in addressing these challenging injuries.

2.5. Rehabilitation and Recovery

Rehabilitation and recovery are inherent components of the treatment of musculoskeletal injuries, particularly glenohumeral ligament injuries. A comprehensive rehabilitation program focuses not only on pain relief but also on range of motion recovery and functional stability. The role of adjunct treatment, such as

Kinesio Taping (KT), in the recovery process has been highlighted by recent studies. KT will seek to modulate pain, improve proprioception, and stabilize the joint, hence permitting an optimal rehabilitation process. Although there have been some short-term benefits of KT documented, current literature is low in terms of strong evidence for its extensive use as a single intervention. All practitioners prefer integrating KT into multimodal therapy that integrates traditional physiotherapy with new approaches, highlighting the need for additional research to demonstrate its role in evidenced-based rehabilitation programs (Zia et al., 2025). Rehabilitation modalities also usually apply additional modalities for enhancing recovery from recurring musculoskeletal trauma, such as an ankle sprain. Rehabilitation has traditionally been underpinned by methods of physical therapy, but more recent additions of low-level laser therapy (LLLT) and KT have been valuable adjuncts. LLLT, in fact, has been shown to be particularly valuable in augmenting pain relief and hastening the course of functional recovery, a point of considerable interest for the athlete. In a clinical trial of randomization comparing both treatments, LLLT scored higher for pain relief and functional recovery compared to KT. The outcomes reflect an increased interest in exploring the complementarities between various treatment methods to improve rehabilitation protocols for ankle sprain and comparable conditions (Yasin et al., 2025). Effective rehabilitation and recovery are not merely a product of the techniques employed, but also of response to treatment and adherence to rehabilitation protocols on the patient's part. Age, extent of injury, and prior history of injury all contribute significantly to the alteration of recovery time. Tailoring rehabilitation programs to meet each patient's individual requirements is key to optimizing outcomes. They should also be educated in their role in the rehabilitation process, including adherence to exercise regimens and follow-up assessment attendance. With the face of musculoskeletal management constantly evolving, ongoing research is imperative to advance rehabilitation methods so that they are evidence-based and aligned with best practice for long-term recovery and minimizing recurrent strain.

2.5.1. Role of Physical Therapy

The role of physical therapy in musculoskeletal injury rehabilitation is pivotal in restoring function and alleviating pain. As an integral component of rehabilitation, physical therapy applies a multidisciplinary model of manual therapy procedures, therapeutic exercises, and patient education to rehabilitate a variety of musculoskeletal disorders. The multidisciplinary approach works best for conditions such as sprains, strains, and tendinitis, where the goal is to enhance mobility, strengthen the affected muscle, and avoid reinjury. Clinical evidence demonstrates that interventions like neuromuscular exercises and personalized physical therapy programs are able to produce notable improvement in pain tolerance and functional capacity. Such rehabilitative approaches not only focus on the management of the injury on a physical basis but also include the psychological aspects to facilitate an integrated process of rehabilitation to the point that the patients' mental well-being is addressed as a vital component of effective recovery (Aabedi et al., 2025). By integrating contemporary advances in diagnostic methods, physical therapy can be amplified with the aid of modalities such as musculoskeletal ultrasound (MSKUS). This imaging modality allows real-time visualization of soft tissue anatomy, which permits therapists to precisely evaluate the degree of injuries, for example, those to the lateral elbow. The ability to detect pathoanatomical alterations using MSKUS profoundly impacts the construction of focused rehabilitation programs. For instance, identification of the injury itself can guide interventions regarding strength training, flexibility, and proprioceptive training as designed specifically for the patient's individual needs. With physical therapists being able to monitor recovery more accurately by using MSKUS, they are able to adjust treatment protocols accordingly for optimal recovery and return to baseline activity levels (Manske et al., 2025).

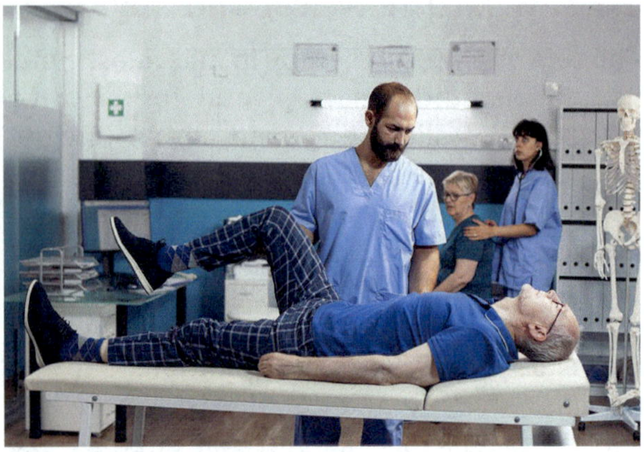

Figure 2.11. A man with a leg muscle injury is receiving orthopedic.

Source: https://www.healthybodiesphysiotherapy.com.au/wp-content/uploads/2022/01/man-with-leg-muscle-injury-receiving-orthopedic-900x600-1.jpg.

Furthermore, the integration of physical therapy with psychotherapy is a novel enhancement in musculoskeletal trauma treatment. As emotional concerns such as pain catastrophizing and anxiety tend to exacerbate physical complaints and prolong recovery, the integration of cognitive-behavioral interventions can facilitate a superior therapeutic outcome. Approaches such as mindfulness-based stress reduction and pain neuroscience education address the affective components of pain, foster resilience, and strengthen coping skills among patients. This hybrid model not only alleviates temporary distress but also renders individuals with wisdom and capabilities to manage pain in the long term. Thus, the blending of psychological care and physical rehabilitation constitutes a holistic model that aligns with the multifaceted nature of musculoskeletal trauma and ultimately leads to improved patient outcomes (Aabedi et al., 2025) (Figure 2.11).

2.5.2. Importance of Gradual Return to Activity

A gradual return to activity following musculoskeletal trauma is crucial in optimizing recovery and preventing re-injury. It is established that brash returns to high intensity activities can exacerbate existing injury or create new ones since the body lacks sufficient time to recover and accommodate the muscles. A progressive process allows one to gradually add stress to the injured site, something that is critical for strength acquisition as well as range of motion increase. This metered recovery process not only encourages physical rehabilitation, but also sustains psychological health by minimizing the apprehensions that otherwise follow being capable of returning to sport or ordinary activity. This is particularly relevant in working settings, where the Health ↔ Work Toolbox provides that gradual return to activity has the potential to empower managers and employees to collaborate on creating positive recovery settings and sustainable work engagement (Kendall et al., 2015). In the case of individual cases, like young athletes, the benefit of having a structured return-to-activity protocol becomes immensely clear. For instance, with a young athlete experiencing anterior knee pain due to activity, allowing recovery time with progressive return to activity is important for long-term joint health as well as athletic function (Formosa, 2006). The younger age group will generally require special care in striking a balance between their interest in sports and the call for medical advice during recovery. An individualized return plan not only enables physical rehabilitation but also encourages a greater appreciation of preventing injury and learning body mechanics, so that young athletes may safely and effectively return to their sport. Thus, an extensive, progressive return plan is vital for physical rehabilitation and the preservation of athletic aspirations. Besides, the generalization of phased return to work has widespread implications in multiple cases of recovery because they are crucial in occupational health management.

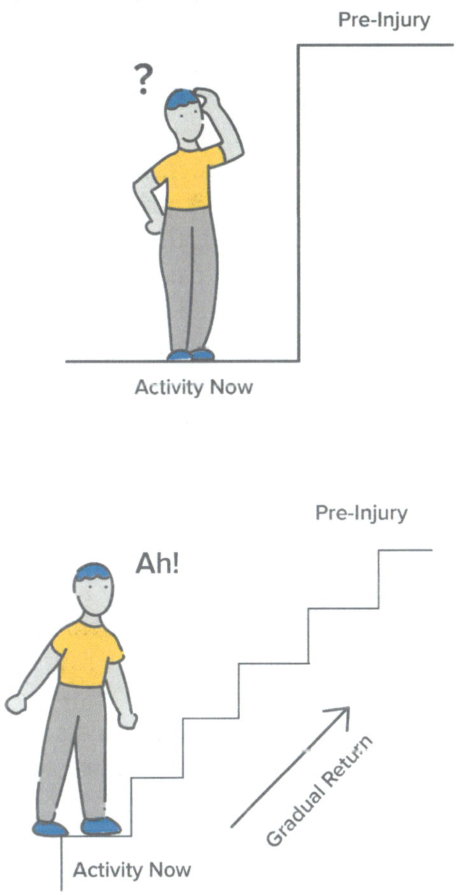

Figure 2.12. Gradual return to activity.

Source: https://concussion.vch.ca/assets/article-img/gradual_return_to_activities.png.

Incorporating phased activity return guidelines into workplace health interventions can minimize the impact of common musculoskeletal injuries on worker productivity and absenteeism. By providing structured, evidence-based models such as the Health ↔ Work Toolbox, organizations can instill a workplace culture conducive to positive health management. This integrated approach not only treats short-term health problems but also highlights the importance of maintaining continuity of work participation. With this, workplace morale as a whole is enhanced, chances of re-injury are minimized, and productivity is increased, ultimately having a healthier workforce (Kendall et al., 2015) (Figure 2.12).

2.5.3. Psychological Aspects of Recovery

Psychological dimensions of rehabilitation from musculoskeletal injury are an integral component of the rehabilitation process. Psychological factors such as motivation, coping, and attitude have a direct bearing on the healing process and the effectiveness of the interventions. Optimistically oriented patients are more likely to engage with physical therapy and adhere to rehabilitation regimens. Furthermore, the presence of stressors such as worry about job security or economic stability is known to enhance pain perception and disrupt recovery. The literature identifies knowledge about these psychological factors as essential for healthcare providers in order to individualize interventions that not just address the physical dimensions of injury but also emotional and cognitive determinants of patient outcomes. This comprehensive approach is in agreement with the biopsychosocial model that incorporates biological, psychological, and social considerations in the management of musculoskeletal disorders and, hence, is most critical for effective rehabilitation. In assessing the effectiveness of the treatment modalities for musculoskeletal trauma, it is critical that the psychosocial factors' contribution is considered. Evidence exists that interventions with a biopsychosocial model are more effective compared to biomedical interventions only. Patients with upper limb disorders, for instance, are enriched by multimodal treatment that includes physical rehabilitation and cognitive behavior with a focus on self-efficacy and emotional health. Employer involvement in constructing adaptive workplaces is also a determinant of recovery promotion because it acknowledges the impact of workplace dynamics on health. Coordination of efforts among patients, employers, and healthcare professionals is key to establishing a common understanding of recovery objectives, thus improving occupational outcomes. Integration of psychosocial aspects into the rehabilitation procedures is thus required for successful musculoskeletal injuries, both physical and psychological recovery. The development of tools facilitating musculoskeletal injury management should also incorporate consideration of psychological recovery. Programs like the Health ↔ Work Toolbox aim to activate line managers and support individuals who have workplace health problems. By using a proactive approach that emphasizes resilience and workplace engagement, these tools aim not only at physical symptoms but also at the stressors that may impede recovery. The toolbox advocates for interventions based on evidence-informed principles that allow employees to work through occupational challenges while overcoming health issues. Such integrated methods are in keeping with the biopsychosocial model of health, adding strength to the imperative of a culturally responsive method to work injury. By strengthening a participative model between employers, workers, and healthcare professionals, we can make real strides in reducing the effects of musculoskeletal injury and recovery outcomes in various areas of a person's life (Kendall et al., 2015).

2.6. Prevention Strategies

Effective prevention strategies are paramount in reducing the risk of musculoskeletal injury (MSI) in high-demand professions such as healthcare and manual labor. Utilizing ergonomic assessments within the working environment can significantly contribute to reducing the incidence of such injuries. Ergonomically designed schemes specific to the job demands can enhance posture, minimize repetitive strain, and limit overexertion upon performing body labor. Regular training sessions that educate workers on proper body mechanics and posture during job tasks can create awareness and encourage preventative measures. In addition, a workplace safety and prevention culture can allow employees to prioritize their overall well-being and health over productivity alone. With the integration of these preventative measures, organizations can not only protect their workforce but also optimize overall job satisfaction and productivity. In addition to ergonomic interventions, the adoption of proactive methods of healthcare, such as regular physical conditioning, is essential in the prevention of musculoskeletal injury. Involvement in the exercises that build strength, flexibility, and endurance can equip individuals with the physical buffers necessary to withstand the rigors of their work. Additionally, the incorporation of formal warm-up routines can acclimatize muscles and joints to resist grueling work, reducing the likelihood of instant injury. According to endoscopic procedure research, years of experience and procedure volume are significant predictors that contribute significantly towards practitioner injuries, making preventive intervention towards the unique occupational demands (Oliveira et al., 2025) very crucial. Embodying physical health programs strategically into company policy not only invests in the physical capabilities of workers but also in long-term health and job retention. Finally, it is necessary that there be a system of feedback wherein employees are able to report discomfort or potential risks on time to provide an active response for the purpose of avoiding injury. Regular communication devices, such as surveys or suggestion boxes, can serve as mechanisms for employees to voice concerns regarding ergonomics and work safety. Additionally, having regular health and safety workshops held can also stimulate the importance of addressing chronic pain or discomfort at an early stage. This aligns with findings indicating that certain interventions, such as altering ergonomics and reducing procedural demands, have been successful in managing injury among healthcare professionals (Oliveira et al., 2025). When employees are supported and well-educated, they will tend to use preventive steps that ultimately reduce the risk of musculoskeletal injuries, providing a healthier and more sustainable work environment.

2.6.1. Importance of Warm-Up and Stretching

Stretching and warm-up cannot be overemphasized in the prevention of musculoskeletal injury. An effective warm-up routine gradually raises blood flow to the muscles and enhances overall body temperature, thus resetting the musculoskeletal system to accommodate greater physical effort. This physiological adjustment is crucial in reducing risk for strains and sprains, usually seen in sports and work environments. Through the use of a warm-up, individuals are able to avoid injuries due to effort or inappropriate movement. Through this warm-up period, there is also a chance for an increased range of motion, producing flexibility that is invaluable in the transition to future activities and reduces the impact on joints and ligaments from stress. Stretching is a valuable component of providing long-term musculoskeletal wellness outside of the use of warm-ups. Stretching every day can make a person more flexible and mobile, and reduce soreness after exercise. Evidence has been supplied by research that proves stretching improves sit-and-reach scores, demonstrating its effectiveness in producing optimal movement patterns. For example, some research, like one that compared aerobic cycling, foam rolling, and stretching, shows that stretching and similar routines can have significant effects on lower extremity flexibility, ultimately re-adjusting muscle for dynamic movement and preventing injury (Bushong, 2011).

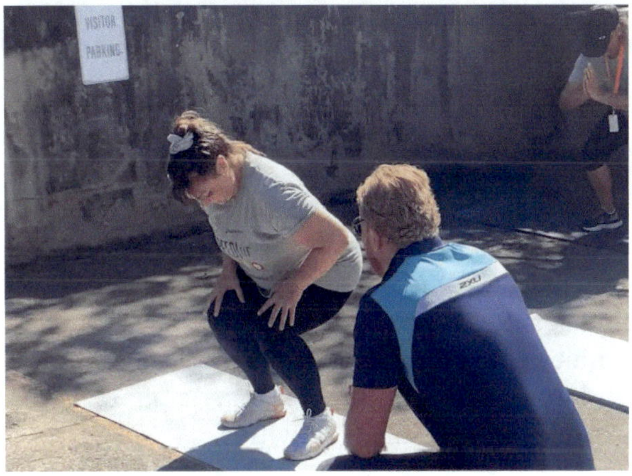

Figure 2.13. Dynamic warm-up.

Source: https://www.employhealth.com.au/nitropack_static/PYDjvDDZFiMBrrGKJpPtAodsXVApnJZW/assets/images/optimized/rev-3f50e18/www.employhealth.com.au/wp-content/uploads/2021/11/28-940x500.png.

Additionally, stretching can also cause an increase in synovial fluid production, which reduces friction with movement and lubricates joints, therefore eliminating the potential for injury and improving overall performance. Particularly in high-risk occupations such as construction, the application of warm-ups and stretching is vital in injury prevention as well as management. Research carried out in the workplace has shown that most injuries, especially sprains, have been a result of inadequate preparation before engagement in physical exertion (Horwitz & McCall, 2004). Since the majority of the workers are not well-endowed with proper warm-up procedures, the likelihood of suffering injuries is greater, especially among the novices or those who have just started working there. Therefore, the incorporation of structured warm-up routines and appropriate stretching procedures is paramount in such settings to assist in reducing injury occurrence and further improving well-being and productivity. Accordingly, enacting such interventions not only mitigates individual performance but also triggers a culture of safety within physically demanding settings (Figure 2.13).

2.6.2. Use of Protective Gear in Sports

Proper use of protective gear in sporting activities is a simple but fundamental component of injury prevention, particularly in contact sports where there is an increased chance of musculoskeletal injuries. Protective gear, ranging from helmets and shin guards to pads and mouthguards, is utilized to dissipate impact forces and minimize the extent of damage sustained through sporting activity. For instance, the absence of adequate protective gear can hugely increase the chances of concussions and fractures, thereby complicating the physical and psychological impacts of sports injuries. Research infers that the effectiveness of such gear largely relies on compliance from the athletes, meaning that frequent and accurate usage is most vital when it involves safeguarding athletes, especially novice participants who are least likely to be experienced with the risks associated with their activities.

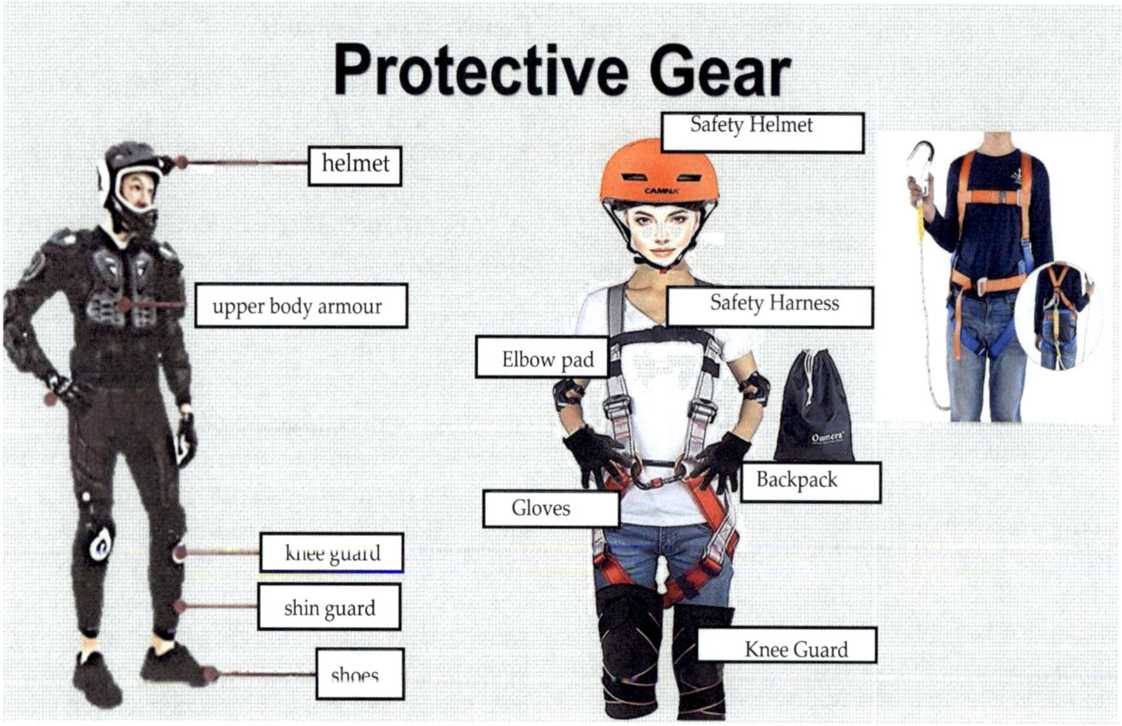

Figure 2.14. Protective gear.

Source: https://i.ytimg.com/vi/6gxTs1Gg3Dk/maxresdefault.jpg.

Therefore, an extensive understanding of the safety precautions offered by gear is fundamental to the proper prevention and management of injury. In sports like martial arts involving intense body contact, protective gear usage has become extremely targeted with rising participation levels and associated injury risks. The benefits of donning protective gear extend beyond merely physical protection in the sense that it also instills a sense of confidence and psychological resilience among participants. Studies examining martial arts training among youth have noted that protective gear not only minimizes the danger of acute injuries but also contributes towards enhanced mental health outcomes by enabling practitioners to focus on mastering skills and self-improvement without the fear of getting injured (de Borja et al., 2025). Nevertheless, the double-edged nature of protective gear must be taken into consideration; while it protects, it may result in a false sense of security, allowing them to engage in unnecessary risk-taking while training and competing. This reality demands rigorous training of athletes on proper techniques as well as the limitations of protective gear. Additionally, addressing assumptions surrounding the wearing of protective gear is crucial in promoting its utilization among young athletes. One such study measuring the junior cricketers' understanding of exertional heat illnesses (EHI) yielded a concerning trend: many youths who engage in sport had minimal perception of the risks of protective gear use, which has the potential to lead to permissive attitudes about safety procedures (Gamage et al., 2019). This erroneous perception underscores the importance of education programs to foster an appreciation for the importance of protective gear as a prevention strategy against injury. Coaches, parents, and sports organizations are pivotal in shaping athlete attitudes so that protective gear is viewed, not as an attractive adjunct, but as a key element of good sporting culture. Encouraging such a culture where protective gear is valued has the potential to minimize the risk of injury and enhance the safety and well-being of young athletes engaged in competitive sport (Figure 2.14).

2.6.3. Education on Proper Techniques and Ergonomics

The relevance of education on correct technique and ergonomics cannot be underestimated when it comes to musculoskeletal injury and therapy. Knowledge of ergonomic principles provides a person with habits that lower the risk of injury from repetitive task exposure and incorrect posture. With the evolving workplace, so does the way workers maintain healthy bodies. Incorporating ergonomics training into occupational safety initiatives not only enhances productivity but also contributes to a broader culture of wellness and health. By teaching employees how to lift, how to set up a workstation, and about body mechanics, organizations enable their employees to take responsibility for maintaining their own physical health, thus reducing the incidence of musculoskeletal disorders associated with ignorance or neglect. Furthermore, the teaching aspect of ergonomics needs to extend past strict compliance with manuals. Effective training needs to create a holistic capacity to absorb the knowledge that physical interaction with tools and equipment can lead to chronic illnesses. Recent studies have indicated that corporations that invest in regular ergonomic training experience huge reductions in employees' compensation claims, which serves to demonstrate the cost benefit as well as health benefit of doing this. Also, informing workers about signs and symptoms of musculoskeletal injury allows them to receive early treatment, and minor problems are not turned into significant disabilities. Overall, preventive education is a crucial line of defense in prevention and management of musculoskeletal injury. Incorporating case studies and examples in ergonomic training programs makes them extremely effective. By studying documented workplace health hazards, companies can illustrate the possible hazards of disregarding ergonomic principles. Such empirical information can be an effective impetus for change, stimulating greater participation by both management and employees. Of special significance is that knowledge garnered from regulatory initiatives and real-world solutions contributes to a more solid ergonomics foundation. Therefore, as stressed in workplace health literature, ongoing evaluations of ergonomics programs are channeled into best practices and provide extremely valuable lessons learned that are relevant to informing future training standards. Ultimately, harmonization of educational efforts with applications in the field achieves a sustained impact favoring healthier workers with reduced injury burden of musculoskeletal disorders and associated management costs (Kriebel et al., 2011; Fauzi & Sabah, 2018) (Figure 2.15).

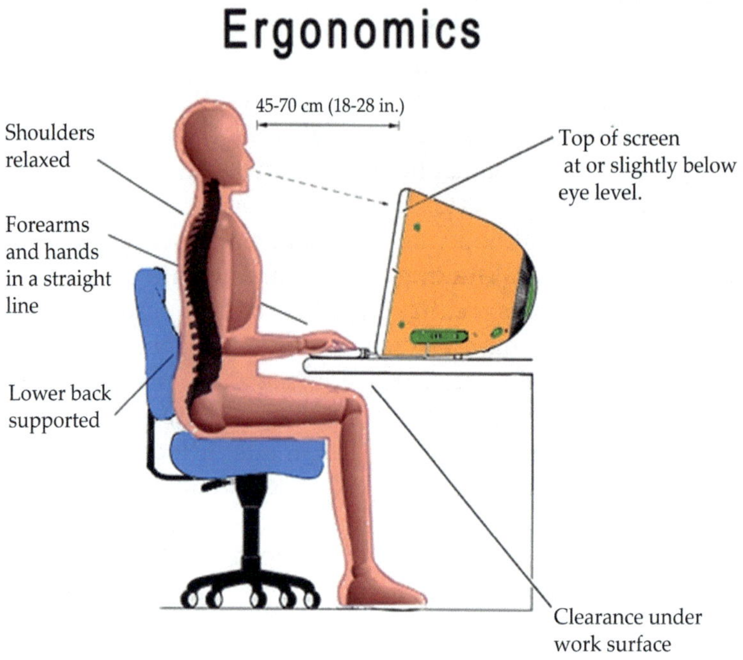

Figure 2.15. Ergonomics.

Source: https://publichealthnotes.com/wp-content/uploads/2018/08/Ergonomics-brochure1.jpg.

SUMMARY

The assessment of musculoskeletal injuries, and more so in runners, is that the injuries are not only prevalent but also complex to manage. With running's popularity on the increase, the risk factors for lower limb injuries necessitate a preventive and curative approach in their management. The systematic review based on a comprehensive literature synthesis demonstrates a high need for particular interventions, such as gait retraining and certain exercises, to prevent the incidence and severity of these injuries. The findings indicate the importance of understanding causes of running-related injuries as fundamental for the formation of effective management strategies. As can be observed from the study, the combined method of treatment can be a cause of improved outcomes for runners' subjects, which includes the relevance to ongoing research on the efficacy of interventions and mechanisms of preventing injury (Firlando & Assyifa, 2024). Additionally, research into novel treatment methods, such as transdermal anti-inflammatory patches, also has massive relevance to the specialty. The more recent meta-analysis that assessed the effectiveness of these patches showed low-certainty evidence but noted the possibilities of delivering immediate and sustained relief from pain in treating musculoskeletal disorders. Although the effect was not clinically significant in certain contexts, the research raises provocative questions concerning the integration of new technology in treatment for patients with acute and chronic musculoskeletal pain. This innovation underscores the need for consistent evaluation of new therapies in clinical practice, prioritizing that effective management of injury must continually adapt to include advancements that enhance patient results and respect heterogeneity in treatment outcomes (Sánchez et al., 2024). Finally, the treatment of musculoskeletal injuries requires an integrative approach that unites prevention, treatment, and ongoing research. The convergence of evidence-based interventions with novel treatment strategies presents a very promising direction towards improving the quality of the care being delivered to the impacted groups. It is recommended that future research target the use of standardized protocols in comparing different interventions, along with longitudinal evaluations to determine the effects of the injuries and their treatment over the long term. By facilitating cooperation between researchers, medical practitioners, and patients, a more effective and supportive environment for managing musculoskeletal trauma can be developed. With increasing maturity of the specialty, attention needs to be placed on education and patient awareness among practitioners and patients to prevent the burden imposed by such injuries and enhance overall musculoskeletal health (Firlando & Assyifa, 2024; Sánchez et al., 2024).

The occurrence of musculoskeletal injuries (MSKIs) in various populations, particularly among the military, highlights an immediate need for preventive care and proper management. High rates of disability and medical discharge attributed to these injuries highlight a need to comprehend the causative factors in depth. The physically demanding tasks of the military have been highly linked with the occurrence of musculoskeletal disorders (MSDs) by studies. There has been a thorough literature review that has identified potential risk factors like physical stress from duties and training, which create a susceptible culture for injury and long-term harm. Understanding the importance of such risk factors is instrumental in designing tailored interventions for lowering rates of injury and enhancing readiness levels overall among military staff (Ramlee et al., 2025). Furthermore, psychological aspects heavily impact musculoskeletal injury development, and thus, a multidimensional approach to its treatment. Stress and mental illness have also been recognized as key factors that accelerate physical conditions. Such psychological variables tend to combine with physical hazards such as poor conditioning and repetitive motion, thus complicating the prevention of injury. Hence, intervention in the mental health domain, in addition to physical training, is critical in achieving holistic care of injury. This combined approach is in line with contemporary sports medicine that demands evidence-based prevention programs prioritizing mental health's role in physical well-being. Wider programs that combine physical and mental testing can have a marked improvement in resistance to musculoskeletal injury in high-risk populations (Ramlee et al., 2025). Effective management of musculoskeletal injuries depends on successful prevention programs. Systematic reviews also emphasize the efficacy of training interventions, ergonomic assessments, and individually designed rehabilitation programs as the key components of successful intervention techniques. By employing methods that consider physical and psychological dimensions in health, it becomes possible to significantly reduce the prevalence of MSDs. Also, guidelines adopted from practice on the management of disorders, such as those formulated by the International Network for Orofacial Pain and Related Disorders, are adopted as blueprints in osteopathic and orthopedic practice. Apart from seeking to improve the knowledge basis of the practitioners, these guidelines also seek to standardize care methods among different healthcare settings towards the goal of enhancing outcomes for musculoskeletal injury patients.

CLOSER LOOK

STRETCHING AND WARM-UP

Stretching and warm-up are essential components of physical activity that prepare the body for exercise, sports, and daily movement. A proper warm-up gradually increases heart rate, blood circulation, and muscle temperature, which helps improve flexibility, coordination, and performance while reducing the risk of injury. Light aerobic activities such as brisk walking, jogging, skipping, or dynamic movements are commonly used during warm-up sessions. Stretching focuses on improving the flexibility and elasticity of muscles and joints. Dynamic stretching, involving controlled movements through a full range of motion, is recommended before physical activity to enhance mobility and readiness. Static stretching, where a position is held for a period of time, is more suitable after exercise to relax muscles, reduce stiffness, and promote recovery. Together, warm-up and stretching help improve posture, balance, and muscle efficiency. Regular warm-up and stretching also support long-term musculoskeletal health by preventing muscle tightness, joint stress, and overuse injuries. They enhance blood flow to working muscles, increase oxygen supply, and prepare the nervous system for coordinated movement. For athletes, proper warm-up and stretching can improve performance, speed, and agility. For non-athletes, they make daily tasks safer and more comfortable. Overall, incorporating stretching and warm-up into any physical routine is a simple yet effective way to promote safety, flexibility, and overall physical well-being.

REFERENCES

1. Aabedi, A., Wang, V., Fraix, M. P., & Agrawal, D. K. (2025). Psychological treatment in the management of pain following musculoskeletal injury. *Journal of Orthopedics and Sports Medicine, 7*, 162–168. https://www.semanticscholar.org/paper/d18ad7f8d1beaf2715dc018924a2bcfbe2dd6a18 (accessed on 26th June 2025).
2. Abdul Khalek, I. M., Mert, Z. N., & Møller, A. M. (2024). Protocol for scoping review: Mapping the landscape of acute pain management in sports-related musculoskeletal injuries. *Acta Anesthesiologic Scandinavica, 69*. https://www.semanticscholar.org/paper/fc69acc71ef5edb18baf2bd1ddee32dbca122516 (accessed on 26th June 2025).
3. Abid, K., & Polo, F. (2024). Narrative review on talent management: Evaluating two decades and exploring future research directions. *Journal of Global Mobility: The Home of Expatriate Management Research*. https://www.semanticscholar.org/paper/bca0146f56a5774b20ea67fd064d91714b1d9737 (accessed on 26th June 2025).
4. Aldanyowi, S., & AlOraini, L. (2024). Personalizing injury management and recovery: A cross-sectional investigation of musculoskeletal injuries and quality of life in athletes. *Orthopedic Research and Reviews, 16*, 137–151. https://www.semanticscholar.org/paper/1015371d48eb7789398bd91d0c9d2603685b971e (accessed on 26th June 2025).
5. Blyth, M., Anthony, I., Francq, B., Brooksbank, K., Downie, P., Powell, A., Jones, B., MacLean, A., McConnachie, A., & Norrie, J. (2015). Diagnostic accuracy of the Thessaly test, standardised clinical history and other clinical examination tests (Apley's, McMurray's and joint line tenderness) for meniscal tears in comparison with magnetic resonance imaging diagnosis. *Health technology assessment (Winchester, England), 19*(62), 1–62. https://doi.org/10.3310/hta19620(accessed on 26th June 2025).
6. Altamimi, T. A., Alkathami, A. A., Al-Awn, R. M., Alkhaldi, M. H., Alhudaithi, M. H., Alqahtani, A., Alzahrani, A., et al. (2024). A narrative review of rotator cuff tear management: Surgery versus conservative treatment. *Cureus, 16*. https://www.semanticscholar.org/paper/94f50169c075db2e8fe7ca47fdd7dbbcc7d570ed (accessed on 26th June 2025).
7. Biz, C., Golin, N., De Cicco, M., Maschio, N., Fantoni, I., Frizziero, A., Belluzzi, E., & Ruggieri, P. (2019). Long-term radiographic and clinical-functional outcomes of isolated, displaced, closed talar neck and body fractures treated by ORIF: the timing of surgical management. *BMC musculoskeletal disorders, 20*(1), 363. https://doi.org/10.1186/s12891-019-2738-2(accessed on 26th June 2025).
8. Bendahan, D. H., Mitchell, C., Chauduri, S., Wing, J., Bird, B., Safeer, S., & Hota, S. (2024). 1805 The importance of ongoing awareness and education for lying and standing blood pressure (LSBP) during hospital admissions. *Age and Ageing*. https://www.semanticscholar.org/paper/119f6c3c1d6911e4820d13d2f9d3afaa06e3e32c (accessed on 26th June 2025).
9. Lansdown, D. A., Bendich, I., Motamedi, D., & Feeley, B. T. (2018). Imaging-Based Prevalence of Superior Labral Anterior-Posterior Tears Significantly Increases in the Aging Shoulder. *Orthopaedic journal of sports medicine, 6*(9), 2325967118797065. https://doi.org/10.1177/2325967118797065(accessed on 26th June 2025).
10. Bin Zia, M., & Kiran, Q. (2025). Rehabilitative role of Kinesio taping in glenohumeral ligament injuries: A narrative review. *Insights–Journal of Health and Rehabilitation*. https://www.

semanticscholar.org/paper/363c74e42bcc52751c1ab66d9abdaccb32e36b65 (accessed on 26th June 2025).

11. Borg, M., & Cachia Pickard, A. (2008). Audit on the use of radiography and the management of ankle sprains in A&E. Malta Medical Journal. 2008, Vol.20(4), p. 12-14. https://core.ac.uk/download/46602202.pdf (accessed on 26th June 2025).
12. Bureau of Labor Statistics. (2014). Occupational injuries and illnesses: A pilot study of job-transfer or work-restriction cases, 2012. https://core.ac.uk/download/20318555.pdf (accessed on 26th June 2025).
13. Kendall, N., Burton, K., Lunt, J., Mellor, N., & Daniels, K. (2015). *Developing an intervention toolbox for common health problems in the workplace.* Health and Safety Laboratory. http://www.hse.gov.uk/research/rrhtm/rr1053.htm(accessed on 26th June 2025).
14. Bushong, J. R. (2011). Foam rolling as a warm-up: The effect on lower extremity flexibility compared to aerobic and stretching protocols. https://core.ac.uk/download/84119765.pdf (accessed on 26th June 2025).
15. Carey, M. R. (2018). An evaluation of the treatment modality and management of acute and chronic low back pain individuals in rural southeast Kansas. https://core.ac.uk/download/217281799.pdf (accessed on 26th June 2025).
16. Clark, A. R., Kulwatno, J., Kanovka, S. S., Klarmann, G., Hernandez, C. E., Natoli, R., McKinley, T. O., et al. (2024). A two-stage approach integrating provisional biomaterial-mediated stabilization followed by a definitive treatment for managing volumetric muscle loss injuries. *Journal of Functional Biomaterials, 15.* https://www.semanticscholar.org/paper/ea60f1479507d8498585a75306c675a10221ba68 (accessed on 26th June 2025).
17. McArthur, K., Jorgensen, D., Climstein, M., & Furness, J. (2020). Epidemiology of Acute Injuries in Surfing: Type, Location, Mechanism, Severity, and Incidence: A Systematic Review. *Sports (Basel, Switzerland), 8*(2), 25. https://doi.org/10.3390/sports8020025(accessed on 26th June 2025).
18. de Borja, C., Ocampo, R., & Teal, A. (2025). Primary Care Considerations for Youth Martial Arts Athletes. *Current reviews in musculoskeletal medicine, 18*(3), 73–78. https://doi.org/10.1007/s12178-024-09942-7(accessed on 26th June 2025).
19. Deokar, A. M., Omar, H. A., & Smith, S. J. (2007). Use of topical NSAIDs in acute musculoskeletal sports injury: A brief review. https://core.ac.uk/download/232571568.pdf (accessed on 26th June 2025).
20. Deokar, A. M., Omar, H. A., & Smith, S. J. (2010). Acute musculoskeletal sports injury and topical NSAID. https://core.ac.uk/download/232583707.pdf (accessed on 26th June 2025).
21. Fauzi, M., & Sabah, M. (2018). E-government services and citizens' satisfaction in the United Arab Emirates: A research agenda. https://core.ac.uk/download/12008290.pdf (accessed on 26th June 2025).
22. Gamage PJ, Fortington LV, Finch CF. Risk perceptions for exertional heat illnesses in junior cricket in Sri Lanka. BMJ Open Sport & Exercise Medicine. 2019;5:e000508. https://doi.org/10.1136/bmjsem-2019-000508(accessed on 26th June 2025).
23. Firlando, A. Y., & Assyifa. (2024). The study of prevalence, management and outcome of musculoskeletal injuries in runners: A comprehensive systematic review. *Journal of Advanced*

Research in Medical and Health Science (ISSN 2208-2425). https://www.semanticscholar.org/paper/0265210f10e5811667eeafb4102b11930fa4419a (accessed on 26th June 2025).

24. Formosa, A. (2006). Knee pain. Malta Medical Journal, 18(4), 32-36.(accessed on 26th June 2025).

25. Giraldo-Vallejo, J. E., Cardona-Guzmán, M. Á., Rodríguez-Alcivar, E. J., Kočí, J., Petro, J., Kreider, R., Cannataro, R., et al. (2023). Nutritional strategies in the rehabilitation of musculoskeletal injuries in athletes: A systematic integrative review. *Nutrients, 15.* https://www.semanticscholar.org/paper/e07b18cc1c169e65f5708a90f997f13a1595928f (accessed on 26th June 2025).

26. Hamad, H., Omer, D., Abdelnabi, R., & Abdelgaleel, A. (2024). Motives and consequences of musculoskeletal injuries management at traditional bone setting centers rather than hospital orthopedic departments in Khartoum, Sudan 2020. *African Health Sciences.* https://www.semanticscholar.org/paper/e7ab096438e32e2f708216efba297754df07e758 (accessed on 26th June 2025).

27. Herring, S. A., Kibler, W., Putukian, M., Boyajian-O'Neill, L. A., Chang, C. J., Franks, R. R., Hutchinson, M., et al. (2024). Initial assessment and management of select musculoskeletal injuries: A team physician consensus statement. *Current Sports Medicine Reports, 233*, 86–104. https://www.semanticscholar.org/paper/ace4792c7974dfe3fc8d0941b274bf845a173277 (accessed on 26th June 2025).

28. Lema MK, Chalya PL, Mabula JB, Mahalu W. Pattern and outcome of chest injuries at Bugando Medical Centre in Northwestern Tanzania. *J Cardiothorac Surg*. 2011;6:7. Published 2011 Jan 18. doi:10.1186/1749-8090-6-7(accessed on 26th June 2025).

29. Kim, D., & Lee, M. (2025). Prevention of hamstring injuries in elite football players: Exercise and load management strategies. *Exercise Science.* https://www.semanticscholar.org/paper/a9f579afd239dfc427f90f7a767bde710cce76d6 (accessed on 26th June 2025).

30. Puhakka, J. , & Koistinen, L.(2014). Akuuttien nilkkavammojen konservatiivisten kuntoutusmenetelmien vaikuttavuus kudostyypeittäin. https://core.ac.uk/download/38103931.pdf (accessed on 26th June 2025).

31. Kriebel, D., Tickner, J., Jacobs, M., & Markkanen, P. (2011). Lessons learned: Solutions for workplace safety and health. Lowell Center for Sustainable Production University of Massachusetts Lowell. https://core.ac.uk/download/71352756.pdf (accessed on 26th June 2025).

32. Kwan, Z., Han, W., Yong, S., Faheem, N. A. A., Choong, R. K. J., Zainuddin, S. I., Lam, C. L., et al. (2023). Dermatological issues among individuals receiving palliative care: A review. *American Journal of Hospice and Palliative Medicine®, 41*, 952–964. https://www.semanticscholar.org/paper/656a47f550bdce57d05db105a9e299d1cc75c6a0 (accessed on 26th June 2025).

33. Lindahl, A. K. (2016). The effect of intermittent pneumatic compression on the management of pain associated with delayed onset muscle soreness. https://core.ac.uk/download/222996030.pdf (accessed on 26th June 2025).

34. Liu, G., Lv, G., & Liu, F. (2024). Suture techniques in the surgical management of flexor tendon, Achilles tendon and cruciate ligament injuries: A systematic review. *BMC Musculoskeletal Disorders, 25.* https://www.semanticscholar.org/paper/8a09432d324a8080f068764f8dca502f773e401d (accessed on 26th June 2025).

35. Manfredini, D., Häggman-Henrikson, B., Al Jagshi, A., Baad-Hansen, L., Beecroft, E., Bijelic, T., Bracci, A., et al. (2024). Temporomandibular disorders: INfORM/IADR key points for good clinical practice based on standard of care. *CRANIO®, 43*, 1–5. https://www.semanticscholar.org/paper/6872d48a634f04904ee405af21357149df90a15f (accessed on 26th June 2025).

36. Manske, R., Wolfe, C., Page, P., & Voight, M. L. (2025). Diagnostic musculoskeletal ultrasound for the evaluation of the lateral elbow: Implications for rehabilitation providers. *International Journal of Sports Physical Therapy, 20*, 137–143. https://www.semanticscholar.org/paper/aa6f2a2c204b57d047f1599da9410c440ceecd51 (accessed on 26th June 2025).

37. Skelton, D. A., & Mavroeidi, A. (2018). How do muscle and bone strengthening and balance activities (MBSBA) vary across the life course, and are there particular ages where MBSBA are most important? *Journal of frailty, sarcopenia and falls, 3*(2), 74–84. https://doi.org/10.22540/JFSF-03-074

38. https://core.ac.uk/download/293863667.pdf (accessed on 26th June 2025).

39. Horwitz, I. B., & McCall, B. P. (2004). Disabling and fatal occupational claim rates, risks, and costs in the Oregon construction industry 1990-1997. *Journal of occupational and environmental hygiene, 1*(10), 688–698. https://doi.org/10.1080/15459620490508787(accessed on 26th June 2025).

40. Oliveira, R., Roseira, J., Estevinho, M., Tavares de Sousa, H., Rolanda, C., Meining, A., & Walter, B. (2025). Endoscopy-related musculoskeletal injuries: A systematic review and meta-analysis on prevalence, risk factors and prevention. *United European Gastroenterology Journal.* https://www.semanticscholar.org/paper/93cffbfa784b71ec10013536b9cfd79eacd15f1d (accessed on 26th June 2025).

41. Parvizi, D., Sahafi, R., Pisarski, T., Kandikattu, S., Aavula, M., & Agrawal, D. K. (2025). Risk factors, incidence, and management of re-injury following repair of shoulder rotator cuff. *Journal of Orthopedics and Sports Medicine, 7*, 179–185. https://www.semanticscholar.org/paper/5eb0e730e28a2788cc4ac051d42f111185b029dc (accessed on 26th June 2025).

42. Paudel, S., Luitel, P., Thapaliya, I., Thapa, A., & Sharma, S. (2024). Successful management of severe scalp avulsion injury: A case report and review of surgical interventions. *Journal of Surgical Case Reports, 2024.* https://www.semanticscholar.org/paper/78f196fe1173d283f83c6b2b5987ad64dc8fc1dc (accessed on 26th June 2025).

43. Pouliakas, K., & Theodossiou, I. (2010). An inquiry into the theory, causes and consequences of monitoring indicators of health and safety at work. https://core.ac.uk/download/177141.pdf (accessed on 26th June 2025).

44. Prakash, S., & Sharma, A. (2025). Non-specific lower back pain in healthcare professionals and students: Diagnosis, management, and prevention strategies. *Middle East Research Journal of Medical Sciences.* https://www.semanticscholar.org/paper/cddc4a0066e0c14a2a7fff78a1e68891cf290ba9 (accessed on 26th June 2025).

45. Ramlee, S. N. S., Tamil Selvan, H. K., Megat Mokhtar, M. A., Rafiudin, N. M., & Nizam, K. (2025). Systematic review of risk factors contributing to musculoskeletal disorders (MSDs) and injuries in military personnel. *International Journal of Education, Psychology and Counseling.* https://www.semanticscholar.org/paper/773e6b773421a53223b6f4aa0492349116a29de6 (accessed on 26th June 2025).

46. Rappaport, E. (2001). Ergonomics in the workplace: Is it time for an OSHA standard? https://core.ac.uk/download/5124662.pdf (accessed on 26th June 2025).

47. Reis, L., Lopes, B., Sousa, P., Sousa, A., Caseiro, A., Mendonça, C., Santos, J. M., et al. (2024). Equine musculoskeletal pathologies: Clinical approaches and therapeutical perspectives—A review. *Veterinary Sciences, 11.* https://www.semanticscholar.org/paper/fbf12d86cdef83691651135d4e7c640edfa0b95a (accessed on 26th June 2025).

48. Sadasivam, A. K., Ayyan, S. M., Sindujaa, S. N., & Manu, S. (2024). Improving door-to-analgesia timing in musculoskeletal injuries in an academic emergency department in India: A quality improvement project. *BMJ Open Quality, 13.* https://www.semanticscholar.org/paper/141a942f11c1577ae53c75e66aa8516de5ad8d03 (accessed on 26th June 2025).

49. Sánchez, M. B., Callaghan, M. J., Selfe, J., Twigg, M., & Smith, T. O. (2024). Efficacy of transdermal anti-inflammatory patches for musculoskeletal pain: A systematic review and meta-analysis. *Pain Management, 14*, 557–569. https://www.semanticscholar.org/paper/0841a6aa26f08e1e9269a4066bcf08e7b68033d5 (accessed on 26th June 2025).

50. Sethi, M., Limaye, R., & Limaye, N. (2024). Is internal brace augmentation (IBA) better than isolated modified Brostrom Gould (MBG) repair for chronic lateral ligament injury? A retrospective analysis. *Orthopedic Proceedings.* https://www.semanticscholar.org/paper/b660543b59afafa3c791cfc54c3ada6161459ab3 (accessed on 26th June 2025).

51. Shoukri, M. (2025). Corticosteroid joint injections in primary care. *InnovAiT: Education and Inspiration for General Practice.* https://www.semanticscholar.org/paper/357c43bdb902855d508272ee0c43ec7880a8ae61 (accessed on 26th June 2025).

52. Soh, T., Lee, H. J., Choi, J., & Oh, J. Y. L. (2025). Iliolumbar vein injuries in preposes lateral lumbar interbody fusion: Strategies for prevention and management. Illustrative case. *Journal of Neurosurgery: Case Lessons, 9.* https://www.semanticscholar.org/paper/67ab9ddbfecc0c3a009b9b439e849a2e234fa28c (accessed on 26th June 2025).

53. Tayyib, N. A. (2024). Advancements in vacuum therapy for musculoskeletal wound care: A comprehensive analysis of chronic wounds and acute injuries. *Journal of Musculoskeletal Surgery and Research.* https://www.semanticscholar.org/paper/914447cec6ab647a80679476b6468064921f2eaf (accessed on 26th June 2025).

54. Yadav, A., & Choudhary, S. (2024). Identification of the most prevalent hypokinetic disorders linked to sedentary lifestyles and their impact on public health. *Sports Science & Health Advances.* 2, 1 (Jun. 2024), 185–192. DOI:https://doi.org/10.60081/SSHA.2.1.2024.185-192. https://core.ac.uk/download/613190434.pdf (accessed on 26th June 2025).

55. Yasin, S., Lakhani, A., Aslam, F., Jalal, M., Hafiza, N. K., Ali, B., Muneeb, S., et al. (2025). A comparative study of laser therapy and Kinesio taping for functional recovery in ankle sprain. *Insights–Journal of Health and Rehabilitation.* https://www.semanticscholar.org/paper/b02715dd5865607cd2b2e21d714df8167695f7cd (accessed on 26th June 2025).

56. Yuan, C., Song, W., Jiang, X., Wang, Y., Li, C., Yu, W., & He, Y. (2024). Adipose-derived stem cell-based optimization strategies for musculoskeletal regeneration: Recent advances and perspectives. *Stem Cell Research & Therapy, 15.* https://www.semanticscholar.org/paper/057f774a9cd0f9fb7579e2f9e1cdbf9e5af469ba (accessed on 26th June 2025).

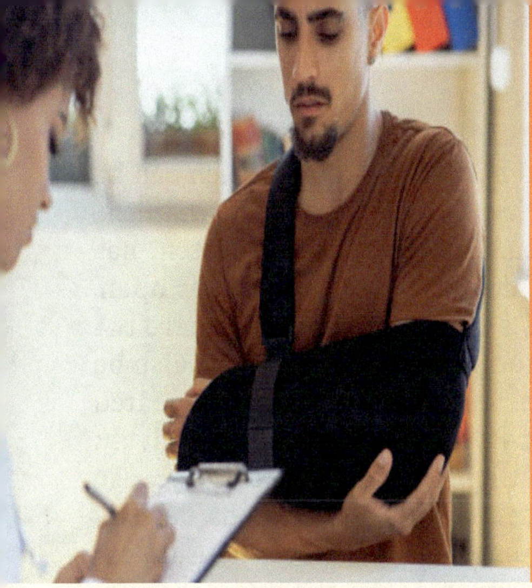

Chapter 3

FRACTURES AND DISLOCATIONS

Contents

Introduction 69

3.1. Types of Fractures 72

3.2. Types of Dislocations 76

3.3. Causes and Risk Factors 80

3.4. Symptoms and Diagnosis 84

3.5. Treatment Options for Fractures 88

3.6. Treatment Options for Dislocations 92

Summary 96

References 99

Introduction

The field of orthopedics is principally delineated by the complexity that attends fractures and dislocations, both having unique challenges in diagnosis and management. Both of these injuries are prevalent across different populations, among sportsmen, active patients, and children, who are placed at unique exposures due to aspects of growth. Fractures can result from repetitive stress or high-energy trauma, disrupting the bone, while dislocations are the complete displacement of bone articulations, ranging from acute to chronic instabilities. It is necessary that healthcare providers understand the mechanisms, types, and consequences of such injuries for the proper application of treatment approaches. Both dislocations and avulsion fractures, unless treated promptly, will have grave complications and therefore necessitate an acute awareness of their long-term implications and clinical features for quality of life and patient mobility. Of fractures, avulsion injuries such as those near the knee are most pertinent, as they frequently occur to young athletes involved in contact sports.

These are caused when forces exceed the tensile strength of a tendon or ligament and result in a fragment of bone that becomes avulsed. Current literature believes that diagnosis is best achieved by radiographic imaging, with newer technologies such as CT and MRI providing additional information regarding soft tissue trauma. Some classifications, such as Meyers and McKeever for the anterior cruciate ligament avulsion, are required for treatment determination. The treatment can comprise conservative care for nondisplaced fractures or more aggressive surgical care for those presented or complicated by instability. Prompt diagnosis of such injury may prevent longstanding disabling complications, including malunion or residual instability, and hence the need to educate healthcare providers on such issues (J-hyun et al., 2025). Dislocations, particularly shoulder dislocations, are another critical element of orthopedic practice that requires thorough study. The shoulder dislocation is further complicated by fractures, as in rare cases of bilateral anterior shoulder dislocations from seizures. Multifaceted conditions like these need careful observation to avoid serious complications such as avascular necrosis. Reducing dislocations on time is especially critical in the prevention of the risks of long-standing displacement, and thereby the focus is on early management. Because medical practitioners are confronted by fractures and dislocations in numerous clinical settings, understanding the various etiologies and presentations will enable them to provide maximal and timely care. This is part of a broader demand for thorough education and sensitization throughout orthopedic medicine for better patient outcomes and avoidance of resulting long-term disability from these injuries (Wilt et al., 2025).

Definition of Fractures

The fracture definition in musculoskeletal trauma focuses on the osseous structure's integrity. A fracture occurs due to excessive trauma or force leading to bone breakdown, which can be classified in various ways, such as by mechanism, severity, or area. The classification system has the words that describe if the fracture is open, where the skin is violated, or closed, where the skin is intact. Additionally, fractures can also be stress fractures, which are created by repeated forces that may weaken the bone progressively. It is worth noting such differences because each of the fracture categories needs various clinical management and interventions. After a consensus arrived at by the International Skeletal Society, there exists a recognized jargon within radiology that is used to describe such conditions and one that aids healthcare professionals in communication and treatment planning (Palmer et al., 2020). In the field of sports medicine, description of fractures gains a new significance due to the peculiar types of injury sport individuals often endure. Fractures in these cases are usually categorized based on their occurrence during training or competition, and fractures can be brought about by acute injury or chronic overuse conditions. The International Olympic Committee has fostered robust definitions and classifications of injuries like fractures for the purpose of enhancing consistency in data collection and research report description (Bahr et al., 2020). The added level of definition is required to track injury patterns among athletes, recognize risk factors, and devise prevention strategies. Defining fractures in the same manner across sports enables stakeholders to better grasp the impact of such injuries on performance and health outcomes. The consistent fracture definitions benefit not only in enhancing treatment strategies but also in informing prevention and rehabilitation strategies effectively. Classification of fracture types enables total assessment of patient needs and rehabilitation program planning for the return of function. In addition, understanding certain aspects of fracture enables clinicians to anticipate potential complications, i.e., rates of healing or re-injury, particularly among the sports population. By utilizing standardized definitions, scientists have the ability to contribute to the overall body of knowledge about fractures, paving the way for new prevention and treatment methods that are tailored to the needs of different groups. The introduction of logical definitions to research and clinical practice ensures that individuals receive full care and have maximum musculoskeletal function (Figure 3.1).

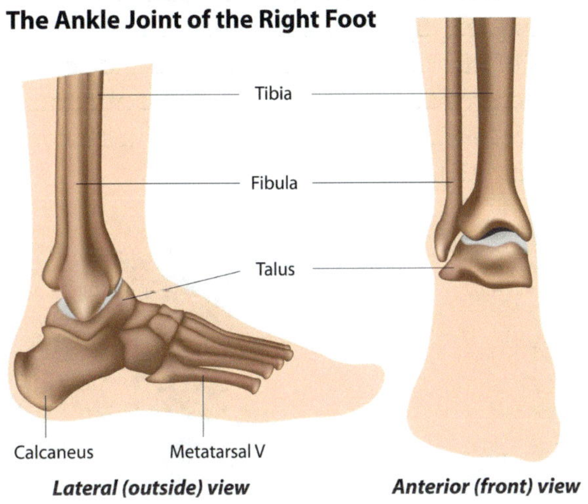

Figure 3.1. The context of musculoskeletal injuries.

Source: https://www.jeffreybergmd.com/wp-content/uploads/2014/08/ankle.jpeg.

Definition of Dislocations

The word dislocation, if applied to the context of musculoskeletal injury, means the complete displacement of a bone outside of its rightful position in the joint. It is most often due to trauma, such as accidents or falls, that cause excessive forces on the joint, which spread the bones participating in the joint apart. Dislocations may occur in various joints, with the shoulder being the most common joint affected. Unlike fractures, in which the bone is fractured, dislocations are more a function of the soft tissues surrounding the joint, including ligaments and tendons, resulting in acute pain, swelling, and inability to move the affected area. An acute dislocated joint, in the initial moment, has a clinical presentation that is characteristically one of apparent deformity that has an unwelcome appearance and deserves immediate medical care. The differentiation between fractures and dislocations is crucial for both diagnosis and treatment. While fractures are characterized by compromised structural bone continuity, dislocations describe the interruption of joint alignment. In diagnosing between the two, imagery in the form of X-rays plays a vital role as it will both demonstrate fractures and the severity of dislocation and associated soft tissue damage. Treatment is highly varied; fractures may at times necessitate immobilization or surgery, but dislocations often must be reduced promptly to replace the bones within the joint. Rehabilitation is thereafter essential to regain function, typically in the guise of physical therapy, to stabilize the joint and enhance the range of motion. Prevalence of dislocation dictates that prevention and knowledge are essential, especially in high-risk activities. Incidental causes include sports and fall injuries, which often result in severe morbidity if left untreated. With the new face of workplace safety, it is indispensable to learn about the hazards of dislocation to make injury prevention even more effective. Patterns of work injuries causing job transfer or limitation according to the nature of injuries are evidenced by studies, necessitating ongoing education and training in proper means to avoid such traumatic events. Utilizing joint stability and safety practices is an intervention that can be applied to minimize dislocation rates, thus improving occupational health and safety levels (Ruser & Wiatrowski, 2013; Brenner et al., 2015).

Importance of Understanding These Injuries

It is of critical importance to comprehend fractures and dislocations, both in relation to proper medical management and in relation to maximizing patient outcomes in a myriad of situations. Acute knowledge of these injuries alerts clinicians to possible complications, which can vary from chronic pain to functional impairment. For instance, following the devastating earthquakes in Türkiye on February 6, 2023, there was a definite relationship between prolonged exposure to traumatic injuries and the incidence of some injuries to the spine, such as compression fractures and burst fractures, according to the findings attributed to the occurrence (Bolukçu et al., 2024). This highlights the significance of ascertaining the mechanical forces involved and their consequences on the human body in trauma. Evaluation of spinal injury with a thorough understanding allows effective management programs that are vital in cases of disasters, where timely and effective treatment is paramount. Moreover, the details of complex dislocations, particularly the elbow, highlight the importance of tailored surgical approaches and rehabilitation. Complex elbow dislocations are notoriously challenging by virtue of the involvement of important anatomical elements and carry a tendency to occur differently among population groups. Retrospective examination comparing outcomes in subjects with such dislocations demonstrated that surgical interventions are able to yield disparate results, with age playing a role in varying patterns of recovery (Bolukçu et al., 2024). Awareness of these injuries gives healthcare practitioners the knowledge to use individual patient-specific techniques for optimal function and recovery. This general awareness also encourages a goal-oriented rehabilitation strategy, by which practitioners can realistically set goals and modify follow-up care to optimize long-term outcomes. Further, the knowledge of dislocations and fractures enhances prevention, where the significance of public awareness on injury risk and safe behaviors is emphasized. With the dissemination of information on the causation of such injuries, health practitioners can help individuals recognize risk factors and employ prevention in sports and daily activities. For instance, the identification of risk patterns among population groups, such as the earthquake victims in Türkiye, enables one to have specific community health programs to reduce occurrences of injury in these disaster cases (Bolukçu et al., 2024). Additionally, the investigation of complex elbow dislocations stretches into sports medicine, too, where the understanding of prevalence and outcome facilitates enhanced training and prevention techniques. By proceeding proactively on the basis of information, the incidence and severity of fractures and dislocations can be minimized, thus resulting in better public health outcomes (Figure 3.2).

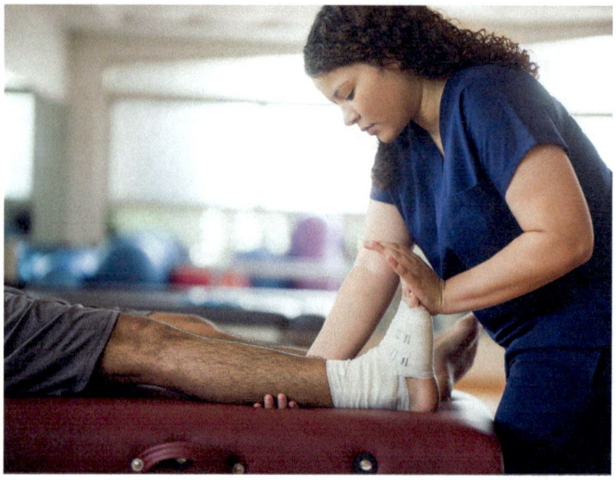

Figure 3.2. The fractures and dislocations.

Source: https://wp02-media.cdn.ihealthspot.com/wp-content/uploads/sites/202/2024/10/iStock-1132546141-1.jpg.

3.1. Types of Fractures

Fractures are also divided into numerous categories based on their nature and the forces that caused them. Two of the most common types are closed and open fractures. Closed fracture is where the bone is cracked but does not exit the skin, whereas open fracture or compound fracture is a break communicating with the external environment and has the potential to cause infection. The management of these fractures also varies, with open fractures tending to require more harsh management. One should identify these variations to facilitate appropriate management, especially in cases where specialist access is low, since most of these injuries will be handled initially by primary care or emergency services, particularly in the military, where rapid treatment is paramount (Hunt et al., 2023). One further significant fracture classification is one based on pattern, including transverse, oblique, and spiral fractures. A transverse fracture occurs straight across the bone, whereas an oblique fracture occurs at an angle, a common type of high-energy trauma. Spiral fractures typically result from twisting motion and can indicate severe injury or abuse in certain populations. Recognition of these patterns enables healthcare workers to establish why the fracture has occurred and how to modify treatment in response. As an example, oblique and spiral fractures may need surgical intervention more frequently than transverse fractures since they are more unstable (Hunt et al., 2023). Correct classification not only influences treatment but also facilitates possible evaluations of healing and rehabilitation. Lastly, specific fractures such as stress fractures and pathologic fractures present unique diagnostic and therapeutic challenges. Stress fractures are most commonly caused by repetitive stress that is built up over a period of time and typically occur in athletes and soldiers engaged in strenuous physical activities. Pathologic fractures, conversely, result from weakened bone structures due to conditions such as cancer and osteoporosis. As indicated by the prevalence of finger and hand fractures in varied settings, it is important to identify the kind of fracture for effective management (Hunt et al., 2023). Effective diagnosis comes with better outcomes and decreased recovery periods, which emphasizes the importance of proper knowledge in trauma assessment, especially in emergency and primary care contexts. In general, identification of the fracture type dictates not just short-term treatment but long-term care essential to complete recovery (Figure 3.3).

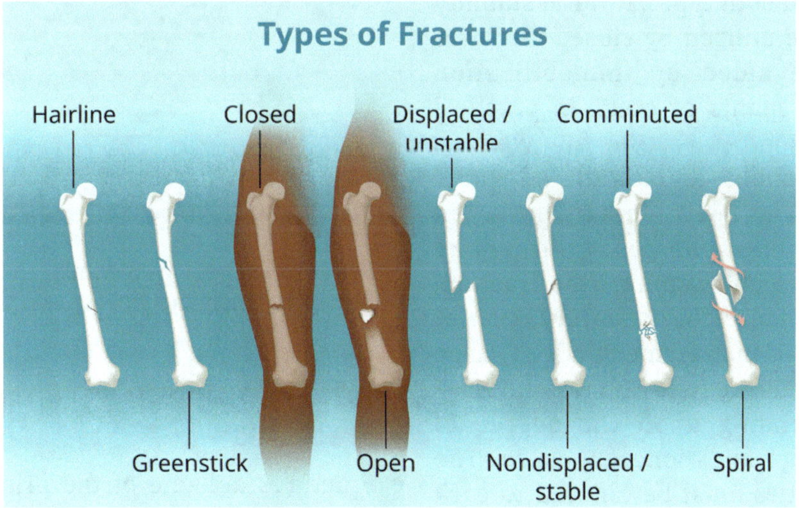

Figure 3.3. Fractures are classified into various types based on their characteristics and the forces that caused them.

Source: https://www.verywellhealth.com/thmb/EDmg42PbTXc83WBVoKl5yzPa8U0=/1500x0/filters:no_upscale():max_bytes(150000):strip_icc()/Fracture-WhattoKnowAboutThisInjury-v2-5936ff9b9dd048e9b8be221450f994d8.png.

3.1.1. Closed vs. Open Fractures

Fractures are normally separated into two main categories: closed and open fractures, both of which reflect the status of the adjacent soft tissue. Closed fractures occur when the line of fracture is internal without crossing the skin, thus they tend to result in fewer infections and tissue damage complications. This fracture is prone to have less complicated treatment modalities, as surgical interventions are usually unnecessary. By contrast, compound or open fractures involve a fracture of the skin, along with the fracture itself, which makes bones exposed and potentially leads to serious complications. Open fractures present an additional challenge to management by clinicians because open fractures have an additional risk of infection and soft tissue damage, complicating recovery. Awareness of these differences is crucial to effective treatment planning and judgment of prognosis in orthopedic care. The repair of open and closed fractures is very different depending on the difference in the integrity of soft tissues around both types. Natural stability and alignment are utilized by closed fractures to heal and are aided by immobilization methods such as splints or casts. In practical terms, closed fractures can be followed up by repeated injections to monitor adequate healing without any need for surgery. Open fractures can require emergency surgery to debride the wound and stabilize the fracture, a necessary procedure for the prevention of infection. Operative management might range from external fixator devices to more invasive techniques, depending upon the degree of soft tissue damage and bone exposure. The treatment modalities must be tailored to each category of fracture, integrating the surgical and non-surgical treatments to provide optimal healing. In addition, implications for recovery and rehabilitation vary between open and closed fractures, leading to distinct recovery courses. In patients with closed fractures, pain relief and progressive return to function through physical therapy can be aimed largely at them, allowing a relatively predictable recovery duration. On the other hand, the process of treating open fractures is more involved and takes longer due to infection and probable side effects of surgery. Customized treatment protocols, as noted in new studies through the observation of patellar dislocation and talus fracture, have to be designed to address the specific anatomical and pathophysiological determinants underlying each group of fracture (Petri et al., 2015; Wijers, 2024). This tailored approach maximizes healing outcomes as well as maximizes overall quality of patient care for patients suffering from such types of injuries (Figure 3.4).

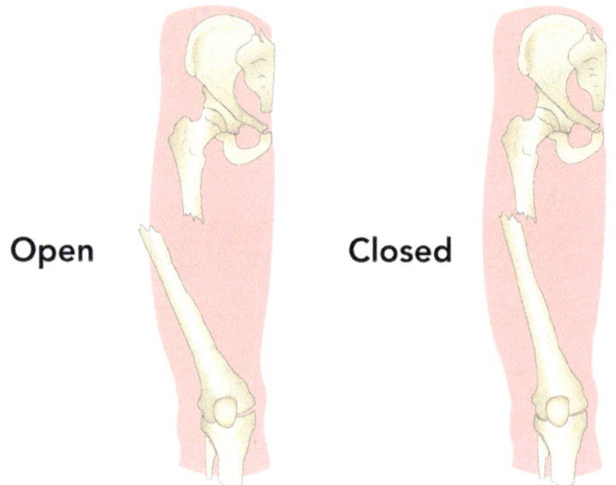

Figure 3.4. Fractures are classified primarily into two categories: closed and open fractures.

Source: https://www.hcortho.sg/wp-content/uploads/2022/12/Types-of-Fractures.png.

3.1.2. Complete vs. Incomplete Fractures

Fractures are one of the prime areas of focus in the practice of orthopedics, and their division into complete and incomplete fractures has significant diagnostic, therapeutic, and rehabilitative implications. Complete fractures consist of a complete separation between the fracture-producing bone and resulting in two discrete fragments that may be displaced or non-displaced. This break typically results in immediate and severe impairment of function as the bone structure is entirely compromised. Complete fractures must be well comprehended because they usually require more aggressive types of treatment, such as surgery or immobilization, to heal and recover function. The urgency of treating complete fractures is brought out by their potential complications, including nonunion or malunion if they are treated inappropriately and in a timely fashion. In contrast, incomplete fractures are defined by partial destruction of the bone structure in which the bone has some continuity. Such fractures, which are typical in children since their bones are softer and more pliable, are visible in several different ways, including blunt forced fractures or buckle fractures. Although incomplete fractures may be less symptomatic initially compared to complete fractures, they must receive proper examination and care to avoid aggravation or complications. Because they tend to heal on their own with conservative management like casting or splinting, recognition of the characteristic features of such fractures is necessary for optimal orthopedic management. Appreciating the subtleties in treatment recommendations and follow-up care indicated for incomplete fractures can lead to optimal patient outcomes. The distinction between incomplete and complete fractures is more than classification; it has implications extending to the treatment processes and mechanisms of healing. The technical complexity of total fractures typically entails problems with surgical technique, reduction, and method of fixation to regain healing and functional return. Alternatively, the relatively uncomplicated nature of incomplete fractures may permit non-surgical management, with emphasis on follow-up and observation for hidden complications that may arise. Significantly, cases such as high-entropy alloys (HEAs) exhibit material response under strain similarities, correlating intrinsic properties with orthopedic condition phenomena such as fractures (Ding et al., 2018). Additionally, mechanochemistry evidence supports ongoing treatment process development, enabling better understanding and optimization of healing in conditions such as fractures and dislocations (Páž et al., 2013). This reciprocity of material science and orthopedic practice will provide the key to new approaches in treating complete and incomplete fractures.

3.1.3. Common Fracture Types (e.g., Transverse, Spiral)

Fractures are also grouped based on their appearance and mechanism of injury, with typical varieties being transverse and spiral fractures. Transverse fractures consist of a perpendicular angle through the bones long axis, frequently due to a direct blow or extreme force that is perpendicular to the bone. These present clinically as stable fractures that may be managed by immobilization with casting or splinting. In cases of instability or when fragments need to be realigned, surgery might be necessary. As an example, a pediatric patient can have a transverse fracture of the tibia that, if not properly treated, can become an issue, and therefore accurate treatment is essential for optimal recovery, as highlighted in available literature (Sleem, 2024). Spiral fractures, on the other hand, have their helical fracture line running around the bone, usually caused by rotational force on the limb. The fractures are most commonly seen in patients who engage in sports or high-impact activities that have twists or abrupt changes in direction. They are perhaps more complex than transverse fractures because of the possibility of widespread displacement and soft tissue injury, often demanding full imaging studies for accurate diagnosis. The mechanism of spiral fracture is crucial in designing suitable treatment interventions, as identified from research that indicates older children and adolescents are at greatest risk of such fractures following greater aggressive activity levels (Sleem, 2024). In practice in veterinary medicine, the study of fractures of long bones in canines reveals consistent patterns of fracture, with transverse fractures again being the most frequently encountered. Examinations verify that the fractures are often caused by trauma, such as road traffic accidents or falls, especially in younger animals. The occurrence is found to be greater in certain breeds and suggests an association between the predisposition of the breed and the nature of fractures observed. The management and surgical methods applied in animal practice are similar to those practiced in human medicine, with the focus remaining on stabilization methodology based on the stability of fractures. Both effective treatment planning and prevention rely on the understanding of these general fracture patterns, reinforcing the importance of careful research in the discipline (Figure 3.5).

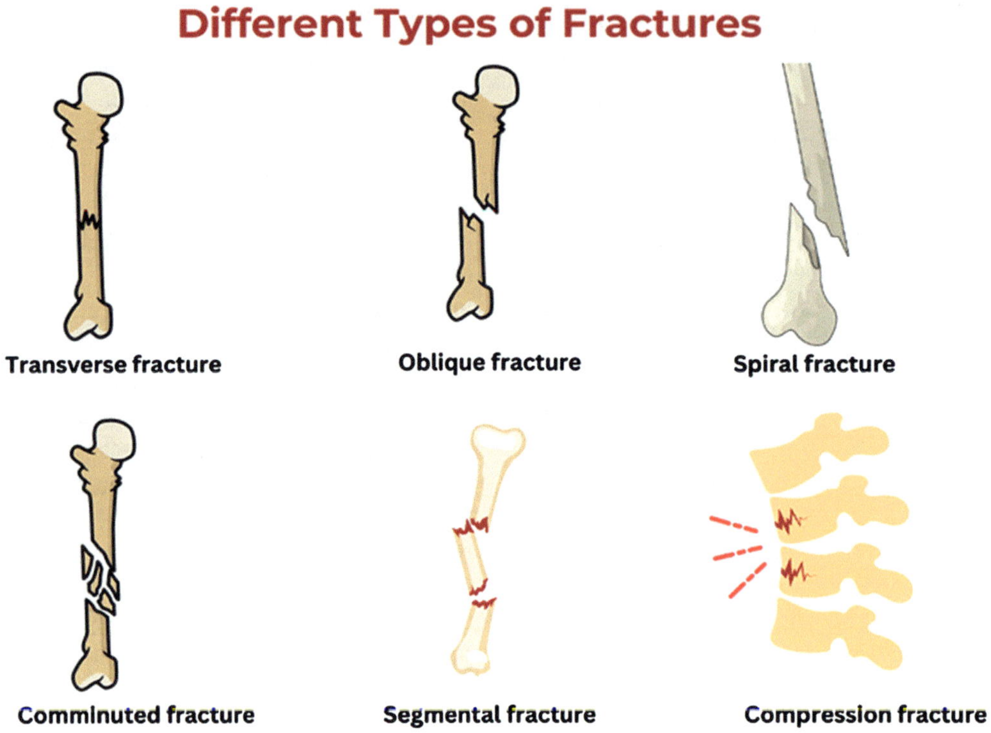

Figure 3.5. Fractures are categorized based on their characteristics and mechanisms of injury.

Source: https://boneandspine.com/wp-content/uploads/2007/08/types-fracture.png.

3.2. Types of Dislocations

The concept of dislocations is the foundation of material deformation learning, particularly structural integrity analysis in many engineering applications. Dislocations can largely be classified into screw and edge dislocations, both distinct mechanisms through which crystals experience strain accommodation. Edge dislocations result from the introduction of an extra half-plane of atoms into a crystal lattice, local distortion, and the consequent ability to slip under stress. Screw dislocations result from a helical arrangement of atoms, permitting deformation along the axis of dislocation. The presence and movement of such kinds of dislocations are the universal reasons for plasticity, which affect material response to external forces, like the behavior of material fracture in engineering materials, as highlighted in the course material in materials science (Bodrova & Kramar, 2017). Understanding the mechanism through which dislocations are moving in materials is crucial in the prediction of failure modes. For instance, edge dislocations tend to interact with such obstacles as precipitates and grain boundaries more easily than screw dislocations, and this can significantly affect the material's yield strength. While in motion, dislocations tend to multiply and interact, leading to work hardening, a phenomenon where materials tend to become harder and resist deformation more as strain increases. This property is of paramount importance in engineering applications, where the strength and longevity of mechanical components must be guaranteed. The engineering relevance of dislocation theory is widespread and far-reaching, influencing alloy and composite design for optimizing their performance under load (Bodrova & Kramar, 2017). Dislocation behavior and structural defects on the nanoscale have been highlighted as key considerations in recent research on ceramics, particularly those that show low-temperature deformability. The flash-sintering process has been shown to create a particular microstructure in ceramics such as TiO2, where the presence of stacking faults and nanotwins aids in their mechanical behavior. The inability of normal dislocation motion in ceramics, leading to brittle failure, makes the possibility of how nanoscale aspects are capable of imparting ductility questionable. From the examination of the behaviors of dislocations in interacting with other defects, scientists are beginning to discover mechanisms that would allow ceramic materials to perform at a higher level in conditions of multiaxial loading. This study further emphasizes the importance of characterization of dislocation kinds and types for advancing material design and utilization in engineering applications (Figure 3.6).

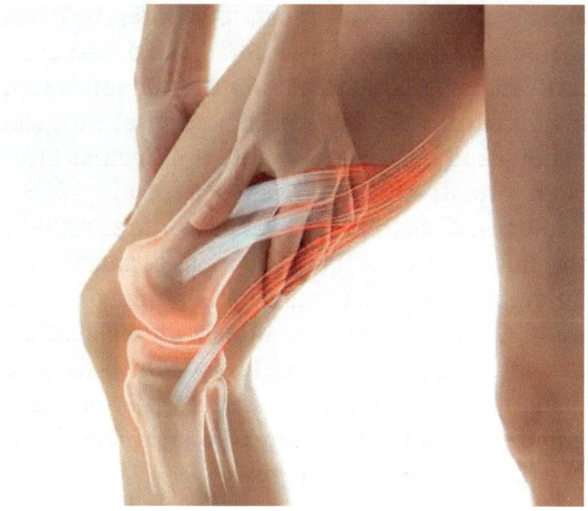

Figure 3.6. Dislocations

Source: https://www.carehospitals.com/ckfinder/userfiles/images/dislocation_b.webp.

3.2.1. Shoulder Dislocation

Shoulder dislocation is a pathological condition and most commonly follows a traumatic injury such as a fall or direct blow to the shoulder. The most frequent is anterior dislocation, where the head of the humerus is displaced in an anterior direction from the glenoid cavity. In addition to acute pain and immobilization, it can even lead to chronic complications such as recurrent dislocations, especially in younger and more active patients. The pathophysiology of injury highlights the precarious balance between joint mobility and stability. Risk factors like exposure to sports and certain occupational hazards augment the incidence of shoulder dislocations, hence the need to use preventive measures among the high-risk group. The management of shoulder dislocation varies significantly based on the level of injury complexity and whether there is associated fracture or soft tissue damage. Normally, the initial management is by closed reduction techniques for the reduction of the humeral head into the glenoid cavity. In more complex cases, particularly fractures such as the reverse Hill-Sachs injury, surgical intervention can be necessary. Advanced-level interventions, including 3D-printed individualized prostheses, indicate promising results in the rehabilitation of joint function and minimization of surgical trauma and hence better patient outcomes after such catastrophic injuries (Hu et al., 2023). Evolution of custom surgical procedures reflects the new face of orthopedic management, with an emphasis on maximizing rehabilitation and mobility of recovering patients with dislocation. Reverse shoulder arthroplasty (RSA) has also gained wide popularity as a successful treatment choice for shoulder dislocations with resultant proximal humeral fractures.

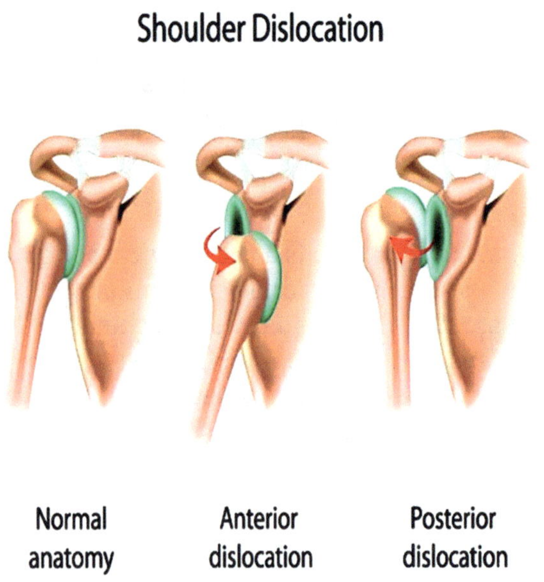

Figure 3.7. Shoulder dislocation represents a significant clinical concern.

Source: https://i0.wp.com/orthobangalore.com/wp-content/uploads/2024/05/Shoulder-Dislocation-treatment-bangalore1818-09-15-15_09_36.jpg?resize=500%2C500&ssl=1.

Evidence indicates that outcomes of RSA in traumatic settings are comparable to outcomes of degenerative conditions such as arthritis, thus warranting its use as a consideration (Ng et al., 2022). As the incidence of shoulder dislocations continues to increase, being aware of the appropriate indications for surgery will be crucial in optimizing functional outcomes. Postoperative analysis of outcomes such as pain measurements and range of motion informs clinicians about the efficacy of intervention. Eventually, technological advances and research will further define the therapeutic scope of shoulder dislocations, enabling improved recovery options for persons who have been afflicted with the condition (Figure 3.7).

3.2.2. Finger Dislocation

Finger dislocation is a significant problem within the broad picture of fractures and dislocations, as much as it pertains to complicated digit anatomy and its very relevance to hand function. Dislocations include the bones of a joint being displaced from their usual position because this causes acute pain, swelling, and apparent loss of movement. It is most common in the realm of sports, when repeated high-impact movements increase the likelihood of injury. Of all finger dislocations, proximal and distal interphalangeal joint dislocations are especially noteworthy due to their frequency and risk of long-term sequelae. The fact that several joints are involved and operative or conservative management modalities are frequently required indicates the necessity for accurate diagnosis and early intervention to reestablish normal function and prevent future complications. Finger dislocation treatment is very variable based on which joint alone is affected, as well as the severity of the injury. Nonoperative methods of treatment, such as closed reduction with splinting, are commonly applied, particularly in cases that are uncomplicated. For more complex situations, particularly with multicampus involvement, like concomitant dislocation of the proximal and distal interphalangeal joints, surgery can become a consideration. A case representative reports a patient with such dislocations treated by closed reduction and splinting, with no pain on range of motion in a 24-month follow-up

(Saglam et al., 2022). This is an indication of the success of conservative treatment in managing most dislocation cases and reflects the necessity of personalized plans to address the unique conditions present in each patient. Despite advancements in management techniques, finger dislocations can lead to long-term complications, including stiffness, pain, and loss of range of motion. Proximal interphalangeal joint injuries are particularly serious because they primarily cause functional loss that disrupts activities of daily living and affects a person's quality of life. Such complications are aggravated when the injury is compounded by intra-articular fractures or significant joint displacement, with difficulty restoring normal function (Nordback & Waris, 2021). Hence, rehabilitation protocols like physical therapy to increase strength and flexibility play a key role in supporting maximum recovery. With ongoing studies, clinicians should keep current with the latest treatment algorithms for finger dislocations to ensure that they treat their patients with the most effective care and improve long-term results in hand function (Figure 3.8).

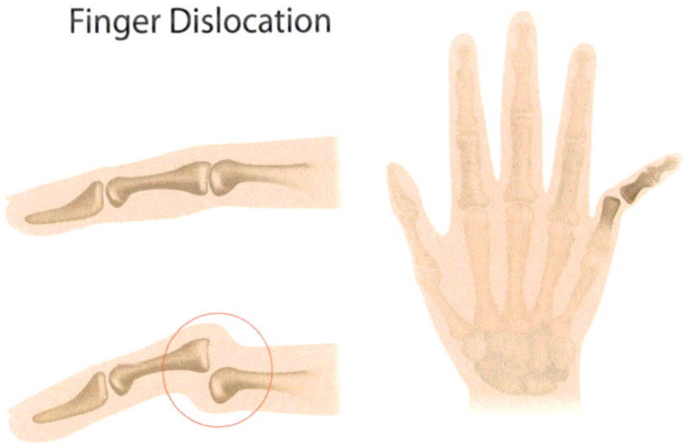

Figure 3.8. Finger dislocation represents a significant concern within the broader context of fractures and dislocations.

Source: https://www.melbournehandtherapy.com.au/wp-content/uploads/2020/08/dislocations.jpg.

3.2.3. Hip Dislocation

Hip dislocation is a severe orthopedic problem that is generally a result of high-energy trauma, and both the immediate and ultimate patient results are impacted. Hip dislocation is comprised of femoral head dislocation from the acetabulum and typically results in related damage such as femoral neck or acetabular fractures. Early recognition and prompt intervention are essential in the management of hip dislocations to prevent complications, such as avascular necrosis or post-traumatic arthritis. The direction of the dislocation, anterior or posterior, can specify treatment modality, as posterior dislocations are more common and typically related to hip fracture patterns. Precise clinical evaluation and imaging are essential to establish the severity of the injury and carry out an optimal management plan, especially in children with anatomical complexities, making the treatment process more challenging (Zomar et al., 2024). Treatment of hip dislocation also varies based on the severity of the injury and the occurrence of a fracture along with it. Closed reduction would usually be the first line of treatment, aiming to re-establish normal alignment without the need for surgery. Surgical options in the form of hip hemiarthroplasty (HHA), however, may be required in some cases, especially those with unresolved instability or associated fractures. Dislocations after HHA present particular issues, as they are associated with high morbidity, as illustrated in current studies on operative outcomes and methods for dislocation management. As an example, one survey assessing patients with hip fractures reported frequent dislocation in the first few weeks following surgery, highlighting the necessity of close observation and possible surgical revision operations in the afflicted (Saxena et al., 2024). By adopting a multi-dimensional treatment strategy, long-term hip dislocation management can be maximized to minimize recurrence and maximize patient quality of life. For instance, orthopedic surgeons, physiotherapists, and geriatricians can play a significant role in post-dislocation rehabilitation, especially in elderly patients who are at risk of developing recurrent dislocations. A successful rehabilitation program is required to restore mobility and function and address intrinsic risk factors that can predispose the patient to future dislocations. Continuing investigation of the outcomes of various treatment methods, such as in large cohort series, is necessary to present evidence-based practices that optimize recovery and patient satisfaction following hip dislocations (Zomar et al., 2024) (Figure 3.9).

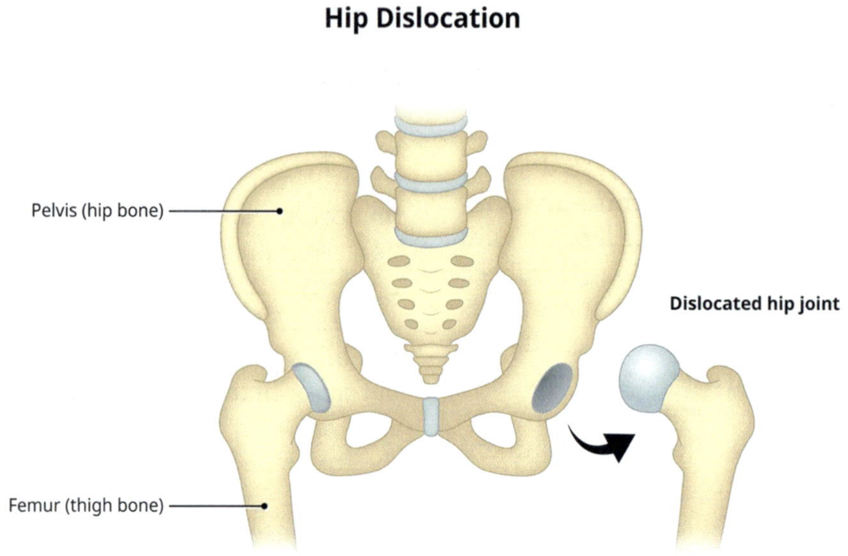

Figure 3.9. Hip dislocation.

Source: https://cdn-assets-eu.frontify.com/s3/frontify-enterprise-files-eu/eyJwYXRoIjoiaWhoLWhlYWx0aGNhcmUtYmVyaGFkXC9maWxlXC9BTWtFbzJ5VnFmTFdIWWs0bXQ5dC5qcGcifQ:ihh-healthcare-berhad:SKEMrJpq54Zbe_rTZCfWt5A2RZ2mfxzXZ0qQIAtUDPY?format=webp.

3.3. Causes and Risk Factors

It is important to understand the etiology and risk factors behind fractures and dislocations in order to manage their occurrence and public health burden. An important cause of such injuries is the epidemiological trend of aging populations. Older people have decreased bone density and muscular strength, so they are more susceptible to falls, which is a primary cause of fractures. Based on data about death from injury, injuries are a significant burden; importantly, they are the fourth most common cause of death in some regions, e.g., Ireland (Scallan et al., 2001). Hence, awareness of age-related changes in body mechanics can initiate directed prevention efforts in the elderly. Lifestyle and environmental factors are also essentially critical in the causation of fractures and dislocations. For instance, exposure to dangerous activities, such as sport or work, significantly raises the chances of such injury. The case of a 65-year-old man who inflicted shoulder pain by painting his house is a sufficient example of the way in which everyday activities can lead to unintentional injury, especially when proper precautions are not taken (Vassallo, 2008). Certain illnesses—such as osteoporosis or other musculoskeletal diseases—also make one more susceptible to fractures. These determinants indicate the importance of individual risk assessment and prevention education programs at the community level. Moreover, underlying systemic factors like socioeconomic status may predispose one to fracture and dislocation as well. Lower socioeconomic individuals tend to have less access to healthcare and preventive services, which contributes further to their risks from risk factors like poor nutrition or inactivity. Public health data point out that variations in rates of injury still persist among various groups in the population, which indicates a need for universal interventions with such differences in mind (Scallan et al., 2001). Such interventions may be in the form of community training programs covering prevention of falls, enhanced workplace safety protocols, and greater availability of healthcare services, particularly for vulnerable populations. By keen consideration of these multifactorial causes and risk factors, healthcare practitioners can develop appropriate interventions to minimize the occurrence and severity of fractures and dislocations.

3.3.1. Sports-Related Injuries

In sports, players are susceptible to a range of injuries that can have a detrimental impact on their performance and overall health in the long term. Amongst these, fracture and dislocation injuries are more serious because, other than the acute medical attention they require, they also involve prolonged periods of rehabilitation. Understanding the mechanisms and environments involved in such injuries is central to effective prevention and management. For instance, athletes in collision sports such as football or gymnastics are more prone to traumatic injury due to the nature of their sport. Secondly, stress fractures happen through overuse injury, whereby repetitive microtrauma outpaces the ability of the body to heal itself, and thus recovery is hampered. Identification of such patterns allows physicians and coaches to offer targeted training programs that are able to neutralize the threat of such injuries for athletes. In particular, in hip and elbow injuries, the spectrum of sports injuries has a multifaceted relationship between acute and chronic injuries. Elbow trauma, such as dislocations and radial head fractures, usually occurs in contact sports and those that excessively fatigue the joint. As seen in Abel & Sutter (2025), most cases of overuse and traumatic injury underscore the importance of prompt assessment and management. Similarly, hip injuries, which are frequent among athletes who participate in running and jumping, can result in severe complications if not properly diagnosed. According to Abel & Sutter (2025), failure to diagnose these injuries will result in a longer recovery time and a higher likelihood of suffering chronic disease, making the importance of early diagnosis and proper medical evaluation necessary. All of this awareness is paramount not just for quick recovery but also in reducing the dangers of long-term disability from such injuries. Treatment of dislocations and fractures has to be treated from a holistic point of view, including both immediate treatment and long-term recovery measures. Early management usually includes stabilizing and immobilizing the affected limb to avoid further damage, and then, through imaging tests, determining the severity of the damage. After diagnosis, treatment can also differ greatly, ranging from conservative methods such as physiotherapy to surgical procedures, based on injury severity. For instance, the player with a dislocated elbow needs to be treated carefully and may even require surgery to repair and restore the proper function, together with reducing the chances of recurrence, as seen in Khalid (2025). On the broader scale, training sessions that teach players proper technique, warm-up, and the importance of cross-training can go a long way towards the prevention of such injuries. Hence, creating a whole strategy that combines the medical method with educational activities is imperative for guaranteeing athlete health and longevity in their sport (Figure 3.10).

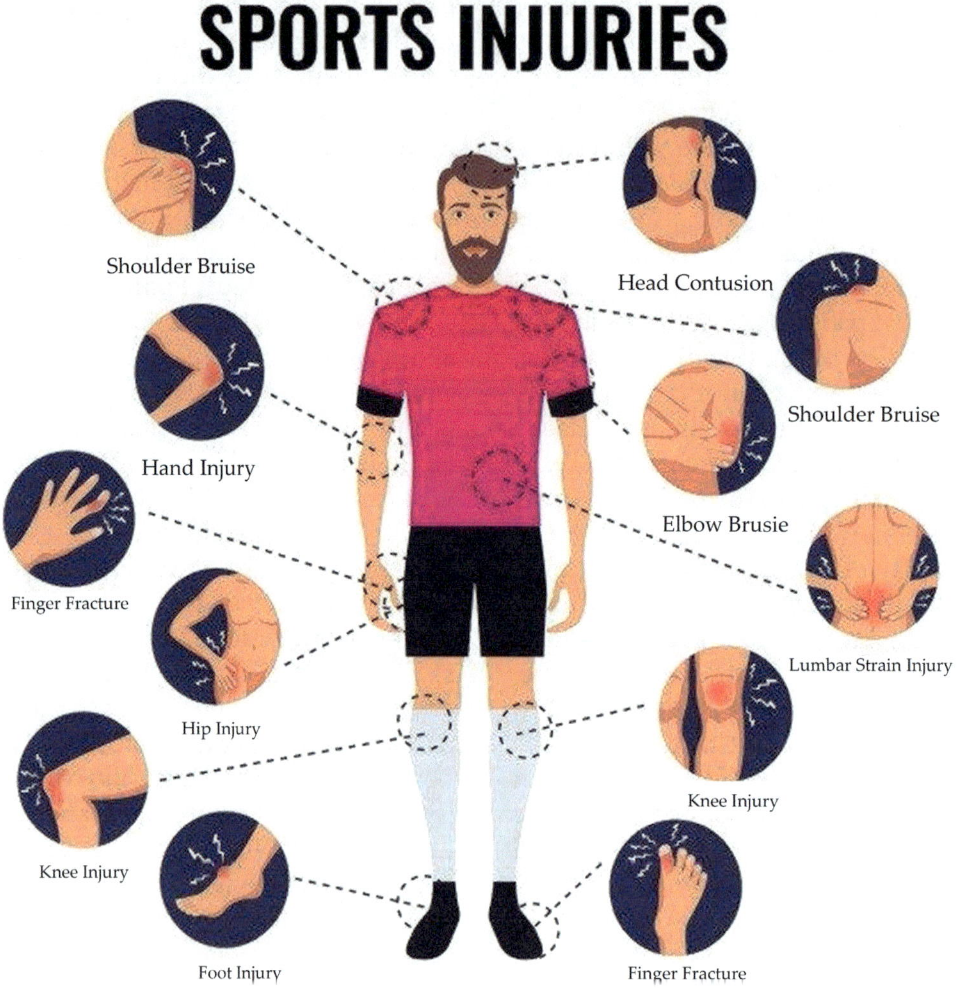

Figure 3.10. The sports-related injuries.

Source: https://bimshospital.com/wp-content/uploads/2021/07/sport.jpg.

3.3.2. Falls and Accidents

Falls and injuries from accidents constitute a high percentage of the cases that lead to dislocations and fractures, particularly in high-risk groups such as young adults and the elderly who engage in recreational activities. Increasing numbers of studies indicate that the etiologies of these kinds of injuries have multifactorial causes based on a combination of environmental and individual risk habits. For instance, the use of stand-up electric scooters, a new form of transport, has revealed shocking statistics regarding accidents; the majority of participants in this activity do not wear helmets as well as other protective gear, which leads to more cases of falls that result in serious injury, i.e., fractures and dislocations of joints (Dunet et al., 2013). Identification of high-risk settings and management of modifiable risk factors are crucial components of prevention strategies for avoiding injury to curtail the occurrence of fractures and dislocations due to such accidents. The rate of falls in adults and older adult patients has the propensity of having serious consequences, of which fractures of various types are a few. Falls have been shown to represent a large proportion of hospital admissions for traumatic injury, particularly for acetabular fractures, which are found to take place at significantly higher rates in older individuals who are defined by lower bone density and poor balance. Research into acetabular fractures indicates the outcome varies greatly based on the nature of the fall and consequent medical intervention, with nonoperative treatment having a tendency to bring long-term complications such as osteoarthritis (Dunet et al., 2013). It is hence essential to understand the causes and consequences of falls in designing effective clinical protocols for assessment and treatment, thereby enhancing recovery and minimizing the need for invasive procedures. Additionally, the impact of extrinsic factors and lifestyle on fall risk cannot be overstated. Engaging in dangerous activities while under the influence of alcohol or drugs significantly increases the risk of injuries from falling. In the case of electric scooter accidents, for example, information shows that a high percentage of injured individuals were under the influence of alcohol at the time of injury, which suggests the possibility of impaired cognition to add to the gravity of accidents (Alwani et al., 2020). Moreover, the probability of individuals disregarding safety measures on recreational activities not only raises their personal risk but also adds a heavier burden on healthcare systems that have to treat the consequences of these accidents. Therefore, certain education protocols aimed at promoting safety awareness could have a perceptible effect in stemming the occurrences of falls and injuries thereto, eventually resulting in improved public health levels.

3.3.3. Osteoporosis and Age-Related Factors

With increasing age, the susceptibility to osteoporosis increases tenfold, a condition that is characterized by weakened bone structure and decreased bone density. The major reason for loss of bone with age is hormonal changes, particularly in postmenopausal women, due to loss of estrogen, leading to rapid bone loss. Apart from hormonal changes, other factors such as reduced physical activity and low dietary intake of calcium further augment susceptibility to osteoporosis in the elderly. The interaction between lifestyle and biological influences requires a general understanding of osteoporosis because its progression typically leads to fragility fractures—serious damage that has the potential to play a major role in the quality of life and independence for older adults. Also, elderly people's awareness of osteoporosis risk factors among them is essential, especially against a backdrop of research pointing to insufficient knowledge regarding the condition and its application to personal health management (Roza et al., 2025). Effective prevention strategies for osteoporosis are based on greater awareness and proactive measures aimed at addressing risk factors associated with age. Age-related screening recommendations, as contained in the Qatar fracture risk assessment tool, offer crucial data for clinicians managing osteoporosis. The recommendations ensure risk stratification guiding treatment strategies based on risk profiles and hence prevent fragility fractures before they occur. As individuals older than 50 years account for an inordinate burden of osteoporosis, intervention in this age group is critical. Such interventions may include lifestyle adjustments, pharmacological treatment, and routine tests to evaluate changes in bone density so that those at higher risk may be given appropriate interventions tailored to their specific needs (Alam et al., 2024). Again, the psychological factors in osteoporosis in the elderly cannot be overlooked. Older people find themselves at variance with various beliefs about their susceptibility to bone weakness. As suggested by research among menopausal and peri-menopausal women, perceived risk, health beliefs, and intention to be tested for osteoporosis have significant correlations. Importantly, better knowledge of osteoporosis could be pivotal in increasing the likelihood of individuals engaging in proactive health behaviors. Educational interventions addressing misconceptions and emphasizing the importance of the early detection and control of osteoporosis can empower the elderly population to engage in osteoporosis screening and prevention interventions (Roza et al., 2025). Consequently, heightened awareness regarding osteoporosis benefits not only individual outcomes of health but also alleviates public health expenditures due to fractures and dislocations (Figure 3.11).

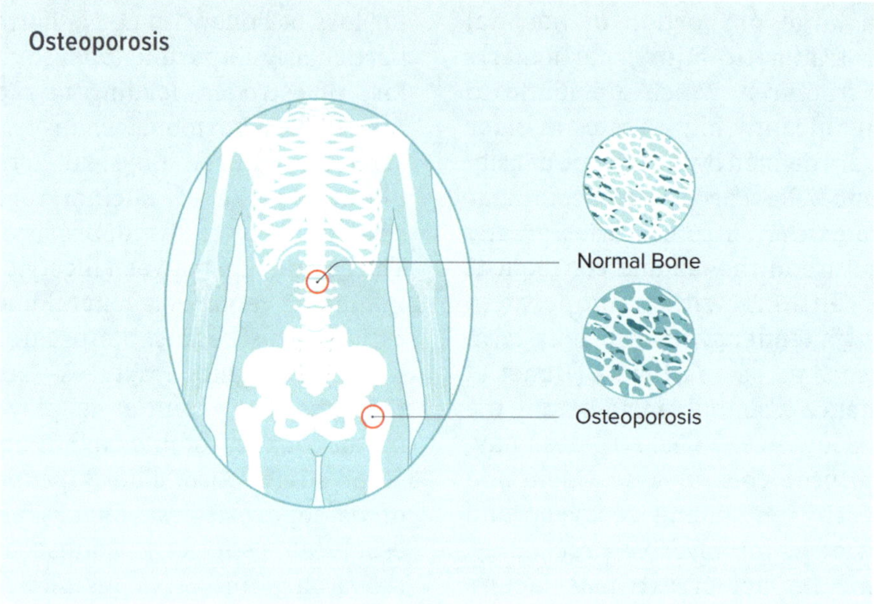

Figure 3.11. As individuals age, the risk of developing osteoporosis markedly increases.

Source: https://post.healthline.com/wp-content/uploads/2021/12/Fotografi%CC%81as-de-osteoporosis.jpg.

3.4. Symptoms and Diagnosis

Fractures and dislocations present a number of signs that are highly crucial for effective diagnosis and treatment. For the most part, the patient will have severe pain in the area of injury, swelling, and obvious deformity, which could indicate a fracture or dislocation. Restriction in movement, such as the inability to move the injured limb, accompanies these signs and usually worsens with movement. Initial assessment by healthcare providers typically involves visual examination and measurement of the range of motion and palpation of the region in question to assess for abnormal alignment or tenderness. Further, an intensive patient history is required because it provides some insight into the mechanism of injury and associated symptoms to aid in making an accurate diagnosis. Early detection of these symptoms is important in determining the management plan and prevention of complications such as chronic pain or joint instability. Diagnostic imaging then becomes essential to confirm fractures and dislocations because clinical assessment alone will not provide a clear indication of the injury. X-rays are the primary imaging modality to visualize the bony structure and identify any fracture, while high-tech imaging modalities such as MRI or CT scans may be employed for better evaluation, especially in complex injuries or if injury to soft tissue is being considered. For instance, hip fractures, which are a common problem among the elderly, must be treated with care and consideration for radiological examination to ascertain the precise location and extent of the fracture (Zhang et al., 2020).

This method of diagnosis ensures effective treatment planning based on the nature of the injury so that recovery potential is maximized. Additionally, understanding the injury mechanisms through imaging facilitates predicting long-term outcomes and complications. Identification of complications of fractures and dislocations is crucial both in diagnosis and in the management of patients. For instance, an undiagnosed fracture can lead to complications of malunion or nonunion, where the bone fails to heal, resulting in chronic pain and loss of function. A failure to diagnose a dislocation can result in compromised blood supply or nerve damage, and so emphasizing the need for urgent and proper treatment. Also, biocompatibility of surgical treatment materials, such as metallic implants, hinges on how the body responds from the patient and the probability of corrosion in the body (Eliaz, 2019). Hence, when conducting diagnosis and treatment of fractures and dislocations, it is important that doctors consider both short-term symptomatology and long-term effects to enhance the treatment of patients and assist in delivering favorable rehabilitation outcomes.

3.4.1. Common Symptoms of Fractures

Fractures, or disruptions in the continuity of bone, generally manifest in a broad spectrum of symptoms that have considerable effects on an individual's mobility and quality of life. Some of the most commonly known symptoms are extreme pain at the location of the injury, inflammation, and bruising. Pain is typically sudden and harsh, which makes immobilization of the affected region necessary, which is a protective reflex. Swelling can rapidly develop as a result of inflammation and of fluid accumulation around the fracture site. Deformity is seen in some instances, e.g., a limb could appear to be displaced or in an abnormal position. These dramatic clinical presentations deserve immediate medical evaluation because untreated fractures can lead to complications or chronic pain, not only impacting physical function but also overall well-being (Xin et al., 2024). Not only is pain and swelling due to fractures a symptom, but patients can also have a limited range of motion, as well as pain with weight-bearing on the affected limb. The impairment of function in performing normal movements can tightly limit customary daily activity, leading to frustration and distress. Depending upon the location and degree of the fracture, this impairment of functioning may be temporary or permanent. For instance, fractures of weight-bearing bones such as the femur or tibia produce more serious issues with mobility compared to fractures of less central locations. Furthermore, associated symptoms such as tingling or numbness can be suggestive of involvement of the nerves and need urgent assessment to prevent irreversible neurological damage. Detection of such symptoms, in this case, is crucial to effective intervention and rehabilitation, enabling the patient to restore a normal condition (Xin et al., 2024). Once again, an important symptom that might be linked to fractures is the development of crepitus, which is a grating sensation typically felt while moving the injured area. This is because of the friction between the shattered tips of the bones against each other or against ruptured soft tissues, with damage. Crepitus also serves as a sign to diagnose and an additional cause of pain for the patient. Besides, fractures can also lead to complications such as compartment syndrome or neurovascular injury, thus further reinforcing the urgency for full and quick assessment. Because all of these signs serve to reflect the complexity of fractures, identification and awareness of them can significantly direct acute treatment and chronic rehabilitation programs (Fitriana et al., 2023) (Figure 3.12).

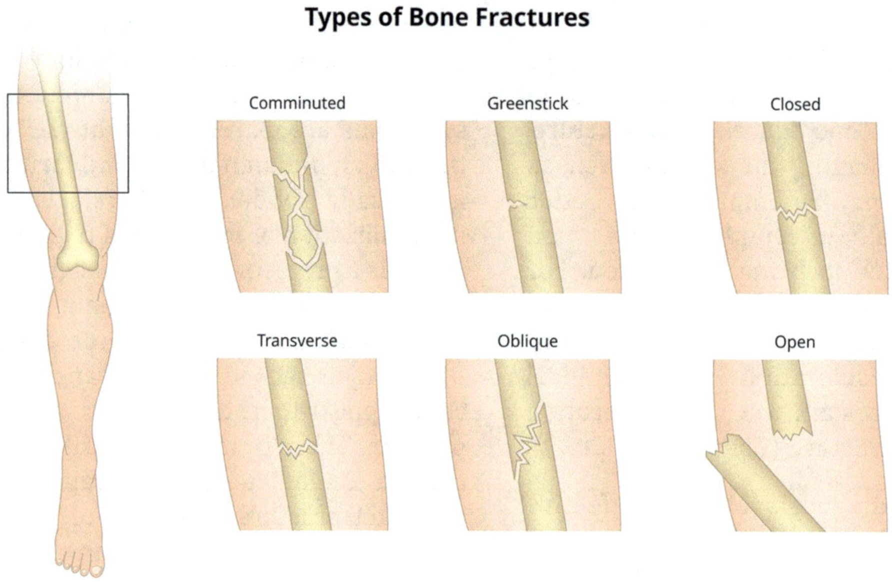

Figure 3.12. Common symptoms of fractures.

Source: https://cdn-assets-eu.frontify.com/s3/frontify-enterprise-files-eu/eyJwYXRoIjoiaWhoLWhlYWx0aGNhcmUtYmVyaGFkXC9maWxlXC9MMjJ2alZZNmZjcWVodnBuTnE0RS5qcGcifQ:ihh-healthcare-berhad:y6ZtjxM6eg2TTzquGiwi40qbsnhhwWThTRDndfx97s0?width=%7Bwidth%7D.

3.4.2. Common Symptoms of Dislocations

Dislocations occur when bones within a joint are displaced from their normal position, resulting in a range of acute signs that typically occur immediately upon the injury. One of the most common signs of dislocations is pain, which typically occurs due to pulling or rupture of ligaments, tendons, and surrounding soft tissue covering these structures. This pain may be exacerbated by motion and typically occurs with aching and an abrupt onset. Besides pain, most patients will also have bruising and swelling of the affected area due to inflammation and damage to blood vessels. These markers of injury are overt signs that can inform diagnosis and treatment. Immediate recognition of these signs is vital for effective management as they directly affect the urgency of visiting a physician to prevent further complications. Another frequent symptom of dislocations is that there is a loss of mobility in the affected joint. It is difficult or impossible for patients to move the dislocated joint, leading to reduced overall function. Immobilization is particularly concerning in the shoulder and knee joints, where range of motion is critical in performing activities of daily living. Besides, certain patients can also say that they feel unstable or as if the joint can slide out of position again. In some cases, the visible presence of a deformity, like an irregular shape or abnormal location of the joint, can be a horrible sign of dislocation. These physical signs indicate the necessity of prompt evaluation and treatment since continued injury to the joint may develop into long-term disability and chronic instability should it not be treated. The physiological responses of the dislocation are often more than local pain and stiffness; they can also be neurological symptoms resulting from potential nerve impingement. The patient can experience numbness, tingling, and limb weakness in the affected joint. For instance, the brachial plexus is more likely to be affected by a shoulder dislocation and cause altered sensation or weakness in the arm. In more severe conditions, such as sternoclavicular dislocation, symptoms such as dyspnea or dysphagia may be experienced due to compression of significant structures in the thoracic region, and therefore, healthcare practitioners need to have a thorough assessment of both musculoskeletal and neurological function (Abrassart & Hoffmeyer, 2011). Recognizing such general symptoms helps not only in early diagnosis and treatment but also highlights the importance of proper follow-up care to prevent long-term effects related to dislocations.

3.4.3. Diagnostic Imaging Techniques (e.g., X-rays, MRIs)

Detection of dislocations and fractures relies heavily on the use of sophisticated imaging techniques, two of which are X-rays and MRIs. X-rays are used as a primary imaging modality due to their immediate availability, cost-effectiveness, and ability to provide instant feedback about bone integrity and positioning. They have the ability to reveal the underlying presence of fractures, dislocations, and related bone deformities. However, X-rays may not detect fine injuries or soft tissue pathologies and hence further examination is necessary. Magnetic resonance imaging (MRI), however, gives better visualization of the overall pathosis, particularly of the soft tissues such as ligaments, cartilage, and muscles surrounding the site of injury. This enhanced functionality is valuable in cases where there may be concomitant soft tissue injury along with bone pathosis, allowing for accurate diagnosis and treatment planning. Practically, the choice of imaging technique can have a great bearing on the outcome in patients. While X-rays are sufficient to detect uncomplicated fractures and dislocations, complex cases often call for the precision of MRI to assess the extent of injury comprehensively. Thus, physicians increasingly emphasize the employment of a strategic approach in selecting imaging modalities based on the specific clinical scenario. As an illustration, clinicians might apply X-rays as a main screening tool and use MRI as a follow-up when soft tissue compromise has been implicated—particularly in such injuries as complex knee injury that may be described by multiple components, with ligament articular compromise being present. This dual approach makes sure that clinicians not only correctly diagnose fractures and dislocations but also create comprehensive treatment plans according to the complexities of the injuries, hence enhancing rehabilitation. Moreover, the addition of developments in imaging technology further enhances diagnostic capability in orthopedics. Technologies such as high-resolution MRI and the development of imaging protocols designed particularly for musculoskeletal evaluation make lesser injuries more detectable that are not able to be seen with X-rays. To provide an example, with the issue of patellofemoral instability prevalent in young athletes, skilled imaging plays an important role in distinguishing between the nature of the injury and determining the proper treatment method. According to Dunet et al. (2013), a significant percentage of orthopedic surgeons recommend MRI for patients with knee effusion after trauma, thus showing the concordance of its use in diagnostics. Lastly, the synergistic combination of X-rays and MRIs provides a solid platform for dislocation and fracture diagnostics that ensures effective treatment on the basis of trustworthy imaging (Figure 3.13).

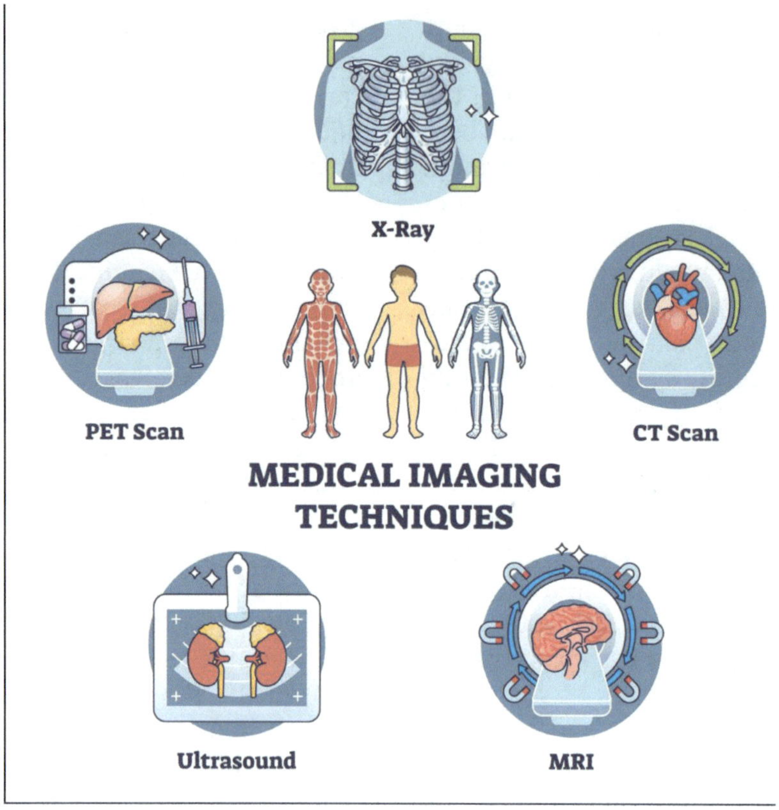

Figure 3.13. The diagnosis of fractures and dislocations relies heavily on advanced imaging techniques.

Source: https://continentalhospitals.com/uploads/Types%20of%20Radiology%20Procedures.jpg.

3.5. Treatment Options for Fractures

Fracture management is a multi-faceted process that is typically dictated by the nature and sophistication of the fracture. Primary management typically involves the stabilization of the fracture to avoid additional trauma and facilitate healing. Stabilization can be achieved by many means, including the application of splints or casts. If the fracture is displaced, surgery might be necessary. Surgical interventions often involve internal fixation methods, such as plate, screw, or intramedullary nail placement, providing strong stabilization and allowing for early mobilization. Moreover, minimally invasive techniques are receiving greater usage because of their advantages, including less soft tissue damage and quicker recovery. By utilizing specialized treatment methods on the basis of unique fracture patterns, practitioners can enhance patient outcomes to a large extent and hasten the rehabilitation process. Even when surgery is optimal, however, conservative treatment is still necessary for some fractures, particularly with no complicating circumstances. Most, for instance, children's fractures can be effectively managed with immobilization without surgical intervention, and therefore, this would be the initial option. Even in adults, fractures where osteoporotic alterations are present may also be treated with a conservative solution with attention to pain relief and progressive mobilization.

Rehabilitation is also key in the recovery process, the key being the use of physiotherapy in the restoration of function, strength, and range of motion after fracture. Patients also receive prevention of the injury, especially those at greater risk of future fractures. With the blending of conservative and rehabilitative measures, healthcare workers can encourage recovery while reducing the risk of complications or re-injury. In some conditions, such as Charcot neuroarthropathy, in which peripheral neuropathy can complicate fractures, one must approach it more subtly. Fractures and dislocations secondary to cumulative trauma from sensory loss are the most common causes of this condition and involve a careful consideration of treatment options. Surgical treatment can be needed to stabilize and protect the affected joint from further injury. A systematic review draws attention to varied surgical management techniques in treating Charcot neuroarthropathy, emphasizing the significance of customized treatment regimens in the context of case complexity. Nevertheless, when it comes to the timing of surgery and fixation technique, they are generally controversial due to a lack of strong evidence, and further prospective research is required to guide best practice. Developing effective management policies for such complex diseases is vital to improve patient outcomes and quality of life (Galhoum et al., 2021).

3.5.1. Non-Surgical Treatments (e.g., Casting, Splinting)

In the case of fractures and dislocations, non-surgical treatments such as splinting and casting remain the foundation practices due to their ability to stabilize injury and provoke healing without the use of surgery. Casting, most commonly applied to immobilize broken bones, facilitates correct positioning and offers the support required for recovery. By restricting motion, casts not only alleviate discomfort but also protect neighboring tissues from reinjury. In addition, splinting is a versatile choice, particularly for temporary stabilization. The process is of specific use in an acute setting or when there has not yet been an ultimate diagnosis reached. Both processes highlight a main principle in orthopedic management: immobilization allows the body to heal naturally, essentially preventing long-term sequelae resulting from erroneous position or motion during the healing process's critical period. Existing literature offers support for the efficacy of these non-surgical interventions, indicating their invaluable role in the management of various fractures and dislocations. Based on studies conducted across multiple studies, evidence exists that, while casting has been accepted worldwide as a method of treatment for stable fractures, splinting can also be effective in specific cases where temporary mobility is to be maintained. Variability of treatment modalities highlights the role of individualized management of the patient, depending on the nature and severity of injury. Furthermore, studies of hand fractures reveal that there is a prevalence of randomized controlled trials, but they also show heterogeneity and limitations in their design. These results underscore the call for a deficit of quality clinical evidence, with casting and splinting being practiced but with an ever-present requirement for quality research to guide orthopedic intervention in a variety of clinical situations (Mousoulis et al., 2020). Examining the character of some fracture types, such as those of the calcaneus, demonstrates the significant variability of outcomes when non-surgical treatment methods are used. For instance, a multicenter study that compared the status of patients who were treated with traditional casting to heel-unloading orthotics depicted differences in functional rehabilitation, demonstrable improvements at three months post-treatment. In accordance with this study, patients receiving the Graffin orthosis had significantly more elevated functional evaluation scores than those who received traditional casting or splinting only (Kagami et al., 2022). These findings indicate that while the traditional methods remain correct, other non-surgical interventions can be advantageous under certain circumstances. In general, this ongoing research into non-surgical interventions within the realm of fractures and dislocations not only enhances our understanding of the effectiveness of interventions but also enhances clinical practice, which leads to enhanced patient outcomes (Figure 3.14).

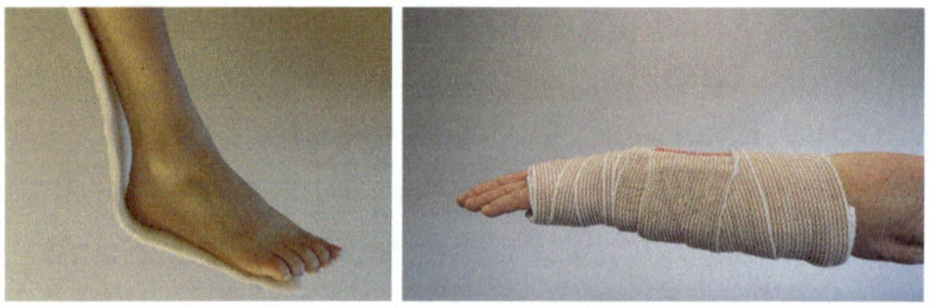

Figure 3.14. Non-surgical treatments.

Source: https://orthoinfo.aaos.org/contentassets/c761f19175ea4a618043620 5aa59934b/a00095f04_ankle-wrist-splint-compressor_resize.jpg.

3.5.2. Surgical Interventions (e.g., Internal Fixation)

Surgical interventions have become a cornerstone in the treatment of fractures and dislocations, particularly when conservative management cannot achieve satisfactory healing or alignment. Internal fixation is one of the principal modalities that employs metal screws, plates, or rods to stabilize fractured bones to achieve optimal healing. This surgical method not only provides immediate mechanical stability to the fracture but also enables early mobilization without the complications of immobilization. Whether internal fixation is applied or not largely depends on a number of factors, including the site, nature of the fracture, and the overall health status of the patient. Such individualized treatment protocols stress the importance of accurate preoperative assessments in order to have optimal outcomes. Thus, the use of internal fixation techniques in everyday orthopedic practice has considerably curbed the incidence of malunion or nonunion in otherwise high-risk injuries for prolonged disability. Among varied surgical strategies for dealing with orthopedic emergencies, the debate between open reduction and internal fixation versus primary arthrodesis has gained prominence, particularly in the case of complex injuries like Lisfranc joint injury. As underscored in current studies, primary arthrodesis has produced outcomes that are comparable or superior to those achieved through open reduction and internal fixation, challenging traditional paradigms in surgical orthopedics. Such a revelation calls for re-examination of surgery procedures in treating some conditions. Such a selection has immediate consequences on patient prognosis and underscores the need to constantly review new evidence to guide surgery procedures. Through close examination of high-level meta-analyses comparing diverse interventions, physicians are better able to make informed decisions, ultimately contributing to furthering patient outcomes in the setting of severe foot and ankle trauma, among other complex fracture patterns. Finally, effective management of fractures and dislocations through surgical methods such as internal fixation requires intimate knowledge of potential risks and complications. Use of internal fixation also carries risks such as infection, hardware failure, or further surgeries to remove implants. The reward, however, is restoration of function and alignment, and these generally are higher than the risks when performed by trained orthopedic surgeons. As orthopedic surgery advances, investigations of new materials and techniques continually improve the safety and efficacy of internal fixation and other treatments. Lastly, the use of such advances in the practice of clinical medicine not only enhances fracture and dislocation surgery but also provides patients with the ability to recover more efficiently and quickly, resulting in a rehabilitation to pre-injury level (Figure 3.15).

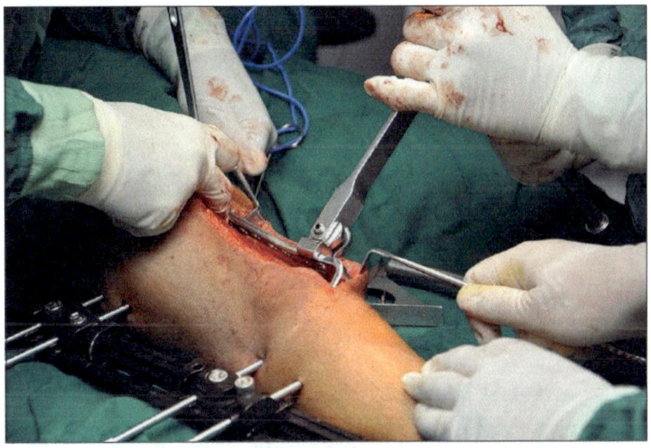

Figure 3.15. Surgical interventions have become a cornerstone in the treatment of fractures and dislocations.

Source: https://www.researchgate.net/publication/266683206/figure/fig4/AS:202719592751115@1425343525204/Clinical-photograph-showing-internal-fixation-is-being-carried-out-while-external.png.

3.5.3. Rehabilitation and Recovery

The recovery and rehabilitation following dislocations and fractures is intricate and requires an interdisciplinary approach to restore function and prevent long-term impairment. Rehabilitation begins with early management, emphasizing the importance of early mobilization and formalized rehabilitation protocol. For instance, with hip dislocation, prompt closed reduction and full rehabilitation protocol can lead to full functional recovery within a few months. Such interventions not only mitigate risks such as avascular necrosis and osteoarthritis post-trauma but also function to highlight the need for personalized care plans that meet each patient's specific needs. The research indicates that an orderly approach, with periodic assessments of progress, significantly enhances the efficacy of the recuperation process, providing better outcomes for patients who experience complex fractures and dislocations (Grupkovic et al., 2025). Continuing to build the science of recovery and rehabilitation, present technology is a necessary component of improving diagnosis and treatment methods. Modalities like magnetic resonance imaging and computed tomography allow accurate diagnoses to direct rehabilitation programs. Such advanced imaging techniques allow clinicians to personalize recovery plans based on the particular characteristics of the injury, including the extent of soft tissue disruption. Moreover, minimally invasive surgery, i.e., arthroscopic stabilization, has revolutionized the management of certain dislocations, with quicker recovery times for patients. Integration of such emerging technologies with rehabilitation systems has demonstrated significant improvement in patient outcomes, as evidenced through comparative studies highlighting enhanced functional recovery through supervised physiotherapy and exercises (Ugli et al., 2025). Therefore, the marriage of surgery with advanced diagnostic methods continues to frame rehabilitation strategies. Ultimately, rehabilitation and healing are successful if there is a high degree of coordination among healthcare providers, patients, and support systems. Communication is essential during the recovery phase on a regular basis to address any physical or mental problems that may arise. Using a multi-disciplinary team incorporating orthopedic surgeons, physiotherapists, and occupational therapists ensures holistic care, which is critical to successful recovery. Patient education also plays an important role in making individuals actively participate in their rehabilitative phase. Lifestyle changes and adherence to recommended exercises are critical for optimal recovery. While studies assist in developing protocols and guidelines, it is increasingly clear that evidence-based and systematic rehabilitative methods come to the foreground in dealing with fracture and dislocation consequences and thereby enhancing quality of life for victims (Grupkovic et al., 2025; Ugli et al., 2025).

3.6. Treatment Options for Dislocations

Treatment of dislocation depends mostly on the severity, location, and nature of the injury. Reduction is often performed as immediate treatment, where the dislocated joint is reduced to its original anatomical position. In cases of acute injuries, this may be accomplished using closed reduction methods, where they utilize their gentle manipulative analogues to restore the alignment of the joint without requiring any surgery.

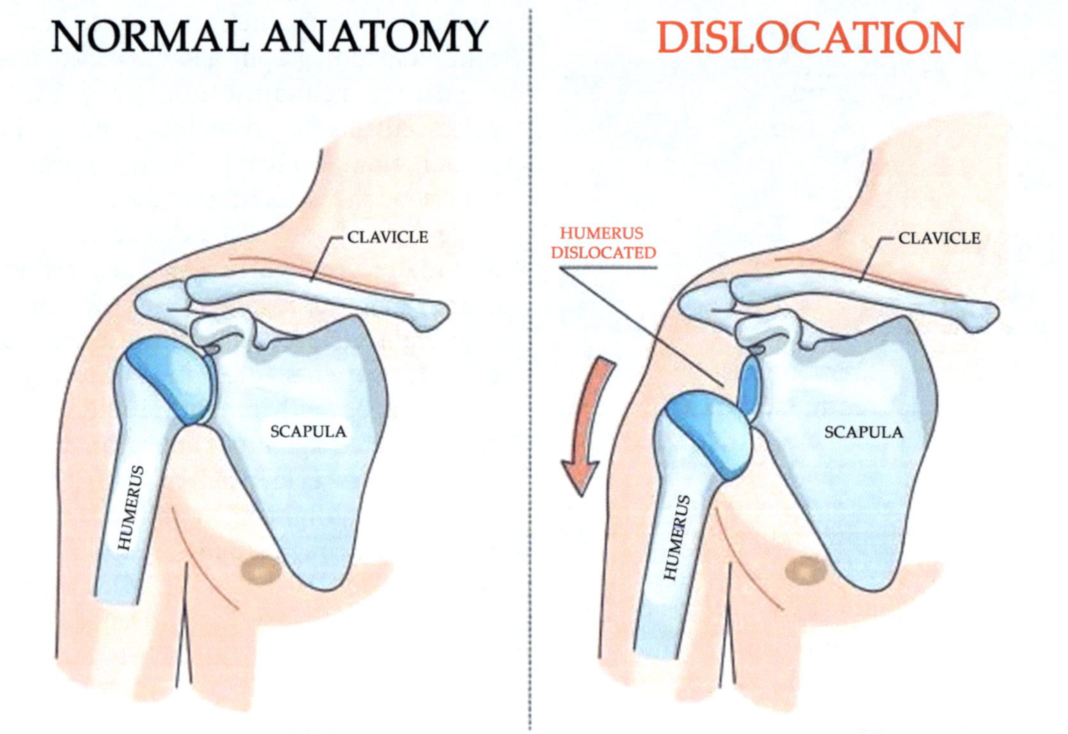

Figure 3.16. Treatment options for dislocations are largely determined by the type.

Source: https://www.carehospitals.com/ckfinder/userfiles/images/dislocation_a.webp.

In posterior shoulder dislocations, proper assessment is required since improper management can lead to chronic instability. Research in recent years emphasizes the need for individualized strategies, wherein patient-related factors like age and level of activity will dictate treatment (Paparoidamis et al., 2020). A treatment pathway has been proposed to help healthcare professionals manage such complicated cases effectively. Therefore, understanding the specifics of dislocation management is essential in obtaining the best results from patients. Once a dislocation is successfully reduced, the next step is to determine post-reduction therapy, whether immobilization, rehabilitation, or even surgery in some cases. Immobilization is usually bracing and slings in immobilizing the joint during healing. This is especially important where there has been extensive injury to soft tissues or bone, as stability will heavily influence recovery time and rehabilitation effectiveness in general. Rehabilitation protocols usually work on the range of motion, strength, and function of the affected joint. In others, such as in complex shoulder dislocation with concomitant fractures, open reduction and internal fixation or even shoulder arthroplasty may be the required surgical options (Paparoidamis et al., 2020). The decision for surgery depends upon the unique nature of the injury as well as the functional demands of the patients. In the situation of hip dislocations, particularly in the elderly, treatment options can be multiple due to comorbidities and high surgical risk. Displaced fractures of the femoral neck, for example, are likely to call for consideration of hip arthroplasty, which may be in the form of total hip arthroplasty (THA) or hemiarthroplasty (HA). Even though THA has shown improved outcomes in pain and function, the higher risk of dislocation requires a strict postoperative protocol, especially in the early postoperative period. Thus, a customized management protocol must not only strive to recover anatomy but also to avoid complications such as dislocation, which can adversely impact rehabilitation outcomes and patient quality of life. Finally, treatment should be chosen based on a person's activity level and general health status to provide a balanced response to dislocation management (Figure 3.16).

3.6.1. Reduction Techniques

Effective methods of reduction play a critical role in the management of dislocation and fracture, aiming to restore anatomical position and function with minimal complications. The most common method employed in orthopedic surgeries is the closed method of reduction, which entails manipulation without opening the skin. This method is optimally suited for certain dislocations and fractures, such as anterior shoulder dislocation, in which immediate and accurate reduction plays a decisive role in the result. Closed reduction can circumvent the need for surgery, thus decreasing the overall morbidity of the patient and easing the recovery process. For example, some patients have had uneventful shoulder reductions without analgesia or anesthesia, which indicates the effectiveness of the skilled health professionals in performing these maneuvers under different clinical scenarios, as witnessed in the recent literature (Quintero et al., 2022). In the field of patellar resurfacing in total knee arthroplasty, the techniques involved in the reduction have evolved considerably over time. The choice of resurfacing the patella lies with surgeons and depends on the balance of the scales between predicted complications and possible benefit in terms of pain relief and functional rehabilitation. Placing a polyethylene dome over the patella has the aim of restoring its articulation with the femur and thus potentially relieving postoperative anterior knee pain by optimizing joint mechanics and more evenly sharing stress along the joint surface. However, although the beneficial effects of patellar resurfacing have been espoused, in many cases, there has been an extremely high incidence of complications like dislocations and patellar fractures. This highlights the importance of the utilization of the appropriate reduction method and attention to the specific needs of each patient in order to maximize outcomes and prevent negative effects (Quintero et al., 2022). Novel methods of reduction continue to arm orthopedic surgeons with new approaches to reducing dislocations. One such approach, recently developed, is characterized by its simple process that does not require the utilization of analgesia, thereby being extremely useful in environments where there is limited availability of resources. This method has proved to have reproducible success rates in different cases, including delayed dislocations, proving that it is a reliable method for use in clinical practice. By leveraging gravitational forces and the positioning of the patient to allow for shoulder reduction, this method highlights the application of biomechanical principles over conventional traction methods. The more clinicians adopt these newer techniques, the more important it is to assess the outcome and patient experience in an evidence-based manner, thereby contributing valuable information to the field of trauma and orthopedics and enhancing the techniques applied in the reduction of fractures and dislocations (Prakash, 2018).

3.6.2. Immobilization Methods

Fracture immobilization is a simple orthopedic intervention that gives stability at the injured site and helps in healing. Various forms of immobilization, such as a cast, splint, and external fixator, are employed depending on the severity and nature of the injury. The most conventional method is the use of a cast, which gives rigid support to broken bones, particularly in lower limb fractures. They are most effective in restricting movement and protecting the injured area from additional damage. However, in the other types of fractures, i.e., those with associated significant swelling or complex dislocations, other methods must be employed. The selection of an immobilization technique is of highest priority because improper stabilization can lead to malunion or nonunion of fractures, which underscores the significance of thorough evaluation in initial treatment. In dislocated fractures, the approach to stabilization is typically anatomical alignment-based and soft tissue condition. Evidence shows that one initial medial clear space with dislocation is a strong predictor for achieving proper reduction on immobilization (Hecht et al., 2025). A case in point is a study of dislocated ankle fractures that emphasized the point that patients with an initial medial clear space greater than 9 mm had a higher risk of unsatisfactory reduction if treated by a cast alone. Based on this, acute external fixation or internal fixation is warranted to prevent secondary dislocation and allow optimal conditions for final operation, especially if, because of subsequent swelling, normal cast application becomes impracticable.

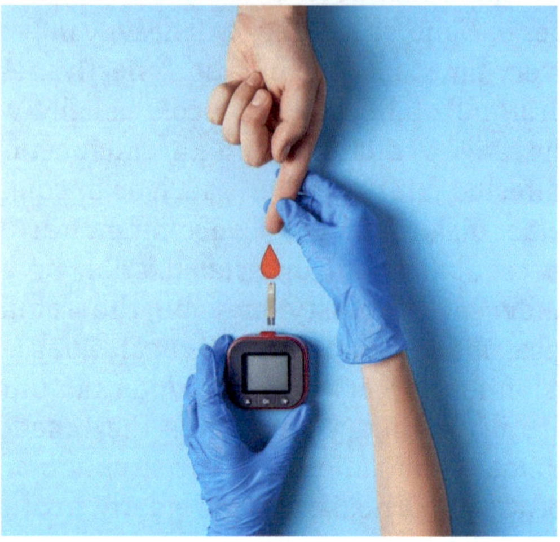

Figure 3.17. The immobilization of fractures is a fundamental aspect of orthopedic treatment.

Source: https://www.azonano.com/images/Article_Images/ImageForArticle_6121_16554703018513976.jpg.

Therefore, the immobilization method of choice must be determined in relation to the nature of each fracture to promote positive healing and minimize complications. Furthermore, immobilization duration also contributes to recovery from fractures and dislocations. Research indicates that over immobilization could have adverse effects in the form of flexion contractures, particularly in injuries of the elbow with some anatomical conditions (Lee et al., 2025). Comparative analysis between coronal shear fracture patients of the distal humerus showed no difference in functionality between the groups immobilized for less than three weeks and those immobilized for longer than three weeks. This implies that while immobilization is necessary, extended length may hinder recovery more than assist. Efforts to determine injury patterns through advanced imaging can guide immobilization length to optimize recovery times and ensure stability to heal effectively. This, therefore, implies that interaction between immobilization strategy and length needs accurate evaluation in fracture and dislocation management (Figure 3.17).

3.6.3. Physical Therapy and Rehabilitation

Physical therapy and rehabilitation are integral parts of recovery for individuals who have experienced fractures and dislocations. Effective rehabilitation measures are planned keeping the type and intensity of injury in mind, which requires an in-depth understanding of the patient's physical capabilities and limitations. For instance, following traumatic lesion of the elbow, rehabilitation protocols have been seen to utilize objective instruments, including DASH and SF-36 questionnaires, to quantify upper limb function and quality of life. Among surgical patients with injuries of the elbow, there has been research evidence of an average DASH score that reflects some limitations in function, which emphasizes the absolute necessity for individualized interventions in recovering limb function and enhancing well-being. As physical rehabilitation progresses, physical therapists implement customized exercise regimens for building strength, flexibility, and coordination, which are essential for the recovery of mobility and independence. Furthermore, the implementation of evidence-based practice in physical therapy also has a significant effect on patient outcomes. Recent studies indicate that the use of specific equipment and education—particularly in the case of total hip replacement—can minimize the occurrence of dislocations with the potential to occur during the healing process. For example, clinician adherence to guidelines for equipment delivery, such as hip precautions and raised toilet seats, indicates patient safety during rehabilitation. Survey results indicate high conformity among therapists in consistently promoting hip precautions as evidence of post-operative continuity of care. Such pre-emptive measures not only aid in physical protection but also enhance patients' faith in the performance of daily tasks, which are otherwise lost after surgery. Therefore, understanding the nuances of rehabilitation procedures becomes a part of efficient healing following fractures and dislocations. The collaborative activity of physiotherapists, occupational therapists, and patients is most crucial to developing successful rehabilitation results. As shown in the example of elbow surgery, multidisciplinary teams often revise and refine rehabilitation plans on an ongoing basis based upon ongoing assessment of patient improvement and feedback. This is particularly beneficial in searching for lapses in patient knowledge or adherence with suggested interventions. Ongoing follow-up and reassessment allow therapists to revisit exercise programs and instruct patients in new strategies or equipment that can aid in recovery. Most prominently, the psychosocial aspects of rehabilitation are addressed by this multidisciplinary configuration, allowing for patients' overall well-being. By addressing not only physical recovery but also psychological well-being, rehabilitation schemes ensure that fracture and dislocation patients can recover social and occupational roles, thereby facilitating an all-around recovery process.

SUMMARY

It is evident that such injuries are complicated, impacting not just physical health but also patients' overall quality of life. The complexities of types of fractures, injury mechanisms, and healing processes underscore the importance of an accurate diagnosis and customized management strategies to optimize patient outcomes. The literature shows that surgical intervention, e.g., operative reduction and internal fixation (ORIF), is of advantage for the majority of fractures, particularly those resulting from high-energy trauma, like femoral head fracture. Proper treatment of such injury involves not only immediate fracture management but also assessment for concomitant complications such as avascular necrosis and post-traumatic arthritis, which can adversely compromise recovery and functionality (Scolaro et al., 2017). Also, identification of associated injuries is crucial in the case of a fracture, especially in a complicated case of trauma such as sacral fractures. Such uncommon injuries can be present concomitantly with significant complications like neurologic impairment and pelvic ring disruption, thus requiring complete evaluations to achieve successful intervention. The interaction of such injuries can influence prognosis and affect therapeutic approaches employed. A careful evaluation of skeletal and systemic injuries avoids missing any complications, which may significantly influence healing. These relationships highlight the importance of interdisciplinary treatment in trauma care, with a focus on rigorous diagnostic routines necessary to ensure desirable outcomes for patients with fractures and dislocations (Rodrigues-Pinto et al., 2017). In summary, dislocations and fractures present peculiar challenges in diagnosis and treatment and require an understanding of their complexity and interdependency. Diversification of the modes of treatment from conservative measures to surgery testifies to the requirement for individualized management based on the inherent characteristics of the injury. Finessing treatment mechanisms and seeking new trends in treatment to enhance outcomes will be the emphasis of research in the coming years. In addition, education for patients and doctors regarding the importance of fractures and dislocations could also improve care planning. Ultimately, an aligned, evidence-based process, with continuous review and revision as new information is published, is necessary to ensure that victims of these kinds of injuries receive the optimal outcomes and regain their level of quality of life.

The subtleties of fractures and dislocations are tremendous both in the clinical and public spheres, especially with regard to comprehending their frequency among different populations. In fact, falls remain a leading cause of fractures, with unusually high frequency among elderly adults. Not only do these conditions impose direct physical consequences, but they also generate chronic complications that adversely affect a person's functional autonomy and overall quality of life. The effects reach far beyond the patient, increasing morbidity and mortality rates and contributing to rising healthcare costs for care and rehabilitation. The identification of such problems underscores the need for standard and updated guidelines for prevention and management strategies. Pre-existing inequalities in such laws demonstrate a dearth of integrated knowledge, foregrounding the requirement for a universally applicable protocol to effectively address such injuries, as reported in Montero-Odasso et al. (2022). One key factor in the management of fractures and dislocations is the multidimensional nature of their treatment. Management of such injuries requires an interdisciplinary approach, involving surgery, rehabilitation, and prevention strategies that are tailored to the unique circumstances of each patient. Surgery may be necessary in the most difficult situations, but post-surgery rehabilitation still has an integral role in a successful recovery. Rehabilitation protocols must consider various factors, including the age of the patient, comorbidities, and the nature and location of the fracture or dislocation. Intensive rehabilitation not only attempts to restore physical function, but also to overcome psychological effects, i.e., fear of re-injury. This holistic strategy is crucial to the enhancement of patient outcomes and needs to be guided by current clinical practices reflecting recent research advancements, as noted in Stein & Leineweber (2020). Preventive strategies are central to the minimization of the incidence of fractures and dislocations, particularly among vulnerable groups such as the elderly. Risk factors, such as falls prevention, can significantly reduce the risk for such injury. Community-based programs for counseling older persons on safe mobility, home adaptation, and muscle strengthening can also have beneficial impacts. Increasing awareness of osteoporosis and its association with fragility fractures is equally important for prompt treatment and prevention. The necessity of having consistent messaging about these preventive practices is most critical in that it helps create an environment conducive to the prevention of falls and associated injuries. In this manner, the combining of preventative practices with targeted treatment can form a comprehensive regime that not only prevents current injury but also promotes long-term health and mobility among the elderly, as discussed in Montero-Odasso et al. (2022).

CLOSER LOOK

MUSCULOSKELETAL TRAUMA

Musculoskeletal trauma refers to injuries affecting the bones, muscles, joints, ligaments, tendons, and surrounding soft tissues, usually caused by accidents, falls, sports injuries, violence, or natural disasters. These injuries range from minor sprains and strains to severe fractures, dislocations, and complex soft tissue damage. Musculoskeletal trauma is a major cause of pain, disability, and reduced quality of life worldwide.

Immediate and accurate assessment is critical in managing musculoskeletal trauma. Clinical examination, supported by imaging techniques such as X-rays, CT scans, and MRI, helps determine the type and severity of injury. Early intervention, including immobilization, pain control, wound care, and sometimes surgical repair, is essential to prevent complications and promote proper healing. Advanced orthopedic p rocedures, such as internal fixation, joint reconstruction, and minimally invasive surgery, have significantly improved outcomes. Rehabilitation plays a vital role in recovery, focusing on restoring strength, flexibility, and functional movement. Physiotherapy, occupational therapy, and gradual return-to-activity programs help patients regain independence and prevent long-term disability. Psychological support is also important, as trauma can cause emotional stress and anxiety. Prevention strategies include road safety measures, protective sports equipment, workplace safety practices, and public awareness programs. Overall, effective management of musculoskeletal trauma requires a multidisciplinary approach that combines emergency care, orthopedic treatment, rehabilitation, and preventive efforts to ensure optimal recovery and long-term well-being.

REFERENCES

1. Abel, F., Schmaranzer, F., & Sutter, R. (2025). Sports-related hip injuries. *Seminars in Musculoskeletal Radiology, 29*, 442–456. https://www.semanticscholar.org/paper/ab21bdc2d45ed12d7471cb97c5b4b060dab9bd06 (accessed on 26th June 2025).
2. Abood, H., Alotibi, M., Alhashim, Z., Alotaibi, E., Alkandari, S., Yousif, R., Almahdi, S., et al. (2024). Emergency surgical interventions: A comparative review of acute cases in general surgery and orthopedic surgery. *International Journal of Medicine in Developing Countries*. https://www.semanticscholar.org/paper/e98194dc3ab2d6190e2a1eaf81af9eee44835c15 (accessed on 26th June 2025).
3. Abrassart, S., & Hoffmeyer, P. (2011). (P2-13) Pitfalls for Upper Limb Injuries in Emergency. *Prehospital and Disaster Medicine*, *26*(S1), s139–s139. doi:10.1017/S1049023X11004572(accessed on 26th June 2025).
4. Alam, F., Alsaed, O., Abdulla, N., Abdulmomen, I., Lutf, A., & Al Emadi, S. (2024). Guidelines for fracture risk assessment and management of osteoporosis in postmenopausal women and men above the age of 50 in Qatar. *Archives of Osteoporosis, 19*. https://www.semanticscholar.org/paper/77cb3717a61d5cbc9255541ddeecc24915b2ad91 (accessed on 26th June 2025).
5. Allen, C. R., Ding, D. Y., Feeley, B. T., Hodax, J., et al. (2019). Tibial tubercle osteotomy and medial patellofemoral ligament imbrication for patellar instability due to trochlear dysplasia. https://core.ac.uk/download/323079207.pdf (accessed on 26th June 2025).
6. Alwani M, Jones AJ, Sandelski M, et al. Facing Facts: Facial Injuries from Stand-up Electric Scooters. *Cureus*. 2020;12(1):e6663. Published 2020 Jan 15. doi:10.7759/cureus.6663(accessed on 26th June 2025).
7. Kagami, Y., Tokutake, K., Takegami, Y., Okui, N., Sakai, T., Inoue, H., Kanemura, T., Hanabayashi, M., Ito, O., Kanayama, Y., Maruyama, K., Yoshida, H., Ando, T., Sugimoto, R., Sugimoto, T., & Imagama, S. (2022). Do heel-unloading orthoses improve clinical outcomes in patients after surgical treatment of calcaneal fracture? A propensity-matched, multicenter analysis of the TRON database. *Prosthetics and orthotics international*, *46*(6), 569–575. https://doi.org/10.1097/PXR.0000000000000168(accessed on 26th June 2025).
8. Bahr, R., Clarsen, B., Derman, W., Dvořák, J., Emery, C. A., Finch, C. F., Hägglund, M., et al. (2020). International Olympic Committee consensus statement: Methods for recording and reporting of epidemiological data on injury and illness in sports 2020 (Including the STROBE extension for sports injury and illness surveillance (STROBE-SIIS)). *Orthopedic Journal of Sports Medicine, 8*. https://doi.org/10.1177/2325967120902908 (accessed on 26th June 2025).
9. Baláž, P., Achimovičová, M., Baláž, M., Billik, P., Cherkezova-Zheleva, Z., Criado, J. M., Delogu, F., et al. (2013). Hallmarks of mechanochemistry: From nanoparticles to technology. *Chemical Society Reviews, 42*, 7571–7571. https://doi.org/10.1039/c3cs35468g (accessed on 26th June 2025).
10. Rodrigues-Pinto, R., Kurd, M. F., Schroeder, G. D., Kepler, C. K., Krieg, J. C., Holstein, J. H., Bellabarba, C., Firoozabadi, R., Oner, F. C., Kandziora, F., Dvorak, M. F., Kleweno, C. P., Vialle, L. R., Rajasekaran, S., Schnake, K. J., & Vaccaro, A. R. (2017). Sacral Fractures and Associated Injuries. *Global spine journal*, *7*(7), 609–616. https://doi.org/10.1177/2192568217701097(accessed on 26th June 2025).

11. Jin Li *et al.* Nanoscale stacking fault–assisted room temperature plasticity in flash-sintered TiO_2.*Sci. Adv.***5**,eaaw5519(2019).DOI:10.1126/sciadv.aaw5519(accessed on 26th June 2025).

12. Dunet, B., Tournier, C., Billaud, A., Lavoinne, N., Fabre, T., & Durandeau, A. (2013). Acetabular fracture: long-term follow-up and factors associated with secondary implantation of total hip arthroplasty. *Orthopaedics & traumatology, surgery & research : OTSR, 99*(3), 281–290. https://doi.org/10.1016/j.otsr.2012.12.018(accessed on 26th June 2025).

13. Bodrova, L. G., & Kramar, H. M. (2017). Notes and laboratory reports on "Technology of structural materials and material science" Part 2. https://core.ac.uk/download/161261279.pdf (accessed on 26th June 2025).

14. Bolukçu, A., Erdemir, A., Idilman, I., Yıldız, A., Coban Cifci, G., Onur, M. R., & Akpınar, E. (2024). Radiological findings of February 2023 twin earthquakes-related spine injuries. *World Journal of Radiology, 16*, 398–406. https://www.semanticscholar.org/paper/f6ee68d8172e5880206cd6a82f3353da39cf14f3 (accessed on 26th June 2025).

15. Petri, M., Ettinger, M., Stuebig, T., Brand, S., Krettek, C., Jagodzinski, M., & Omar, M. (2015). Current Concepts for Patellar Dislocation. *Archives of trauma research, 4*(3), e29301. https://doi.org/10.5812/atr.29301(accessed on 26th June 2025).

16. Brenner, E., Chirculescu, A. R. M., Reblet, C., Smith, R., et al. (2015). Assessment in anatomy. Eur. J. Anat. 19 (1): 105-124 (2015) . https://core.ac.uk/download/30611187.pdf (accessed on 26th June 2025).

17. Papp MR, Souza RC, Lima SM, Matsumoto MH, Chamliam TR, Santos JB. Comparison between Dash and SF-36 of the injured elbow rehabilitated in occupational therapy. Acta Ortop Bras. [online]. 2011;19(6):356-61. Available from URL: http://www.scielo.br/aob. (accessed on 26th June 2025).

18. De Roza, J. G., Koh, D. H. M., & Goh, L. J. (2025). Impact of health beliefs and risk perception on willingness to undergo osteoporosis assessment among perimenopausal and menopausal women in primary care: A descriptive cross-sectional study. *BMC Primary Care, 26*. https://www.semanticscholar.org/paper/952cd279c902909c26d08161d011af60f4f12e6f (accessed on 26th June 2025).

19. Mousoulis, C., Thomas, K., Leighton, P., Deshmukh, S., Grindlay, D., & Karantana, A. (2020). Treatment interventions for hand fractures and joint injuries: a scoping review of randomized controlled trials. *The Journal of hand surgery, European volume, 45*(2), 111–118. https://doi.org/10.1177/1753193419865897(accessed on 26th June 2025).

20. Ding, J., Yu, Q., Asta, M., & Ritchie, R. O. (2018). Tunable stacking fault energies by tailoring local chemical order in CrCoNi medium-entropy alloys. *Proceedings of the National Academy of Sciences, 115*, 8919–8924. https://doi.org/10.1073/pnas.1808660115 (accessed on 26th June 2025).

21. Smith, T. O., & Sackley, C. M. (2016). UK survey of occupational therapist's and physiotherapist's experiences and attitudes towards hip replacement precautions and equipment. *BMC musculoskeletal disorders, 17*, 228. https://doi.org/10.1186/s12891-016-1092-xEliaz, N. (2019). Corrosion of metallic biomaterials: A review. *Materials, 12*, 407–407. https://doi.org/10.3390/ma12030407 (accessed on 26th June 2025).

22. Scolaro, J. A., Marecek, G., Firoozabadi, R., Krieg, J. C., & Routt, M. L. C. (2017). Management and radiographic outcomes of femoral head fractures. *Journal of orthopaedics and traumatology*

: *official journal of the Italian Society of Orthopaedics and Traumatology, 18*(3), 235–241. https://doi.org/10.1007/s10195-017-0445-z(accessed on 26th June 2025).

23. Fitriana, N. F., Estria, S. R., Nitiprodjo, A. H., Nandia, J. R. D., Juwita, D. R., Aprilina, H. D., Anggraeni, A. D., et al. (2023). Optimalisasi keterampilan pertolongan pertama cedera otot menggunakan metode REST, ICE, COMPRESS and ELEVATE (RICE management). *Journal Abdi Masyarakat.* https://www.semanticscholar.org/paper/ca416984bbe8c399266edad8fc145c4d2b6b84b6 (accessed on 26th June 2025).

24. Scallan, E., Fitzpatrick, P., Kelly, A., Laffoy, M., et al. (2001). Injury in Ireland. https://core.ac.uk/download/11309290.pdf (accessed on 26th June 2025).

25. Fizazi, K., Shore, N. D., Tammela, T. L. J., Ulys, A., Vjaters, E., Polyakov, S., Jievaltas, M., et al. (2020). Nonmetastatic, castration-resistant prostate cancer and survival with darolutamide. *New England Journal of Medicine, 383*, 1040–1049. https://doi.org/10.1056/nejmoa2001342 (accessed on 26th June 2025).

26. Galhoum, A. E., Trivedi, V., Askar, M., Tejero, S., Herrera-Pérez, M., Alrashidi, Y., & Valderrábano, V. (2021). Management of ankle Charcot neuroarthropathy: A systematic review. *Journal of Clinical Medicine, 10*, 5923–5923. https://doi.org/10.3390/jcm10245923 (accessed on 26th June 2025).

27. George, J., Wilt, E., Sharma, S., & Burke, C. D. (2025). Bilateral anterior shoulder dislocations with greater tuberosity fractures: A case report. *Journal of Orthopedic Case Reports, 15*, 141–145. https://www.semanticscholar.org/paper/aa76be204254bcb460fd0d28348785d31a7cd16c (accessed on 26th June 2025).

28. Giai Via, R., Faccenda, C., Artiaco, S., Dutto, E., Lavia, A. D., Massè, A., & Battiston, B. (2024). Functional and subjective outcomes after surgical management of complex elbow dislocations: A retrospective study. *European Journal of Orthopedic Surgery & Traumatology, 34*, 4027–4036. https://www.semanticscholar.org/paper/e90e0129b41783d1e89dc3b89b05f0127c6ea6fa (accessed on 26th June 2025).

29. Grupkovic, J., Dabetić, U., Bogosavljević, N., Aleksandric, D., Milanovic, M., Savicevic, D., & Zagorac, S. (2025). Traumatic bilateral asymmetrical hip dislocation with acetabular fracture: A case report and review of current evidence. *Life, 15*. https://www.semanticscholar.org/paper/fd38cb3905fe85a3f68cab2e7e53b1039565080b (accessed on 26th June 2025).

30. Hatzell, K. B., Chen, X. C., Cobb, C. L., Dasgupta, N. P., Dixit, M., Marbella, L. E., McDowell, M. T., et al. (2020). Challenges in lithium metal anodes for solid-state batteries. *ACS Energy Letters, 5*, 922–934. https://doi.org/10.1021/acsenergylett.9b02668 (accessed on 26th June 2025).

31. Hecht, V., Mosimann, E. S., Krause, F., Kurze, C., Lustenberger, T., & Anwander, H. (2025). The medial clearspace is a risk factor for secondary dislocation following cast immobilization after closed reduction in closed ankle fracture dislocations. *European Journal of Trauma and Emergency Surgery, 51*. https://www.semanticscholar.org/paper/3602142db0231fa0a9c94b3c0391d96d4adbf344 (accessed on 26th June 2025).

32. Hu, Y., Yang, K., Liu, H., Wang, L., Wang, S., Zhang, X., Qu, B., et al. (2023). 3D-printed custom implant for the management of "locked" posterior dislocation of the shoulder joint with reverse Hill-Sachs lesion: A case report. *Frontiers in Bioengineering and Biotechnology, 11*. https://www.semanticscholar.org/paper/05ff08208a6dd5b3b9f850e72d1f49aa76c19e38

(accessed on 26th June 2025).

33. Hunt, T. J., Powlan, F. J., Renfro, K. N., Polmear, M., Macias, R. A., Dunn, J. C., & Wells, M. (2023). Common finger injuries: Treatment guidelines for emergency and primary care providers. *Military Medicine, 189*, 988–994. https://doi.org/10.1093/milmed/usad022 (accessed on 26th June 2025).

34. Khalid, M. (2025). Sports-related elbow injuries. *InnovAiT: Education and Inspiration for General Practice.* https://www.semanticscholar.org/paper/1679f80abf9435e73e9b96b407c859557ae8773a (accessed on 26th June 2025).

35. Koh, J. H., Song, H. K., Cho, W. T., Sakong, S., & Lim, S. (2025). Treatment of avulsion fractures around the knee. *Journal of Musculoskeletal Trauma.* https://www.semanticscholar.org/paper/ae415a0a9f1b939e82f554d0bf0f5e6ad51abaed (accessed on 26th June 2025).

36. Lee, J. H., Jenkins, C. W., Park, G. C., Ahn, K., & Rhyou, I. (2025). Impact of immobilization period and anterior capsular injury on flexion contracture in distal humerus coronal shear fractures. *Clinics in Shoulder and Elbow, 28*, 187–195. https://www.semanticscholar.org/paper/bb80be37ca5eeca030011d12afbfa6f907630cab (accessed on 26th June 2025).

37. Liu, Y., Chen, X., Zhang, P., & Jiang, B. (2020). Comparing total hip arthroplasty and hemiarthroplasty for the treatment of displaced femoral neck fracture in the active elderly over 75 years old: A systematic review and meta-analysis of randomized control trials. *Journal of Orthopedic Surgery and Research, 15.* https://doi.org/10.1186/s13018-020-01725-3 (accessed on 26th June 2025).

38. Montero-Odasso, M., van der Velde, N., Martin, F. C., Petrović, M., Tan, M. P., Ryg, J., Aguilar-Navarro, S. G., et al. (2022). World guidelines for falls prevention and management for older adults: A global initiative. *Age and Ageing, 51.* https://doi.org/10.1093/ageing/afac205 (accessed on 26th June 2025).

39. Ng, J., Tham, S. Y. Y., Kolla, S., Kwan, Y. H., Tan, J., Teo, T. D., Wee, A., et al. (2022). Short-term comparative outcomes between reverse shoulder arthroplasty for shoulder trauma and shoulder arthritis: A Southeast Asian experience. *Clinics in Shoulder and Elbow, 25*, 210–216. https://www.semanticscholar.org/paper/6d16f85cc3b6bc2a0c0ec8bea244bf323d205700 (accessed on 26th June 2025).

40. Nordback, P., & Waris, E. (2021). Percutaneous intramedullary reduction technique for impacted middle phalanx base fractures. *Techniques in Hand & Upper Extremity Surgery, 26*, 2–6. https://www.semanticscholar.org/paper/b8c770b4bc5261d77f0fe82c5624e5f9bfd05b82 (accessed on 26th June 2025).

41. Palmer, W. E., Bancroft, L. W., Bonar, F., Choi, J. A., Cotten, A., Griffith, J. F., Robinson, P., et al. (2020). Glossary of terms for musculoskeletal radiology. *Skeletal Radiology, 49*, 1–33. https://doi.org/10.1007/s00256-020-03465-1 (accessed on 26th June 2025).

42. Paparoidamis, G., Iliopoulos, E., Narvani, A., Levy, O., Tsiridis, E., & Polyzois, I. (2020). Posterior shoulder fracture-dislocation: A systematic review of the literature and current aspects of management. *Chinese Journal of Traumatology, 24*, 18–24. https://doi.org/10.1016/j.cjtee.2020.09.001 (accessed on 26th June 2025).

43. Prakash, L. (2018). A new method for reduction of shoulder dislocations. *1*, 1–5. https://www.semanticscholar.org/paper/eb1551593d56ba0f145ba4ed1ee965590f4e09b3 (accessed on 26th June 2025).

44. Quintero, D., Allegra, P. R., Cardoso, F. N., McNamara, C. A., Martín, A. R., Ezuddin, N., Carvajal, J., et al. (2022). Imaging findings of patellar sparing total knee arthroplasty. *JBJS Journal of Orthopedics for Physician Assistants, 10*, e22.00009. https://www.semanticscholar.org/paper/8dcc1639659ba3fa95575d9b1560aff12c4982d1 (accessed on 26th June 2025).

45. Ruser, J. W., & Wiatrowski, W. J. (2013). Restricted work due to workplace injuries: A historical perspective. https://core.ac.uk/download/19958954.pdf (accessed on 26th June 2025).

46. Ruziev, S. O. U., & Shorustamov, M. T. (2025). Clinical and surgical aspects of treating fractures and dislocations of the acromial end of the clavicle. *World Journal of Biology Pharmacy and Health Sciences*. https://www.semanticscholar.org/paper/e7c9df75a38c44bcd1862fbeaafc3e09c3b30d13 (accessed on 26th June 2025).

47. Saglam, F., Baysal, Ö., Sağlam, S., Şirin, E., & Sofulu, Ö. (2022). Floating phalanx: Simultaneous double dislocation of the interphalangeal joint in a finger: A case report and literature review. *Turkish Journal of Trauma & Emergency Surgery, 28*, 876–878. https://www.semanticscholar.org/paper/50f5ff34ac7155257f6d846bbd8a468590fa2f74 (accessed on 26th June 2025).

48. Saxena, P., Amanullah, N., Rajagopalan, S., & Ashwood, N. (2024). Outcomes and management of dislocated hip hemiarthroplasty. *Cureus, 16*. https://www.semanticscholar.org/paper/2ebc83278c4fc1631202fc3711e74c2490018877 (accessed on 26th June 2025).

49. Sleem, B. (2024). Pediatric tibial shaft fractures: A comprehensive review. *Journal of Surgery Research and Practice*. https://www.semanticscholar.org/paper/be7fc4d759145eba7b0f55666a710ba3553baf26 (accessed on 26th June 2025).

50. Sriharsha, G. V., Kumaresan, A., Kokila, S., Arulmozhi, A., K. S., & D. S. (2024). A retrospective study on the incidence of long bone fractures in dogs. *International Journal of Veterinary Sciences and Animal Husbandry*. https://www.semanticscholar.org/paper/1de9b7a704f6612dd3a710871ce5181849e676df (accessed on 26th June 2025).

51. Stein, F., & Leineweber, A. (2020). Laves phases: A review of their functional and structural applications and an improved fundamental understanding of stability and properties. *Journal of Materials Science, 56*, 5321–5427. https://doi.org/10.1007/s10853-020-05509-2 (accessed on 26th June 2025).

52. VandenBerg, C., Sarkisova, N., Pace, J. L., Rhodes, J., & Green, D. W. (2019). Current practice trends in the surgical management of patellofemoral instability: A survey of the Pediatric Research in Sports Medicine (PRiSM) Society. *Orthopedic Journal of Sports Medicine, 7*. https://doi.org/10.1177/2325967119s00090 (accessed on 26th June 2025).

53. Vassallo, K. (2008). Shoulder pain in general practice. https://core.ac.uk/download/46602184.pdf (accessed on 26th June 2025).

54. Vesely, B. D., Michels, L., King, M., Gangopadhyay, P., & Scott, A. T. (2024). Primary arthrodesis versus open reduction and internal fixation for Lisfranc joint fracture-dislocations in adults: A systematic review. *Journal of the American Podiatric Medical Association, 114*(1). https://www.semanticscholar.org/paper/61564987577ec9105a493eb878d35ee0c1c9fc04 (accessed on 26th June 2025).

55. Watts, R. E., Gorbachova, T., Fritz, R. C., Saad, S. S., Lutz, A. M., Kim, J., Chaudhari, A., et al. (2023). Patellar tracking: An old problem with new insights. *Radiographic, 43*. https://doi.org/10.1148/rg.220177 (accessed on 26th June 2025).

56. Wijers, O. (2024). Fractures of the talus: Diagnostics, management and outcome. https://core.ac.uk/download/604744532.pdf (accessed on 26th June 2025).

57. Xin, G. D., Liu, X. Y., Fan, X. D., & Zhao, G. J. (2024). Exosomes repairment for sciatic nerve injury: A cell-free therapy. *Stem Cell Research & Therapy, 15.* https://www.semanticscholar.org/paper/f4432d3e28beb5a105024c431e486b277bc82bce (accessed on 26th June 2025).

58. Zhang, C., Feng, J., Wang, S., Gao, P., Xu, L., Zhu, J., Jia, J., et al. (2020). Incidence of and trends in hip fracture among adults in urban China: A nationwide retrospective cohort study. *PLoS Medicine, 17,* e1003180–e1003180. https://doi.org/10.1371/journal.pmed.1003180 (accessed on 26th June 2025).

59. Zomar, B., Chen, M., Schaeffer, E., Mulpuri, K., & Joeris, A. (2024). Management of long bone fractures and traumatic hip dislocations in pediatric patients: Study protocol for a prospective global multicenter observational cohort registry. *BMJ Open, 14.* https://www.semanticscholar.org/paper/7ea4cafed0f46a55765ab9c9e7d6d7387a8872ba (accessed on 26th June 2025).

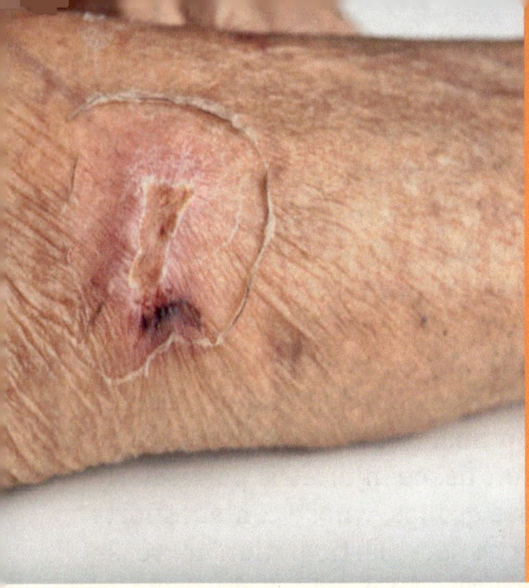

Chapter 4
SOFT TISSUE INJURIES

Contents

Introduction 105
4.1. Types of Soft Tissue Injuries 109
4.2. Causes of Soft Tissue Injuries 112
4.3. Symptoms of Soft Tissue Injuries 115
4.4. Diagnosis of Soft Tissue Injuries 119
4.5. Treatment Options for Soft Tissue Injuries 122
4.6. Prevention of Soft Tissue Injuries 126
Summary 130
References 133

Introduction

The topic of soft tissue injury is quite wide-ranging and encompasses a number of conditions involving the body's supportive, connective, and protective tissues such as muscles, tendons, and ligaments. Soft tissue injuries are significant not only because they are prevalent across various populations of people, particularly athletes and the elderly, but also because they can result in long-term functional impairment and lowered quality of life. An understanding of the mechanisms and nature of such injuries, together with their underlying physiological processes, is of paramount importance in the design of proper prevention and treatment measures. With any other disease, proper diagnosis and therapy are of prime importance to facilitate recovery and prevent recurrence of soft tissue injuries. One of the most significant areas of concern within the genre of soft tissue injuries is the effect of trauma on the pelvic floor and associated structures. For example, trauma accrued during the act of parturition can result in pelvic floor dysfunction and fecal incontinence (FI). Research has indicated that injury to the external anal sphincter (EAS) is often linked with such conditions and highlights the critical need for efficient interventions to manage the complications arising due to these injuries (Siddiqui et al., 2025). A variety of treatment modalities, including conservative and surgical, are available, but most of the existing standard interventions fail to efficiently avert long-term side effects and overall quality-of-life improvement in individuals affected by them. Current advances in therapeutic medicine offer promising possibilities for the treatment of soft tissue injury, particularly in problematic conditions. For instance, regenerative therapeutic interventions, like platelet-rich plasma (PRP) injections, are gaining popularity due to their ability to enhance healing in damaged tissues. Current clinical practice has demonstrated that PRP treatment is able to lead to significant improvement in EAS injury patients, resulting in symptom resolution and enhanced functional capabilities (Siddiqui et al., 2025). Chiropractic care has also been explored for the management of, for instance, pudendal nerve entrapment, and it has been demonstrated that certain therapeutic modalities directed towards soft tissues can be effective. These novel techniques point toward the direction of less invasive and more effective treatment for victims of soft tissue injuries, and as such, the central position that current research and development within this field plays.

Definition of Soft Tissue Injuries

Soft tissue injury is a broad spectrum of injury that encompasses numerous different musculoskeletal structures, including muscles, tendons, ligaments, and fascia. It is divided further into three primary types: strains, sprains, and contusions. A strain is a pull or tear of muscle fibers, often as a result of excess force or persistent repetition, and a sprain is an overpulling or tear of the ligaments that connect bones to each other at joints. Contusions, also known as bruises, occur when muscle tissue is compressed or directly struck, leading to localized inflammation and bleeding. Presentation of these types of injuries can vary widely in severity, with minor injuries often causing only brief pain, while severe ones necessitate surgery or serious rehabilitation. A clear appreciation of these types of injuries is essential for accurate diagnosis and optimal treatment measures. The prevalence of soft tissue injuries is particularly common in active groups, whose contact sports and high-impact sport participation increase the vulnerability to trauma. As highlighted in research, certain groups, such as adolescents who engage in contact sports such as football, basketball, and martial arts, face exposure to heightened vulnerability from these activities' physical nature (Aoude, 2013). Also, causative factors such as inadequate conditioning, poor warm-up, or substandard protective equipment enhance soft tissue injury prevalence. Treatment is according to the RICE principle—rest, ice, compression, and elevation—to alleviate initial pain and swelling. Rehabilitation programs, however, for individual needs, focus on strengthening surrounding muscles, flexibility improvement, and reestablishing function. This two-stage approach emphasizes the importance of a complete and combined understanding of immediate treatment and long-term healing. While fairly straightforward in nature, soft tissue injuries are often misjudged in terms of severity and treatment, which can severely affect healing and lead to long-term complications. One of the most prevalent misconceptions is that all soft tissue injuries are self-healing and don't involve professional care, which can lead to inadequate healing and long-term complications. Multidimensional by nature, such injuries may also require not only the physical therapy but also an understanding of the biomechanics of the affected area (Donya et al., 2014). Sensitization and education of coaches, athletes, and healthcare providers on the nuances of soft tissue injuries allows for a better resource plan of prevention, treatment, and rehabilitation. Lastly, an integrated understanding of soft tissue injury is central to achieving optimal athletic performance and minimizing the risk of re-injury, affirming the necessity for continued research and evidence-based practice in managing such prevalent conditions (Figure 4.1).

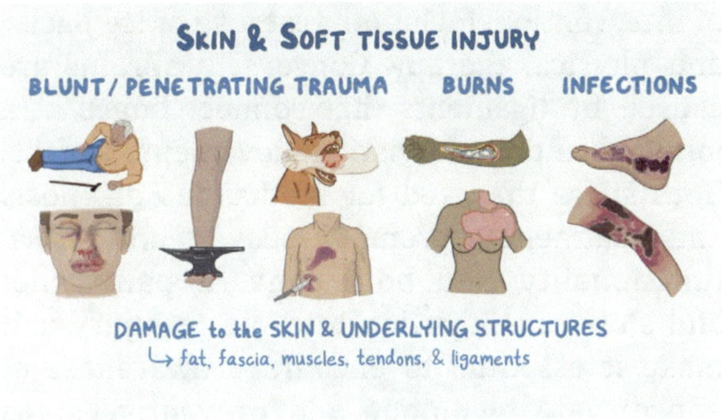

Figure 4.1. Soft tissue injuries represent a significant category of trauma that affects various structures.

Source: https://www.osmosis.org/_next/image?url=https%3A%2F%2Fd16qt3wv6xm098.cloudfront.net%2FZtjFyLu8Sye8ACUc4OlQcoh-TJOH_Xsf%2F_.jpg&w=3840&q=75.

Importance of Understanding Soft Tissue Injuries

Understanding of soft tissue injuries is of vital significance to effective treatment and rehabilitation, both on the individual level but also with long-term health implications. Soft tissue injury involving muscles, tendons, ligaments, and fascia makes up a significant proportion of sports injuries. They can induce acute pain, swelling, and loss of function for which a full appreciation of their pathomechanisms is necessary. An educated strategy enables medical practitioners to implement appropriate therapy regimens, which may include physical therapy, medications, or surgery. Treatment of such injury and diagnosis can avert the onset of chronic disease, thereby enabling an earlier return to normal activities and potentially reducing healthcare costs attributed to prolonged recovery periods. Also, understanding the biomechanics of soft tissue injury makes healthcare professionals able to tailor prevention strategies individually. The consequences of neglecting soft tissue injury are tremendous, such as chronic pain and long-term functional impairment. For instance, a lateral ankle sprain, a common soft tissue injury, causes chronic ankle instability (CAI) if it is not properly treated. CAI is characterized by recurrent sprains, chronic pain, and instability, which have a profound impact on one's quality of life. 40% of individuals experiencing a first-time lateral ankle sprain will develop CAI, making it pertinent to the implications of the injury and requiring a complete clinical evaluation and rehabilitation process to combat the intricacies of these injuries effectively (Hertel & Corbett, 2019). Therefore, a good background in soft tissue injuries is imperative to provide better care and prevent long-term sequelae, again favoring continued education programs for both patients and practitioners. In addition, a firm understanding of soft tissue injuries optimizes prevention measures, which are necessary in athletic and non-athletic populations. Prevention of injury benefits the patient by reducing the likelihood of re-injury, but also benefits public health and resource utilization. Education programs for improving techniques of physical training, as well as strength and conditioning methods, can significantly reduce the incidence of these injuries. For instance, awareness of risk factors such as poor biomechanics or poor footwear can be used to make changes to minimize the risk of injury. In addition, an understanding of conditions like osteoporosis is also important in the treatment of soft tissue injury, given that patients with lower bone density are at high risk of fracture and accompanying complications (LeBoff et al., 2022). Hence, an investment in knowledge regarding soft tissue injury not only enhances healing and recovery but also contributes to public health by way of a greater practice of safe exercise.

Overview of Common Types of Soft Tissue Injuries

Soft tissue damage encompasses a range of conditions that target the connective tissue, muscles, tendons, and ligaments and are most frequently the result of trauma or overuse. The most prevalent of these are lacerations and abrasions, which result when the skin is scraped or sliced and produce a degree of bleeding and risk of infection. Lacerations, due to their deep cuts, can have a significant impact on the tissues that lie beneath them and must be very carefully assessed and managed to avoid complications.

Abrasions are not as profound and are usually limited to the epidermis, although they tend to need attention to avoid further irritation or infection. Such injuries are commonly noted in sporting environments, as noted in oral and maxillofacial injuries, where external force is instrumental in creating such conditions, with emphasis on proper wound care and management during initial treatment phases (Kileo, 2012). Contusions, or bruising, is another common form of soft tissue injury due to blunt trauma resulting in bleeding beneath the skin without fracture. The injury is characterized by discoloration, swelling, and pain over the affected area.

Although commonly regarded as trivial, contusions can in some cases be manifestations of more severe underlying injuries, like muscle tears or strain, that must receive a careful assessment to direct treatment procedures. In high-impact sports, individuals tend to develop contusions as a result of falls and collisions and these heal slowly with the right treatment. How important it is to diagnose and treat contusions cannot be overemphasized because the wrong treatment will definitely lead to continued pain and dysfunction of the injured muscles, so that immediate treatment and rehabilitative methods in the long run are essential for athletes (Yamasaki, 2019). Another significant category of soft tissue injury is strains and sprains which essentially involve the muscles and the ligaments, respectively. Strains are produced through overstretching or muscle fiber tear, most often during physical activities involving sudden force or change in movement. Strains can vary in severity from mild overstretching to muscle tearing and thus need varying degrees of intervention, including rest, use of ice packs, and physical therapy. Conversely, sprains are caused by ligaments that connect bones at a joint, often due to twisting movements or falls. Both share the need for meticulous diagnosis and treatment to promote recovery and return functionality, and both concern pain relief and slow rehabilitation to avoid re-injury and make it essential to encourage awareness of appropriate technique and preventive steps in both recreational and competitive sports environments (Figure 4.2).

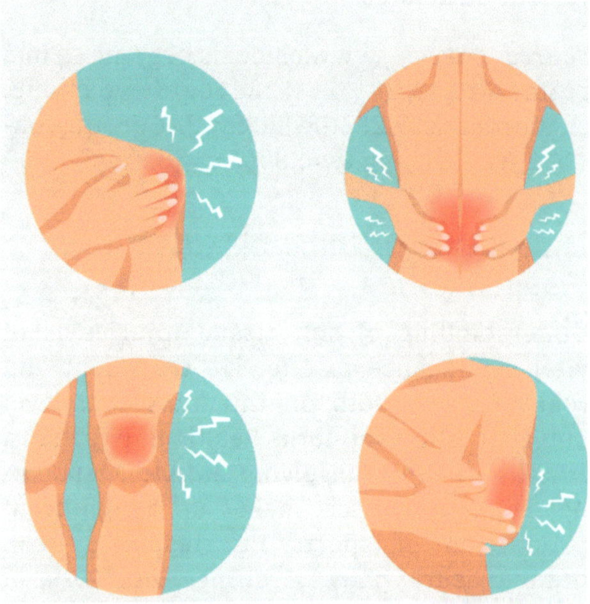

Figure 4.2. Soft tissue injuries encompass a range of conditions affecting the connective tissues.

Source: https://images.ctfassets.net/eexbcii1ci83/54WslpdtlshBhD5Q6DshOv/ad00a42d6393f2a51988b058ec9eb3f2/What_are_the_types_of_soft_tissue_injuries.png.

4.1. Types of Soft Tissue Injuries

Soft tissue injury encompasses a variety of harm to connective tissues like tendons, muscles, ligaments, and skin. Some of the more familiar ones are contusions, abrasions, lacerations, and avulsions. Contusions or bruises occur due to blunt trauma, resulting in localized bleeding beneath the skin. This type of injury is typically characterized by discoloration and soreness but rarely requires severe medical intervention. Conversely, abrasions involve scraping away the superficial layer of the skin with exposure of underlying tissue. While they tend to heal normally, they are at risk of infection. Lacerations represent deeper cuts that may extend beyond the skin itself and often require suturing for optimal healing.

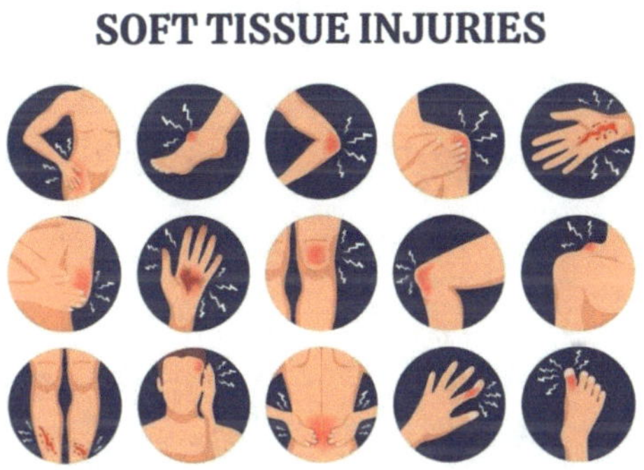

Figure 4.3. Soft tissue injuries encompass a variety of damage to connective tissues.

Source: https://external-content.duckduckgo.com/iu/?u=https%3A%2F%2Fwww.lezdotechmed.com%2Fblog%2Fwp-content%2Fuploads%2F2021%2F11%2FPictures-explaining-about-soft-tissue-injuries-on-parts-of-the-human-body-1024x683.jpg&f=1&nofb=1&ipt=c6c840ad9c2b8997a885109d0d9c449c8f88ef65ed12835d0f96c7449e50b7ea.

Last but not least, avulsions occur when a part or tissue is forcibly torn off, leaving both functional and cosmetic complaints, particularly in extremity injuries. Particularly with athletes, the mechanism of injury can be very varied, making specific types of soft tissue damage more probable. For instance, studies of surfing populations show that skin trauma and injury from one's own surfboard are relatively common, indicative of the kinematics of high-impact sports (McArthur et al., 2020). Acute injury is typically categorized according to its etiology and affected body area, since some sports predispose athletes to certain kinds of injuries.

For this purpose, the identification of patterns of injury reinforces the merit of preventive measures, such as cushioning sporting equipment or protective gear that lessens the risk of disastrous injuries. Coaches and players thus need to know about some sporting injuries to design proper training as well as safety routines to maintain enhanced overall performance as well as health. Besides these common forms of soft tissue injury, the location and circumstances of occurrence also determine their presentation and the way they should be treated. For example, soft tissue injury in the oral and maxillofacial region, often a result of road traffic accidents or domestic violence, can make recovery and treatment complicated (Kileo, 2012). These injuries may range from minor abrasions to complex lacerations requiring surgical intervention. Knowing the most prevalent type of injury occurring in certain settings directs treatment practices toward addressing the distinct requirements of those injured. Because soft tissue injury is often neglected with respect to more visible hard tissue injury, appropriate treatment and monitoring are essential in preventing such complications as chronic pain or impairment of function, highlighting the significance of an educated and systematic approach to treatment and rehabilitation (Figure 4.3).

4.1.1. Sprains

Among the many classes of soft tissue trauma, sprains, in which ligaments are stretched beyond their limits or ruptured, are a common issue both in sports and in everyday life. Sprains often occur in joints and are most vulnerable in the ankle in sports activities that involve sudden changes of direction, jumping, or landing. The symptoms are typically instantaneous and can include pain, swelling, and reduced mobility, which can significantly impair a person's capacity to perform physical activities. Mechanisms for sprains can be multifactorial in nature, such as awkward landings or slipping when exercising physically.

It is important to learn about these dynamics as early identification allows for direct treatment, which can forestall further complications and enhance recovery, underlining the importance of education and awareness for the prevention of sprains among groups of interest, including athletes and those who work in high-risk occupations. The prevalence of sprains among groups of interest underlines the importance of special measures for preventing injury. For instance, a study of part-time soldiers in the Australian Army established that a high percentage of soft tissue trauma was associated with combat training exercises, and the knee was one of the most frequent sites of injury. Specifically, soft tissue injuries with no traumatic or known cause accounted for a large percentage of knee injuries and thus need tailored interventions that address the individual needs and activities of this population (Schram et al., 2018). Educating individuals on correct warm-up and cool-down processes, along with conditioning exercises aimed at assisting ligament strengthening, can significantly eliminate the occurrence of sprains. These injury prevention techniques are not just essential in military settings but also in sporting competitions and leisure activities. Besides, a sprain is not a single incident but has been attributed to cumulative stress associated with a specific activity. For example, research on injuries to surfers has revealed several soft tissue injuries with varying rates of prevalence based on the activity involved (McArthur et al., 2020). Analyses of the type of injury in relation to mechanism—e.g., being struck by a surfboard or falling—may also identify trends and inform prevention. The employment of protective gear or adaptive techniques may also decrease sprain risk further in higher-risk situations like surfing. Consequently, an integrative strategy involving education and adaptive interventions is essential in dealing and preventing sprains in all groups, enhancing performance and safety in a vast array of physical tasks (Figure 4.4).

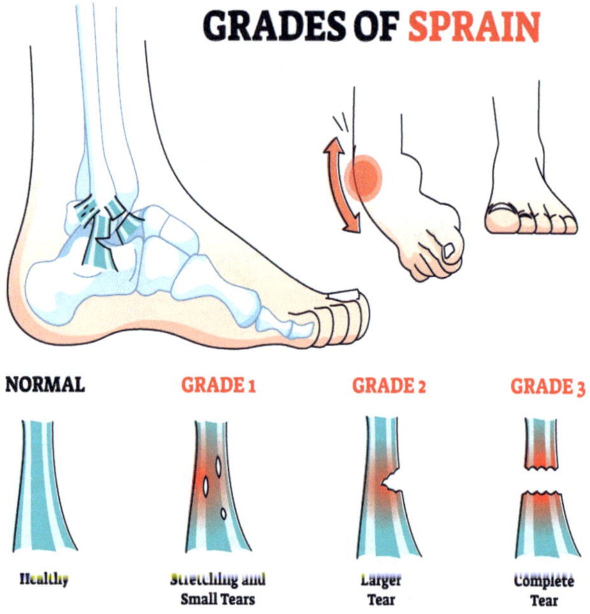

Figure 4.4. The various classifications of soft tissue injuries.

Source: https://external-content.duckduckgo.com/iu/?u=https%3A%2F%2Fimages.squarespace-cdn.com%2Fcontent%2Fv1%2F5ee2540d1675086c7c750894%2F367e64ca-ac81-4a71-bd1d-a7f6b3dc57bf%2FPicture4.jpg&f=1&nofb=1&ipt=711e076a7c6719bf9b5ee8c3d84fc748b2953c0cc8319bc23f42eba82c47a8cb.

4.1.2. Strains

Strains, brought about by overstretched or torn muscles or tendons, are a widespread problem in the realm of soft tissue injuries. The etiology of strains commonly consists of acute changes in movement or force, frequently occurring in sport or physical activity demanding explosive power or rapid acceleration. It is important to note the grading of strains, graded into three types: Grade I, involving mild stretching; Grade II, indicating partial tears; and Grade III, indicating complete tears. Each type has a distinct clinical presentation with differential pain, swelling, and dysfunction. Proper and early management of strains is important to prevent long-term damage and to provide optimal healing. In managing strains, treatment modalities must be tailored according to the degree of injury and subsequent impact on functional capacity. Early treatment protocols usually begin with the R.I.C.E. principle (Rest, Ice, Compression, Elevation), addressing relief of pain as well as a decrease in swelling. As healing progresses, rehabilitative techniques can involve physical therapy modalities for recovery of range of motion and strength. In this regard, new treatments such as cupping have also been gaining traction, demonstrating positive outcomes in enhancing flexibility and improving pain in injured groups. In an interesting twist, the application of cupping as a therapeutic intervention for muscular strains expands the vista of traditional treatment approaches (Schafer, 2018). While such interventions are yet to accumulate evidence, it is an amalgamation of multi-faceted interventions that form a holistic recovery plan. The effectiveness of the various passive physical modalities in treating strains is a virtue that awaits discovery. A systematic review of the intervention for soft tissue injury emphasizes the need for scientific assessments of therapy methods (Ameis et al., 2015). Unlike conventional therapies such as splinting or acupuncture, newer modalities such as Kinesio taping and laser therapy hold promise as adjunct therapies in the symptomatic treatment of strains. Furthermore, understanding the interplay between different treatment methods can enhance the management of strains, with influences on outcomes for recovery time and return to activity. As research progresses, knowledge of the intricate dynamics of healing soft tissues will allow clinicians to maximize treatment regimens, ultimately improving patient outcomes as it relates to musculoskeletal health.

4.1.3. Contusions

Contusions, or simply bruises, are caused by the formation of blunt trauma to the skin, which causes bleeding beneath the surface. The injury is marked by discoloration, swelling, and tenderness, showing the resultant disruption of small blood vessels beneath. Contusions can significantly impact an athlete's performance and recovery from soft tissue injury. While small contusions are occasionally self-limited, more significant contusions have the potential to jeopardize patients with complications. Understanding the pathophysiology that results in contusions and how the body responds to this type of injury is thus paramount. Both prompt evaluation and appropriate management are paramount in achieving successful recovery and allowing patients to return to their own sports activities or jobs in a safe and timely manner. Contusions are often clinically assessed, though imaging tests can be useful in determining the degree of the injury. Radiologic imaging tests, such as MRI, are particularly useful in distinguishing from other types of soft tissue injury and fractures, and clarifying the degree of the injury. To have knowledge of the effectiveness of these modalities can be extremely beneficial to practitioners in developing an individualized treatment plan. For under-evaluated or mismanaged contusions, the risk of prolonged recovery and potential chronic pain is high, necessitating informed clinical practice. In addition, coaches, health professionals, and athletes need to recognize signs and symptoms of contusions at an early stage so that early treatment can be administered and complications can be prevented. In sports medicine, the prevalence of contusions cannot be exaggerated in high-impact and collision sports. Athletes may suffer both acute contusions from single trauma and chronic contusions from recurrent abuse to a specific area of the body. There is much variability of symptoms that makes diagnosis difficult in the presence of other associated injuries. Functional tests and appropriate imaging modalities then come into focus in differentiating between contusions and other soft tissue injuries. The multifaceted nature of such injuries makes their accurate assessment and treatment crucial to the return of athletes to competitive play without risking injury to their conditions. Through the integration of clinical data with the latest imaging approaches, clinicians can enhance diagnostic accuracy and implement overall therapy, thereby supporting swifter recoveries in athletes suffering from contusions (McSweeney et al., 2012; Zhou, 2024) (Figure 4.5).

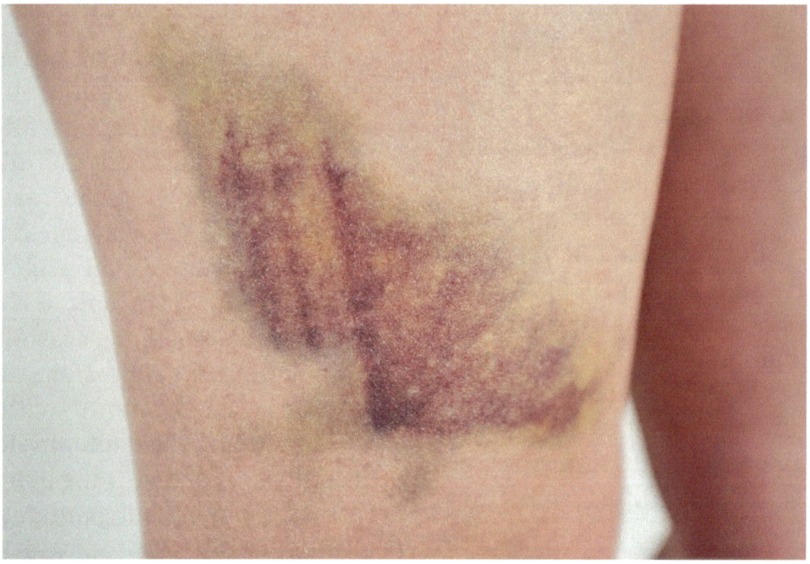

Figure 4.5. Contusions.

Source: https://external-content.duckduckgo.com/iu/?u=https%3A%2F%2Fphysioflowpt.com%2Fwp-content%2Fuploads%2F2022%2F05%2FContusion-2-scaled.jpg&f=1&nofb=1&ipt=7365b6d29448c624375f6426be68e2d56fa9900cb1a03baca08d83829e447032.

4.2. Causes of Soft Tissue Injuries

Soft tissue injuries are most frequently caused by various extrinsic and intrinsic reasons, attributing the etiology as complex. For example, participation in intensive physical training is among the prominent causes. This is particularly prevalent in high-demand environments such as the military. Research shows that a high percentage of part-time military personnel have higher rates of injury compared to their full-time counterparts, despite similarities in the nature of employment. Such injuries primarily affect the knee, where incidents occur predominantly in combat training or physical exercises. This is a trend that suggests that dedicated efforts at enhancing physical readiness and promoting injury prevention initiatives are needed to minimize the risk of soft tissue injuries during strenuous efforts, underlining the necessity for complete conditioning programs tailored to specific contexts (Schram et al., 2018). In addition, car accidents are among the major causes of soft tissue injury, especially in urban areas. A study of oral and maxillofacial trauma in a large hospital revealed that road traffic accidents were the culprit behind a staggering 64.2% of the cases, with lacerations and bruises being the most common soft tissue injuries. Such injuries are likely to occur when there is a fall or an impact, and it is because of the injury to the tissues and the skin. The importance of such evidence cannot be emphasized enough since it focuses on greater road safety measures as well as public campaigns against the incidence of such accidents. Consequently, an understanding of the effects of road accidents on soft tissue injury rates can inform both prevention strategies and treatment of such injuries (Kileo, 2012). Sporting activity is also linked with a major cause of soft tissue injury, revealing a link between sport and vulnerability to injury. The competitive environment of sports also involves repetitive movements, impact collisions, and insufficient warm-up or conditioning, all of which enhance the risk of injury in the form of strains, sprains, and contusions. Further, the absence of proper protective gear can enhance these risks during competition. Coaches and competitors need to appreciate the importance of fitness training and prevention of injuries, employing the best warm-up techniques and strength conditioning strategies to increase body resistance. By appreciating the determinants of soft tissue sports injuries as multifactorial, stakeholders are able to facilitate safer sport participation and optimize overall sport performance while reducing the injury burden on athletes (Schram et al., 2018).

4.2.1. Sports-Related Activities

Involvement in sports activities is inherently linked to a variety of physical consequences, particularly soft tissue injuries, which are typical among players and participants. As the body of a human being remains active, i.e., running, jumping, and swift turns, there are high risks of injury to muscles, tendons, and ligaments. For example, researchers have revealed that knee injuries are the most frequent events during combat training contexts, being most frequently induced by techniques that impose excessive stress on such soft tissues. Specifically, statistics collected by the Australian Army Reserve reveal that knee injuries, particularly soft tissue trauma injury, comprise a great percentage of total injuries. Above all, these kinds of injuries often occur in scenarios of fighting and physical activity, highlighting the importance of understanding the circumstances under which injuries will occur and the necessity for personalized injury prevention strategies aimed at responding to risk from sport participation (Schram et al., 2018). The ramifications of soft tissue injuries extend beyond tangible pain and rehabilitation; they are potentially able to impact the performance and willingness to compete in activities on behalf of an athlete. For instance, individuals who participate in contact sports or certain recreational activities may experience fear of reinjury, subsequently altering their levels of participation as well as overall experience. Adolescents and teens who are highly involved in sporting activities are particularly susceptible to such injuries, which affect their physical development and mental well-being. The frequency of injuries such as cuts to soft tissue and muscle strains supports the implementation of preventative measures. The use of proper protective gear, including mouthguards, not only protects teeth but also serves as a mental defense against fear of injury. Therefore, the comprehension of the multi-faceted implications of injury upon sportsmen is paramount in an attempt to promote a sound sporting environment (Aoude, 2013). Additionally, an expenditure in novel protective gear, particularly within high-risk sporting activities, represents a preemptive action for reducing injury incidence. The effectiveness of mouthguards designed to support shock absorption and force distribution has also been observed to significantly reduce the incidence of traumatic dental injury in athletes. Evidence shows that mouthguard wearers are nearly three times less susceptible to dental trauma compared to non-users, which emphasizes the significance of such technologies in ensuring health. With the developers moving into new materials and technology, the top priority is to maximize protection without compromising on comfort or performance. For instance, technological developments in mouthguard technology, in which material improvements are achieved by utilizing ethylene vinyl acetate (EVA) and adding air cell structures, reflect the advancement in safety items intended to cater to the needs of athletes. The incorporation of such features into sporting-related activities not only enhances safety but also encourages long-term participation and commitment to sports (Aoude, 2013) (Figure 4.6).

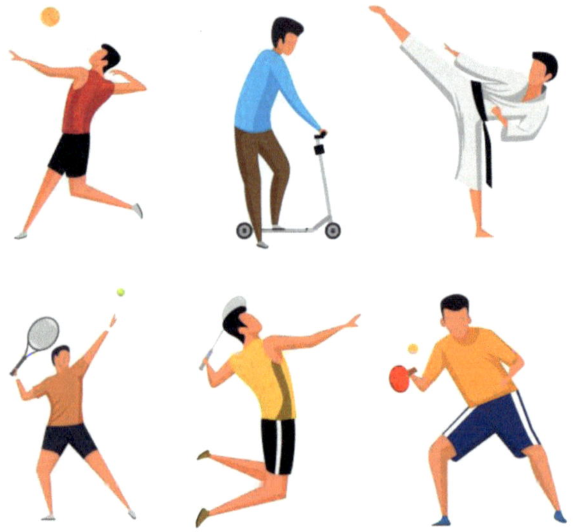

Figure 4.6. Engagement in sports-related activities.

Source: https://i.pinimg.com/736x/a4/46/74/a4467413c9e2e7a33ab781390cb38e4f.jpg.

4.2.2. Accidents and Falls

Falls and accidents are common causes of soft tissue injury, especially in the emergency medical setting. The dynamic environment of daily life tends to create conditions in which patients are more likely to slip, trip, or fall and sustain serious trauma. Statistics show that these accidents are responsible for a high percentage of emergency room visits, making it a public health problem of some significance. For instance, studies indicate that facial trauma which is usually associated with accidents and falls, is responsible for the predominant pathology that warrants immediate treatment under the emergency services. The outcomes range from superficial cuts to severe damage of soft tissues, and they illustrate the variability of the health and wellness impact such an accident can have (Kileo, 2012). Demographic patterns that are involved in accidents and falls recognize a particular susceptibility in certain groups. Both male and female young adults aged between twenty and thirty years are found to have a high level of susceptibility to facial trauma as a result of accidents, contributing to the overall number of soft tissue injuries. Other than age and gender, environmental determinants, including urban locations, affect the incidence of injuries. The excessive use of recreation activities and work responsibilities tends to produce situations where one may experience falls, frequently facilitated by a lack of implementation of sufficient safety provisions. Notably, findings from numerous studies create a strong link between violent incidents, including interpersonal altercations and accidents, pointing to the need for targeted prevention interventions (Kileo, 2012). Prevention of falls and accidents is imperative to curtail the disease burden of soft tissue injuries in our communities. Effective interventions have to target individual behavior change and more encompassing social interventions. Education in safety protocols, proper footwear, and awareness of the environment will significantly reduce the number of falls. Furthermore, the inclusion of safety devices in public spaces, such as handrails and non-slippery floors, can foster a safer environment, eventually minimizing the occurrence of traumatic injuries. Healthcare systems bear instant consequences in the form of reduced medical costs and improved patient outcomes because initial preventive approaches might decrease injury severity caused by accidents and falls, reasserting the importance of addressing this issue as an entire entity (Azcue et al., 2025) (Figure 4.7).

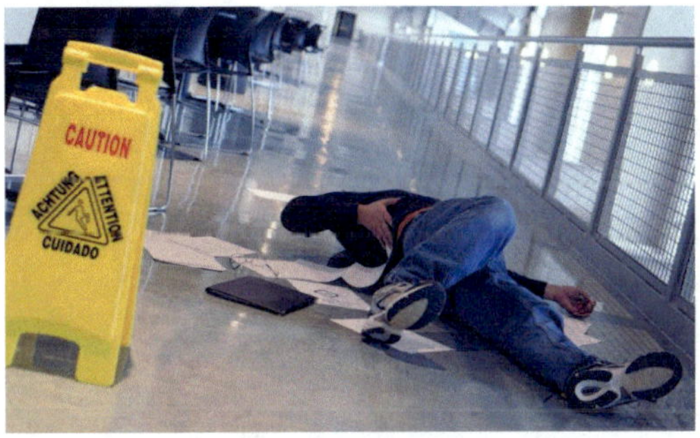

Figure 4.7. Accidents and falls are prevalent contributors to soft tissue injuries.

Source: https://www.spektorlaw.com/wp-content/uploads/2022/06/slip-fall-accidents-main.webp.

4.2.3. Repetitive Motion and Overuse

Repetitive motion injury is increasingly prevalent in modern society, particularly among individuals engaged in activities involving repetitive physical movements over a prolonged duration. The injuries, characterized by a progressive build-up of pain, inflammation, are due to the overuse of tendons or muscles. Daily tasks common in work and play contexts—typing, assembly line work, or athletics—are repetitively stress-inducing with limited provision for recovery. Such repetitive strain can ultimately lead to conditions like tendinitis, bursitis, and stress fractures. An example is plantar fasciopathy, which is most frequently induced by repetitive strain on the soft tissues of the foot, illustrating the multifactorial causes of such conditions as internal and external forces intersect (Beeson, 2014). Moreover, Medial Tibial Stress Syndrome (MTSS) is another severe outcome of repetitive motion and overuse in athletes. It feels like chronic pain along the shinbone, which gets worse upon use in sports such as running or jumping. The subtlety of MTSS is in its causes, which may comprise biomechanical flaws, inadequate shoe choice, or faulty training methods. The issue with treating MTSS is that no definite knowledge exists of how it can be prevented and what treatment measures can be employed for it. However, the evidence suggests that a proactive strategy with a focus on preventive measures is more effective than attempting to rehabilitate once the injury has occurred (Yamasaki, 2019). An accurate understanding of how repetitive motion and overuse result in soft tissue injury emphasizes the importance of preventive measures that minimize risks. Training in the proper ergonomic practices, frequent breaks during repetitive tasks, and changing movement patterns have a high potential for reducing the occurrence of overuse injuries. Physical conditioning tailored to the requirements of specific activities also enhances muscle resilience and stamina, therefore reducing the risk of injury. Establishing a correct understanding of the potential impact of repetitive movements on the individual is crucial to both the individual and the healthcare provider. This information brings about a culture where preventive measures are appreciated and, in the end, result in overall musculoskeletal health in populations.

4.3. Symptoms of Soft Tissue Injuries

Understanding the symptoms of soft tissue injuries is critical in ensuring timely diagnosis and best treatment. Soft tissue injuries, such as damage to muscles, ligaments, and tendons, are typically characterized by a range of symptoms that arise immediately or develop over time. Localized pain, swelling, bruising, and a reduction in range of motion are common symptoms that can prevent the affected region from functioning. For active individuals and athletes, early identification of these symptoms is critical in order not to worsen the injury. Failing to treat such symptoms can result in chronic illnesses, making recovery more difficult and raising chances of reinjury. Attention in symptom identification is thus vital for anyone who is physically active since it directly affects the management and rehabilitation stages required to recover completely. Symptoms may vary in severity based on the extent and type of soft tissue injury. Acute ones such as sprains or strains are of immediate and severe type followed by swelling and bruising shortly after injury. Chronic forms of injury such as tendinitis are gradual in development, and patients are likely to overlook initial symptoms as they could be subtle in onset. They can develop chronic pain or stiffness, particularly on exertion, which can be easily dismissed as normal overuse or fatigue. Being familiar with these varied presentations is also relevant in the instance of injury-specific management. For instance, where acute injuries would react to immediate rest and ice application, chronic injuries would call for a more general strategy, involving strengthening and rehabilitation of affected tissues as well as preventing recurrence. Practically, accurate assessment of soft tissue injury is based on proper identification and interpretation of symptoms. Careful scrutiny of the patient's symptomatology and history allows clinicians to ascertain the type of injury and guide appropriate management. Particularly in children, as in the case of growth plate injuries, extreme suspicion must be exercised to avoid issues like angular deformities and arrest of growth. The controversy surrounding such injuries emphasizes the necessity for specific treatment programs, which are essential to optimizing patient outcomes. As the literature would indicate, attention to early diagnosis and proper care is critical to minimizing long-term morbidity that occurs from soft tissue injuries. This procedure facilitates rapid return to function, emphasizing education regarding symptoms within sporting communities and the population at large (Sabharwal & Sabharwal, 2018; Yamasaki, 2019) (Figure 4.8).

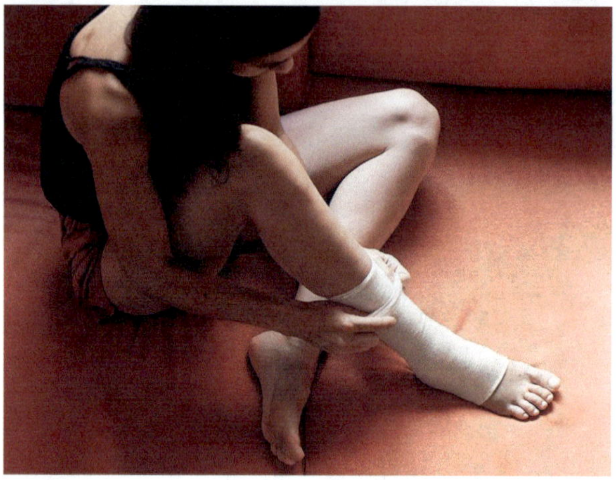

Figure 4.8. The symptoms of soft tissue injuries are crucial for timely diagnosis and effective treatment.

Source: https://media.post.rvohealth.io/wp-content/uploads/sites/3/2024/03/MNT-person-wrapped-ankle-732x549-thumbnail.jpg.

4.3.1. Pain and Tenderness

Pain and tenderness are prominent telltale signs among the range of soft tissue injuries, and they represent urgent markers for internal harm that requires healthcare treatment. Pain is intrinsically subjective and varies significantly between patients as a function of physiological and psychological factors. Tenderness, as indicated by pain on palpation, is relatively typical of muscle strain, ligament sprain, or tendon rupture. This combination of pain and tenderness is indicative of inflammation and derangement of tissue. Diagnosis and optimal course of treatment are contingent upon assessment of these signs. An understanding of the pathophysiology of pain perception is enhanced by clear comprehension, which can enhance therapeutic intervention, guiding practitioners in the management of soft tissue injury. For instance, in inguinal disruption (ID), a name coined to distinguish from standard hernia terminology, there are specific pain patterns of tenderness that are accounted for. ID leads to the lack of a true hernia but with undue tension in the groin area, and tenderness occurs around the site where the inguinal ligament becomes attached. Its multifaceted definition gives significant weight to pain control as part of its treatment protocol.

Evidence from expert conferences highlights that management of tenderness with personalized physiotherapy is capable of producing effective relief and aiding in recovery. Therefore, identification of the interrelations among pain, tenderness, and underlying pathology constitutes the key to optimizing the treatment of patients, particularly sporting populations, where groin injuries are prevalent (Sheen et al., 2013). In addition, clinical cases often suffer from issues of addressing pain and tenderness successfully.

For example, a case in a 65-year-old man illustrates the complexity found when pain does not respond to conservative therapy. Following a bout of activity such as painting, this patient complained of shoulder pain accompanied by tenderness under the acromion, which is consistent with an acute soft tissue sprain. Despite paracetamol, the nominal relief obtained illustrates the heterogeneity of response in pain control. This case emphasizes the need for systematic physical examination to identify areas of tenderness and intervene accordingly. In this manner, ongoing observation of pain and tenderness with soft tissue injury not only facilitates accurate diagnoses but also directs treatment to maximize patient outcomes (Vassallo, 2008).

4.3.2. Swelling and Inflammation

Swelling and inflammation are normal responses to trauma of soft tissues, and both are a necessary part of the healing process. When tissues are damaged, the body responds with an increase in blood supply to the site of injury, an occurrence facilitated by the release of inflammatory mediators such as histamines and cytokines. This vascular response creates high permeability of blood vessels, leading to the fluid movement to interstitial spaces and resulting in swelling. While this inflammation is desirable to induce repair mechanisms, excessive swelling or swelling over a long period can lead to other problems, hindering recovery as well as causing pain to the patient. A delicate balance of useful and detrimental reduction of inflammation is essential for effective soft tissue injury management. Also, the process from swelling to inflammation can be complicated by an array of factors, like the nature of the trauma and the overall health status of the person. For instance, long-term traumas like Medial Tibial Stress Syndrome (MTSS) are examples of how persistent swelling can lead to self-destructive inflammation. In such a case, inflammation can become a reaction leading to further tissue degeneration and chronic pain. In addition, swelling management with ice or compression may prevent inflammation and induce a more favorable healing environment. Therefore, it is essential to develop methods not only for symptomatic relief but also for the resolution of causes to ensure long-term recovery (Yamasaki, 2019). Recent studies emphasize the importance of exact measurement of inflammation to enhance treatment strategies for soft tissue injury. Early Wound Healing Score (EHS) is proposed as a new tool for the evaluation of healing in soft tissues through a quantification of clinical signs of inflammation and other factors. With such scoring systems, clinicians can follow the healing process more efficiently and make optimal decisions for intervention methods. This approach emphasizes that a focus on inflammation is not as a symptom but an essential element that impacts results in healing for soft tissue injury. Managing and learning about inflammation can improve the effectiveness of treatment measures, producing maximum healing and returning individuals to their activity with less possibility for recurrence (Marini et al., 2018) (Figure 4.9).

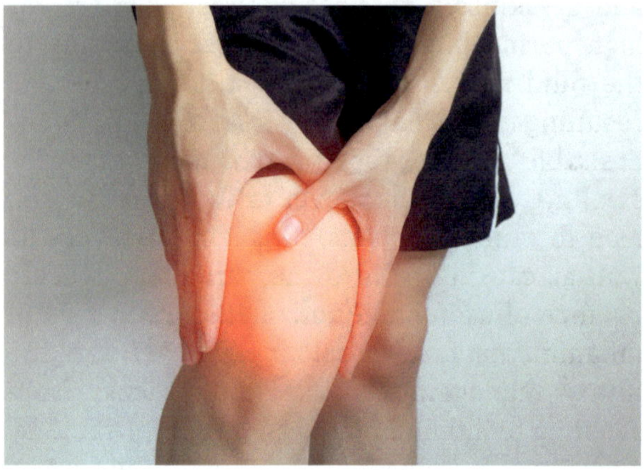

Figure 4.9. Swelling and inflammation are common responses to soft tissue injuries.

Source: https://www.healthdigest.com/img/gallery/the-real-difference-between-inflammation-and-swelling/l-intro-1636734169.jpg.

4.3.3. Limited Range of Motion

The state of limited range of motion (ROM) significantly affects individuals with soft tissue injury, underlining the intricate interplay between flexibility and bodily health. When tissues such as tendons, ligaments, and muscles get injured, they have the tendency to become stiff and less flexible and capable of stretching or contracting normally. Their stiffness often results in a reduced ability to perform daily activities, increasing pain and limiting general function. Poor flexibility in scientific research has been reported to increase injury risk, and there is evidence that indicates an issue of causality in that currently existing limitations are within a feedback loop that creates further dysfunction. In addressing these problems, it is necessary to explore intervention for improving ROM, a significant rehabilitation aspect for soft tissue damage, because improved flexibility can minimize pain and promote healing through function restoration and mobility. Cupping therapy, a historical intervention that has caused Western medicine to take notice, has shown promise in boosting flexibility, thereby improving ROM in individuals with soft tissue injuries. Cupping therapy is conducted by applying suction cups on areas of the body where blood flow is needed, allowing for the healing process to occur. Research evaluating the efficacy of cupping therapy indicates it can yield quantifiable improvement in flexibility, helping patients regain ROM necessary for everyday function as well as sports participation. The therapy is beneficial specifically in terms of disability restricting movement, as increased ROM is a foundation upon which more comprehensive treatment plans can be based and aimed at physical rehabilitation and pain management. Although more studies need to be done, cupping is a promising tool in the arsenal for reversing patient mobility with soft tissue injury (Schafer, 2018). For instance, rotator cuff injury is one of the most definitive examples of the ill effects of limited range of motion on an individual's quality of life. With tears of the rotator cuff increasingly frequent, especially in the older adult, the resulting loss of motion at the shoulder joint may compromise day-to-day function, i.e., reaching or lifting. Pain and loss of strength resulting from the injuries tend to render patients inactive, which further exacerbates the issue of limited ROM. Conservative management modalities like focused physical therapy play a pivotal role in the management of such injuries, allowing for flexibility while concurrently offering pain relief and restriction from functional restriction. As scientists explore new avenues of therapy, including platelet-rich plasma (PRP) therapy, the focus is placed on effective facilitation of ROM through biologic approaches. Lastly, understanding the intricacies of restricted ROM in soft tissue injuries is vital to the development of effective treatment plans so that patients may recover their bodily functions (Loccisano, 2016).

4.4. Diagnosis of Soft Tissue Injuries

Diagnosis of soft tissue injuries is also a process that is complex and one that typically calls for good clinical evaluation and knowledge of the history of the patients. The clinicians will typically begin by evaluating in detail the mechanism of injury, the level of pain, and prior injuries that can impact the current condition. Observational findings, such as bruising, swelling, and impaired range of motion, provide valuable evidence of the extent and quality of injury. Specifically, clinical manifestations such as disproportionate pain and pain with passive stretch have been identified as valuable markers of acute injuries (Ali et al., 2014). These symptoms, in conjunction with a complete physical examination, bring healthcare practitioners to a more accurate diagnosis and a tailored treatment regimen. Imaging studies become a key player in diagnosing soft tissue sprains, particularly where clinical examination findings are nondiagnostic. Techniques such as ultrasound and magnetic resonance imaging (MRI) are typically employed to image the extent of soft tissue damage, including tears, sprains, and other muscle damage. MRI, in most instances, is now a gold standard for evaluating complex soft tissue injuries due to its superior tissue differentiation and ability to detect minor pathologies (Loccisano, 2016). Use of such novel imaging modalities not only enhances diagnostic specificity but also allows for a delineation of possible complications, crucial in planning effective management and establishing realistic expectations for recovery by the patient. Furthermore, standardized assessment tools may significantly increase the consistency and reliability of the diagnosis of soft tissue injury. These tools can include functional outcome measures that score the impact of injury on overall mobility and daily activities. These metrics not only inform clinicians of the extent of the injury but also provide a baseline for measuring patient improvement throughout the course of rehabilitation. By developing a systematic approach to diagnose and follow up, physicians can better manage the multi-factorial pathophysiology of soft tissue trauma and thereby produce better clinical outcomes and optimal recovery routes (Ali et al., 2014; Loccisano, 2016). Ultimately, proper diagnosis unlocks avenues for evidence-based management and enhances patients' quality of life following trauma (Figure 4.10).

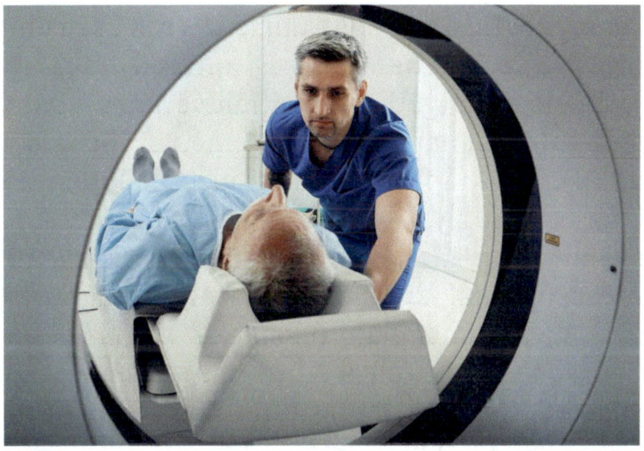

Figure 4.10. The diagnosis of soft tissue injuries.

Source: https://www.johnfoy.com/wp-content/uploads/2024/04/Man-begins-test-that-are-used-to-diagnose-soft-tissue-injuries-scaled.jpg.

4.4.1. Physical Examination

A complete physical examination is the basis upon which soft tissue injuries are diagnosed. The assessment involves a number of methods used to determine the integrity of fascia, ligaments, tendons, and muscles. Flexibility plays an important part in diagnosing predisposition towards such injuries; its absence can predispose one to strain and tearing. Evidence has shown that practices like cupping therapy will enhance flexibility, possibly affecting injury prevention (Schafer, 2018). Adding a series of assessments enables clinicians to gain a precise understanding of the patients' physical condition, which is advantageous to tailored treatment plans as well as rehabilitation algorithms. A judicious physical examination, then, extends beyond the straightforward identification of injuries; it also focuses special notice on pre-injury status and functional abilities that influence recovery trajectories. In addition to the measurement of flexibility, the physical examination also includes various clinical tests to evaluate joint stability and functional range of motion. For example, knee laxity standardized tests allow clinicians to measure the integrity of collateral ligaments directly proportional to the degree of soft tissue damage in the knee joint. Clinicians can use non-invasive techniques, such as infrared tracking technology, to gather quantitative knee laxity and joint behavior measurements (Schafer, 2018). This approach minimizes subjective bias commonly associated with conventional examination methods, enabling clinicians to make optimal decisions regarding diagnosis and treatment plan formation from data. Consequently, the physical examination not only enables diagnosis of soft tissue injuries but also serves as a paradigm for measuring the progress of rehabilitation and directing further clinical interventions. Secondly, physical examination is instrumental in educating patients about their injuries and ensuring a collaborative treatment process. Through clear descriptions of the examination results, treatment professionals are able to educate patients regarding the nature of injuries, the benefits of rehabilitation, and steps towards the prevention of future accidents. Informing patients motivates them towards adherence to treatment protocols and participation in the healing process. Therefore, in addition to its diagnostic and therapeutic functions, the physical examination essentially plays a part in an integrated approach to the treatment of soft tissue injuries. This integrated approach guarantees that not only the physical recovery but also the psychological health of patients is considered, resulting in better outcomes and well-being (Figure 4.11).

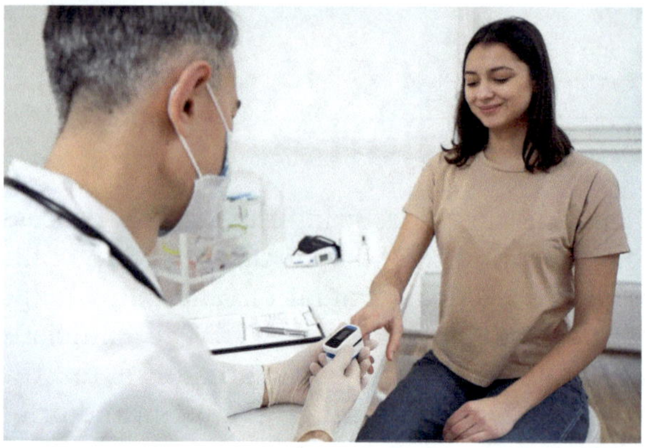

Figure 4.11. The physical examination serves as a cornerstone for diagnosing soft tissue injuries.

Source: https://windermeremedical.com/wp-content/uploads/2025/02/2149281059.webp.

4.4.2. Imaging Techniques (X-rays, MRI)

The assessment and diagnosis of soft tissue trauma require high-fidelity imaging techniques that are able to capture the subtleties of varied tissues. While X-rays have been employed in medical imaging for decades, they are not primarily used to describe bone structures. Their failure to properly assess soft tissue, such as muscles, ligaments, and tendons, is noteworthy since X-rays lack sensitivity to detect subtle injury or internal bleeding. Secondly, X-rays are not capable of providing functional information about the tissue or establishing biomechanical properties, which are critical in the assessment of the severity of soft tissue injuries. This is the setback that has seen the focus on other imaging modalities that complement the diagnostic value of such injuries, the shift to more advanced procedures like MRI, which offer better resolution, particularly in the soft tissues, thus facilitating better treatment regimens. The invention of Magnetic Resonance Imaging (MRI) has revolutionized the examination of soft tissue injury by enabling unparalleled resolution of soft tissue anatomy. Unlike X-rays, which rely on the use of ionizing radiation to image the body, MRIs utilize strong magnetic fields and radio waves to create high-definition images that can identify issues in tendons, ligaments, and cartilage, making MRI an invaluable instrument in sports medicine. Its ability to image soft tissue in various planes allows for a complete evaluation of injuries like tears, sprains, and inflammation. However, despite its usefulness, MRIs are not endlessly useful; they are costly, time-consuming, and need patient stillness during scanning, which can be difficult in actual situations. Therefore, while as valuable as MRI itself is to proper diagnosis of soft tissue trauma, clinicians need to weigh its utility against such limitations on an individual basis. With future advances in medical imaging technologies now on the horizon, innovative new technologies such as photoacoustic imaging (PAI) pose exciting alternatives to current standard methods such as X-rays and MRI. PAI is a combination of optical imaging and ultrasound techniques, providing high-resolution images of soft tissues without any risk factor related to ionizing radiation. The potential of PAI to assess the metabolic condition of tissues and image vasculature distinguishes PAI from other imaging technologies. This new imaging method evaluates tissue oxygenation and metabolic functions essential in the tracking of soft tissue injury healing, finally providing a better-rounded insight into injury rehabilitation. Additionally, the lack of invasiveness may complement conventional imaging techniques, solving some of their limitations, potentially improving injury diagnosis and resulting treatment plans for patients and sportsmen. With more research available to validate its application, PAI can be a leading figure in the future of sports medicine and soft tissue injury evaluation (Donya et al., 2014; Ma et al., 2025) (Figure 4.12).

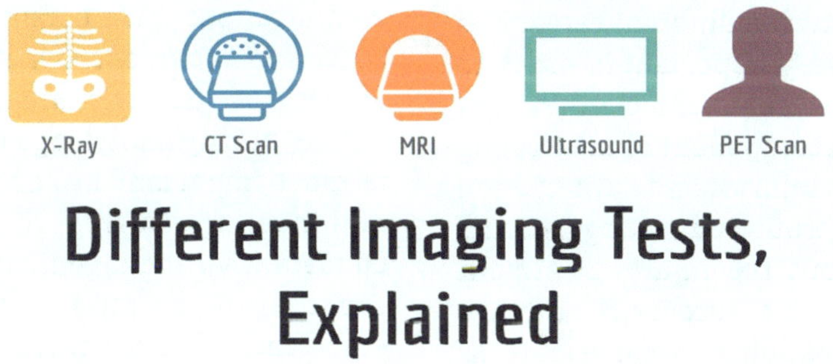

Figure 4.12. Imaging techniques (X-rays, MRI).

Source: https://blog.radiology.virginia.edu/wp-content/uploads/2019/09/header-2_compressed.jpg.

4.4.3. Patient history and Symptom Assessment

A thorough patient history is the foundation of the assessment for soft tissue injuries because it helps providers appreciate the context and circumstance of the injury. This type of history typically includes the mechanism of injury, previous injuries, and overall general state of health, including any systemic conditions that may affect healing. As an example, knowing whether the injury was the result of acute trauma, repetitive strain, or medical conditions directs further treatment and evaluation.

Understanding a patient's activity level before being injured also informs the treating physician on how to tailor rehabilitation intervention. Adding this comprehensive history results in a more comprehensive evaluation and ultimately better treatment in terms of optimizing recovery and returning function. Evaluation of symptoms is also another important function in the diagnosis and treatment of soft tissue injuries. Not only must clinicians evaluate the nature and location of the pain, but also evaluate associated symptoms such as bruising, swelling, and impairment of function. This is followed by physical examinations where the range of motion and any deformity that is representative of the severity of the injury can be noted. Symptoms can also provide information about the injury mechanism; for example, pain that is sharp is usually a tear, whereas pain that is dull or sore could be indicative of inflammation. Through careful evaluation of these parameters, clinicians are able to sequence interventions on the basis of the individual needs of the patient to best optimize their recovery pattern. Effective symptom assessment also facilitates the differentiation between different categories of injuries, which is very important in order to apply the appropriate treatment plan. Patient education is a critical component of the healing process for soft tissue injuries and optimization of recovery results. Through educating patients in intense detail about the injury, treatment options, and expectations of recovery, healthcare providers empower patients to participate as active partners in their care. This covers details concerning symptom management, activities to be avoided or modified, and return times to normal activities. It is crucial for patients to understand that even if drugs relieve symptoms, they do not circumvent the need for body rehabilitation and adjustment of activity. The study emphasizes that early involvement in self-care activities can significantly decrease the degree of disability and improve healing, particularly with illnesses like back pain where long-term symptoms develop. Thus, integrating patient education into routine evaluation will not just improve better management of soft tissue injuries but also promote long-term health and injury prevention initiatives (Banning, 2008; Lee et al., 2021).

4.5. Treatment Options for Soft Tissue Injuries

The treatment of soft tissue injuries is multifaceted, with treatments varying depending on the severity, location, and overall status of the patient. Treatment could first involve sticking to the R.I.C.E. principle—Rest, Ice, Compression, and Elevation—designed to prevent initial pain and swelling. More serious injuries tend to need more vigorous treatment. Surgical techniques, such as Open Reduction and Internal Fixation (ORIF), Minimally Invasive Plate Osteosynthesis (MIPO), and external fixation (EF), have individual strengths depending on the nature of the injury. Besides the recovery of function, they also address potential secondary injury complications, thus maximizing overall patient outcomes as evidenced in studies evaluating the efficacy of such treatments (Biz et al., 2018). Hence, having knowledge of what is to be done is most important in successful rehabilitation and healing. During the recovery process, conservative management gains significance, especially for soft tissue strains such as rotator cuff tears. Conservative management could include physical therapy, oral medications, corticosteroid injection, or newer modalities like Platelet-Rich Plasma (PRP) therapy, which uses the patient's own body material to stimulate healing (Loccisano, 2016). Research has shown that conservative treatments can result in significant improvement in pain and function in patients with partial rotator cuff tears, preventing surgery. In consideration of the factors stated above, the decision-making process in undertaking surgical or conservative management still remains complex and greatly dependent on factors such as age, level of activity, and degree of the injury. In conclusion, treatment for soft tissue injury ranges from a spectrum of therapy, from conservative to surgical. There are a variety of factors for clinicians to consider, ranging from the type of injury and the specific patient situation, when developing a treatment plan. Ongoing research into biologic therapies, such as PRP, indicates a promising future with potentially less invasive options with positive results (Loccisano, 2016). Ultimately, successful management of soft tissue injuries hinges on a personalized approach that gives top priority to both healing and functional needs of the patient, providing a solid basis for long-term rehabilitation and quality of life (Figure 4.13).

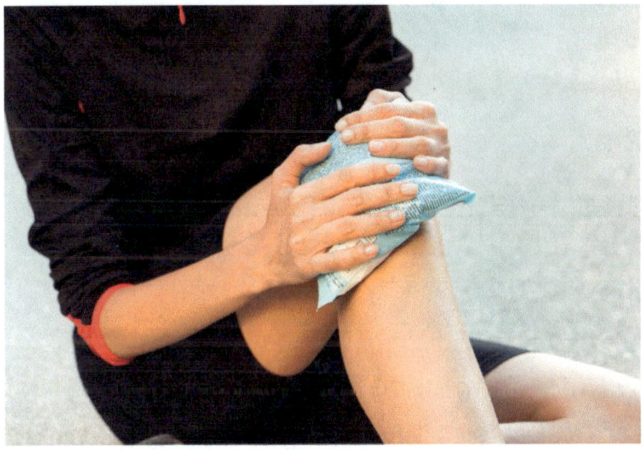

Figure 4.13. The management of soft tissue injuries.

Source: https://milehighspine.com/wp-content/uploads/SoftTissue1.jpg.

4.5.1. Rest, Ice, Compression, Elevation (RICE)

The RICE procedure, consisting of Rest, Ice, Compression, and Elevation, is a major treatment approach for soft tissue injury. Traditionally applied following acute trauma such as sprains and strains, RICE operates to diminish pain, swelling, and further damage to the damaged tissue. Each procedure within the protocol plays an individual role; Rest prevents ongoing strain on the area of injury, and Ice reduces inflammation and has analgesic effects. Clinical practice has long reinforced this strategy as a first response, due to its simplicity and ease of administration. Evidence supports compliance with RICE principles to enhance recovery, with return of function and mitigation of the risk of further injury in athletes and active people. While historically significant, more recent evidence has spawned controversy regarding the effectiveness of the RICE protocol. Certain studies indicate that while RICE can control immediate symptoms effectively, it might not be able to optimally assist the underlying cause of soft tissues. A new sports medicine concept proposes alternatives such as P.E.A.C.E. & L.O.V.E. protocols, which are designed to maximize natural healing without the risk of anti-inflammatory interventions. This shift in emphasis demonstrates a rising recognition of the intricacies of tissue healing and the limitations of RICE as an isolated treatment strategy. In addition, the low level of awareness of these new techniques among athletes only serves to demonstrate the need for education programs about present-day injury management practices, which can significantly influence recovery trajectories. To complement research into the RICE method, the synergy of cold and compression suggests the necessity of therapeutic intervention for soft tissue injury. From the studies, coupling cold with compression has been found to augment the therapeutic reduction of temperature needed for pain relief and reduction of edema. Specifically, more recent studies indicated that traditional ice packs were as effective as newer cold compression units, such as Game Ready. This finding means that while RICE remains an important factor in injury management, research into the integration of new strategies could possibly be able to bring more optimality to recovery outcomes in athletes. With the integration of knowledge from new research, practitioners can better assist athletes with evidence-based practices to manage recovery, which can lead to improved performance and well-being in their sporting careers (McCarthy et al., 2018; Rizvi et al., 2025) (Figure 4.14).

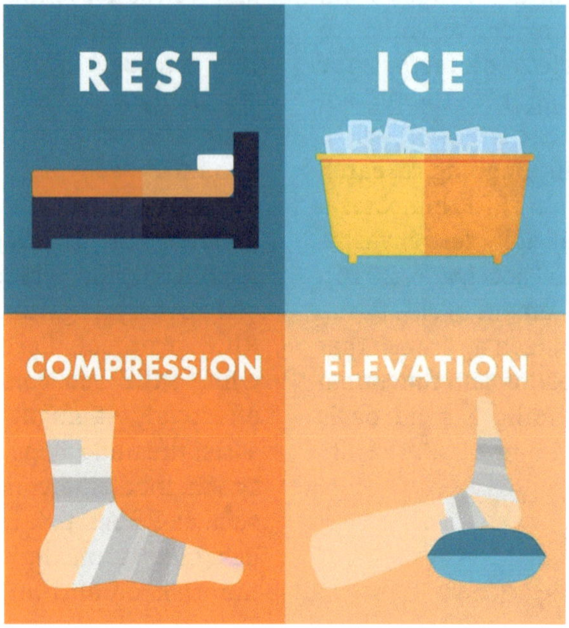

Figure 4.14. Rest, ice, compression, elevation (RICE).

Source: https://www.verywellhealth.com/thmb/ML1jw4V5NleI8om7I7Ipo-uKX5Q=/1500x0/filters:no_upscale():max_bytes(150000):strip_icc()/what-is-rice-190446_FINAL-5bc5fcebc9e77c005135258d.png.

4.5.2. Physical Therapy and Rehabilitation

Effective physical therapy and rehabilitation play a critical role in the management of soft tissue injury, which has a direct influence on an individual's mobility and quality of life. These injuries commonly involve muscles, tendons, ligaments, and fascia, and hence need a comprehensive therapeutic approach. Physical therapists employ a variety of modalities, including manual therapy, exercise prescription, and patient education, to facilitate healing and restore function. A fundamental aspect of rehabilitation is measuring flexibility since impairments in this regard will likely increase the susceptibility to injury. Techniques such as cupping therapy, which have gained popularity for improving flexibility, are increasingly being incorporated into rehabilitation protocols. However, there is a necessity of investigating the efficacy of these treatment techniques in evidence-based practice settings to ascertain their actual value for the group of injured people, particularly in terms of recovery enhancement (Schafer, 2018). Myofascial release is yet another applicable physical therapy technique treating soft tissue injury by focusing on the fascia, a form of connective tissue surrounding muscles and organs. Traditionally considered a passive structure, the fascia is now recognized as an active participant in physiological body function, influencing movement and pain perception. Myofascial release techniques aim to eliminate inhibitions in fascial tissue and enhance its elasticity, with the ultimate outcome being enhanced stability and range of motion. Research has demonstrated the efficacy of these techniques in musculoskeletal pain, a common consequence of soft tissue trauma. With the incorporation of myofascial release in rehab treatment, physical therapists can provide a more holistic treatment that addresses not only certain injuries but also promotes generalized fascial function and health, leading to improved patient outcomes (Hetherington, 2019). The application of a combination of therapeutic modalities underscores physical therapy's adaptability and responsiveness in addressing the complexity of soft tissue trauma. A multimodal treatment approach, often with incorporation of treatment by other healthcare practitioners, ensures that rehabilitation programs are tailored to an individual's needs. For instance, the utilization of modalities like cupping therapy with myofascial release can improve the overall efficacy of treatment by attending to different aspects of soft tissue well-being. Secondly, the inclusion of patient education in rehabilitation facilitates self-management methods, which allow individuals to take an active role in their recovery. Lastly, the overall physical therapy and rehabilitation program not only facilitates the healing process but also informs patients on how to prevent future injury, thereby ensuring long-term physical well-being.

4.5.3. Surgical Interventions

Management of soft tissue injury is often in the form of surgeries, particularly when the injury is extensive or complex. Certain of these surgical options, such as debridement, repair, and reconstruction, are most crucial to restore the structural integrity of injured tissue, reduce the possibility of infection, and provide optimal healing. Deciding to proceed with surgery is often based on factors such as the severity of trauma, whether there is foreign material involved, and the patient's condition. Interestingly, in traumatic cases, where cases present in war settings, the risk of complications—such as invasive fungal infection—can actually push surgery very high. As pointed out in Kronen et al. (2017), surgical debridement is typically identified as the gold standard treatment, highlighting the importance of high-quality surgical practices to facilitate better outcomes for patients with severe soft tissue injury. A proper understanding of the mechanism driving soft tissue injuries is at the core of the need for surgical interventions. Varied injuries, ranging from lacerations to penetrating trauma, differ significantly in their management strategy. For instance, patients presenting with blast trauma or severe limb injury may require a damage control orthopedic strategy, as purported in Ng et al. (2015). This includes aggressive wound care and early stabilization of fractures to prevent secondary complications such as infection or necrosis. Surgical interventions in these scenarios are not just reactive; they are an integral part of a comprehensive treatment strategy focused on optimal recovery with removal of the immediate dangers associated with complicated trauma. Surgical interventions are, more likely than not, multidisciplinary in scope, given the requirement for coordination of specialties to optimize patient management in traumatic contexts. Also, outpatient treatment of soft tissue injuries is normally behind the demands from more severe cases that require surgical intervention. After an initial evaluation, the patient can be placed on a continuum of care that includes rehabilitative therapies, which are invaluable in the prevention of long-term disability and restoration of function. Extensive postoperative planning may be necessary for surgical interventions, as infection risk and patient mobility are important factors to consider. For example, a study by Kronen et al. (2017) reveals that patients who undergo surgical debridement for invasive fungal infection following trauma face an elevated risk, including amputation risk and delayed healing, highlighting the complexity of surgical decision-making. Thus, effective surgical management of soft tissue trauma not only entails direct repair but also requires an assessment of each patient's specific risk factors and ability to recuperate and ultimately affects long-term outcomes of surgical intervention in such patients (Figure 4.15).

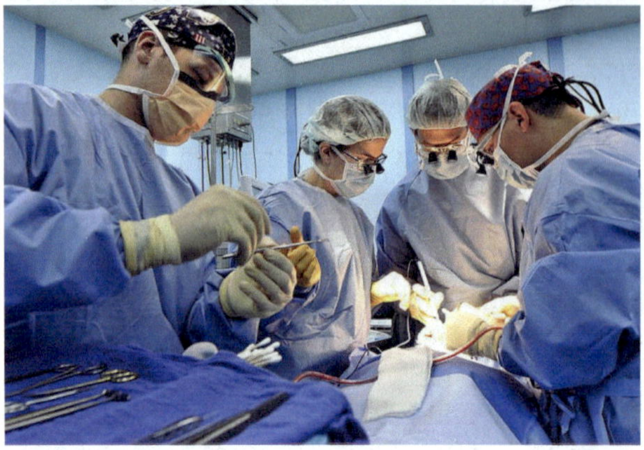

Figure 4.15. Surgical interventions.

Source: https://bonesmart.org/wp-content/uploads/2010/10/bonesmart_image_articles_knee_surgical_interventions_1024x680.jpg.

4.6. Prevention of Soft Tissue Injuries

Prevention of soft tissue injury is the most important for athletes and active players who aim to maximize performance and minimize recovery time. Prevention of injury must include a general strategy to training, warm-up protocols, and training in injury awareness. Effective training programs must emphasize progressive overload, where individuals can progressively develop their physical requirements to prevent overloading of the musculoskeletal system. A systematic method to a warm-up can effectively condition muscles and connective tissue for use, enhancing blood circulation and flexibility and prevention against strains or sprains. Furthermore, the education of coaches and players about common factors of risk and warning signs that lead to injury can result in the early stages of intervention, ultimately fostering a culture of safety and prevention of injury in training environments. Beyond training and equipment, equipment and protective equipment cannot be forgotten when considering prevention from soft tissue injuries. Good footwear, for instance, can make a great difference in altering risk factors associated with particular actions. Sport shoes facilitate the support and traction that are required to maintain balance, in addition to distributing excessive stress on the body. Protective bracing and padding may also enhance safety in high-contact sports by spreading shock and preventing hyperextension or over-torsion of the limb joints. Nonetheless, it is crucial to check the fitness of such equipment regularly so that it remains safe, since faulty gear cannot always offer adequate protection. By ensuring that athletes utilize the appropriate equipment, sporting bodies can do their best to minimize the incidence of soft tissue injury among them. Lastly, rehabilitation and recovery protocols are also vital to avoiding recurrent soft tissue injury. Adopting a regular regime of strengthening exercises and flexibility exercises as an athlete's norm not only helps in the recovery process but also makes the body more resilient against future injury. Alternating active recovery techniques with and without rest can enable healing without loss of gains. Furthermore, application of evidence-based prevention programs for injuries, such as addressing specific biomechanical issues, can be very rewarding. For example, teaching movement patterns and core stability, which are optimal, can improve resistance to injury. These prevention methods call for interdisciplinary collaboration between physical therapists, coaches, and athletic players to construct individualized schemes that efficiently treat individualized needs and provide a platform for long-term prevention (Meyers et al., 2012; Aber, 2016).

4.6.1. Proper Warm-Up and Stretching Techniques

The significance of proper warm-up exercises before exercise cannot be stressed enough, as it is essential to bring about flexibility and reduce the risk of soft tissue injury. A good warm-up goes in stages that typically consist of low-intensity aerobic activity and dynamic stretching. The initial stage enhances circulation to muscles and increases total body temperature, preparing the cardiovascular and musculoskeletal systems for more demanding work. Evidence also indicates that involvement in warm-up regimens, such as foam rolling and aerobic cycling, greatly increases flexibility compared to a control group withholding such actions. Participants also evidenced greater sit-and-reach flexibility after foam rolling warm-ups, further indicating its capacity to mitigate risk of injury related to high-performance events (Bushong, 2011). Thus, an understanding and application of appropriate warm-up protocols is critical to the injury prevention mechanism in physical conditioning. Stretching, when employed as part of a warm-up regimen, represents a critical mechanism for enhancing muscle flexibility and overall physical function.

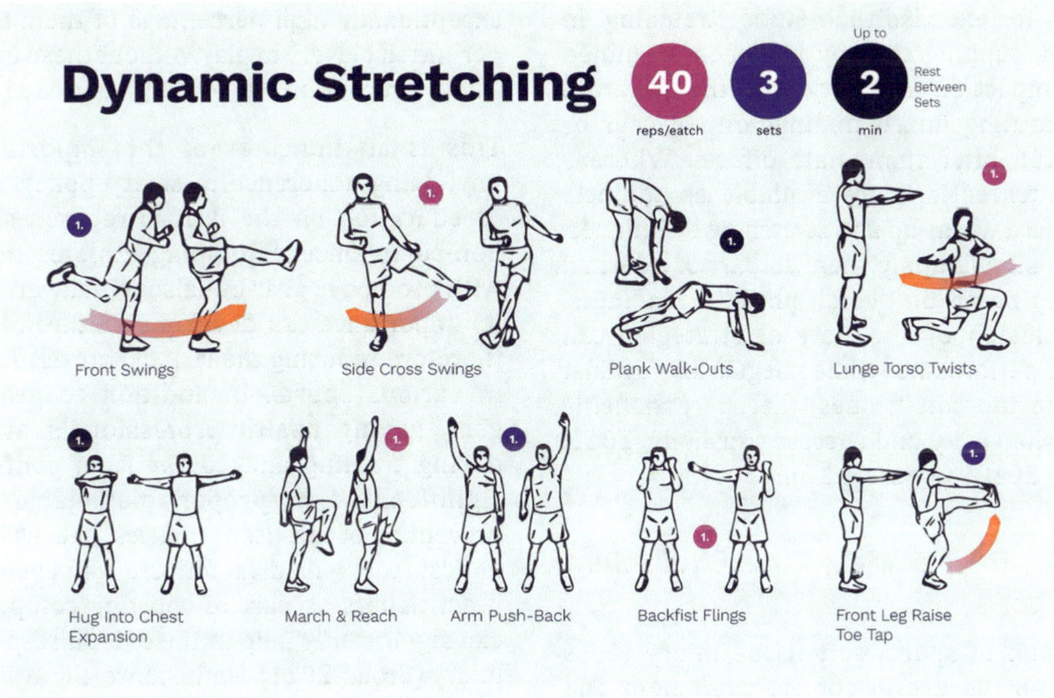

Figure 4.16. The significance of proper warm-up techniques before physical activity cannot be overstated.

Source: https://external-content.duckduckgo.com/iu/?u=http%3A%2F%2Fhealthandbeautystuff.com%2Fwp-content%2Fuploads%2Fdynamic-stretching-exercise.png&f=1&nofb=1&ipt=01316cafa1b492cb405d502eec5db38e5ebe05237dd58bbb72deb3be795bb939.

Static and dynamic methods of stretching are involved in the elongation of muscle fibers, with therapeutic effects upon the range of motion and reduced muscle stiffness. Current literature highlights the use of a combination of such methods as superior to each in isolation, and the requirement for an overall flexibility training program. While static stretching has long been viewed as being useful in the recovery stages after exercise, it now appears that it is critical before athletic competition in the form of dynamic stretching. By effectively conditioning muscles through directed movements, dynamic stretching primes the body to accommodate the stress of intense action, thereby reducing the risk of tears or strains (Schafer, 2018). Therefore, incorporating diverse stretching methods in warm-ups can be beneficial in minimizing soft tissue injury. The role of advanced techniques such as foam rolling and cupping therapy has been questioned in the context of warm-up and injury prevention. Foam rolling, a new method of self-myofascial release, has been shown to improve flexibility and decrease muscle stiffness before exercise. The modality is suggested to increase the range of motion and possibly more effectively prepare muscles for exercise than static stretching. In addition, cupping therapy has been examined for its impact on flexibility, with the literature demonstrating mixed findings on whether or not it can offer immediate effects. Whereas these interventions are available as adjuncts to standard warm-up and stretching techniques, athletes should apply them as part of a formal warm-up based on overall physical readiness. The inclusion of a variety of strategies can enhance performance while safeguarding against injury to the soft tissues, thereby enhancing athletic longevity and success (Bushong, 2011; Schafer, 2018) (Figure 4.16).

4.6.2. Use of Appropriate Equipment and Gear

Prevention of sports soft tissue injury relies mainly on the use of correct equipment and protective gear. This can be observed in various sporting scenarios, where the utilization of specialized gear reduces injury potential. In sports involving contact, the utilization of mouth guards serves a basic role. Research confirms that mouth protection is able to decrease notably the incidence of dental trauma, and thus the importance of using such gear to enhance athletes' oral health (Broad, 2011). Moreover, access to proper headgear and padded apparel can also able to reduce impacts and abrasions, which are common in sports that involve physical contact. Wearing properly fitted protective equipment regularly is not just a protective health approach but also an organizational policy in the majority of sporting organizations, prioritizing a collective responsibility for players' safety. In addition, a multi-component approach towards the proper equipment involves not just the reduction of hazards but also prompting conformity among players. Protective equipment rules significantly influence players' actions on training and match days. A Scottish Rugby Union club research study found that although most clubs had a policy or guided the utilization of mouth protectors, an exceptionally high percentage of them actually permitted players to play without these essential safety precautions in place (Broad, 2011).

This is an indicator of the importance of unyielding adherence to safety policy, as well as education on the drastic repercussions of non-compliance. Equipping athletes not only with protective gear but also with awareness of its importance can develop a culture of safety, therefore reducing the risk of soft tissue injury in various sports. In addition to protective gear, having health professionals available during training and competition contributes significantly to proper management and prevention of soft tissue injuries. The availability of first aiders, medical officers, and even dental practitioners as part of sporting competitions can significantly help in the overall response to injury (Broad, 2011). For instance, the availability of professional personnel can facilitate early examination and treatment, something crucial in avoiding long-term damage associated with soft tissue injuries. Sporting organizations need to attend not just to the provision of protective gear but also to the readiness of medical staff at practice sessions and games.

Through this double-barreled approach of conditioning players physically and being present professionally, the occurrence of soft tissue injuries can be significantly reduced, registering an holistic approach to player safety.

4.6.3. Education on Body Mechanics and Ergonomics

Education on body mechanics and ergonomics is significant in the prevention of soft tissue injuries, particularly in environments of repetitive motion or prolonged posture, such as in the office setting. Education in these areas equips one with knowledge that enables one to acquire proper ways of doing things in a manner that maximizes physical positioning and reduces unnecessary stress to muscles and ligaments. For instance, training laborers to arrange their workstations in a way that enhances their posture causes huge reductions in the occurrence of musculoskeletal disorders. Not only does this prevention establish a safer workplace, but it also increases productivity since workers experience less pain and fatigue in the long term. Therefore, incorporation of ergonomic discipline into regular training enhances the alertness of employees and encourages individuals to actively participate in healthcare, a clear indication of the linkage between education, mechanistic experience, and injury prevention. Incorporation of well-structured ergonomics training demonstrates the true benefits that derive from educated intervention procedures. A successful ergonomics program, with effective implementation, can effectively minimize the occurrence of soft tissue injury, as observed through various studies. These interventions typically involve surveying employees' workspaces, identifying factors of injury risk, and training employees on appropriate body mechanics during tasks such as lifting, typing, and sitting. Moreover, according to the literature, the training instills the practice of regular training to reinforce best practices and adapt to developing workplace challenges. Among the key findings is that an educated workforce is more likely to regulate itself and maximize its work habits, which could significantly account for the overall health and work performance. This reflective learning process promotes safety and health culture and is hence critical in companies that aim to prevent soft tissue injury. It can lead to considerable long-term benefits for employees as well as employers. These actions not only reduce the rate of accidents resulting in soft tissue injuries but also reduce workers' compensation costs by substantial amounts. Reframing the importance of ergonomics, public awareness campaigns can debunk myths surrounding office work, showing that even sitting tasks have potential for musculoskeletal disorders. As cited in literature, an effective program commonly includes approaches that make provision for adapting workspaces and tasks to ergonomic principles, hence fostering an adaptive work culture. Through the empowerment of employees with the information and resources needed to recognize and remove risks, organizations can create an environment supportive of health and efficiency. Lastly, the synergy of body mechanic education and ergonomics is a foundation of the elimination of soft tissue injury and of occupational health and safety in general (Figure 4.17).

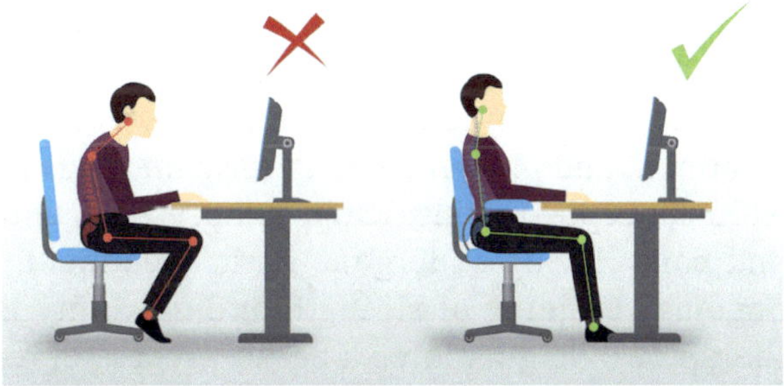

Figure 4.17. Education on body mechanics and ergonomics.

Source: https://ptclinic.com/img/photos/ergonomics-computer.png.

SUMMARY

In conclusion, soft tissue injury research exhibits a multifaceted problem that not only encompasses the physical impacts but extends to the socioeconomic problems of such injuries. Soft tissue injuries among certain populations, such as young adults involved in road traffic accidents, pose an important target for public health intervention. Evidence confirms that the majority of oral and maxillofacial injuries are precipitated by such accidents, thereby supporting increased regulation of security measures and enforcement of law to arrest transportation-induced risk. These findings from research confirm the call for stakeholders like policymakers and health authorities to address the causes of these injuries with speed, particularly among high-risk groups (Kileo, 2012). Furthermore, the results after treatment of soft tissue injuries call attention to the significance of efficient and timely medical interventions. The evidence suggests that the utilization of proper medical treatments on time, such as surgical debridement and wound therapy, enhances recovery patterns to a great extent. Notably, patients with severe presentations develop complications, including infection, which prolong healing time and necessitate more medical intervention. The need for comprehensive management plans with pain management and rehabilitation services becomes a prominent conclusion from the literature, further highlighting that an integrated approach is necessary to ensure optimal patient outcomes. Management of such complexities not only benefits individual health but also assists in reducing the overall burden of healthcare in coping with the same injuries (Schafer, 2018). Lastly, the therapeutic potential of novel therapeutic modalities such as cupping therapy for the healing of soft tissue injury needs further clarification. Ancient treatments have gained appeal in modern treatment paradigms, but the scientific rationale behind their clinical value is conflicting. Current research indicates that its application may not be followed by significant increases in flexibility in healthy individuals, which may necessitate a reevaluation of its value in injury recovery. Hence, further research is needed to elucidate the potential benefits of integrative treatments in rehabilitation, and thus, the necessity of further studies into alternative treatment approaches that augment standard care. Emphasizing a multidimensional system with evidence-based practice will ultimately enhance the effectiveness of treatment for soft tissue injury, thus advancing the practice of orthopedic medicine and enhancing patient treatment (Schafer, 2018).

Proper treatment and prevention of soft tissue injuries are most crucial for full recovery and recurrence prevention. A combination treatment is most typically most successful, with both instant treatment and preventive long-term methods being emphasized. Treatment typically adheres to the RICE concept—resting, icing, compressing, and elevating—and aids in preventing further swelling and pain. Having undergone initial treatment, conducting rehabilitation exercises that emphasize ongoing regaining of strength and flexibility is most critical. Additionally, incorporating physical therapy would guarantee a better process of recovery, particularly for those suffering from chronic symptoms following an injury. The holistic approach treats not only the short-term symptoms but also the basis for long-term recovery. In the case of prevention efforts, determining the particular risk factors for soft tissue injury in its entirety would be vital. Research has highlighted that reserve troops, for instance, may have a greater prevalence of injury due to lower physical fitness than their full-time counterparts (Schram et al., 2018). The application of personalized conditioning programs can hence effectively minimize the occurrence of injuries. Training in correct techniques and body mechanics for activities such as combat training and exercise is also equally significant. Furthermore, pre-participation testing and strength assessments can identify individuals at higher risk and enable tailor-made prevention procedures to be established. Furthermore, certain injury types, such as Medial Tibial Stress Syndrome (MTSS), put the utmost importance on appropriate preventative actions, claiming that preventative measures before injury may be more beneficial than treatments post-injury (Yamasaki, 2019). This underlines the necessity for a shift of focus towards preventive initiatives, including progressive progressive exacerbation of training, appropriate footwear, and cross-training modalities to assist in reducing repetitive strain. Research into less conventional forms of treatment, such as biomechanical assessment and individually tailored training schemes, also indicates a shifting injury management environment. Therefore, the coordination of preventive and treatment protocols on an integrated basis will significantly help in the control of soft tissue injury, ensuring better results for the victims.

CLOSER LOOK

SPRAIN

A sprain is a common musculoskeletal injury that occurs when a ligament, the strong band of tissue connecting bones at a joint, is stretched or torn. Sprains typically result from sudden twisting movements, falls, sports activities, or accidents that force a joint beyond its normal range of motion. The most frequently affected areas include the ankle, wrist, knee, and thumb. Sprains are classified into three grades based on severity. Grade I involves mild stretching of the ligament with slight pain and swelling. Grade II includes partial tearing, leading to moderate pain, swelling, bruising, and limited joint movement. Grade III is a complete ligament tear, causing severe pain, significant swelling, instability, and loss of joint function. Common symptoms of sprains include pain, swelling, bruising, tenderness, and difficulty moving the affected joint. Diagnosis is based on physical examination and may involve imaging tests such as X-rays or MRI to rule out fractures and assess ligament damage. Initial treatment follows the RICE principle: Rest, Ice, Compression, and Elevation. Pain relievers, braces, and physiotherapy are often used to support healing.

Rehabilitation exercises help restore strength, flexibility, and stability, reducing the risk of re-injury. Preventive measures include proper warm-up, stretching, use of protective gear, and maintaining good muscle strength and balance. With appropriate care, most sprains heal fully, allowing individuals to safely return to normal activities.

REFERENCES

1. Aber, R. (2016). Improving health literacy: Parental medical decisions regarding lower extremity amputations. https://core.ac.uk/download/84402968.pdf (accessed on 26th June 2025).
2. Marini, L., Rojas, M. A., Sahrmann, P., Aghazada, R., & Pilloni, A. (2018). Early Wound Healing Score: a system to evaluate the early healing of periodontal soft tissue wounds. *Journal of periodontal & implant science*, *48*(5), 274–283. https://doi.org/10.5051/jpis.2018.48.5.274c(accessed on 26th June 2025).
3. Ali, P., Santy-Tomlinson, J., & Watson, R. (2014). Assessment and diagnosis of acute limb compartment syndrome: A literature review. https://core.ac.uk/download/151161255.pdf (accessed on 26th June 2025).
4. Ameis, A., Brown, C., Carroll, L. J., Cox (Dresser), D., et al. (2015). The effectiveness of passive physical modalities for the management of soft tissue injuries and neuropathies of the wrist and hand: A systematic review by the Ontario Protocol for Traffic Injury Management (OPTIMa) Collaboration. https://core.ac.uk/download/pdf/82645232.pdf (accessed on 26th June 2025).
5. Biz, C., Angelini, A., Zamperetti, M., Marzotto, F., Sperotto, S. P., Carniel, D., Iacobellis, C., & Ruggieri, P. (2018). Medium-Long-Term Radiographic and Clinical Outcomes after Surgical Treatment of Intra-Articular Tibial Pilon Fractures by Three Different Techniques. *BioMed research international*, *2018*, 6054021. https://doi.org/10.1155/2018/6054021(accessed on 26th June 2025).
6. Aoude, G. Y. (2013). Mouthguards for contact sports: Current state of use. https://open.bu.edu/bitstream/2144/12045/6/Aoude_George_2013_nosig_nocv.pdf (accessed on 26th June 2025).
7. Araujo Azcue, A. F., Renteria, J. M. M., Chang, E. O., Bonilla, S. Y. H., Lopez, R. L. R. L. Y., & Vitelly, J. A. U. (2025). Violence in our country as a public health issue, prevalence of facial trauma at the hospital general de Mexico from 2020-2024. *International Journal of Research in Medical Sciences*, *13*(2), 669–672. https://doi.org/10.18203/2320-6012.ijrms20250235(accessed on 26th June 2025).
8. Rizvi, A., Fatima, T., Khan, W., Asthana, S., & Naqvi, Z. A. (2025). Holistic approach to managing acute soft tissue injury: PEACE and LOVE protocol-observational research. *International Journal of Research in Orthopaedics*, *11*(3), 530–534. https://doi.org/10.18203/issn.2455-4510.IntJResOrthop20251129(accessed on 26th June 2025).
9. Beeson P. (2014). Plantar fasciopathy: revisiting the risk factors. *Foot and ankle surgery : official journal of the European Society of Foot and Ankle Surgeons*, *20*(3), 160–165. https://doi.org/10.1016/j.fas.2014.03.003(accessed on 26th June 2025).
10. Banning, M. (2008). Topical diclofenac: Clinical effectiveness and current uses in osteoarthritis of the knee and soft tissue injuries. https://core.ac.uk/download/335727.pdf (accessed on 26th June 2025).
11. Kronen, R., Liang, S. Y., Bochicchio, G., Bochicchio, K., Powderly, W. G., & Spec, A. (2017). Invasive Fungal Infections Secondary to Traumatic Injury. *International journal of infectious diseases : IJID : official publication of the International Society for Infectious Diseases*, *62*, 102–111. https://doi.org/10.1016/j.ijid.2017.07.002(accessed on 26th June 2025).
12. Ng, C., Mifsud, M., Borg, J. N., & Mizzi, C. (2015). The Libyan civil conflict: selected case series of orthopaedic trauma managed in Malta in 2014. *Scandinavian journal of trauma,*

resuscitation and emergency medicine, 23, 103. https://doi.org/10.1186/s13049-015-0183-2(accessed on 26th June 2025).

13. Brantigan, O. C., Ikuma, H., Insall, J. N., Krackow, K. A., Miyasaka, K. C., Saragaglia, D., van Damme, G., et al. (2012). Standardizing the clinical assessment of coronal knee laxity. https://core.ac.uk/download/9039947.pdf (accessed on 26th June 2025).
14. Broad, M. T. (2011). Mouth protectors in junior rugby in Scotland. https://core.ac.uk/download/370584.pdf (accessed on 26th June 2025).
15. Bushong, J. R. (2011). Foam rolling as a warm-up: The effect on lower extremity flexibility compared to aerobic and stretching protocols. https://core.ac.uk/download/84119765.pdf (accessed on 26th June 2025).
16. Ma C, Chadha AN, Wu C, Giannoudis PV, Guo JJ. Is There a Role of Photoacoustic Imaging in Sports Medicine: Evidence Today. *Orthop Surg*. 2025;17(6):1589-1603. doi:10.1111/os.70031(accessed on 26th June 2025).
17. McArthur, K., Jorgensen, D., Climstein, M., & Furness, J. (2020). Epidemiology of Acute Injuries in Surfing: Type, Location, Mechanism, Severity, and Incidence: A Systematic Review. *Sports (Basel, Switzerland)*, *8*(2), 25. https://doi.org/10.3390/sports8020025(accessed on 26th June 2025).
18. Sheen, A. J., Stephenson, B. M., Lloyd, D. M., Robinson, P., Fevre, D., Paajanen, H., de Beaux, A., Kingsnorth, A., Gilmore, O. J., Bennett, D., Maclennan, I., O'Dwyer, P., Sanders, D., & Kurzer, M. (2014). 'Treatment of the sportsman's groin': British Hernia Society's 2014 position statement based on the Manchester Consensus Conference. *British journal of sports medicine*, *48*(14), 1079–1087. https://doi.org/10.1136/bjsports-2013-092872(accessed on 26th June 2025).
19. Lee SW, Nguyen D, Mack D, Aguila E, Thomas M, Doddy K. Conservative Management of Low Back Pain. *HCA Healthc J Med*. 2021;2(5):319-328. Published 2021 Oct 29. doi:10.36518/2689-0216.1261 (accessed on 26th June 2025).
20. Meyers, W. C., Yoo, E., Devon, O. N., Jain, N., Horner, M., Lauencin, C., & Zoga, A. (2012). Understanding "Sports Hernia" (Athletic Pubalgia): The Anatomic and Pathophysiologic Basis for Abdominal and Groin Pain in Athletes. Operative Techniques in Sports Medicine, 20(1), 33–45. https://doi.org/10.1053/j.otsm.2012.03.005 (accessed on 26th June 2025).
21. Schram B, Orr R, Pope R. A Profile of Knee Injuries Suffered by Australian Army Reserve Soldiers. *Int J Environ Res Public Health*. 2018;16(1):12. Published 2018 Dec 20. doi:10.3390/ijerph16010012(accessed on 26th June 2025).
22. Donya, M., Radford, M., ElGuindy, A., Firmin, D., & Yacoub, M. H. (2014). Radiation in medicine: Origins, risks and aspirations. *Global cardiology science & practice, 2014*(4), 437–448. https://doi.org/10.5339/gcsp.2014.57 (accessed on 26th June 2025).
23. Hertel, J., & Corbett, R. O. (2019). An updated model of chronic ankle instability. *Journal of Athletic Training, 54*, 572–588. https://doi.org/10.4085/1062-6050-344-18 (accessed on 26th June 2025).
24. Hetherington, C. S. (2019). Myofascial release. https://core.ac.uk/download/289198166.pdf (accessed on 26th June 2025).
25. James, J. (2022). How diversity, equity, inclusion and belonging impacts student recruitment and admission practices within education: An examination of the Department of Occupational

Therapy at Western New England University. https://core.ac.uk/download/619720949.pdf (accessed on 26th June 2025).

26. Kileo, B. F. (2012). The pattern of oral and maxillofacial injuries among patients attending Muhimbili National Hospital, Dar es Salaam, Tanzania. https://core.ac.uk/download/pdf/11307821.pdf (accessed on 26th June 2025).

27. LeBoff, M. S., Greenspan, S. L., Insogna, K., Lewiecki, E. M., Saag, K. G., Singer, A., & Siris, E. S. (2022). The clinician's guide to prevention and treatment of osteoporosis. *Osteoporosis International, 33*, 2049–2102. https://doi.org/10.1007/s00198-021-05900-y (accessed on 26th June 2025).

28. Loccisano, A. (2016). Platelet-rich plasma for the treatment of partial rotator cuff tears. https://open.bu.edu/bitstream/2144/14355/9/Loccisano_bu_0017N_10415.pdf (accessed on 26th June 2025).

29. McCarthy, M. S. (2018). Determining skin temperature differences between three cold compression modalities. https://core.ac.uk/download/267589271.pdf (accessed on 26th June 2025).

30. McSweeney, S. E., Naraghi, A., Salonen, D., Theodoropoulos, J., & White, L. M. (2012). Hip and groin pain in the professional athlete. *Canadian Association of Radiologists journal = Journal l'Association canadienne des radiologistes, 63*(2), 87–99. https://doi.org/10.1016/j.carj.2010.11.001 (accessed on 26th June 2025).

31. Olson, H. (2016). Diagnosis and conservative chiropractic care of chronic idiopathic pudendal nerve entrapment causing saddle-like paresthesia and restless genital syndrome: A case study. *Journal of Spine, 2016*, 1–4. https://www.semanticscholar.org/paper/a8e0996088c7417858ed3f83f67d0bbf7705434c (accessed on 26th June 2025).

32. Sabharwal, S., & Sabharwal, S. (2018). Growth plate injuries of the lower extremity: Case examples and lessons learned. https://core.ac.uk/download/305124253.pdf (accessed on 26th June 2025).

33. Schafer, M. (2018). The acute effects of cupping therapy on hamstring range of motion compared to sham. https://digitalscholarship.unlv.edu/cgi/viewcontent.cgi?article=4327&context=thesesdissertations (accessed on 26th June 2025).

34. Siddiqui, I. J., Probst, J., Mahadevan, S., Desronvilles, R. J., & Dineen, K. J. (2025). Treating external anal sphincter injury with platelet-rich plasma to resolve post-partum fecal incontinence caused by birthing trauma: A case report. *Journal of Case Reports and Images in Obstetrics and Gynecology*. https://www.semanticscholar.org/paper/12e89c0863818512c9173fbf3cdfd2f5c3efa758 (accessed on 26th June 2025).

35. Van der Westhuizen, G. (2009). Quad bike injuries and injury prevention opportunities. https://core.ac.uk/download/185400142.pdf (accessed on 26th June 2025).

36. Vassallo, K. (2008). Shoulder pain in general practice. https://core.ac.uk/download/46602184.pdf (accessed on 26th June 2025).

37. Yamasaki, S. (2019). A review of the treatment and prevention options for medial tibial stress syndrome. https://core.ac.uk/download/213464302.pdf (accessed on 26th June 2025).

38. Zhou, X. (2024). Radiologic diagnosis and differential diagnosis of traumatic fractures. https://core.ac.uk/download/617192030.pdf (accessed on 26th June 2025).

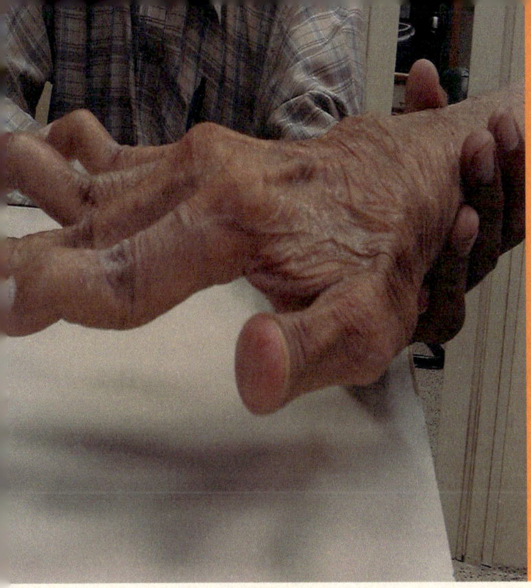

Chapter 5
ORTHOPEDIC CONDITIONS

Contents

Introduction 137
5.1. Osteoarthritis 140
5.2. Rheumatoid Arthritis 144
5.3. Fractures 148
5.4. Tendonitis 152
5.5. Bursitis 156
5.6. Sports Injuries 160
Summary 164
References 167

Introduction

Orthopedic disorders comprise a broad range of conditions that lead to musculoskeletal system disorders, including bones, joints, ligaments, tendons, and muscles. The disorders can arise as a result of various reasons, like trauma, degenerative disorders, infections, or congenital defects. Fractures, osteoarthritis, rheumatoid arthritis, and tendinitis are some of the common disorders that can have a significant impact on the mobility and quality of life of a patient.

In these situations, it is significant to observe the basic role that diagnoses play in determining the proper treatment options. Preemptive diagnosis and proper diagnosis can prevent complications and provide early intervention that will enhance pain management as well as restore function. In addition, with increases in medical technology, the diagnosis of orthopedic diseases has become more proficient, enabling more individualized methods of treatment to be used based on the specific needs of each patient and therefore leading to a general improvement in orthopedic care outcomes.

Orthopedic conditions are sometimes treated with a multidisciplinary treatment plan involving orthopedic surgeons, physical therapists, and pain management professionals. Treatment methodologies can vary significantly, ranging from conservative treatment, such as medication and physical therapy, to surgical intervention, depending on the nature and severity of the condition. Conservative and surgical treatments share identical objectives, such as pain relief, enhanced function, and improvement in the quality of life in patients. Rehabilitation is also an important step following treatment, particularly in surgical patients, because recovery of strength and movement depends upon it.

An understanding of the specifics of these treatments is of utmost significance to healthcare professionals, as each patient's response can differ dramatically depending upon such specifics as age, general health, and the nature of the orthopedic condition. New technologies like 3D printing are beginning to revolutionize the orthopedic field by enabling new methods of creating patient-specific models and implants. This technology not only improves the precision of surgical procedures but also allows for enhanced preoperative planning, which is important in complex cases. With 3D printing, it offers surgeons accurate replicas of anatomy, which gives them a better knowledge of the patient's own anatomy, thus resulting in improved surgical outcomes.

Aside from this, these technologies hold much in store for the future of orthopedic treatment since they usher in the possibility of individualized implants and, in the not-so-distant future, even 3D-printed organs that could be used to treat complicated musculoskeletal disorders. And as the technology develops further, such integration will also enhance the treatment of orthopedic disease further, as per ongoing trends toward personalized medicine and innovative solutions to patient care.

Definition and Scope of Orthopedics

Orthopedics is a branch of medicine that involves the diagnosis, treatment, and prevention of diseases that are linked to the musculoskeletal system, such as bones, joints, ligaments, muscles, and nerves. One of the unique characteristics of orthopedics is that it is a multidisciplinary field since specialists apply various approaches, from traditional surgery to innovative technologies such as arthroscopy and minimally invasive procedures. The frontiers of this specialty have expanded significantly in the last few years to encompass the most recent innovations, like the augmented and virtual reality systems that increase the accuracy of surgeries and training. The innovations have not only improved surgical results but also extended the avenues through which patients receive care, offering orthopedics as an evolving specialty responsive to progress in medical technologies as well as patient requirements. Also, the use of artificial intelligence (AI) in orthopedics represents a groundbreaking shift in research and clinical application. The ability of AI to analyze vast amounts of data and enhance diagnostic accuracy is particularly pertinent when handling musculoskeletal injuries and diseases. By employing machine learning algorithms, clinicians are able to more accurately predict patient outcomes and individualize treatment regimens, and thereby optimize overall patient care. Use of AI also addresses pressing concerns in the healthcare field, such as optimizing surgical procedures and decision-making. However, effective implementation of AI towards orthopedics necessitates a good understanding of potential biases and ensuring human oversight to ensure safety and ethics, hinting at increasing sophistication in this respect. The training aspect of orthopedics is equally important since ongoing development and innovation in technologies greatly affect practitioners' ability. Surgeons are required to know new tools and techniques, and therefore, it is imperative that broad-based training programs incorporate virtual reality in order to enhance spatial awareness and confidence in surgery. This focus on learning brings a culture of continuous development, enabling professionals to meet the rapidly changing nature of orthopedics. Because the frontiers of this specialty continue to expand, the intersection of novel training models and leading-edge technologies positions orthopedics at the forefront of medical specialties, ultimately resulting in improving the quality of care rendered to patients suffering from varied musculoskeletal diseases.

Importance of Studying Orthopedic Conditions

The significance of learning about orthopedic conditions goes well beyond the simple knowledge of bone and joint disease; it is a complete vision of human function and health. Given that musculoskeletal disorders are a leading cause of disability worldwide, they take a considerable toll on people's quality of life as well as on national productivity. The study of these conditions not only facilitates the development of successful therapies but also the development of preventive measures for the reduction of incidence rates. Moreover, due to the aging population, age-dependent orthopedic diseases such as osteoarthritis become more prevalent, and as such, there is an urgent need for research as well as education in the area. By empowering healthcare professionals through intensive education, learning about orthopedic conditions ultimately leads to improved patient outcomes as well as superior healthcare systems. Moreover, the interdisciplinary nature of learning about orthopedic conditions emphasizes its applicability across a range of disciplines, including biomechanics, rehabilitation, and emergency medicine. Innovative developments in each of these fields contribute meaningfully to our understanding and the management of musculoskeletal disorders. For instance, the novel consensus on management of intra-abdominal hypertension and abdominal compartment syndrome is an answer to growing awareness regarding the complexities of handling orthopedic emergencies and presenting the need for precise diagnosis and high-profile treatment protocols for high-risk patients. Such interdisciplinarity encourages the development of combined treatment protocols that can address the multidimensionality of orthopedic issues and ensure better functional recovery and quality of life for the patient. In addition, studying some of the orthopedic disorders, such as hereditary multiple exostosis (HME), draws attention to orthopedic genetics and tailored treatment. The case of a 28-year-old female nurse with HME illustrates that heterogeneous symptoms need an individual approach to management and rehabilitation by means of orthopedists and physiotherapists. This example not only shows the heterogeneity of orthopedic diseases but also emphasizes the importance of making healthcare professionals aware of such rare diseases. Increased awareness means early diagnosis and improved therapeutic regimens, ultimately leading to improved patient satisfaction and outcomes. As more findings arise in orthopedic diseases, the importance of systematic education in this field becomes more obvious, to the benefit of professionals and their clients alike.

Overview of Common Orthopedic Conditions

Orthopedic conditions are a very wide spectrum of musculoskeletal issues, greatly impacting one's mobility and overall lifestyle. Osteoarthritis, rheumatoid arthritis, fractures, and tendon injuries are some of the most prevalent orthopedic conditions, each with its own difficulties for healthcare professionals as well as patients. Osteoarthritis, in the majority of instances, results from cartilage loss, leading to long-standing pain and stiffness, particularly of weight-bearing joints. On the other hand, rheumatoid arthritis is an autoimmune disorder that causes joint inflammation, which may result in permanent joint damage. Knowledge of the individual presentation and ramifications of such diseases is most crucial to orthopedic physiotherapy since it influences the selection of appropriate remedial interventions based on specific situations. Fractures are a prevalent orthopedic condition, with their impact varying significantly by age and activity level. For instance, hip fractures are common among the elderly and can potentially lead to significant morbidity and additional healthcare costs. Emerging research reports a disturbing deficit of knowledge regarding recovery experiences for younger individuals who sustain such fractures following trivial falls, pointing out the overlooked long-term consequences that follow fractures in this subgroup. Fracture healing is typically a multifaceted process, and thus, requires multidisciplinary treatment, in which orthopedic physiotherapy plays an important role in encouraging the process of rehabilitation and restoration of function. Effective management with physiotherapy can avoid complications, restore motion range, and overall recovery outcomes, and thus make specialized treatment essential in managing common orthopedic conditions like fractures (Janes et al., 2018). Tendinopathies such as tendinitis and rotator cuff tears occur in active patients and older age groups. They are most often due to overuse, repetitive strain, or acute trauma and cause pain and inflammation that may restrict function. The management of tendon injury has evolved, with emphasis on a combination of rest, specific physiotherapy, and strengthening exercises in a progressive manner. Understanding the mechanisms of tendon damage allows physiotherapists to develop optimal treatment plans that support the recovery of movement and pain relief. As additional conditions are unveiled through research, practitioners are optimally placed to apply evidence-based physiotherapy treatments that respond to the needs of patients with such common injuries (Samoy et al., 2016). Lastly, a comprehensive overview of these conditions can enhance patient outcomes as well as the overall quality of physiotherapy practice (Figure 5.1).

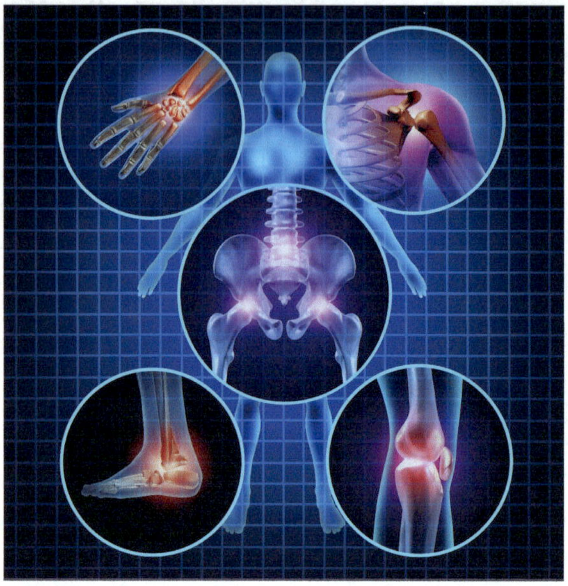

Figure 5.1. Common Orthopedic conditions.

Source: https://images.squarespace-cdn.com/content/v1/65d14a429377d32bcd210237/1708309296801-74SCHF9UTALY5T8OT8T8/GettyImages-497801477.jpg.

5.1. Osteoarthritis

Osteoarthritis (OA) is a degenerative joint disease that predominantly affects elderly individuals and consequently is a frequent complaint in orthopedic physiotherapy. It is characterized by the deterioration of cartilage and subsequent bone loss and typically leads to significant pain and disability, particularly in weight-bearing joints such as the knees and hips. The impacts of these diseases on mobility and quality of life are substantial, and patients frequently experience limitations in physical activity due to related stiffness and pain. They are significant because early diagnosis and conservative management can indeed delay the progression of OA and diminish its disabling effects. In understanding the disease's pathophysiology and what it entails in terms of implications, orthopedic physiotherapists can formulate more efficient intervention strategies that guarantee maximum function and maximization of patients' overall well-being (Lemons et al., 2012). In physiotherapy, the rehabilitation of patients with osteoarthritis is typically centered on strengthening, particularly of the lower extremities. Interventions aimed at strengthening the quadriceps have been shown to significantly enhance patients' functionality and pain alleviation. A pilot study demonstrated that a rehabilitative lower extremity strengthening regimen resulted in marked improvement in quadriceps strength and function in women aged 55 to 65 years with knee OA. Such programs typically include progressive exercises tailored to each patient's ability and joint stability and mobility. These findings illustrate the importance of evidence-based practice in physiotherapy as successful strengthening protocols translate into better control of the condition and enhance the quality of life for OA patients (Lemons et al., 2012). Moreover, the complexity of osteoarthritis also makes a holistic treatment strategy involving education and lifestyle modification, as well as physiotherapy, indispensable. Health professionals must collaborate with patients to maximize adherence to exercise programs and educate them on disease management. Conservative strategies, such as weight control and activity modification, succeed in reducing the effects of osteoarthritis. In addition, early physiotherapy referral has been determined to facilitate early intervention and improve outcomes through effective pain and functional impairment management. With the aging population, an understanding of the subtleties of OA will be essential for healthcare providers to develop patient-specific plans of care that not only manage symptoms but optimize functional capacity and quality of life (Oluchukwu, 2018) (Figure 5.2).

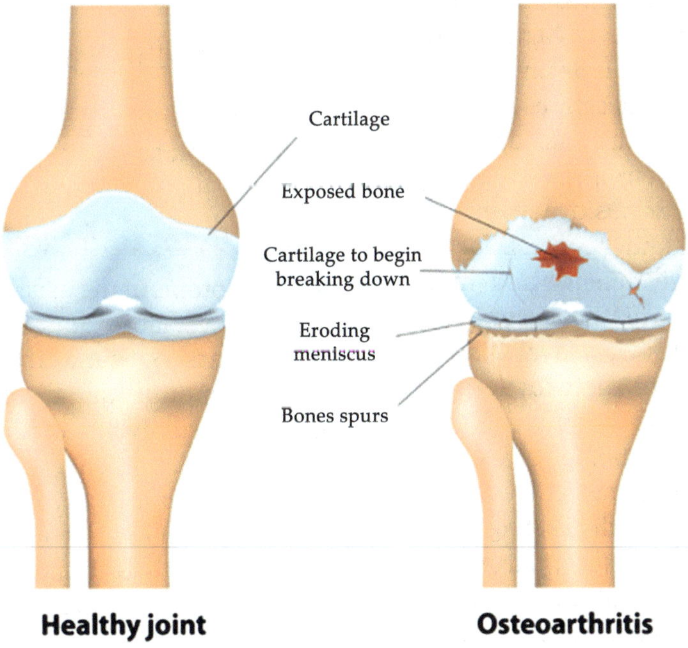

Figure 5.2. Osteoarthritis (OA).

Source: https://novusspinecenter.com/wp-content/uploads/2019/02/osteoarthritis_1500x1386.jpg.

5.1.1. Definition and Causes

Orthopedic disorders constitute a broad category of conditions that affect the bones, joints, ligaments, and tendons. They can be caused by many factors, including acute trauma, chronic disease, and degeneration. Acute trauma typically occurs as a result of injury, such as fractures or ligament tears, often after sudden impacts or repeated stress. Chronic disease, such as osteoarthritis, is caused by prolonged wear and tear, which leads to degeneration of cartilage and overlying tissue. In addition, genetic susceptibility, age-related susceptibility, and lifestyle all contribute predominantly to the causation of these orthopedic issues, which emphasizes their multi-factorial nature of causation. Lifestyle is one of the causative factors for orthopedic disorders and, in particular, is significant when it comes to activity level and ergonomics. Sedentary lifestyle increases the chances of getting ailments such as musculoskeletal disorders, as insecurely positioned joints and weak muscles can lead to injuries while performing even light activities. Conversely, excessive exertion or improper use of technique while exercising can result in acute injuries. Considerations such as ergonomic designing of working environments can avert these risks and also ensure a positive environment to maintain Orthopedics under control. For older adults, the typical bone density and muscle mass loss can exacerbate these conditions, as illustrated in studies with a relationship between age, orthopedic disturbances, and secondary complications (Ponciano et al., 2020). Moreover, the psychological aspect of orthopedic conditions must not be overlooked, for the mind will influence the feeling of pain and the success of rehabilitation. Chronic pain syndromes can lead to debilitating depression and anxiety, once again making it more difficult to rehabilitate. Techniques such as the mind sound resonance technique (MSRT) have been shown to deliver complementary benefits to curing illnesses like ordinary neck pain, aiding not only physical healing but also coping with associated psychological distress (Ebnezar & Ebnezar, 2015). Therefore, the interplay between psychological well-being and physical health must be recognized within Orthopedics management plans, focusing on the necessity of a holistic approach to orthopedic physiotherapy (Figure 5.3).

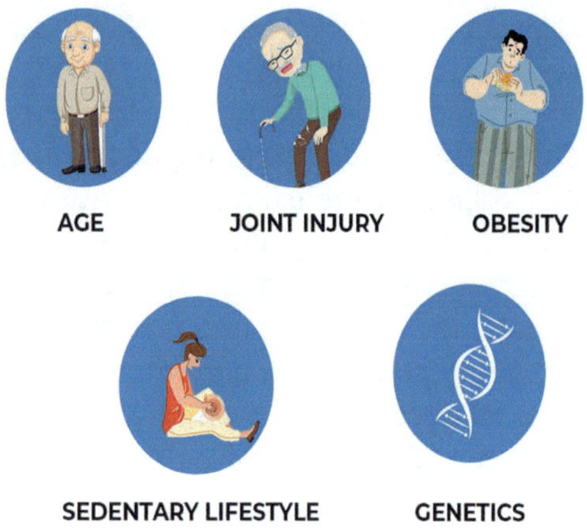

Figure 5.3. Causes of osteoarthritis (OA).

Source: https://mjnaiduhospitals.com/wp-content/uploads/2023/02/07-3.jpg.

5.1.2. Symptoms and Diagnosis

The symptoms of the usual orthopedic conditions may be variable and severe, with common complaints of pain, inflammation, reduced range of motion, and disability. For instance, in lateral epicondylalgia, otherwise referred to as tennis elbow, patients will report episodic pain over the lateral elbow that descends down the forearm. Pain usually aggravates with gripping, lifting, or wrist extension movements. A good understanding of the symptoms is paramount since the symptoms guide clinicians to formulate the right diagnosis. If they are not treated, the progression of these symptoms may lead to chronic pain and significant interference with activities of daily living, stressing the importance of an early and effective management approach. In diagnosing, orthopedic physiotherapy also largely relies on clinical assessment alongside specialty diagnostic procedures to differentiate various orthopedic conditions. The clinician usually employs a blend of patient history, physical assessment, and, in some instances, imaging tests to determine the specific pathology underpinning the patient's symptomology. For instance, the mechanical diagnosis and therapy (MDT) technique, as exemplified by recent case reports, is a systematic process of classifying and treating disorders like lateral epicondylalgia. The process has been successful, as it associates patterns of symptoms with ideal treatment mechanisms. By accurately determining the diagnostic category of conditions such as lateral epicondylalgia, physiotherapists can develop specific therapy interventions to correct the very causes of the patient's pain and dysfunction (Maccio et al., 2016). Effective treatment plans are the result of accurate diagnoses and symptom awareness. Literature finds that employing the MDT strategy is capable of substantially enhancing patient outcomes in lateral epicondylalgia. Patients who receive this therapy not only indicate an immediate reduction of symptoms, but also indicate enhanced functionality within a short course of therapy sessions. The implication of the findings underscores that physiotherapists need to adopt such evidence-based treatments in their professional practice. Overall, the promotion of patient self-management skills also allows patients to become more accountable for their own recovery, illustrating the trend in general orthopedic physiotherapy towards holistic and patient-centered care (Oberlander, 1960).

5.1.3. Physiotherapy Treatment Options

In orthopedic physiotherapy, an array of treatments is used in order to address common disorders in an attempt to provide personalized techniques for individual patient needs. Among these procedures, the function of therapeutic exercise is very important, which enhances strength, flexibility, and endurance, aiding in recovery from injuries such as ligament sprains or fractures. Modality such as ultrasound and electrical stimulation are also frequently used in an attempt to manage pain and inflammation, providing a conducive environment for healing. It is vital that physiotherapists assess the individual situation of each patient, so they can develop a successful treatment plan considering factors like the severity of the condition and the general state of the patient. Evidence-based practice is the foundation of this, since the clinician can adjust his or her choice of treatment in accordance with the latest evidence and promote long-term success for the patient. Manual therapy, including joint mobilization and soft tissue manipulation, is another cornerstone of physiotherapy interventions. Both are focused on restoration of typical joint mechanics, alleviation of pain, and range of motion enhancement, thereby managing musculoskeletal diseases prevalent in various populations. An example is for osteoarthritis (OA), where manual therapy can be particularly effective to alleviate symptoms and promote functional mobility. Studies highlight the importance of conservative management pathways in the initial stages of OA, with the application of physiotherapy interventions holding the promise to hinder disease progression and decrease disability (Oluchukwu, 2018). Physiotherapists often combine these manual therapy approaches with patient education in self-management techniques, which enables individuals to become proactive participants in their rehabilitation process. Apart from conventional physiotherapy modalities, newer techniques such as aquatic therapy and virtual rehabilitation are increasingly being used in the treatment of orthopedic conditions. Aquatic therapy, where exercises are performed in water, reduces joint stress to a large extent and is an excellent option for patients with severe pain or mobility restrictions. It is particularly useful for post-operative recovery or patients with chronic conditions. Moreover, virtual rehabilitation exploits technology to carry out exercise schemes and monitor patients remotely, promoting patient compliance with treatment planning and enhancing involvement (Howard-Wilsher et al., 2016). With the evolution of the physiotherapy practice, such decisions increase accessibility and personalization, generating a comprehensive means of managing common orthopedic disorders that may lead to improved patient outcomes (Figure 5.4).

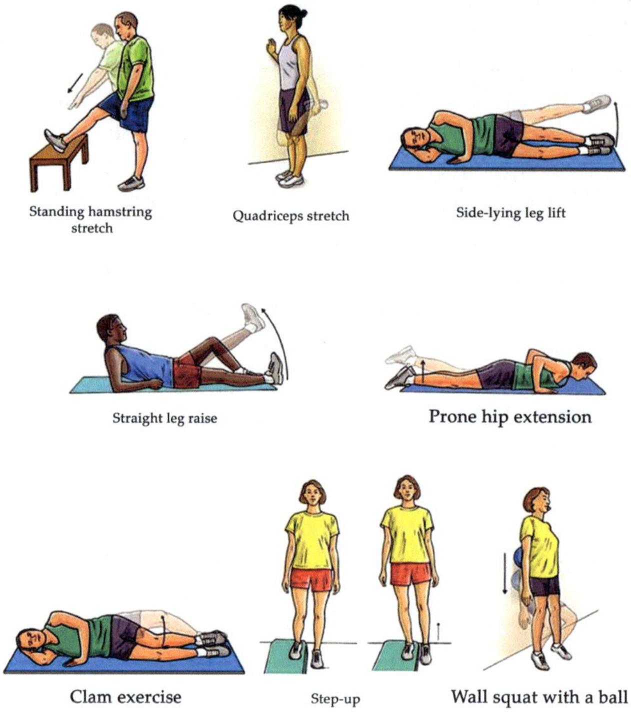

Figure 5.4. Physiotherapy in the management of osteoarthritis of the knee.

Source: https://blogger.googleusercontent.com/img/b/R29vZ2xl/AVvXsEj-tR7RTTu6rv8InrxUlEuTRl9TcmKqe99ZGcXkyDpnCRKjwTakMJGBdrvjMoqHXq7Dv6x5SI-XTQDohbv7moNo7C8UOl-Uu5K3jaqUQ_Ya8acr2Ns6P8XkjqV2T66Rvpe1YGs1bxxCYFr_/s1600/OA4.jpg.

5.2. Rheumatoid Arthritis

Rheumatoid arthritis (RA) is an auto-inflammatory, chronic condition that primarily affects the synovial joints and results in intense pain, inflammation, and ultimate cartilage and bone loss. The intricate pathophysiology of RA is an autoimmune reaction whereby the body's immune system attacks the tissues of the body in error, in this instance, the synovium. This inflammatory response not only destroys the joints but also may affect other systems, such as the cardiovascular and respiratory systems. This makes patients with RA have less mobility and increased functional impairment, for which overall rehabilitation methods become necessary. Orthopedic physiotherapy plays a crucial role in the treatment of these symptoms, providing patients with personalized exercise regimens to improve joint function and reduce stiffness (Crouch, 1947). Furthermore, physiotherapy interventions can enhance the lifestyle of people with RA by fostering independence and engagement in activities of daily living. Rheumatoid arthritis treatment with orthopedic physiotherapy normally encompasses a range of modalities, including pain-relief modalities, education, and therapeutic exercises. Physiotherapists work in close association with the patient to develop individualized exercise programs that treat strength and flexibility so that they are able to maintain activity levels despite joint disability.

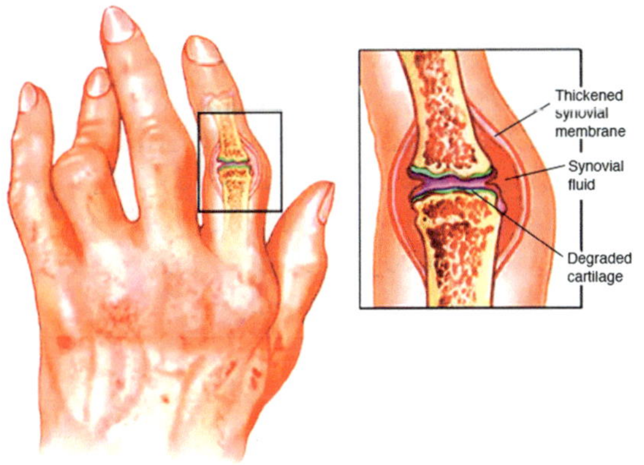

Figure 5.5. Rheumatoid arthritis.

Source: https://www.mayoclinic.org/-/media/kcms/gbs/patient-consumer/images/2013/08/26/10/47/ds00020_im02689_r7_rheumatoidarthritisthu_jpg.jpg.

Cardiovascular health can be improved and comorbidities, typically seen in those with chronic disease such as RA, minimized through aerobic exercises and range-of-motion exercises. Furthermore, educational elements of the therapy are able to make the patients more confident in their disease state, learn how to deal with their symptoms, and undertake self-care strategies (Arge et al., 2012). Such multi-dimensional approaches are required in long-term compliance with treatment protocols and enhanced outcomes for the patients. Despite the progress in treatment and management, rheumatoid arthritis patients have difficulty with joint deformity-related issues, particularly in the hands and feet. These deformities would be most likely to significantly compromise functional ability and adversely affect a patient's quality of life. In the more advanced stages, orthopedic physiotherapy would include interventions aimed at reversing the results of these structural changes, such as orthotic care and increased stretching protocols to ensure joint mobility. Regular review and reassessment by medical professionals are necessary in altering treatment interventions based on changing disease status. Emphasis on personalized physical therapy interventions not only assists in the healing of the immediate physical limitations but also concentrates on generating a feeling of independence and psychological wellness among patients afflicted with rheumatoid arthritis (Crouch, 1947). The role of Orthopedics physiotherapy in the treatment of RA, thus, transcends the physical rehabilitation, eventually culminating in all-around care of the patient (Figure 5.5).

5.2.1. Overview of the Condition

The Orthopedics conditions spectrum features a broad range of musculoskeletal disorders with unique approaches in Orthopedics physiotherapy. They include common conditions like osteoarthritis, fractures, tendon injury, and back pain, each presenting with its own clinical complexities. Osteoarthritis, for instance, is characterized by the breakdown of joint cartilage, leading to pain and stiffness, particularly in weight-bearing joints such as the knees and hips. This condition not only impacts physical function, but quality of life as well, routinely requiring multidimensional rehabilitation. The increased prevalence of such conditions, particularly in the older population, underscores the necessity for effective treatment through interventions that can restore mobility and alleviate pain. Fractures are a prevalent orthopedic condition, commonly resulting from acute trauma or chronic stress. Therapy for fractures is not only effective through surgical intervention but also by other physiotherapeutic methods to promote healing and reduce complications such as stiffness and muscle atrophy. Mobilization and certain exercises are very crucial in rehabilitation, the latter facilitating functional recovery and the overall outcome of the patient.

This aspect of rehabilitation is particularly vital in the recovery of strength and range of motion for the injured extremities to avoid possible future injuries. Some, like tendinous injuries, which are prevalent among sportspeople, also require specialized rehabilitation methods that are intended to promote healing without sacrificing an active lifestyle. The economic implications of orthopedic conditions also cannot be dismissed, with implications for healthcare systems and quality of patient life. Effective rehabilitation programs have been shown to be cost-effective through reduced hospital stays and improved patient outcomes, as demonstrated by systematic reviews of health-related rehabilitation (Howard-Wilsher et al., 2016).

The integration of evidence-based practice, i.e., physiotherapy, into treatment plans has been found to contribute to enhancing functional recovery as well as addressing the unique needs of patients with orthopedic conditions. Besides, recent developments, i.e., the implementation of the DMAIC Lean Six Sigma methodology in Orthopedics services, demonstrate innovations to enhance patient pathways and reduce waiting times, thus enhancing access and efficiency in Orthopedics care (Pierce et al., 2023). These advancements highlight the significance of holistic approaches to treating orthopedic conditions in treatment, in light of clinical as well as economic factors in orthopedic physiotherapy (Figure 5.6).

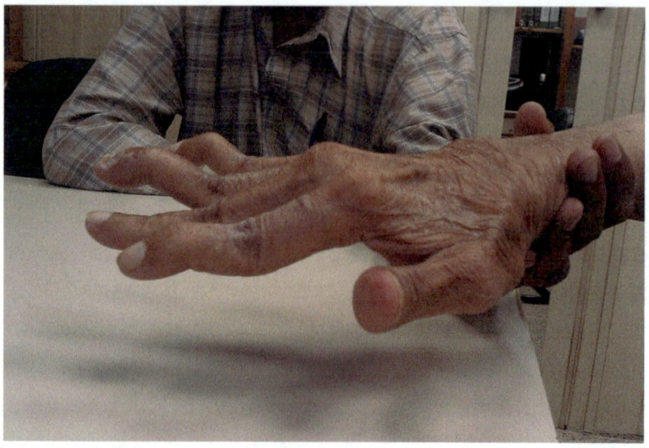

Figure 5.6. Hand deformity, sometimes called a *swan deformity*, in an elderly person with rheumatoid arthritis.

Source: https://upload.wikimedia.org/wikipedia/commons/thumb/8/83/Swan_neck_deformity_in_a_65_year_old_Rheumatoid_Arthritis_patient-_2014-05-27_01-49.jpg/1280px-Swan_neck_deformity_in_a_65_year_old_Rheumatoid_Arthritis_patient-_2014-05-27_01-49.jpg.

5.2.2. Impact on Mobility and Daily Activities

Orthopedic disorders greatly affect an individual's mobility and activities of daily living, traditionally leading to decreased functionality and increased dependency on support. One such example of this effect is the widespread condition, osteoarthritis (OA). Research shows that OA is a common cause of pain and functional disability in any age group, but most so in individuals under the age of 45 years. The progressive aspect of OA can hinder locomotion and lead to disability in normal activities such as walking, climbing stairs, or participating in recreational activities. Conservative management and early intervention not only alleviate pain but also are accountable for maintaining functionality, hence enhancing the general quality of life in the Orthopedics-affected patient, as brought out in clinical studies emphasizing the benefit of early Orthopedics physiotherapy intervention

(Silva, 2011). The functional loss brought about by orthopedic conditions also entails mental and emotional stability and hence is a comprehensive challenge to the patient. As witnessed in large-scale studies, patients with physical therapy for orthopedic complications most often also have psychological stressors that hinder their willingness and compliance with rehabilitation treatment. For instance, having psychiatric disorders, as is common in older adults, was found to be associated with lower functional outcomes in physical therapy. In spite of null findings for the direct association between psychiatric diagnosis and success of physical therapy (Silva, 2011), the dynamics of treatment intensity dictate that constant engagement in physiotherapy is imperative to achieve maximum mobility and satisfy personal rehabilitative goals. Accordingly, understanding these associated factors is essential to the development of effective treatment plans for addressing both the physical and psychological facets of recovery. Furthermore, the consequences of loss of mobility due to orthopedic conditions resonate in virtually every area of life, also including social contacts and working activities. The patient will be further withdrawn from social activities because of the loss of mobility in being able to participate in general social activities, which exacerbates depression and anxiety frequently accompanying physical illness. The rehabilitative function of orthopedic physiotherapy is especially germane here, as pain reduction and functional independence are achieved through specially designed programs, which can be highly effective in promoting participation and occupational performance. Hence, the all-important link between physical rehabilitation and improved quality of life highlights the relevance of successful orthopedic physiotherapy interventions, which, in addition to solving the restoration of mobility, aim to reintegrate patients into normal activities and daily routine in a meaningful manner (Oluchukwu, 2018).

5.2.3. Role of Physiotherapy in Management

Treatment of classic orthopedic conditions chiefly relies on the role of physiotherapy, since it is a key component in obtaining the optimal outcome of recovery and maximizing functional capacity. Physiotherapy employs various techniques aimed at restoring movement patterns, relieving pain, and maximizing physical function. For patients suffering from diseases such as osteoarthritis or ligament sprain, physiotherapists create individual rehabilitation programs that include therapeutic exercises and manual therapy.

Through a focus on the restoration of range of motion and exercise of associated musculature, physiotherapy is able to help patients become independent and improve their quality of life. Furthermore, ongoing physiotherapeutic treatment keeps complications commonly linked to immobility at bay, such as muscle atrophy and joint stiffness, and ultimately leads to an enhanced long-term prognosis in patients suffering from orthopedic disorders. In the management framework of osteoarthritis, physiotherapy is an important component both in delaying disease progression and symptom relief. Scientific research highlights the potential of non-operative management strategies, particularly at the onset of osteoarthritis. Physiotherapy intervention addresses improving joint function and pain reduction through targeted exercise programs and education on joint protection strategies.

By addressing the biomechanical aspects of the condition, physiotherapists can facilitate improved patterns of movement, therefore facilitating a reduction in pain and improvement in overall functional ability. In addition, management is meant to facilitate patients using self-management techniques, which can be of significant influence in reducing the resort to the use of pharmacological mechanisms for pain management. Thus, physiotherapy not only resolves short-term orthopedic problems but also contributes to the general long-term health and general well-being of osteoarthritis patients (Oluchukwu, 2018). Multidisciplinary management of complex cases highlights the significance of physiotherapy. For example, in Moquino A syndrome, an illness characterized by skeletal deformities, a multidisciplinary treatment approach with various healthcare specialists—physiotherapists being part of them—can yield improved management outcomes.

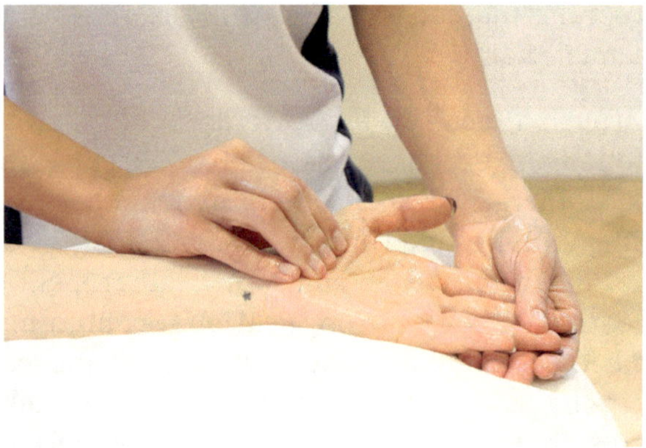

Figure 5.7. Physiotherapy for rheumatoid-arthritis.

Source: https://www.physio.co.uk/images/rheumatoid-arthritis/rheumatoid-arthritis1.jpg.

Physiotherapists contribute by prescribing exercise programs that are tailored to the individual needs of such patients, so as to maximize mobility in a way that takes into consideration the challenge of respiratory engagement and potential spinal cord compression (Hendriksz et al., 2015). Such personalized intervention maximizes functional autonomy and quality of life so that physiotherapy is not only corrective but preventive as well. Through an integrated approach treating both body and other comorbidities, physiotherapists play a central part in overall patient care continuity, establishing a model for improved health outcomes in orthopedic treatment (Figure 5.7).

5.3. Fractures

Fractures are a common Orthopedics condition that poses some of the specific difficulties of diagnosis and management. Fractures are classified according to the kind of break they are, such as simple, compound, and stress fractures, each of which needs customized assessment and intervention strategies. Fractures may occur in various population groups; however, the impact amongst young adults is not yet fully researched despite the increased incidence with low-energy falls, particularly amongst those under 60 years. The research has revealed that recovery experience amongst young adults often varies from what occurs amongst older adults, particularly concerning the psychological and social impacts of their injuries. The multidisciplinary approach to the management of such fractures means that orthopedic surgeons, physiotherapists, and mental health professionals need to address both the physical needs of convalescence and the psychological effects of the injury (Janes et al., 2018). Physical therapy is very crucial in the recovery process following a fracture, concentrating on reclaiming movement and function. It encompasses evidence-based techniques aimed at soft tissue injury, joint stability, and strength recovery. A comprehensive physiotherapy protocol may encompass mobilization techniques, strengthening exercises, and functional assessments as a function of the type of fracture and patient activities. Of interest, an awareness of the various patient experiences of younger participants, as increasingly documented in the more recent literature, can guide physiotherapists to develop more appropriate rehabilitation interventions. Rehabilitation not only seeks physical recovery but also considers potential complications, such as post-traumatic stress symptoms, that may affect the patient's motivation and overall prognosis of recovery. Overall recovery outcome can be considerably improved with the use of individualized interventions (Samoy et al., 2016). Long-term effects of fracture on society, particularly among younger patients, are far-reaching but sometimes undervalued. Since fractures are more likely to cause long-term issues, including economic strain and interference with lifestyle, there must be more effective treatment beyond the initial medical care. The need for healthcare systems to adapt and provide long-term care from the moment of recovery is invoked by such evidence. The results in recent studies show that inadequacies in existing care pathways inevitably lead to negative outcomes, and therefore, there is a critical need for strengthened strategies targeted towards younger groups (Janes et al., 2018). By facilitating interdisciplinary collaboration, integrating psychological support into the practice of physiotherapy, and enhancing communication along the healthcare continuum, a more integrated model of care can be developed that minimizes the long-term sequelae of fracture and allows for a successful return to daily function and well-being (Samoy et al., 2016).

5.3.1. Types of Fractures Commonly Treated

Fractures are classified based on their nature and mode of injury, and common examples are simple, compound, and comminuted fractures. A simple fracture or a closed fracture occurs when the bone breaks without piercing the skin, often resulting in less infection risk and simpler treatment. Compound fractures, on the other hand, expose the broken bone via an open wound, compromising the risk of infection and requiring aggressive surgical management to stabilize the bone and debride the wound. Comminuted fractures are made up of several pieces of bone and typically occur with high-energy trauma, as they represent certain challenges for fixation due to the complexity of the alignment and stabilization needed. Understanding these differences is most important in orthopedic physiotherapy as they determine treatment and rehabilitation programs with the goal of restoring mobility and function. Another significant type of fracture frequently encountered in the clinic is the pathologic fracture, which is due to underlying pathologies such as osteoporosis or malignancy and leads to diminished bone density. They are more susceptible to these fractures, often secondary to minor falls or activities of daily living, in elderly patients.

Treatment of pathologic fractures not only involves the repair of the immediate fracture but also includes starting long-term interventions to strengthen the bone and prevent its recurrence. Physiotherapy is also crucial in this rehabilitation process, using techniques to enhance muscle strength, balance, and coordination, thus reducing opportunities of more fractures. The role of incorporation of physiotherapy, therefore, becomes critical not just in rehabilitation but in addressing underlying vulnerabilities that make an individual susceptible to such fractures. Pelvic fractures are another kind of injury that is commonly seen in the domain of Orthopedics clinics, typically caused by high-energy forces such as accidents or falls.

Pelvic fractures are also a cause for concern since there may be associated complications such as injury to nearby organs or major vessels. Physiotherapy rehabilitation for pelvic fractures is essential since an organized rehabilitation program can significantly impact recovery times and overall functionality. Healing also calls for a combination of conservative therapy and active mobilization procedures to restore mobility and strength in the damaged area. Some of the physiotherapeutic modalities provide relief from pain, improve circulation, and aid in safe movement during healing, noting the important contribution of physiotherapy to the management of such complex injuries as pelvic fractures (Samoy et al., 2016) (Figure 5.8).

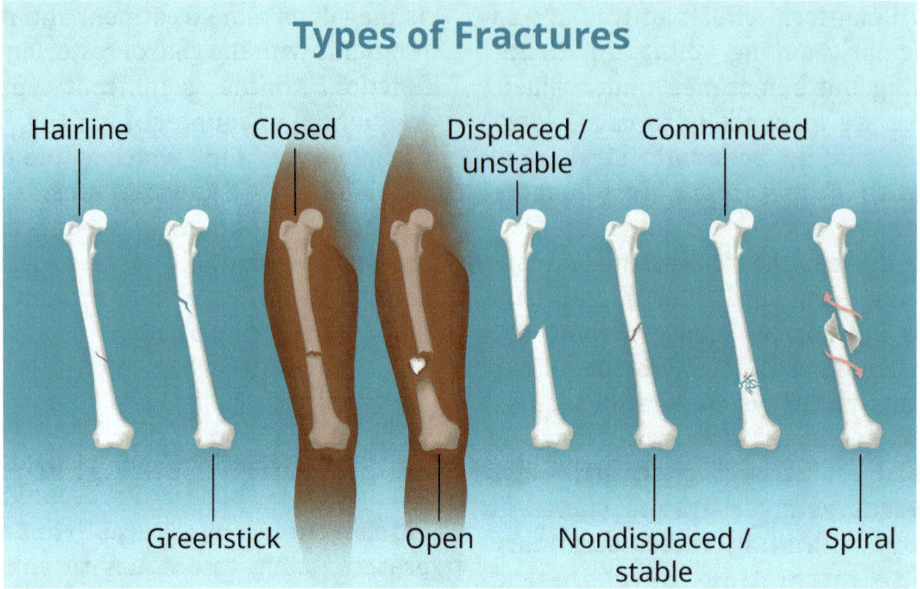

Figure 5.8. Types of fractures.

Source: https://www.verywellhealth.com/thmb/EDmg42PbTXc83WBVoKl5yzPa8U0=/1500x0/filters:no_upscale():max_bytes(150000):strip_icc()/Fracture-WhattoKnowAboutThisInjury-v2-5936ff9b9dd048e9b8be221450f994d8.png.

5.3.2. Healing Process and Rehabilitation

The rehabilitation process following orthopedic trauma or surgery is a three-staged process involving physical, psychological, and social dimensions. Effective rehabilitation is critical for restoring function and maximizing the quality of life for patients. Physiotherapy forms the core component of the process, employing evidence-based techniques to alleviate pain, improve mobility, and augment strength. Tailored rehabilitation protocols typically consist of exercises for specific musculoskeletal abnormalities, with educational components so patients can learn about their ailments and take better care of themselves. As per recent research, an evidence-based practice in physiotherapy can facilitate personalized care, optimizing the highest level of recovery pathways for varying orthopedic conditions. Attention to both the physical and psychosocial aspects ensures an overall treatment plan necessary for optimal results during the process of healing, especially in complicated cases with prolonged rehabilitation (Samoy et al., 2016). Moreover, postoperative pain management is an intrinsic element of the recuperation process, most notably in orthopedic procedures. Effective pain management not only relieves discomfort but also enables early mobilization, a crucial component of rehabilitation. Various methods are employed in managing postoperative pain, from pharmacological methods such as nonsteroidal anti-inflammatory drugs (NSAIDs) and opioids, to non-pharmacological methods such as physical therapy and cryotherapy. Research has shown that a thoughtful integration of these interventions can lead to improved patient satisfaction and compliance with the rehabilitation protocol (Górka et al., 2024).

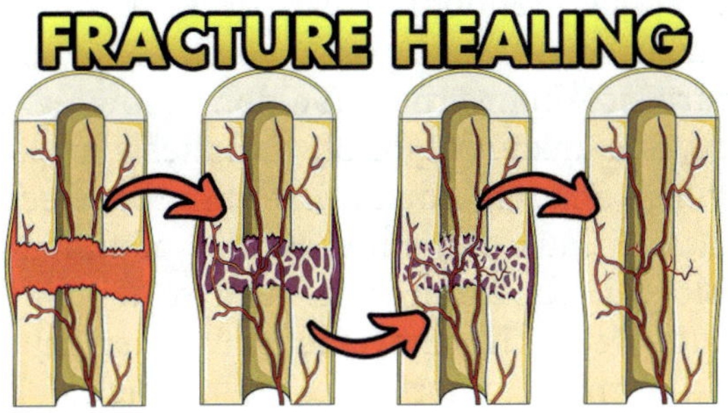

Figure 5.9. Fracture healing.

Source: https://i.ytimg.com/vi/ZD_5Why69IM/hq720.jpg?sqp=-oaymwEhCK4FEIIDSFryq4qpAxMIARUAAAAAGAElAADIQj0AgKJD&rs=AOn4CLDuRzFoMKO-73q4MLdOVNfKbu9Hgw.

Control of pain at the onset of recovery is very important, as its neglect may result in complications that include immobilization for an extended period and delayed healing, ultimately affecting the rehabilitation process of orthopedic patients. In addition to formal rehabilitation processes and effective pain control, the healing process is largely based on patients' emotional and psychological conditions. Orthopedic trauma can result in frustration, anxiety, and depression, which have negative effects on motivation and rehabilitation participation. Therefore, it becomes critical to address these psychological issues through motivational interventions and supportive counseling. Those patients who are given coping strategies along with their physical rehabilitation program are more likely to demonstrate greater adherence to their recovery program. The combination of psychological intervention with physiotherapy can optimize outcomes and offer a more comprehensive rehabilitation program, addressing not only the physical but also the emotional barriers to recovery. Finally, a systems approach that factors in physical rehabilitation as well as mental wellness is crucial in facilitating the effective healing process of orthopedic care, which emphasizes the interconnected nature of such factors toward patient recuperation (Samoy et al., 2016) (Figure 5.9).

5.3.3. Physiotherapy Interventions Post-Fracture

Following a fracture, physiotherapy intervention is necessary to regain function and manage pain. Rehabilitative phases typically begin shortly after immobilization, restoring range of motion and strength to the injured segment. Early mobilization may contribute to healing by increasing circulation, a requirement for healing. Physiotherapists employ varied techniques, including graded exercise programs and joint mobilizations, that are intended to gradually improve load-bearing abilities. Research is indicative of more intensive rehabilitation, especially at weekends, which has increased functional independence and quality of life. A study reveals that participants on the weekend who performed more rehabilitation demonstrated improved functional independence measures and indicate the effectiveness of regular and continued regimes of physiotherapy (Peiris et al., 2013). In addition, individualized plans of treatment are essential to addressing the specific needs of individual patients, particularly in post-fracture rehabilitation. These programs typically involve modalities such as heat treatment, stimulation with electricity, and isolated strength exercise at the fracture site. After mobilization of patients, physiotherapists assess continued functional capacity, adjusting programs to avoid setbacks if necessary. Incorporation of cutting-edge technologies, such as virtual reality (VR), adds more enrichment to the rehabilitation process. VR provides interactive spaces for the practice of movements and neuromuscular re-education, thereby maximizing engagement and adherence of patients (Paladugu et al., 2025). The personalized intervention, aside from restoring the physical function, also breaks down psychological obstacles created by immobility to help regain overall quality of life. As the rehabilitation continues, interventions via physiotherapy also target the prevention of complications commonly associated with immobilization. These may include muscle wasting, joint stiffness, and risk of re-injury. Preventive measures like proprioceptive rehab and balance are integral components of a comprehensive rehabilitative program following a fracture. Incorporating flexibility and strengthening exercises within the protocol of recovery not only provides functional mobility recovery but is also desirable for long-term joint health. Furthermore, education of patients empowers patients to be actively involved in their own rehabilitation, facilitating compliance with exercises and alterations as recommended. Thus, with an awareness of the multifaceted aspect of post-fracture physiotherapy interventions, practitioners can significantly maximize the recovery process of patients, limit long-term complications and maximize optimal function results (Peiris et al., 2013) (Figure 5.10).

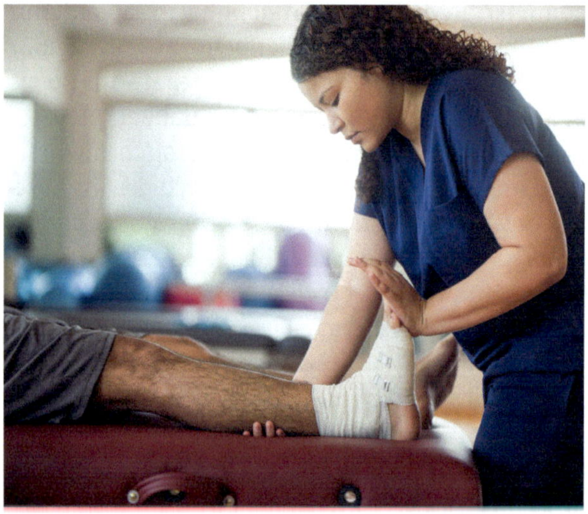

Figure 5.10. Post-fracture physiotherapy.

Source: https://www.glmc.ae/wp-content/uploads/2022/12/iStock 1132546141-1024x768.jpg.

5.4. Tendonitis

Tendonitis is a general orthopedic disorder resulting from tendinous inflammation. Tendons are fibrous tissues connecting muscles and bones. Tendonitis can occur in almost all anatomical sites, with common sites of occurrence being the shoulder, elbow, wrist, knee, and ankle. It typically manifests as pain, swelling, and limited movement in the affected area and causes significant loss of function. Etiological conditions that lead to tendonitis include repetitive movement, overuse injury, and internal biomechanical deficiencies. The disorder is usually seen in athletes as well as in workers who perform jobs that require repetitive action. Understanding the etiology and clinical presentation of tendonitis holds significant value in orthopedic physiotherapists, as it directs the personalized interventions that are needed for effective rehabilitation and recovery. Orthopedic physiotherapy plays a crucial role in the treatment of tendonitis, with the focus being placed on symptom relief as well as functional return. Treatment approaches usually consist of a combination of manual therapy, exercises, and modalities such as ultrasound or electrical stimulation to reduce pain and inflammation. Exercise programs are individualized to strengthen impaired muscles, enhance flexibility, and re-establish the range of motion. In the treatment of tendonitis, physiotherapists consider patient-related factors, such as functional impairment and activity levels. Recent studies have highlighted various determinants of treatment outcomes, particularly for various populations. For instance, evidence indicates that patients who are sedentary and do not work have greater disability and pain levels than those who participate in actual physical work (McArthur et al., 2020). Furthermore, a thorough understanding of the rehabilitation process is critical for effective management of tendonitis. Interventions must consider the particular presentation of the condition among different populations depending on age, gender, and level of activity. Older individuals, for example, may require more conservative interventions due to related medical comorbidities or age-related changes in connective tissue. Moreover, self-management techniques increasingly form the core of the rehabilitative process, empowering patients with skills to minimize the effects of tendonitis on their lifestyle. Incorporating self-management training enhances patient engagement and produces a sense of ownership towards recovery, significantly affecting end outcomes (Carlson et al., 2014). By a focus on patient-specific treatment and evidence-based interventions, Orthopedics physiotherapists are capable of optimizing recuperation for tendinitis sufferers, ultimately promoting amplified functional sustainability and quality of life.

5.4.1. Common Types of Tendonitis

Tendonitis is an orthopedic condition that is common, characterized by inflammation of a tendon and is most often due to overuse, repetitive strain, or trauma. One of the most common types is Achilles tendonitis, which is inflammation of the tendon connecting calf muscles to the bone on the back of the heel. Most susceptible are athletes and runners because of the immense force the Achilles must endure during the state of running and jumping or sprinting. Symptoms tend to comprise pain and inflammation along the tendon, which can remarkably disable mobility and sporting performance.

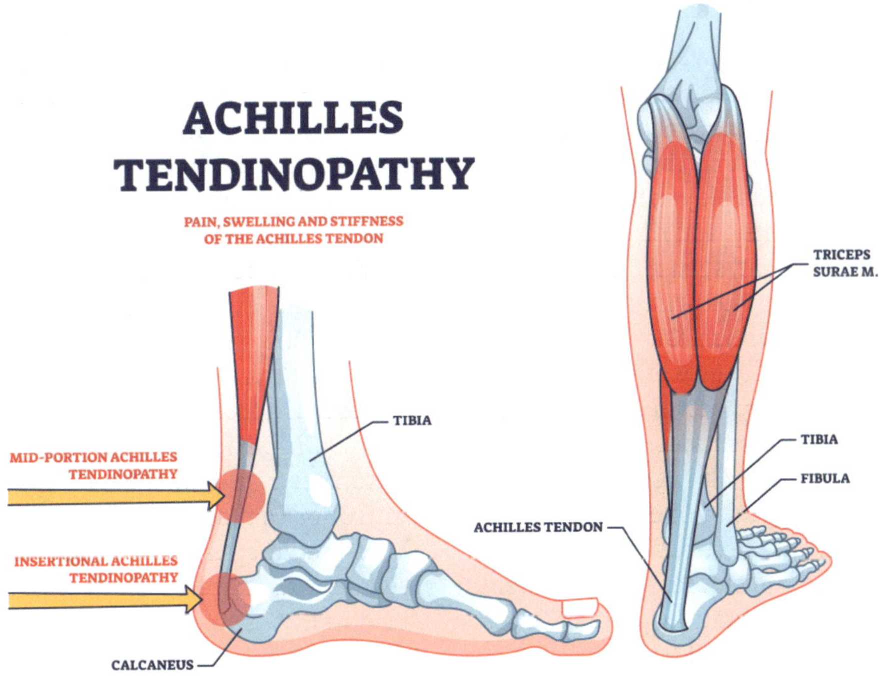

Figure 5.11. Achilles tendonitis.

Source: https://sa1s3optim.patientpop.com/assets/images/provider/photos/2619175.png.

Conservative management, such as rest, ice, and physical therapy, can be successful in reducing pain and allowing healing. For patients like those in the shoulder injury studies, being aware of the precise condition and its implications is paramount for correct treatment and rehabilitation (McArthur et al., 2020). Another type of tendonitis is rotator cuff tendonitis, which occurs in the shoulder. It results from repetitive overhead motions like throwing or lifting, causing irritation or inflammation of the rotator cuff tendons. Individuals whose occupational or sporting activity involves constant use of the shoulder are particularly prone to this. Symptoms most often present themselves as shoulder pain and limited range of motion, which can be extremely debilitating to normal activities and work-related duties. Effective treatment usually involves individualized physiotherapy for stabilizing and strengthening the muscles around the shoulder, with added modalities for pain relief and decreasing inflammation. Occupation and incidence of this illness remind us of the importance of certain rehabilitation strategies in recurrence prevention and optimization of recovery (McArthur et al., 2020). Tennis elbow or lateral epicondylitis is another illustration of tendonitis in the elbow region. It results from cumulative overuse of muscles that are attached to the lateral epicondyle of the humerus, leading to pain on the lateral side of the elbow. Although it is most commonly associated with the tennis player, it can happen to anybody who is doing activities involving repetitive wrist movement, such as carpentry or working on a computer. The primary symptom is pain and tenderness, which can radiate down the forearm and hinder grasping or lifting functions. Treatment for lateral epicondylitis is usually achieved with rest, ice, and accurate exercises to enhance the strength of forearm muscles. Understanding this condition's impact on both recreational and occupational activities emphasizes efficient physiotherapy treatment in managing and rehabilitating patients with tendonitis (McArthur et al., 2020) (Figure 5.11).

5.4.2. Symptoms and Risk Factors

The symptom presentation of orthopedic conditions is usually variable based on the specific malady, but areas of commonality exist among an enormous number of diagnoses. Pain is generally the most frequently reported symptom and it comes with all the features of severity, location, and duration. In osteoarthritis (OA), patients normally complain of joint stiffness, particularly following periods of inactivity, accompanied by swelling and a seeming decrease in range of movement. Such conditions tend to significantly affect daily functioning and quality of life, and as such, patients will look for physiotherapeutic care with a view to pain relief and restoration of function. Early identification of these symptoms may be crucial in developing a successful treatment plan, maximizing the chance of better patient outcomes and satisfaction during the rehabilitation process. Risk factors are the key in the causation and aggravation of orthopedic conditions, the development of which is caused by intrinsic and extrinsic factors. Intrinsic factors may be age, genetic predisposition, and co-morbidities, while extrinsic factors are generally lifestyle factors, occupational hazards, and environmental factors. For instance, research has shown osteoarthritis to be particularly prevalent among the elderly population, yet individuals below 45 years of age are also afflicted by factors like obesity or joint trauma. The relationship between such risk factors not only decides the occurrence of orthopedic disease but also the intensity and progression of the condition. Therefore, identification and control of these risk factors in the clinical environment can avail better preventive measures and customized physiotherapy programs. High control of Orthopedics conditions, particularly OA, is reliant on the control of symptoms as well as associated risk factors. Conservative treatments, such as physical therapy, have been shown to minimize symptoms and halt disease advancement, thereby enhancing patient function and quality of life (Oluchukwu, 2018). In particular, early intervention is critical because prompt referral to physiotherapeutic management can avert pain, decrease stiffness, and improve joint function in general. Therefore, there is a need for healthcare professionals to keep in mind the comprehensive symptom evaluation as well as concomitant risk factors while devising individualized intervention plans.

This approach not only optimizes the treatment of the patient but also builds an active management strategy, which could reduce the risk of severe disability from common orthopedic conditions (Figure 5.12).

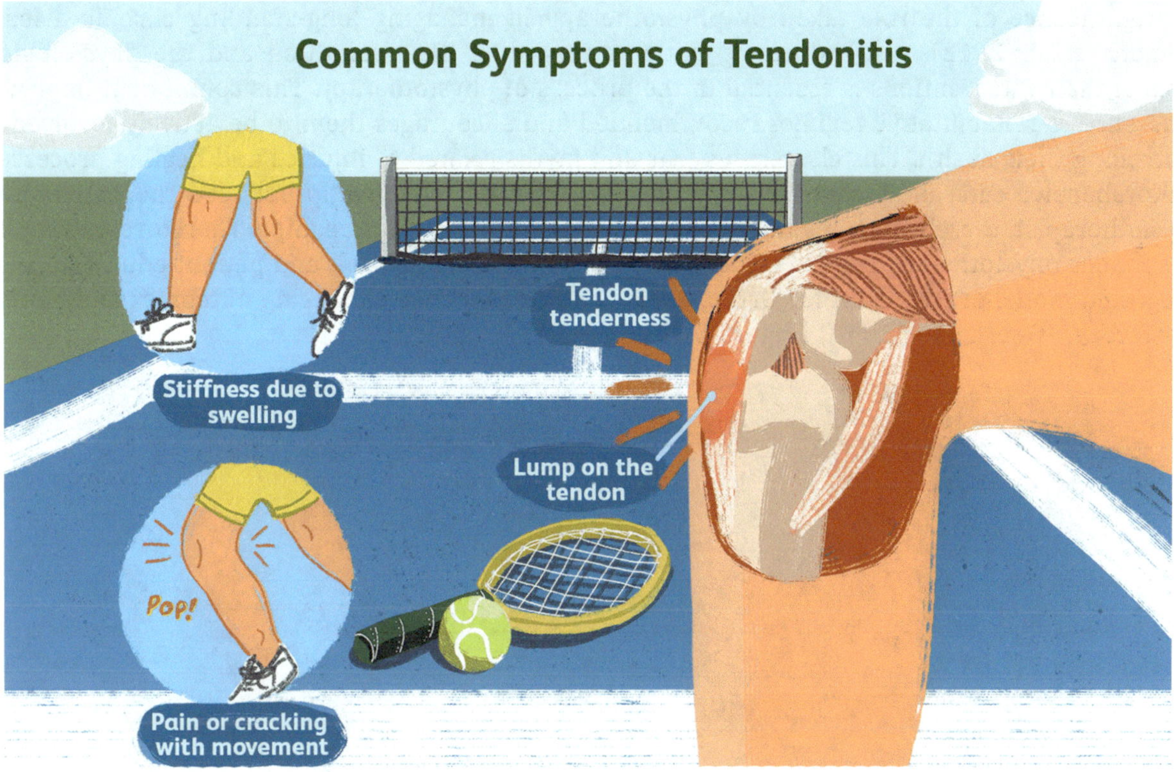

Figure 5.12. Common symptoms of tendonitis.

Source: https://www.verywellhealth.com/thmb/V_ip78GtKa-lvhOd5zh3E_zvvfc=/1500x0/filters:no_upscale():max_bytes(150000):strip_icc()/tendonitis-definition-causes-treatment-2696478-v21-5c77259146e0fb0001a9830f.png.

5.4.3. Physiotherapy Approaches for Treatment

Under orthopedic physiotherapy, diverse interventions are used to treat common conditions that impact musculoskeletal health. Physiotherapists use manual therapy intervention, exercise and education, and patient instruction to create comprehensive treatment plans tailored to individual patients' needs. Manual therapy is made up of expert hands-on skills used to mobilize or manipulate joints and soft tissues and thereby reduce pain and restore mobility. In addition, the exercise role within physiotherapy cannot be overemphasized; certain exercises help to regain function and strength, particularly after surgery or during rehabilitation following injuries. An approach that combines these methods not only helps to manage the symptoms but also proactively involves the patient in the recovery process. Of particular note is the application of structured exercise programs in patients with knee osteoarthritis (OA), a prevalent orthopedic condition. One pilot study set out to develop a home-based regimen of strengthening of the lower extremities for women over fifty years of age, and the outcomes were positive findings. Women completed a 14-week regimen of stepping and walking protocols in phases with incremental increases in step height to progressively challenge their strength and stability. Significant improvements were noted on several measures, including WOMAC scores and quadriceps strength. These outcomes indicate the efficacy of exercise interventions aimed at overcoming functional impairments in knee OA and identify the significance of the role taken by physiotherapy in managing long-standing chronic disease (Lemons et al., 2012). Also, educating patients regarding their condition and the physiological basis of their interventions is essential in the process of physiotherapy. This component improves adherence to rehabilitative regimes recommended and encourages them to be actively involved in controlling their health. This also erases fear and myths related to injuries and healing processes. Comprehensive care allows the development of a trusting relationship between the patient and physiotherapist, thereby opening doors to effective therapeutic relationships. Therefore, this multi-component physiotherapy service combining exercise, manual therapy, and patient education is an integrated model of treatment for Orthopedics conditions, hence enhancing outcomes and patient satisfaction (Oberlander, 1960) (Figure 5.13).

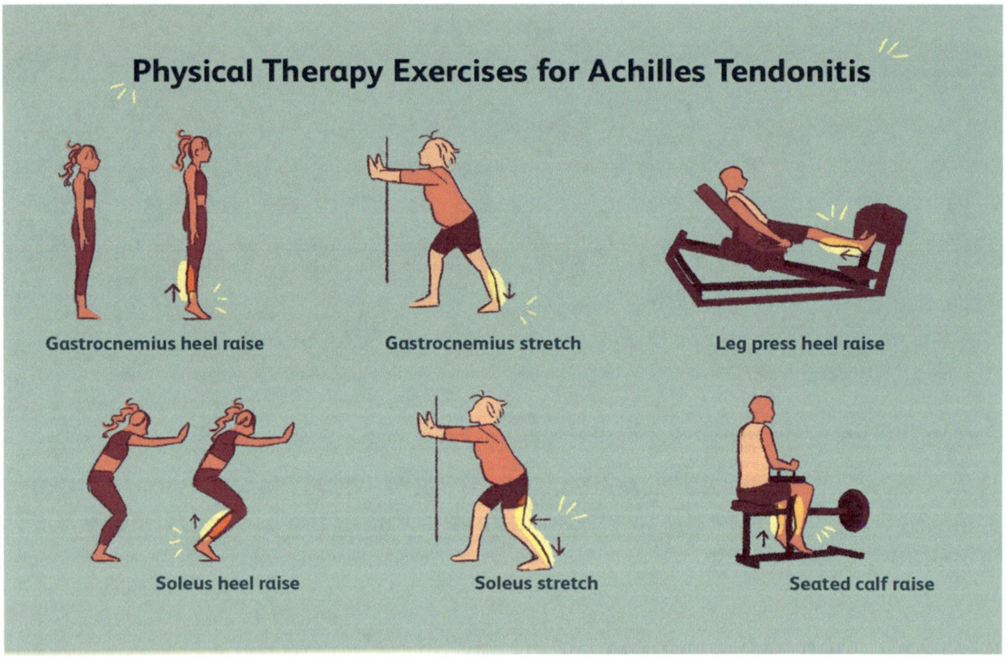

Figure 5.13. Physical therapy exercises for Achilles tendonitis.

Source: https://www.verywellhealth.com/thmb/LVjoKguQiReL9ynVtzI8kvlGYh8=/1500x0/filters:no_upscale():max_bytes(150000):strip_icc()/pt-exercises-for-achilles-tendonitis-5202656_final-a2c745a0e3f6429bb68a6fe068b757a3.jpg.

5.5. Bursitis

Bursitis is a condition commonly encountered in orthopedic physiotherapy, where the bursa becomes inflamed. The bursa is a liquid-filled sac that reduces friction between tissues in joints. The areas involved are the shoulder, elbow, hip, and knee, where repetitive movement or constant pressure causes irritation. The condition is typically encountered in individuals engaging in sporting or occupational activities of repetitive motion, such as throwing or kneeling. The bursitis pain can be functionally impairing, decreasing the capacity to move and engage in sporting and daily activities. Therefore, understanding the etiology and biomechanics underlying the etiology of bursitis is essential for effective therapeutic interventions, such that physiotherapists are able to apply targeted rehabilitation strategies aimed at the causative mechanisms for bursa inflammation. The diagnosis of bursitis often incorporates clinical assessment and more advanced imaging techniques, which are now more accessible. Techniques such as ultrasound or MRI allow physiotherapists to observe intra-articular and extra-articular tissues, which are important in providing an impression of the nature of the condition. For instance, in hip bursitis, imaging can reveal peri-articular pathologies that might complicate treatment (Aprato et al., 2014). Furthermore, differential diagnosis is essential, since bursitis may present like tendonitis or arthritis. This complexity highlights the need for detailed evaluation procedures to guide physiotherapists in designing appropriate management protocols. Thus, with the use of high-tech diagnostic equipment, practitioners can accurately diagnose bursitis and implement successful interventions that alleviate pain as well as restore customary joint function. Therapeutic interventions for bursitis most commonly employ both conservative and rehabilitative methods. Initially, physiotherapy may involve rest, application of ice, and anti-inflammatory medication to manage swelling and pain. After this, therapeutic exercises serve a critical function in restoring musculature about compromised joints, re-establishing stability, and optimizing range of movement. More contemporary literature documents the success of introducing precise rehabilitation programs that are specific to individual patient needs, which may incorporate management by manual therapy and localized stretching exercises (Oberlander, 1960). Towards rehabilitation advancement, functional training is promoted by physiotherapists to re-establish movement patterns with a gradual return to function. Lastly, acknowledging the multifactorial nature of bursitis allows the physiotherapist to implement a successful treatment program that not only controls symptoms but also prevents recurrences (Figure 5.14).

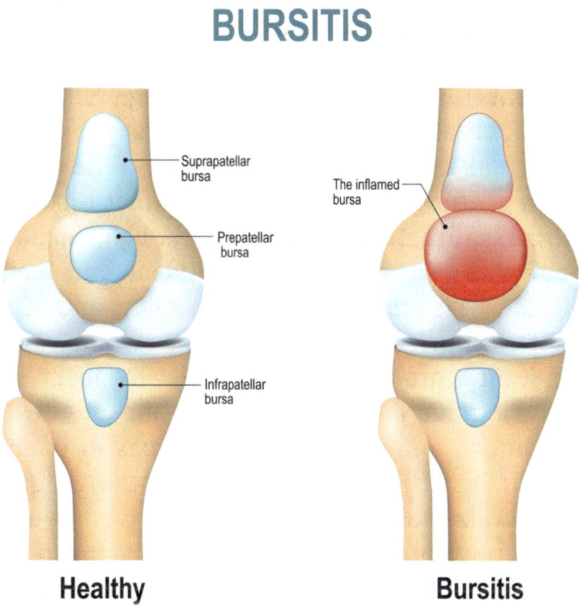

Figure 5.14. Bursitis.

Source: https://wp02-media.cdn.ihealthspot.com/wp-content/uploads/sites/393/2022/09/iStock-654812694.jpg.

5.5.1. Definition and Common Sites Affected

Understanding orthopedic conditions necessitates an entire description and identification of the common locations affected. Orthopedics, essentially, is the diagnosis, care, and prevention of musculoskeletal illnesses that can affect bones, joints, muscles, tendons, and ligaments. Among the many conditions that are managed by Orthopedics physiotherapy, osteoarthritis (OA) is among the most prevalent and specifically occurs in older adults and individuals under 45 years. Degenerative joint disease resulting from the wearing down of cartilage over time causes pain, stiffness, and loss of range of motion of affected joints, where the hips, knees, and hands are the most involved. OA not only limits individual mobility but also carries marked impacts on quality of life, necessitating effective management strategies, particularly at the onset (Oluchukwu, 2018). In addition to OA, other common orthopedic conditions include rheumatoid arthritis (RA), fractures, and sports injuries, each of which presents unique challenges in diagnosis and care. RA is an autoimmune disease that primarily occurs in the small joints of fingers and toes, often leading to crippling inflammation and stiffness. Fractures can occur, though, in any bone due to trauma, excessive wear and tear, or disease, such as in the wrist, ankle, and hip. Sports injuries such as sprains, strains, and tendonitis are frequent locations to occur at the shoulder and knee. Recognition of these conditions and their respective areas of effect is crucial for orthopedic physiotherapists, who utilize targeted rehabilitation techniques to restore function and alleviate symptoms (Oluchukwu, 2018). Lastly, recognition of sites most typically affected by orthopedic conditions offers understanding of prevention and rehabilitation strategies that can be utilized. Conditions such as OA predominantly involve load-bearing joints, and that reflects the importance of population-based management interventions aimed at the maintenance of joint function. As an illustration, interventions in physiotherapy based on strength training and flexibility can delay the loss of function that is typical among these conditions. For OA, early physiotherapy referral has been shown to maximize the outcomes from treatment through pain reduction and enhanced functional ability. Similarly, in sports injuries, rehabilitative intervention is called for to enable the recovery of mobility and re-injury avoidance, emphasizing the need for early intervention in orthopedic physiotherapy (Oluchukwu, 2018).

5.5.2. Causes and Symptoms

A good knowledge of the etiology and symptoms of common orthopedic conditions is essential for effective physiotherapy intervention. Conditions can have many causes, from lifestyle choices to workplace hazards and underlying medical conditions. For instance, repetitive strain injury often relates to specific activities involving prolonged periods of physical exertion, such as typing or lifting. In addition, conditions like osteoarthritis can also occur as a result of the natural wear and tear of joints over time, which is aggravated by factors like obesity and previous injuries. Identification of the root causes becomes paramount in developing specific therapeutic interventions that not only cure the symptoms but also prevent further deterioration of the patient's condition. To this end, a thorough scrutiny of the patient's history and daily habits maximizes the effectiveness of physiotherapy sessions. Symptoms of orthopedic disorders tend to be rather varied but are generally dominated by pain, swelling, and a decrease in range of motion. As an example, in hallux valgus, a common foot deformity, patients tend to complain of pain, swelling, and restriction in undertaking typical day-to-day activities related to mobility of the foot. Moreover, the pain that has occurred may tend to worsen while undertaking weight-bearing activities, leading to further difficulties in walking or standing for extended durations. Symptoms can severely affect quality of life, and therefore, such symptoms motivate people to undergo physiotherapeutic treatment. Home exercise programs have been known to reduce joint mobility and foot pain, enhance overall functional abilities, in the late stage of hallux valgus. Tackling such symptoms is extremely crucial to restore normal function and improve the daily lives of patients (Arge et al., 2012). Further, recognizing the multifaceted nature of symptoms can lead to closer prognostic assessments by physical therapists. Additional symptoms, such as stiffness or weakness of a joint, may be present in some patients, which would represent a more difficult underlying condition and a multidisciplinary treatment regimen. For example, conditions such as rheumatoid arthritis not only cause inflammation in the joints but also yield systemic symptoms that affect additional body systems. Early intervention through physiotherapy can help decrease the progression of such conditions and improve the outcomes of patients. Effective symptom control through targeted exercises, pain management techniques, and education further helps make patients active players in their recovery. Such holistic approaches are essential in addressing the full gamut of causes and symptoms that accompany standard Orthopedics conditions (Oberlander, 1960).

5.5.3. Physiotherapy Strategies for Relief

The management of common orthopedic conditions typically demands an integrated approach to pain relief and restoration of function. A role for physiotherapy practice is central to this scenario, involving a blend of manual therapy and individualized exercise prescription. For instance, patients with conditions such as OA can benefit from local strengthening exercises and improvement in joint stability. This conservative therapeutic strategy is critical in the early stages of OA to retard disease progression and reduce loss of function. By preserving musculoskeletal integrity and educating the patient in proper movement mechanics, physiotherapy not only offers pain relief but also enables the patient to be more participatory in their activities of daily living, enhancing their quality of life, as the literature in the subject describes (Oluchukwu, 2018). Complementing standard physiotherapy methods with complementary therapies can increase effectiveness. Yoga interventions in the guise of the mind sound resonance technique (MSRT) have shown tremendous potential in managing chronic neck pain (CNP). According to the studies, it is recommended that including such therapy can bring holistic relaxation effects, which help in relieving pain and anxiety levels associated with chronic conditions. MSRTs emphasis on resonance with sound is an innovative platform for inducing deep relaxation that can be very effective after a general treatment of physiotherapy. Integration of traditional practices and yoga therapies not only facilitates physical relief but also supports emotional health, thereby reflecting the holistic aspect of effective physiotherapy measures (Ebnezar & Ebnezar, 2015).

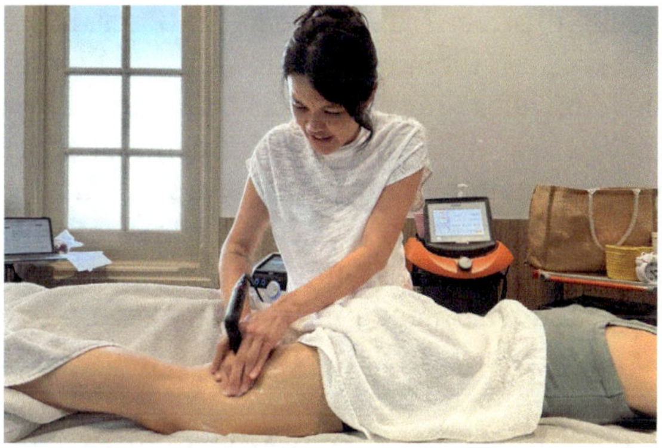

Figure 5.15. Physical therapy for bursitis restores mobility and relieves pain.

Source: https://www.hellophysio.sg/wp-content/uploads/2024/12/bursitis-physical-therapy.jpg.

Ultimately, inclusion of various strategies in physiotherapy reflects a transformational image of patient needs in orthopedic treatment. Since clinicians implement evidence-based therapies, the focus lies more on personalized treatment plans, taking into account the intricacy of each condition. It entails precise assessments and adjustments based on the progress of the individual, not just physical symptoms, but also the psychology involved in recovery. By establishing an environment that facilitates patient participation and education, physiotherapists are able to make treatment more responsive. As outcomes reveal the success of such multi-faceted strategies, the final goal becomes clear: to enhance functionality and allow for long-term freedom from the ills of orthopedic disorders, eventually enhancing the quality of life in patients of various age groups (Figure 5.15).

5.6. Sports Injuries

Sports injuries are a significant area of concern in orthopedic physiotherapy as they encompass a wide range of musculoskeletal injuries that may affect athletes at every level of competition. These injuries, from sprains and strains to fractures and tendinitis, not only adversely affect physical performance but also disrupt an athlete's way of life. Determinants of sports injuries include faulty warm-up, technique flaws, and even overtraining. The intricate presentation of these injuries necessitates an integrated treatment approach that covers both the initial injury and longer-term rehabilitation interventions to prevent further recurrence. Psychological impact of sports injuries, such as fear of re-injury, also becomes an integral part of the recovery process, bringing to the fore the need for holistic management combining physical and emotional care. The most prevalent types of sports injury are those to the knee, such as torn anterior cruciate ligaments (ACL) and osteoarthritis of the knee. Sudden change-of-direction type sports, such as soccer and basketball, are likely to result in such an injury, which can severely disable an athlete. It has been found that programs with progressive exercise protocols can considerably enhance rehabilitation outcomes. For example, a study highlighted that walking exercises significantly improved function and quality of life in patients with knee osteoarthritis (Carlson et al., 2014). Being that sports individuals typically experience long periods of physical stress, having such rehabilitation programs tailored is essential to optimize healing and return to sport. Tailoring can contribute significantly to improving the success of rehabilitation and minimizing the chance of future injury. In addition, integration of advanced technologies in physiotherapy, such as virtual reality (VR), is redefining rehabilitation protocols for sports injuries. Virtual reality environments allow for real-time, individualized feedback, which can help in learning suitable biomechanics and movement patterns required for recovery. Notably, research has demonstrated that applications of VR not only improve functional recovery but also control pain and reduce anxiety associated with immobility (Paladugu et al., 2025). However, even with such promising technologies, challenges remain to be overcome in their adoption, primarily in terms of cost, regulatory licensing, and further proof-of-concept through strong clinical trials. Ultimately, the application of these frontier devices in orthopedic physiotherapy is a shining future for sports injury management, enhancing both patient engagement and treatment effectiveness.

5.6.1. Common Sports-Related Orthopedic Injuries

In athletics, players are prone to numerous orthopedic injuries that can drastically alter their performance and career. Among the frequent ones are sprains, strains, fractures, and tendonitis, which vary in the rehabilitation challenges they present. The prevalence of these afflictions is particularly noteworthy in high-impact sports such as football, where it's common to have sudden collisions and body clashes that increase the chances of sustaining injuries. For example, ligament sprains of the knee and ankle are common among footballers and can easily lead to long recovery periods if they are not promptly and adequately treated. Such injuries bring the demand for cheap sports and exercise medicine (SEM), particularly in those regions where physiotherapy centers are few, such as in certain regions in Kenya. Treatment of these types of injury using proper rehabilitation methods can prevent long-term consequences for the involved athletes (Patel,

2015). Overuse injury is also a significant problem in repetitive motion sports like running or swimming. Tendonitis, bursitis, and stress fractures can develop after some time and are most commonly brought about by improper training programs or technique. The effects of such injuries go beyond the immediate physical pain; they also affect the psychological well-being of an athlete, as prolonged absences from competition can lead to anxiety and loss of drive. Notably, the effectiveness of physiotherapy to cure such injuries hinges on early diagnosis and treatment. Integrated rehabilitation plans that are centered on strength training and flexibility exercises can form the basic part of recovery to allow athletes to return to sport safely. The prevalent rate of turnovers of athletes in competitive environments indicates a critical necessity for increased awareness and implementation of SEM and physiotherapy protocols for developing healthier sporting careers (Setuain et al., 2017). Moreover, prevention of injury cannot be overstressed. Education and familiarity with common sports injuries permit a proactive action by athletes, coaches, and doctors. The integration of specialized warm-up routines, proper technique training, and ongoing physical conditioning can dramatically reduce injury potential. For football, as an example, where frequency and severity of injury are heightened, it is crucial to integrate training programs with injury prevention components. In the absence of such interventions, many athletes have been exposed to career-risking injuries that are largely preventable, even considering the lack of access to quality physiotherapy for most of the world. A push for awareness of orthopedic conditions and emphasis on preventive procedures in sports communities is critical to enhancing longevity and performance among various categories of athletes (Patel, 2015) (Figure 5.16).

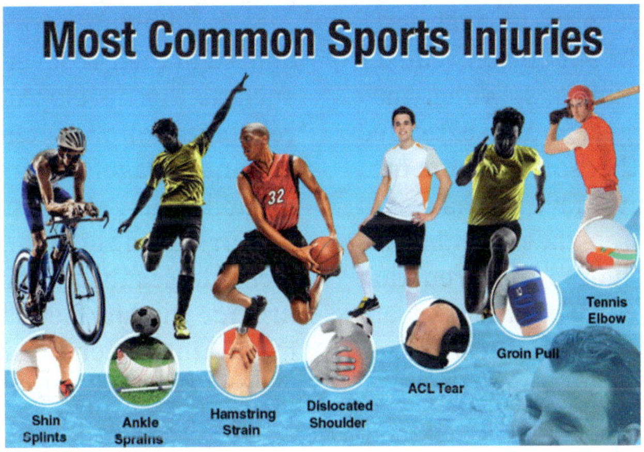

Figure 5.16. Common sports injuries.

Source: https://orangecountyOrthopedicscenter.com/wp-content/uploads/2018/12/Most-Common-Sports-Injuries-by-Orange-County-Orthopedics-Center-1.jpg.

5.6.2. Importance of Early Intervention

Early intervention of orthopedic conditions is crucial in the control of pain and the enhancement of functional outcomes. If patients are treated early after the presentation of symptoms, particularly for conditions such as OA, the alleviation of pain and enhancement of their quality of life is immense. As pointed out in a blog that addresses conservative management of OA, early intervention not only slows disease progression but also reverses secondary effects like diminished functional ability and disability (Oluchukwu, 2018). By adding physiotherapy at an early point in treatment, patients can be empowered to acquire skills to effectively control their symptoms, maintain their independence and mobility, and avoid the chance of requiring more extreme interventions in the future. One of the primary benefits of early intervention is the potential for increased patient participation in their rehabilitation. For instance, digital platforms that enable patients to self-manage their own post-surgery recovery, such as total knee replacement (TKR), identify the importance of education and active participation as part of the earliest stages of treatment (Hussain et al., 2017). Patients can better adhere to rehabilitation timetables and learn about their recovery processes using mobile apps and wearable technology. These attempts also increase communication among patients and clinicians, thus establishing a cooperative healthcare environment that highlights the significance of early intervention in providing desired outcomes. Early intervention may also lead to significant cost benefits to healthcare systems. Delayed treatment often causes increased orthopedic conditions, which may lead to complicated surgeries and extended rehabilitation times. With rapid response to initial symptoms, patients have a chance of avoiding costly procedures that could arise from advanced disease. It is discovered that the economic benefits of early intervention are enormous since they reduce healthcare costs related to long-term care and chronic disability (Oluchukwu, 2018). Against this backdrop, it is clear that prioritizing early intervention not only maximizes patient outcomes at an individual level but also improves healthcare efficiency at a broader level by reducing the necessity for more resource-hungry and multifaceted interventions.

5.6.3. Rehabilitation Techniques in Physiotherapy

Rehabilitation techniques in physiotherapy play a pivotal role in healing patients suffering from typical orthopedic disorders. Rehabilitation techniques include various procedures like exercise therapy, manual therapy, and patient education that are patient-specific. Exercise therapy is the most common technique of rehabilitation and is applied in the management of pain, improved movement, and recovery of function. Physiotherapists can assist patients in slowly regaining their flexibility and strength, both of which are needed for complete recovery, through specialized exercise regimens. Joint mobilization and soft tissue manipulation are also often used as manual therapy methods to decrease pain and improve joint function. All these techniques, when combined, not only cover physical recovery but also instill empowerment amongst patients so that they can actively participate in their rehabilitation (Samoy et al., 2016). Rehabilitation techniques are most salient in the case of total knee replacement (TKR) surgeries because of the complexities involved in recovery. A structured rehabilitation program is of prime importance in optimizing results following surgery and ensuring patients adhere to their recovery plans. Recent advances, such as the development of online orthopedic rehabilitation websites, have proven to enhance patient engagement and adherence to ordered rehabilitation exercises. Such systems typically comprise mobile programs and wearable technologies that monitor the activity levels and provide instant feedback, which is essential in motivating patients during the recovery process. Technology in rehabilitation practice illustrates an extensive shift towards personalized care that allows physiotherapists to deliver patient-tailored interventions while fostering patient responsibility in their recovery (Hussain et al., 2017). Lastly, the effectiveness of rehabilitation techniques in physiotherapy relies on the interactive relationship between the patient and the therapist. Good communication and regular assessment are important to guide treatment plans as patients go through their rehabilitation. Such a perpetual dialogue allows physiotherapists to identify barriers to recovery and tailor interventions to meet the unique needs of their patients. Studies demonstrate that the results of rehabilitation are significantly enhanced when patients are made to feel engaged and informed about their care. Thus, the inclusion of evidence-based methods along with individualized patient care not only allows for recovery at the physical level but also improves the psychological preparedness of patients to adhere to their rehabilitation process. With the advancement of physiotherapy, physicians must remain current on novel rehabilitation modalities so that they are able to treat a wide variety of orthopedic disorders effectively (Samoy et al., 2016) (Figure 5.17).

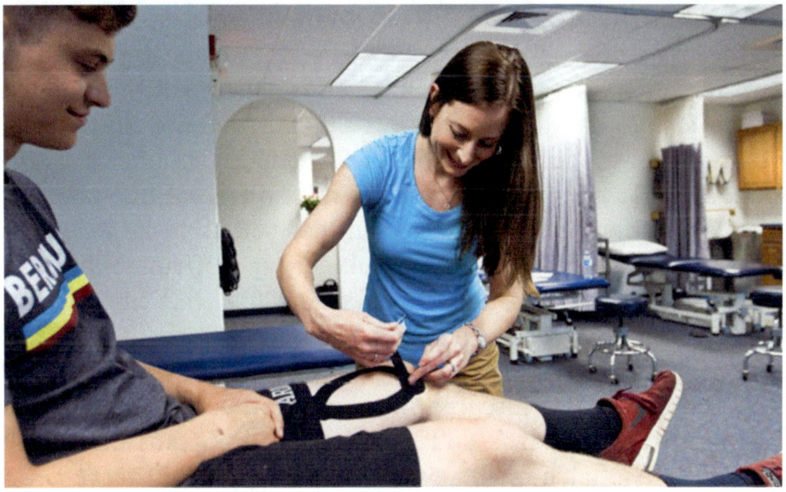

Figure 5.17. Sports injury rehabilitation.

Source: https://rehabconceptspt.com/wp-content/uploads/2017/10/rehab-concepts-Orthopedics-rehabilitation.jpg.

SUMMARY

The research on common orthopedic conditions demonstrates the significant contribution orthopedic physiotherapy can make in the process of rehabilitation. The patients suffering from conditions such as osteoarthritis, tendonitis, and fractures can significantly benefit from special interventions of physiotherapy. These not only reduce pain and increase mobility but also improve the quality of life of the patient. Through the use of evidence-based practice, physiotherapists can tailor their intervention to specific patient needs, maximizing the potential for recovery. The individualized care treats both physical and psychological health, and again highlights the relevance of incorporating physiotherapy into orthopedic regimes of care. Inherent to successful orthopedic physiotherapy is ongoing research that informs practice. Scientific studies have substantiated the effectiveness of many of the physiotherapeutic modalities for the treatment of orthopedic conditions and thereby strengthened the foundation of treatment protocols. With observations pouring in from scientific studies, the possibility of refining therapeutic techniques seems to be a reality. Fresh techniques and fresh technologies are gradually changing the landscape of rehabilitation, leading to better patient outcomes and increased professional standards. This shift highlights the importance of keeping current with research discoveries so that therapies are both effective and pertinent. Lastly, as orthopedic attention is required increasingly, so too is the responsibility of physiotherapists to provide high-level treatment. The integration of physiotherapy into conventional orthopedic practice serves to maximize patient care and address an important deficit in rehabilitation. By recognizing the multi-dimensional benefits of physiotherapy, healthcare practitioners are in a position to collaborate in developing interdisciplinary treatment plans. Through this collaboration, in conjunction with professional growth and research, is essential in advancing the practice. As exemplified, the results of Oberlander, 1960, (1960) on inventive practice solutions and the growing literature concerning physiotherapy's benefit, as mentioned in Samoy et al. (2016), also underscore the importance that orthopedic physiotherapy holds in an integrated recovery process. Orthopedic disorders encompass a wide range of musculoskeletal illnesses that have significant effects on mobility and quality of life. One of the most prevalent disorders is osteoarthritis, the cartilage and bone degeneration within joints, commonly leading to pain and stiffness. It is most often seen in older adults and affects such joints as knees, hips, and hands, leading to extensive functional impairments. Treatment of osteoarthritis is highly involved and encompasses physical therapy, medication, and lifestyle modification with the aim of reducing symptoms as well as enhancing functionality. The pathophysiology of osteoarthritis has to be comprehended to formulate specific physiotherapy interventions that can facilitate the reduction of pain and improve mobility, thereby enabling enhanced independence in activities. Determining these factors is paramount for the Orthopedics physiotherapists treating affected populations and allows for more tailored rehabilitation (Oberlander, 1960). Rheumatoid arthritis is another significant disorder in Orthopedics, which is an autoimmune condition that predominantly affects joint tissues, resulting in inflammation, pain, and the destruction of joints. Compared with osteoarthritis, this disorder is more prevalent in young individuals and can also extend to the body to yield systemic complications. The chronic condition of rheumatoid arthritis calls for global management techniques involving both medication and physical therapy. Physiotherapists contribute greatly to reducing the functional impacts by fostering joint stability and enhancing the range of motion with special exercises. Moreover, the psychosocial impacts of managing a chronic disease call for therapeutic intervention to optimize patients' global well-being. Treating the unique issues of rheumatoid arthritis is of highest significance to the practice of orthopedic physiotherapists endeavoring to improve the quality of life for individuals suffering with this debilitating disease (Howard-Wilsher et al., 2016). Lastly, sports injury is an important subcategory of orthopedic conditions, typically occurring through acute trauma or cumulative overuse. Common injuries are sprains, fractures, and tendonitis that may occur in different sporting environments. As competitive and recreational sports gain popularity, there has also been a raised awareness about injury prevention as well as rehabilitation measures among physiotherapists. It is imperative to have an in-depth understanding of the biomechanics of the musculoskeletal system so that effective intervention programs can be formulated to return athletes to their pre-injury levels of play. Rehabilitation programs typically consist of pain management, restoration of strength and flexibility, and gradual return to sporting activities. By applying evidence-based practices, orthopedic physiotherapists are central to optimizing recovery and minimizing recurrent injury, hence enhancing athletes' long-term performance and health (Oberlander, 1960).

CLOSER LOOK

OSTEOARTHRITIS

Osteoarthritis is the most common form of arthritis, characterized by the gradual breakdown of cartilage that cushions the ends of bones in joints. As cartilage wears away, bones begin to rub against each other, leading to pain, stiffness, swelling, and reduced joint mobility. It most commonly affects weight-bearing joints such as the knees, hips, spine, and also the hands. The condition usually develops slowly and is associated with aging, but factors such as obesity, joint injuries, repetitive stress, genetics, and poor posture can increase the risk. Early symptoms include joint discomfort after activity, mild stiffness, and reduced flexibility. As osteoarthritis progresses, pain may become persistent, joints may swell, and daily activities such as walking, climbing stairs, or gripping objects can become difficult. Diagnosis involves clinical evaluation and imaging techniques like X-rays or MRI to assess cartilage loss and bone changes. Management focuses on relieving symptoms and improving joint function. Treatment includes lifestyle modifications, weight management, physiotherapy, pain-relieving and anti-inflammatory medications, and supportive devices such as braces. In severe cases, surgical options like joint replacement may be recommended. Regular exercise, proper nutrition, and joint protection strategies play a key role in prevention and long-term management. Overall, early diagnosis and comprehensive care can significantly reduce discomfort, maintain mobility, and enhance quality of life for individuals living with osteoarthritis.

REFERENCES

1. Setuain, I., Gonzalez-Izal, M., Paularena, A., Luque, J. L., Andersen, L. L., & Izquierdo, M. (2017). A protocol for a new methodological model for work-related shoulder complex injuries: From diagnosis to rehabilitation. *BMC musculoskeletal disorders*, *18*(1), 70. https://doi.org/10.1186/s12891-017-1435-2(accessed on 26th June 2025).

2. Aprato, A., Jayasekera, N., Bajwa, A., & Villar, R. N. (2014). Peri-articular diseases of the hip: emerging frontiers in arthroscopic and endoscopic treatments. *Journal of orthopaedics and traumatology : official journal of the Italian Society of Orthopaedics and Traumatology*, *15*(1), 1–11. https://doi.org/10.1007/s10195-013-0253-z(accessed on 26th June 2025).

3. Arge, A., Gapeyeva, H., Lenzner, A., Pääsuke, et al. (2012). Range of motion and pain intensity of the first metatarsophalangeal joint in women with hallux valgus deformation after two-month home exercise programmed. https://core.ac.uk/download/25069006.pdf (accessed on 26th June 2025).

4. Hendriksz, C. J., Berger, K. I., Giugliani, R., Harmatz, P., Kampmann, C., Mackenzie, W. G., Raiman, J., Villarreal, M. S., & Savarirayan, R. (2015). International guidelines for the management and treatment of Morquio A syndrome. *American journal of medical genetics. Part A*, *167A*(1), 11–25. https://doi.org/10.1002/ajmg.a.36833(accessed on 26th June 2025).

5. Hussain, M. S., Li, J., Brindal, E., van Kasteren, Y., Varnfield, M., Reeson, A., Berkovsky, S., & Freyne, J. (2017). Supporting the Delivery of Total Knee Replacements Care for Both Patients and Their Clinicians With a Mobile App and Web-Based Tool: Randomized Controlled Trial Protocol. *JMIR research protocols*, *6*(3), e32. https://doi.org/10.2196/resprot.6498(accessed on 26th June 2025).

6. Maccio, J. R., Fink, S., Yarznbowicz, R., & May, S. (2016). The application of mechanical diagnosis and therapy in lateral epicondylalgia. *The Journal of manual & manipulative therapy*, *24*(3), 158–165. https://doi.org/10.1080/10669817.2015.1110303 (accessed on 26th June 2025).

7. Carlson, T., Edvalson, D., Peck, T., Robison, et al. (2014). The effects of a progressive exercise program on functional activity and quality of life for older overweight women with knee osteoarthritis. http://digitalscholarship.unlv.edu/cgi/viewcontent.cgi?article=3456&context=thesesdissertations (accessed on 26th June 2025).

8. Caterina, V. C., Geddes, C., Boljanovic, D., Razmjou, H., Macritchie, I., Richards, R. R., & Lincoln, S. (2015). Examining outcome of early physician specialist assessment in injured workers with shoulder complaints. https://core.ac.uk/download/208804758.pdf (accessed on 26th June 2025).

9. McArthur, K., Jorgensen, D., Climstein, M., & Furness, J. (2020). Epidemiology of Acute Injuries in Surfing: Type, Location, Mechanism, Severity, and Incidence: A Systematic Review. *Sports (Basel, Switzerland)*, *8*(2), 25. https://doi.org/10.3390/sports8020025 (accessed on 26th June 2025).

10. Crouch, M. J. (1947). A course in orthopedics nursing to be used in the basic nursing program of "X" School of Nursing. https://open.bu.edu/bitstream/2144/18794/1/courseinorthoped00crou.pdf (accessed on 26th June 2025).

11. Pierce, A., Teeling, S. P., McNamara, M., O'Daly, B., & Daly, A. (2023). Using Lean Six Sigma in a Private Hospital Setting to Reduce Trauma Orthopedic Patient Waiting Times and Associated

Administrative and Consultant Caseload. *Healthcare (Basel, Switzerland)*, *11*(19), 2626. https://doi.org/10.3390/healthcare11192626(accessed on 26th June 2025).

12. Ebnezar, Y. J., & Ebnezar, J. (2015). Complementary effect of yogic relaxation technique on pain, disability and anxiety in patients with common neck pain. https://core.ac.uk/download/333809381.pdf (accessed on 26th June 2025).
13. Howard-Wilsher, S., Irvine, L., Fan, H., Shakespeare, T., Suhrcke, M., Horton, S., Poland, F., Hooper, L., & Song, F. (2016). Systematic overview of economic evaluations of health-related rehabilitation. *Disability and health journal*, *9*(1), 11–25. https://doi.org/10.1016/j.dhjo.2015.08.009(accessed on 26th June 2025).
14. Ponciano, V., Pires, I. M., Ribeiro, F. R., Marques, G., Garcia, N. M., Pombo, N., Spinsante, S., & Zdravevski, E. (2020). Is The Timed-Up and Go Test Feasible in Mobile Devices? A Systematic Review. *Electronics*, *9*(3), 528. https://doi.org/10.3390/electronics9030528(accessed on 26th June 2025).
15. Górka, D., Kozioł, M., Kupczak, A., Palacz, et al. (2024). Methods of managing postoperative pain in orthopedics. https://core.ac.uk/download/636385492.pdf (accessed on 26th June 2025).
16. Janes, G., Serrant, L., & Sque, M. (2018). Fragility hip fracture in the under 60s: A qualitative study of recovery experiences and the implications for nursing. https://core.ac.uk/download/160276072.pdf (accessed on 26th June 2025).
17. Lemons, J. B., Sheesley, D. C., & Sutton, P. R. (2012). Supervised lower extremity strengthening program to improve function in women over fifty with knee osteoarthritis: A time series design. http://digitalscholarship.unlv.edu/cgi/viewcontent.cgi?article=2329&context=theses dissertations (accessed on 26th June 2025).
18. Paladugu, P., Kumar, R., Ong, J., Waisberg, E., & Sporn, K. (2025). Virtual reality-enhanced rehabilitation for improving musculoskeletal function and recovery after trauma. *Journal of orthopaedic surgery and research*, *20*(1), 404. https://doi.org/10.1186/s13018-025-05705-3(accessed on 26th June 2025).
19. Peiris, C. L., Shields, N., Brusco, N. K., Watts, J. J., & Taylor, N. F. (2013). Additional Saturday rehabilitation improves functional independence and quality of life and reduces length of stay: a randomized controlled trial. *BMC medicine*, *11*, 198. https://doi.org/10.1186/1741-7015-11-198(accessed on 26th June 2025).
20. Oberlander, B. (1960). An exploratory study of the characteristics of chronic returnees to the rehabilitation and physical medicine department of the Massachusetts Memorial Hospitals. https://open.bu.edu/bitstream/2144/27265/1/Oberlander_Beatrice_1960_web.pdf (accessed on 26th June 2025).
21. Oluchukwu, O. C. (2018). Perceptions and experiences of health professionals regarding conservative management of osteoarthritis at a tertiary hospital in Nigeria. https://core.ac.uk/download/199461276.pdf (accessed on 26th June 2025).
22. Patel, M. (2015). Sports and exercise medicine for athletes and footballers: The case of Kenya. https://core.ac.uk/download/232736983.pdf (accessed on 26th June 2025).
23. Samoy, Y., Saunders, J., & Van Ryssen, B. (2016). Physiotherapy in small animal medicine. https://core.ac.uk/download/154408470.pdf (accessed on 26th June 2025).

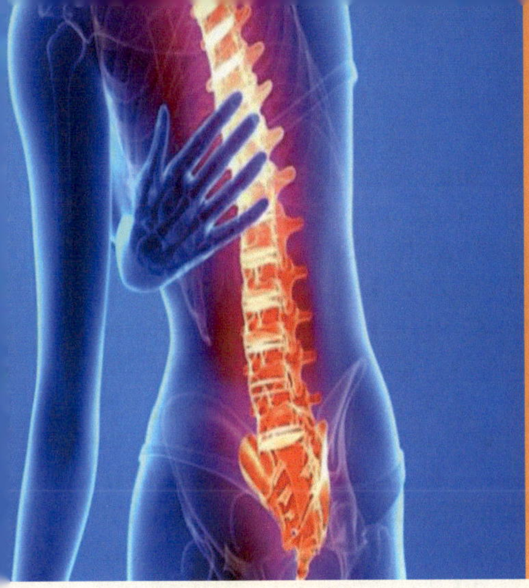

Chapter 6
SPINAL DISORDERS

Contents

Introduction 169
6.1. Anatomy of the Spine 172
6.2. Common Types of Spinal Disorders 175
6.3. Causes of Spinal Disorders 179
6.4. Symptoms of Spinal Disorders 182
6.5. Diagnosis of Spinal Disorders 186
6.6. Treatment Options for Spinal Disorders 189
Summary 194
References 197

Introduction

The history behind spinal disorders is a vital foundation for understanding the subtleties of this health specialty. Spinal disorders are a series of conditions that affect the spine and its associated structures to produce severe pain and disability. Spinal disorders can be grouped under degenerative diseases, injury, and congenital abnormalities, each with inherent difficulties in diagnosis and treatment. Furthermore, the incidence of such conditions is staggering, considering that they significantly impact quality of life, productivity, and overall health. When we place into perspective the context of spinal disorders, we can better appreciate the need for research and proper management strategies that are urgently needed. Defining the nature of the complexity of these conditions will make it possible to understand their physical and psychological effects on people more accurately, thus putting more importance on this subject in the broader healthcare context. Spinal disorders do more than lead to pain and limitation on the physical level; they have long-term consequences for individuals and the health system as a whole. As stated, most common musculoskeletal disorders, including spinal disorders, are resistant to conventional treatment methods, creating the need for new solutions and more targeted research activity (Poltawski et al., 2008). Economic burdens of spinal disorders are also substantial, with estimates indicating that treatment and management costs amount to billions annually. From these statistics, healthcare providers and researchers must prioritize spinal disorders during the allocation of resources for research and treatment programs. Being aware of health disparities when it comes to the control of such diseases is able to further shed light on the gaps that still exist in terms of care accessibility and results, ultimately calling for action. The impact of spinal illness can even be experienced by others, and not only the patient, with consequences affecting families and communities as well. The mental disturbances of depression and anxiety are possible in chronic spinal patients and contribute to their recovery and management workload (Jeffries, 2016). Caregivers also have a higher emotional and physical workload, a factor that cannot be ignored while discussing spinal health. As we delve deeper into the complexities of spinal disorders in this essay, we aim not only to concentrate on the medical and physiological aspects but also on the social and emotional aspects that are involved in these disorders. The establishment of this holistic picture will be important in advocating for such disorders in research, treatment, and policy discussion, thus establishing a more realistic understanding of healthcare in the field of spinal disorders.

Definition of Spinal Disorders

Spinal disorders represent a broad category of disorders that affect the spinal column, its associated muscles, and the associated neural structures. They are present due to various etiologies, including congenital malformations, degenerative changes, trauma, infection, and tumors. An understanding of spinal disorders is important in diagnosing these disorders and their management correctly. Clinically, the disorders present with disparate symptoms, ranging from localized pain and stiffness to catastrophic neurological deficits, depending on the affected structure and severity of the basic condition. As a result, spinal disorder classification often includes terms such as degenerative disc disease, spinal stenosis, herniated disc, and spondylolisthesis, reflecting the heterogeneity of the disorders and necessitating a multidisciplinary treatment strategy. In addition, the effects of spinal disorders extend beyond their physical impacts and have a profoundly disabling influence on the quality of life and functional ability of people. Such chronic disorders as low back pain are frequent and can produce significant disability and influence not only personal well-being but also economic output. Research has determined that spinal disorder treatment often requires a high degree understanding of surgical and non-surgical methods to facilitate effective treatment planning. As an example, posterior spinal fusion (PSF) has emerged as a common surgical procedure for the treatment of certain spinal disorders, indicating the need for accurate prediction of surgical outcomes. Involvement with predictive modelling can enhance decision-making in the clinical setting of spinal surgery, further distinguishing the complexity of spinal disorders and strategies for treatment (Babaee et al., 2017). The evolving nature of medical evidence regarding spinal disorders is central to guiding treatment protocols. For instance, there has been the creation of new guidelines to enhance the management of specific spinal disorders like Moquino A syndrome, which reflects the need for individually tailored care strategies that are patient-specific (Akyol et al., 2019). These reflect the importance of including expert consensus and evidence-based recommendations in an effort to deliver comprehensive care to spinal disorder management. As healthcare providers continue to grapple with the problems posed by spinal disorders, the recognition of the need for solutions beyond medicine will enhance treatment outcomes and effectiveness. Ongoing research and advances in diagnostic as well as treatment modalities continuously emerge, increasing the understanding of spinal disorders that prepares the way for improved patient care solutions (Figure 6.1).

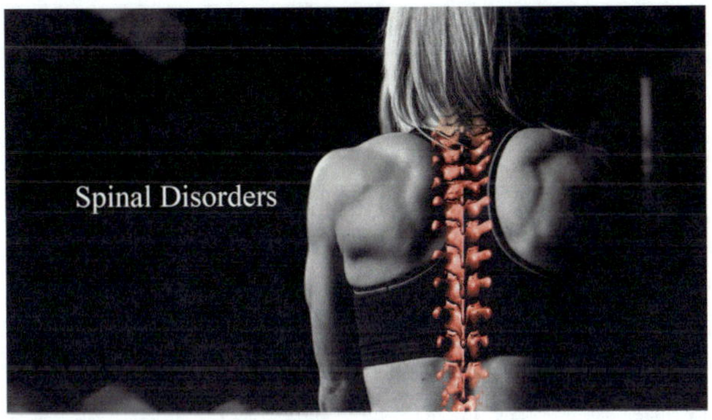

Figure 6.1. Spinal disorders encompass a broad spectrum of conditions that affect the spinal column.

Source: https://external-content.duckduckgo.com/iu/?u=https%3A%2F%2Fwww.spinedoctor33.com%2Fwp-content%2Fuploads%2F2024%2F06%2F8.Spinal-Disorders-1024x576.png&f=1&nofb=1&ipt=df8e16fccf9c5048caa9624562d22b8eb7f5d4433915e9377dfb5e3dfb95b18a.

Importance of Studying Spinal Disorders

The significance of studying spinal disorders is their significant contribution to impairment of quality of life and overall health of the affected. Spinal disorders are a wide spectrum of disease that encompasses herniated discs, spinal stenosis, and degenerative disc disease, all of which can lead to chronic pain and impairment of mobility. Knowledge of the pathophysiology of these diseases is crucial to the manufacture of therapeutic and intervention measures that work. Research in this area not only aims to alleviate pain but also aims to restore function and improve the well-being of the patients. Further, advances in understanding spinal disorders can aid in planning prevention measures, thereby reducing the incidence of these conditions in the population. Greater awareness and knowledge can enable patients to come forward early for treatment, thereby preventing potentially serious consequences of untreated spinal disease. Moreover, scientific investigation of spinal disorders is the driving force behind the development of medical practice and new technologies. The confluence of biomedical engineering and neuroscience has led to novel approaches like minimally invasive surgery and regenerative treatments that improve recovery. For example, researchers are still exploring the role of neuroimmunology and stem cells in spinal health since both fields may reveal new ways of regeneration and repair of spinal tissues (DeLong et al., 2008). On the other hand, understanding the biopsychosocial substrates of spinal conditions is essential in successful treatment programs, which often include physical therapy, psychological counseling, and lifestyle changes. Thus, ongoing research enhances not only medical science but also improved models for healthcare delivery that can meet individual patients' needs, thus improving the face of healthcare among patients with spinal disorders. Finally, the social dimensions of spinal disorders emphasize the need for research in the field. Those with chronic spinal disorders frequently report employment, mental health, and social issues, and these are reasons why model-based care for integrated models that respond to such complex issues is crucial. The Department of Veterans Affairs, for instance, is engaged in expansive research initiatives to enhance the lives of veterans living with spinal disorders, particularly regarding traumatic injuries sustained while serving (Sivhugwana, 2021). By focusing on the rehabilitation and reintegration of such veterans, researchers can develop models that can be applied in non-military contexts. The significance of conducting research into spinal disorders, then, is not just for clinical outcomes but also for its ability to benefit society as a whole, encouraging an evidence-based system to help individuals grappling with the effects of spinal ill health.

6.1. Anatomy of the Spine

The spinal anatomy is a complex and intrinsic component of the musculoskeletal system of the human body, offering both support and protection to the central nervous system. The spine consists of 33 vertebrae and five distinct areas: cervical, thoracic, lumbar, sacral, and coccygeal. All of these areas perform distinct functions and possess distinct features that collectively ensure the flexibility and stability of spines. The intervertebral discs, which are found between the vertebrae, act as a shock absorber and allow movement and flexion and rotation, among other movements. This elaborate structure not only provides the spine with strength but also indicates its susceptibility to illness, with disc degeneration and herniation being some of the chief disorders associated with the spine, which introduce disabling symptoms and affect quality of life. Understanding spinal anatomy is important in the diagnosis and treatment of spinal disorders because a variety of pathologies can arise from structural malformations or trauma. For example, disc problems such as herniation, bulging, and internal disc disruption can cause significant pain and dysfunction of mobility. These pathologies are often caused by age-related degeneration, trauma, or repetitive stress. Their diagnoses are heavily dependent on the proper understanding of spinal biomechanics, which entails studying the interaction between the vertebrae, the intervertebral discs, and the surrounding soft tissues. The intricacy of these interactions further buttresses the importance of full-range diagnostic methodologies, including advanced imaging technologies that can portray spinal dynamics. As seen, a majority of studies have been concerned with mechanical disorders of the spine, noting the burden and impact of such diseases on healthcare in the modern era (Zheng et al., 2001). Treatment of spinal disorders is commonly interdisciplinary in nature, involving medical, physiological, and sometimes surgical approaches.

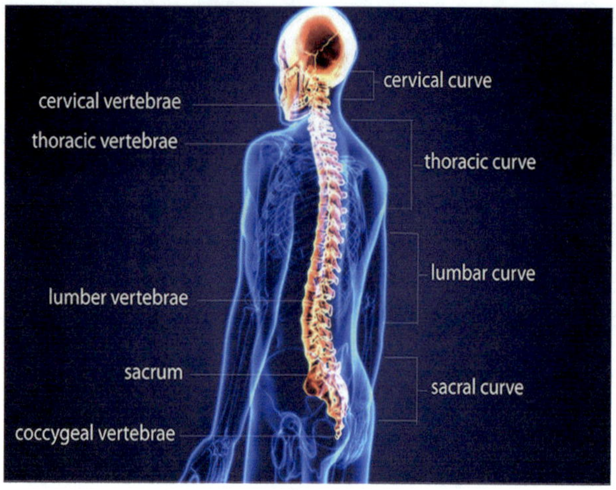

Figure 6.2. The anatomy of the spine is a complex and vital component of the human musculoskeletal system.

Source: https://external-content.duckduckgo.com/iu/?u=https%3A%2F%2Ftse4.mm.bing.net%2Fth%3Fid%3DOIP.dfs0Qk9SAJMuJp_fc9Xr4wHaEK%26pid%3DApi&f=1&ipt=f01029bda214b69b40064ef78c4b50f7cd7806a2e09bea1d66fa130549a7e2b5.

Conservative treatment typically begins with physical therapy to strengthen abdominal muscles, improve flexibility, and alleviate pain. Severe or progressive disc disease or structural abnormalities, if treated conservatively, may call for consideration of more advanced therapy such as spinal injection or surgery. Improved vertebral positioning and motion measurements with new imaging abilities have significantly enhanced diagnostic accuracy and treatment planning. For instance, the use of digital video fluoroscopy (DVF) enables clinicians to capture dynamic images of the spine in motion and facilitate a better understanding of the pathologies that affect spinal mechanics. The new technique is beneficial in tailoring interventions according to a patient's anatomical and pathological type and thereby improving therapeutic efficacy and quality of life for the patient (Walker, 1993) (Figure 6.2).

6.1.1. Structure of Vertebrae

Vertebrae anatomy forms the core of spinal pathology because it tells us about the spine's mechanical and physiological functions. A vertebra consists of several components, like the vertebral body, spinous process, and neural arch, that collectively allow for flexibility, stability, and neurologic protection of the spinal cord. The vertebral body is the weight-carrying component, designed to resist compressive loading with exercise and activity. Surrounding this structure are transverse and spinous processes, which offer areas of attachment for muscles and ligaments to enable movement and support of the spinal structure.

The functioning among these factors makes up the overall health of the spine and regulates the emergence and development of spinal disorders, primarily conditions such as disc disease, which can lead to extreme pain and mobility issues (Walke, 1993). Intervertebral discs occupy the area between vertebrae and act as shock absorbers and aid in spinal flexibility. Both disk contains an outer fibrous ring called the annulus fibrosus and a center filled with gel called the nucleus pulposus. This particular structure allows the discs to absorb various forces in executing motions from everyday bending to high-impact motions. However, with time and usage, such discs degenerate, herniate, or bulge and consequently compress adjacent spinal nerves, leading to radiculopathy or chronic back pain. Taking into account the structure and function of intervertebral discs anatomically, clinicians can better diagnose as well as treat disc degenerative conditions, as well as related disorders, which encompass a wide range of symptoms and treatment options (Walker, 1993). Ankylosing spondylitis (AS) is a good example that shows the structural impact of spinal disease.

The autoimmune condition results in the fusion of vertebrae, severely restricting spinal mobility and deforming the usual curvature of the spine. Pathological processes involved in AS are intricate and include an interplay between exogenous factors and genetic susceptibility that culminates in chronic inflammatory disease that deeply impacts the spine structure. Since the vertebrae eventually join, the patients start to have a vast array of symptoms other than musculoskeletal pain, like cardiovascular, neurological, and reproductive system effects. Not only pharmacologic treatment to prevent inflammation, but also certain exercises for keeping spinal flexibility and function, are also effective for treating AS. Hence, learning about the spinal anatomy gives significant insight into complications and treatment techniques necessary for the management of ankylosing spondylitis and other conditions of the spine (Figure 6.3).

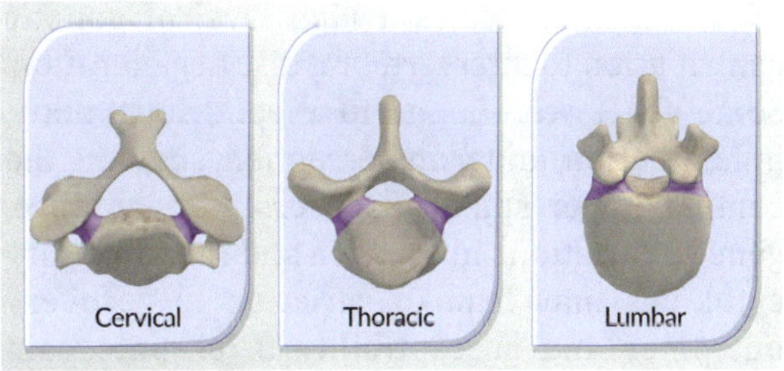

Figure 6.3. The structure of vertebrae.

Source: https://external-content.duckduckgo.com/iu/?u=https%3A%2F%2Fcloudfront.jove.com%2Ffiles%2Fmedia%2Fscience-education%2Fscience-education-thumbs%2F14037.jpg&f=1&nofb=1&ipt=0b8651a366db0d6a5752e14c2f3f282201d4be743de779b5b89ccd37ebec5b93.

6.1.2. Intervertebral Discs and Their Function

Intervertebral discs play a very critical role in the structural support and function of the vertebral column. The discs exist between the vertebrae and serve as a shock absorber, absorbing shocks established during everyday exercises such as walking, running, and lifting. The disc has a gel-filled core known as the nucleus pulposus, which is enclosed within a fibrous outer ring known as the annulus fibrosus. This unique matrix enables the discs to absorb compressive and torsional stresses, both of which are essential for the maintenance of proper posture as well as mobility. When intervertebral discs are compromised due to either degeneration or trauma, they are unable to dissipate forces, leading to pain and suffering, usually manifesting as chronic back pain or sciatica. Understanding the anatomy and physiology of the discs is central to learning about most spinal disorders that originate with disc problems. The health of intervertebral discs is in part genetically determined, which might expose individuals to degenerative disc disease. Research has indicated that heritability estimates of back pain are between 30% and 45%, which indicates a high level of genetic contribution to intervertebral disc degeneration. Some genes were found to affect disc stability, inflammation, and pain perception, showing the complexity of spinal disorders. For instance, genetic variations in collagen and inflammatory cytokines may lead to variation in recovery outcomes and susceptibility to chronic pain between individuals. As such, effective pain management must consider such genetic variation, striving for tailored treatment programs with respect to both symptomatic relief and long-term spinal health. This genetic strategy is essential to the understanding of spinal disorders' multifactorial etiology and their management. Surgical interventions, such as lumbar discectomy, are most often indicated when nonoperative treatments don't alleviate severe pain due to herniated discs. Discectomy effectively removes herniated disc tissue that presses against nerve roots, which alleviates symptoms for the majority of patients. However, certain conditions, such as those involving extensive disc protrusions with minimal degeneration, have high recurrence rates of herniation following surgery. Thus, the need for improved results from surgery has led to the search for insight into biological annular repair techniques. Novel approaches, such as the development of tissue-engineered implants, emphasize improving the repair of damaged annulus fibrosus through the reestablishment of mechanical integrity. These advances highlight the importance of interdisciplinarity in solving the multifaceted problems of spinal disorders, ultimately leading to improved patient outcomes and a reduced rate of recurrent disc herniation (Pandit et al., 2013).

6.1.3. Spinal Cord and Nerve Roots

The spinal cord, a part of the central nervous system, plays the role of facilitating communication between the brain and other parts of the body. Protected by the vertebral column, the spinal cord extends from the brainstem to the lower back, comprising various segments correlating with specific areas of the spine. Each segment is associated with paired roots of nerves that emerge from the spinal cord to provide specific areas of the body. Nerve roots can be divided into anterior roots, which are motor, and posterior roots, which are sensory. Disruption or injury to the spinal cord or its nerve roots can lead to profound motor deficit, sensory loss, and a severely devastating impact on the quality of a person's life, emphasizing the necessity of a comprehensive knowledge of such structures in the context of spinal disease. Normal body function is dependent on the integrity of the spinal cord and nerve roots. Spinal disease, such as herniated discs or spinal stenosis, unfortunately, will lead to compressive forces against nerve roots that are painful and functionally impairing. For instance, patients will create sciatica—a catch-all term for a wide range of symptoms caused by radiating pain, paresthesia, or weakness—due to irritation of the nerve root by mechanical stressors. Evidence shows that while many experience episodes of back pain, serious medical complications requiring surgery are rare.

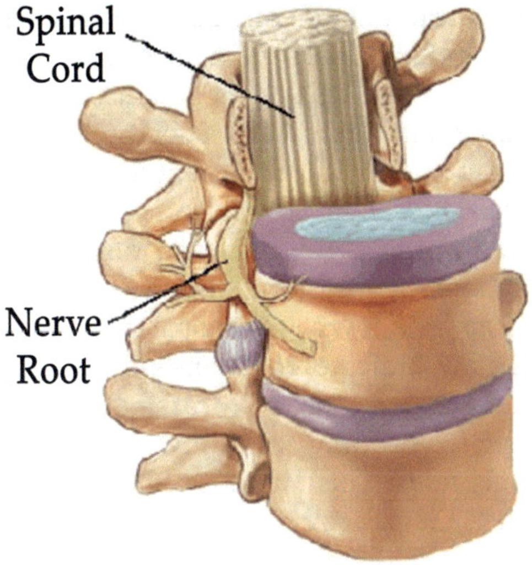

Figure 6.4. The spinal cord, a critical component of the central nervous system.

Source: https://www.researchgate.net/profile/Ian-Gibson-10/publication/221923246/figure/fig4/AS:305191871107075@1449774820906/Nerve-roots-and-spinal-cords.png.

Characteristically, current management approaches stress self-management and return to normal life, facilitated by medication and physiotherapy (Lee et al., 2021). Recovery is thus a significant focus, reflecting the physiological and psychological components of spinal disorders with a substantial influence on the outcome for patients. Clinical case histories illustrate the far-reaching influence of spinal diseases on the lives of patients, which highlights the importance of early treatment and diagnosis. A case in point is a 26-year-old man who gradually developed incapacitating symptoms related to his spinal cord dysfunction. His course began with frightening episodes involving electric shock-type pains and growing weakness of the lower limbs, ultimately making him wheelchair-bound over a few years. Such incidents reiterate the importance of active assessments in patients with spinal complaints, as delay can lead to irreversible damage and a low quality of life. Comprehensive assessment with physical and psychosocial elements is important in providing appropriate therapeutic interventions and support mechanisms to victims (Keddie et al., 2018). This integrated model is a big step forward in spinal disorder management, understanding the relationship between the structural health and the mental welfare of the patients (Figure 6.4).

6.2. Common Types of Spinal Disorders

Spinal diseases encompass a wide range of conditions of the vertebral column and related structures, most often causing pain, loss of mobility, and impaired quality of life. They are one of the most prevalent, including herniated discs, which are due to the displacement of the central gel-like part of intervertebral discs via a tear in the peripheral shell. It can result in compression of nerves and ensuing pain, numbness, and weakness of limbs. Disabling conditions, such as stenosis of the spinal canal, which narrows, can exacerbate symptoms by causing even more pressure on neural structures. Stenosis of the spine and bulging discs are common in individuals, especially those aged 50 and above, a fact that makes the relevance of degeneration of the spine with age in causing them clear. Another significant group of spinal disorders is degenerative disc disease and osteoarthritis, both of which involve progressive wear and tear on the intervertebral discs and spinal joints, respectively (Boardman, 2014). As age progresses, the discs dehydrate and lose their elasticity, leading to diminished shock absorption and increased loading on the vertebrae. This can trigger a pain and stiffness syndrome, typically exacerbated further by the occurrence of bone spurs. These conditions affect physical function but also damage one's psychological well-being in the form of chronic pain. Conservative management, such as lifestyle modifications, medications, and physical therapy, may be enough for most victims, although surgical interventions are warranted in extreme cases where conservative treatment fails to improve symptoms. Other than degenerative conditions, spinal disorders may also be due to congenital or structural abnormalities. Diseases such as scoliosis, a lateral spinal curvature, can be manifest in adolescence and lead to a variety of functional impairments. Scoliosis is not only associated with physical morbidity but also with social impairment due to concern regarding body image. Furthermore, spinal muscular atrophy, a genetic condition that targets motor neurons, is a disorder that directly impacts spinal health since it can lead to progressive weakness in the muscles and deformity of the spine. The complexity of the treatment of such disorders points towards the need for a comprehension that is multi-faceted in respect of physiological as well as psychosocial factors influencing outcome after treatment, as pointed out by the variability in experience with respect to reproductive choice in similar genetic contexts (Morris et al., 2011).

6.2.1. Herniated Discs

Slipped or bulging discs, also known as herniated discs, occur when the soft, inner gel of a spinal disc protrudes through an opening in the thicker outer layer. This typically occurs due to wear and tear associated with aging or as a result of a violent injury and causes pressure on adjacent spinal nerves and a range of debilitating symptoms, including pain, numbness, and weakness in involved areas. The lumbar region is the most susceptible due to its role and the stresses it bears from gravity when one is active. Moreover, the condition can also impact quality of life, and each task proves arduous for them. An understanding of the pathology and mechanics underlying the condition becomes necessary in order to implement useful treatment and management plans with the long-term aim of rehabilitating function and relieving pain for the individual concerned. Effects of herniated discs also include body pains, extending to psychological function and social relationships. Patients report frustration and unhappiness with chronic pain, risking mental disorders such as anxiety and depression. Such presentations emphasize the interconnected nature of physical and mental health, since chronic pain can erode self-worth and disrupt social interactions. A questionnaire with the SF-36 health survey shows that the patients with disc herniations indicate considerable impairment on self-reported health scores in the areas of physical functioning, role-physical, and body pain subscales. This is evidence of the double burden of the patient: chronic pain to deal with, and the psychological impact of having the condition, thereby compromising their quality of life significantly (Pahl et al., 2006). Treatment for herniated disks ranges from conservative treatment, such as pain medication and physical therapy, to more invasive measures such as spinal surgery. Whether to seek treatment depends, in large part, on symptom severity and degree of nerve impingement. While surgery may alleviate symptoms in those who are unresponsive to conservative treatment, it carries risks and must be predicated on a clear comprehension of the patient's individual clinical presentation. Evidence indicates that all four common lumbar spinal disorders, including herniated discs, significantly affect health status (Pahl et al., 2006). This makes the need for individually focused management strategies not only to address the physical components of the disorder but also to consider social and emotional problems to offer an integrated recovery process to the individuals involved (Figure 6.5).

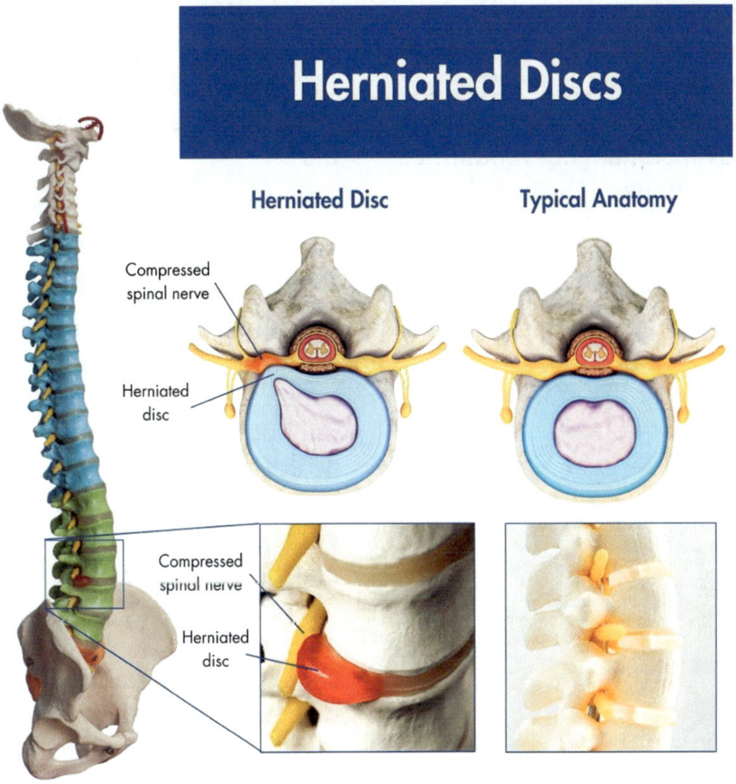

Figure 6.5. Herniated discs.

Source: https://prospinepain.com/wp-content/uploads/2024/04/herniated-discs.jpg.

6.2.2. Spinal Stenosis

As one of the commonest spinal conditions, spinal stenosis involves narrowing of the spinal canal, which may lead to severe neurological impairments. The condition often arises due to degenerative changes that occur with aging, but it can also be precipitated by genetic factors or trauma. With narrowing of the spinal canal, it can compress the spinal cord and nerve roots, leading to chronic pain, weakness, and numbness of the limbs. All these symptoms greatly impair daily activity and decrease the quality of life in patients with the condition. Doctors must record the variations in symptom intensity and onset, which can be quite different from one patient to another. The variability calls for individualized treatment strategies to treat spinal stenosis best and mitigate its impact on the lives of patients. The decision-making process for the treatment of lumbar spinal stenosis (LSS) is typically complex and multidimensional. Conservative management in the form of drugs and physiotherapy is normally recommended as the first line of treatment, but surgery is resorted to when conservative measures fail to alleviate symptoms. Neurosurgeons generally recommend posterior spinal fusion (PSF) surgery as a definitive treatment for the condition in those with advanced neurologic deficits or deteriorating symptoms. It is important to have an accurate prediction of surgical results since they directly influence treatment decisions of patients and surgeons. In a study, a prediction model was developed from many clinical and radiologic factors to predict the probable success rates of PSF. This way, treatment decisions are based on empirical data, and opportunities for successful outcomes are increased among patients with spinal stenosis (Babaee et al., 2017). As the frequency of spinal stenosis increases, especially among the elderly, there is a need to advance imaging modalities as well as treatment options.

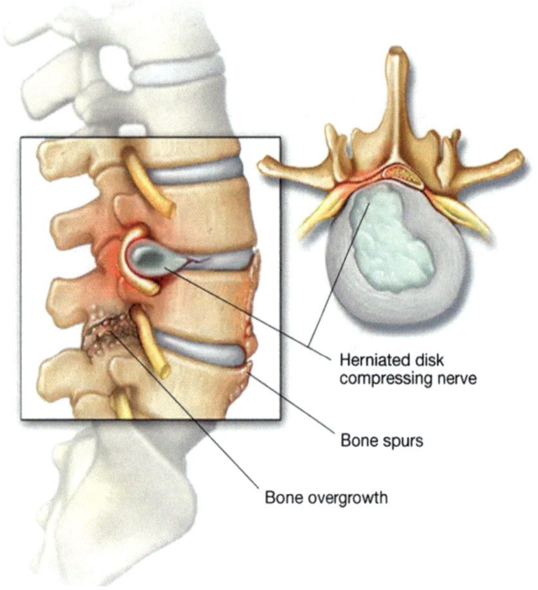

Figure 6.6. The most common spinal disorders.

Source: https://www.mayoclinic.org/-/media/kcms/gbs/patient-consumer/images/2017/05/19/16/32/herniated-disk-bone-spurs-8col.jpg.

Advances in radiological science, and particularly magnetic resonance imaging (MRI), have improved the ability of medical professionals to localize and quantify the degree of stenosis effectively. A new algorithm was devised in an effort to find the exact location of lesions on the spinal nerves in MRI scans and thus have a more accurate diagnosis and individualized treatment plan. With the integration of clinical information and automated analysis, healthcare providers can make more informed decisions, ultimately resulting in improved patient outcomes for LSS (Abbati et al., 2017). Such technological advancements not only improve the diagnostic process but also can have the capacity to standardize the treatment protocols for spinal stenosis and thus equip arm practitioners with the proper tools to deal with this potentially complicated spinal condition effectively (Figure 6.6).

6.2.3. Scoliosis

Scoliosis, which is an unusual lateral curvature of the spine, may appear in childhood or adolescence but also manifests as an adult condition. The spinal condition may appear in degrees, from mild deviation that may hardly impact physical health to severe curvatures that are significantly risky, such as pain and restricted mobility. The etiology of scoliosis remains heterogeneous; it may be idiopathic, without an identifiable cause, or secondary to congenital malformations, neuromuscular diseases, or degenerative changes associated with aging. It is essential to note the multifactorial etiology of scoliosis because it will dictate treatment and patient management strategies for those diagnosed with scoliosis. The health consequences of scoliosis extend beyond mere physical deformity and significantly influence quality of life. Recent literature has put into context how symptomatic adult spinal deformity (SASD), such as scoliosis and other spinal deformities, adversely affects patients' health status compared to the general population. In particular, there is evidence that PCS scores of the patients are considerably lower than the normative U.S. population and demonstrate severe disability with scoliosis. For example, PCS scores in patients with very severe spinal deformities secondary to scoliosis may be comparable to PCS scores in patients with chronic conditions. This discrepancy emphasizes the importance of early diagnosis and concentrating therapeutic efforts to minimize the disabling effects of scoliosis on individual quality of life (Bess et al., 2016). Treatment of scoliosis includes both surgical and non-surgical interventions, with treatment typically based on the degree of the curvature and the patients' age. Some of the non-surgical interventions that serve as a foundation to treat mild to moderate types or preoperative treatment include bracing, physical therapy, and pain control. Severely affected cases, either with or without neurological signs, may need surgical intervention to correct and stabilize the spine alignment. New technology in surgical techniques, i.e., circumferential minimally invasive surgery (cMIS), has been introduced, which has significant benefits, i.e., shorter recovery times and reduced postoperative rates of complications in certain patient populations with scoliosis (Chou et al., 2018). Still, treatment plans need to be individually specialized according to the patient's specific condition, overall health status, and desired results to obtain maximal outcomes and enhance quality of life (Figure 6.7).

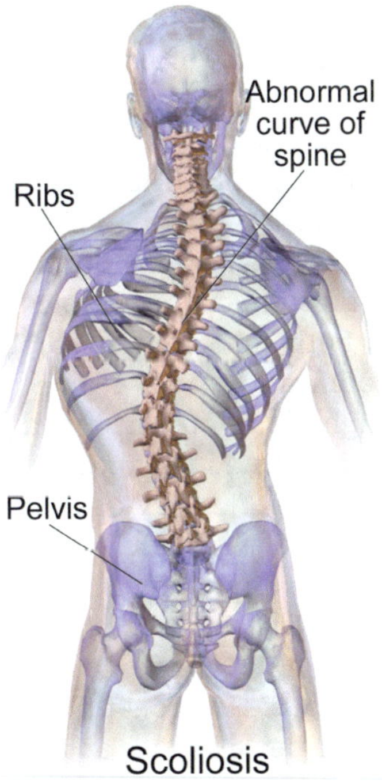

Figure 6.7. Scoliosis, defined as an abnormal lateral curvature of the spine.

Source: https://upload.wikimedia.org/wikipedia/commons/a/a7/Blausen_0785_Scoliosis_01.png.

6.3. Causes of Spinal Disorders

The multifactorial etiology of spinal disease encompasses a wide array of biological, mechanical, and psychological factors. The primary biological determinants are genetic susceptibilities that influence susceptibility to conditions such as herniated discs and spinal stenosis. Furthermore, age-related degeneration has a significant impact on spinal health, as intervertebral discs lose fluid and become less compliant with advancing age, resulting in increased risk for injury as well as for chronic pain. Also, metabolic disease and inflammation can aggravate these disorders, so systemic health does play a key role. The complexity of these relationships demonstrates why understanding the etiology of spinal disorders needs an integrated strategy, with considerations not only of anatomy but also of the overall physiological environment in which they occur. Mechanical trauma is also a significant etiological factor of spinal disorders, most often from acute trauma or repetitive strain. Occupations involving heavy lifting, sitting, or abnormal body mechanics are primary causes of the development of low back pain and spondylosis. These types of injuries can lead to alterations in spinal biomechanics and alignment, which create a pain and dysfunction feedback cycle. Secondly, sport activities are a two-sided sword; while they keep spine health in check if performed correctly, improper form leads to injury. The interconnectedness of physical activity, injury, and consequent spinal disorders reinforces the necessity of education in adequate body mechanics and injury prevention and the incorporation of rehabilitation programs to address deficits. The psychological factors of spinal disorders, all too often overlooked, also play a significant role in the development and sustenance of these disorders. Both anxiety and stress are not only found to heighten sensations of pain but are also said to speed underlying medical illnesses. Research highlights the dynamic interdependence of psychological well-being and somatic health, revealing that chronic pain disorders, like those of the spine, are susceptible to emotional and cognitive effects. Further, maladaptive coping and poor mental health can hinder recovery, cultivating a cycle whereby pain fuels increased distress, further leading to physical limitation. Management of these psychological issues through holistic treatment—combining traditional medical treatments with psychological treatment—offers the promise of a more effective means of spinal disorder control, seeking finally to maximize patient outcomes (DeLong et al., 2008; Larauche et al., 2011) (Figure 6.8).

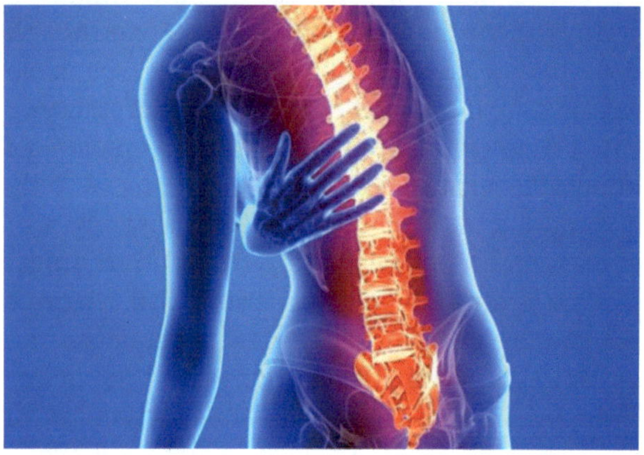

Figure 6.8. The multifactorial etiology of spinal disorders encompasses a wide array of biological factors.

Source: https://www.gncdubai.com/wp-content/uploads/2020/08/Spinal Cord Disorders-600x402.jpg.

6.3.1. Genetic Factors

Genetic factors are the main determinants of causation and expression of spinal disorders, as evidenced by an abundance of studies indicating the influence of hereditary effects on spinal conditions. Such studies have established that some genetic mutations can predispose an individual to conditions such as herniated discs, spinal stenosis, and degenerative disc disease. Such genetic effects can affect collagen synthesis and other structural proteins, which are critical to the maintenance of the integrity of spinal tissues. This inherited predisposition not only alerts clinicians to potential dangers but also allows for the prediction of the course of the disease. Information regarding such inherited traits allows for prevention in a directed manner and personalized therapeutic management, aligned with the growing emphasis on the concept of personalized medicine for the treatment of complex spinal disorders. Beyond obvious genetic influences, gene-environment interaction is important in the determination of the course of spinal disorders. Genetically predisposed individuals are more prone to being affected by extrinsic stressors, and these may trigger or exacerbate spinal conditions. For instance, certain stressors have been identified to initiate changes in the process of pain perception by dysregulation of the brain-gut axis, as seen in the recent literature emphasizing co-integration of psychological distress and physical health (Larauche et al., 2011). The interplay between the genetic and environmental factors points to the intricate nature of spinal disorders, suggesting that effective treatment will need to address both inherited susceptibility and lifestyle modification. This type of integrative therapy might lead to improved outcomes, particularly in populations where there is an established familial history of spinal issues. In addition, emerging research within the field of neurogenetics offers potential directions for investigating spinal disorders on a molecular basis. Technological gains in neuroimmunology and genetics elucidate genetic differences on neuromuscular performance and pain pathway transmission, which play a central role in spinal health (DeLong et al., 2008). For example, certain genetic profiles may determine the effectiveness of treatments such as non-invasive electrical stimulation or deep brain stimulation. Elucidating these genetic determinants will not only contribute to patient-specific treatment response knowledge but also direct subsequent research into new treatments aimed at diminishing the progression of spinal disease. As the understanding of genetic contributions further increases, it is also realized that a multidimensional, patient-oriented approach is essential for optimizing care in spinal health.

6.3.2. Lifestyle Choices

The impact of lifestyle factors on spinal health is large and multifaceted. Physical fitness is arguably the most basic predictor of spinal integrity. Exercise both strengthens muscles that protect the spine as well as heightens flexibility, thereby reducing the risk of injury. Sedentary behavior, conversely, is linked with various spinal ailments, from chronic pain and degenerative disease. Also, maintaining a healthy weight is crucial since excessive body weight causes undue stress on the spine and can lead to issues such as a herniated disc or sciatica. Considering these results, it is beyond doubt that adopting preventive lifestyle modifications has the potential to significantly decrease the risk of spinal disorders and allow individuals to enhance the quality of their well-being, along with that of their functional status. Diet plays an important role in the preservation of spinal health and the prevention of disorders. The proper consumption of basic nutrients such as calcium, vitamin D, and omega-3 fatty acids directly correlates with bone density and general spinal health. Inadequate nutrition causes an individual to be vulnerable to vertebral fractures and other spinal issues, justifying the importance of dietary choices. Moreover, patients with spinal disorders are prone to secondary complications, such as constipation, that compromise their quality of life. Evidence indicates that lifestyle interventions, such as diet modification, can effectively alleviate these complications in patients with conditions such as Parkinson's disease, validating the need for tailored lifestyle advice in the management of spinal disorders (McClurg et al., 2016). By promoting nutritional awareness and healthier dietary habits, health practitioners can prevent and control spinal disorders. Stress management is also a critical aspect of lifestyle that could have effects on spinal well-being. Chronic stress has been found to impair body functions like muscle tension and inflammation, which can exacerbate spinal disease. Such stress management strategies have been found to reduce muscle tension and improve spinal health (Estrine & DeLisle, 2006). They also result in a holistic model of self-care, addressing mental and physical health. The more mindful individuals become in their practices and engage in regular exercise, the relief from spinal discomfort, as well as improved functional outcomes, is possible for them. Lastly, due to prioritizing stress management over lifestyle choices, the body can be dramatically improved with a straighter spine despite dealing with spinal disorders (Figure 6.9).

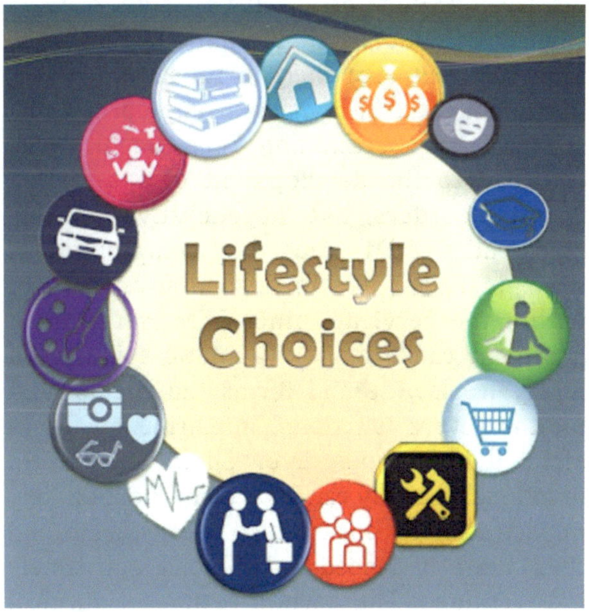

Figure 6.9. The impact of lifestyle choices on spinal health.

Source: https://lh6.googleusercontent.com/proxy/pc5vaymGmYPmDVWVCOVsbmITXBF20b_wgkhFg24WjPfaZAhgMrlpug-mogO5RqYnoY5DDRXLTfYZjrdZb6LQcAQL9NkyYiEG.

6.3.3. Age-Related Changes

With increasing age, the spine experiences a progressive series of alterations that significantly influence the general spinal health and function. One of the most important changes related to aging is the loss of height of the intervertebral discs and disc bulging due to their degeneration. These changes are responsible for the instability of the spine and may result in conditions like spinal stenosis, where spinal canal narrowing is due to disc herniation or vertebral hypertrophy. These changes in anatomy are followed by a decrease in the pliability of the adjacent soft tissues, jeopardizing the biomechanical stability of the spine. They make clinical assessment more difficult because similar morphological outcomes are also seen in asymptomatic individuals, casting doubt about the applicability of such results in diagnosing some spinal disorders (Elliott et al., 2018). Aging-related changes in spinal health are not only structural in nature but also include functional losses that manifest as a restricted range of motion, strength, and coordination. These impairments can lead to the development of age-related spinal disorders, like degenerative cervical myelopathy (DCM), caused by compression of the spinal cord due to degenerative changes within the cervical spine. DCM is the most prevalent cause of nontraumatic spinal cord injury worldwide and forms the background for the severe functional impairment seen in affected individuals. Even slight declines in functional capacity can have disproportionately impactful effects on activities of daily living, and thus, there is a need for effective and timely interventions. Thus, while results of surgical intervention for DCM are optimal, success is significantly predicated on preoperative conditions like functional evaluation, which may be exacerbated by the multidimensional nature of impairment due to age (Stricsek et al., 2018). The interplay between aging changes and diagnosis, and treatment of spinal conditions requires a comprehensive comprehension of dynamic imaging technology. Standard imaging modalities are prone to revealing findings that are inadequately correlated with clinical presentation since degenerative features are ubiquitous even in asymptomatic patients. This discrepancy necessitates the integration of developing imaging modalities, including sophisticated magnetic resonance applications, to improve diagnostic specificity and clarify the intricate interplay between changing anatomy and clinical manifestations. By incorporating advanced imaging with adequate clinical assessments, clinicians are better able to select modifiable risk factors and personalize treatment approaches based on individual patient needs. These advancements not only hold the promise to enlighten the pain and disability mechanisms but also towards improvement in general outcomes in patient treatment in spinal disorders caused by aging (Elliottet al., 2018).

6.4. Symptoms of Spinal Disorders

Spinal disorder symptoms can have multiple presentations, a reflection of the intricate relationship between the spine and nervous system. An example of such is pain presented as radiating to the spine and extending to the legs or arms, depending on the location involved in the spine. This form of referred pain is often indicative of nerve root irritation and allows us to explore inherent pathologies like herniated discs or stenosis. Numbness or tingling sensations can also be encountered by patients, which can significantly impact everyday living. The intertwined characteristics of these symptoms indicate the need for a comprehensive diagnostic workup to establish the specific spinal disorder in question, thus facilitating effective and timely intervention measures targeting both pain management as well as recovery of motility (DeLong et al., 2008). In addition to pain and sensory impairment, patients with spinal disorders may also present with motor impairment. This can range from weakness of discrete muscle groups to incomplete or complete paralysis, typically based on the extent and location of spinal injury. These impairments can be secondary to direct mechanical disruption of spinal tissue or compressive forces interrupting the neurological pathways responsible for voluntary movement. Spinal disorders also usually compromise posture and balance and thus predispose toward subsequent falls and secondary injury. The understanding of these symptoms is crucial for clinicians in formulating rehabilitation programs that go together with physical therapy goals and consider the psychological impact of motor impairment, as they have a great impact on the patient's quality of life (Larauche et al., 2011). Psychological symptoms such as depression and anxiety usually follow physical symptoms of spinal disorders, and this means a complex interaction and complicates treatment. Chronic pain and physical impairment can induce frustration or helplessness, creating a feedback loop that can further increase the subjective report of pain. Additionally, disability stigma as well as chronic illness stigma can dissuade patients from seeking care on a timely basis. It is therefore critical to treat these psychosocial issues in constructing an interdisciplinary care plan involving pain management, physical rehabilitation, and psychiatric care. Thus, medical doctors ought to exercise caution not only towards the physiological symptoms but also towards the emotional and psychological conditions of their spinal disorder patients, to embrace a more holistic therapy practice (DeLong et al., 2008) (Figure 6.10).

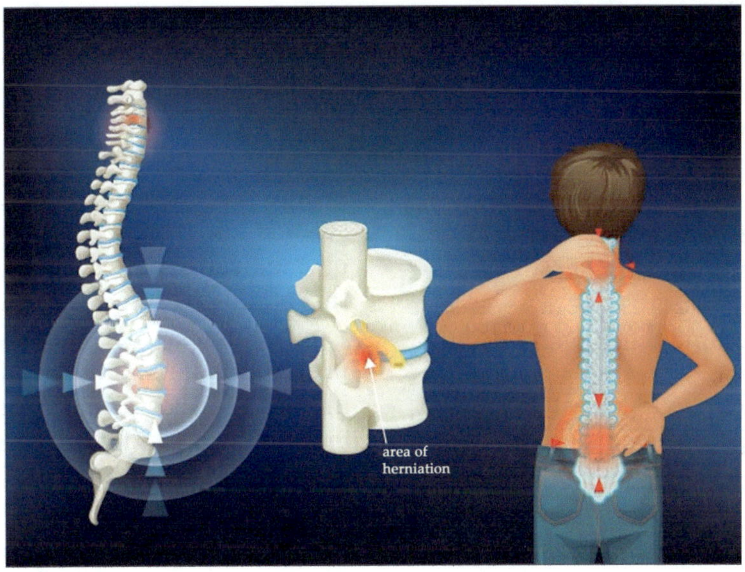

Figure 6.10. The symptoms of spinal disorders can manifest in a variety of ways.

Source: https://www.ibshospitals.com/blogthumb/660d28af6cb55All%20You%20Should%20Know%20About%20Spinal%20Cord%20Injury.webp.

6.4.1. Pain and Discomfort

Discomfort and pain are paramount among the complications of dealing with spinal disorders, which fundamentally impact the quality of life of the individuals involved. Disorders of the spine occur as pain that is acute to chronic, often radiating down the limbs and along the back due to nerve involvement. Understanding how the pain happens is crucial in coming up with effective treatment. Neuropathic pain typically develops due to nerve root irritation or compression, which is typical in diseases like a herniated disc or spinal stenosis. Such disease conditions not only produce physical pain but can also cause psychological distress, thereby complicating the clinical scenario. Faced with such a complex presentation of pain, it requires a multifaceted strategy that addresses physical as well as emotional aspects, highlighting the need for holistic care in the management of spinal health. Chronic pain due to spinal disorders also frequently leads to functional impairment, which further adds to the discomfort of the patients. The psychological impact of spinal diseases increases as day-to-day life becomes difficult for the patients. A study that examined non-ambulant children indicates that physical and social disability due to neuromuscular disorders has profound impact on mental health, exhibiting the ripple effects of chronic discomfort on psychological health (Travlos et al., 2018). In spinal disorders, mobility restriction not only exacerbates the physical sensation of pain but can also lead to social isolation and frustration. This reciprocity between physical and psychological health highlights the need for interventions that address both to ensure optimal patient outcomes. Interventions that enhance social support and engage patients in goal-oriented activities may be beneficial in preventing these adverse effects. In treating spinal disorders, effective pain management strategies are central to reducing pain and improving overall health in patients. Interventions range from pharmacological to non-pharmacological interventions, such as analgesics and anti-inflammatory medications and physical and cognitive-behavioral therapy. New emerging technologies in medical science, including minimally invasive surgery and technological developments in imaging technology, hold promising potential in addressing the causes of pain (Camilleri, 1999). Moreover, patient education plays a major role in equipping them with self-management skills to cope with pain more effectively. By attaining greater knowledge regarding their diseases and lines of treatment, patients are empowered to take active roles in their recovery process, which leads to enhanced levels of satisfaction as well as reduced pain and discomfort associated with spinal disorders. This integrated approach not only treats the symptoms of the condition but also allows individuals to live more actively in their lives.

6.4.2. Numbness and Tingling

Numbness and tingling, paresthesia for short, are neurological symptoms that are most frequently observed in conjunction with spinal disease. They are typically felt when nerves are compressed or injured, which can occur due to herniated discs, stenosis, or degenerative disc disease. As the architecture of the spine deteriorates, it can cause increased pressure on the spinal nerves, resulting in the characteristic numbness and tingling. Such sensations are usually transient and caused by transient compression of nerves in most cases; chronic or recurring symptoms may, however, be related to more serious underlying conditions to be addressed by medical experts. Hence, the knowledge of the etiology of such symptoms is relevant in diagnosing and managing spinal disorders. The prevalence of numbness and paresthesia is very important in cases where there is a deficiency of vitamin B12 and is emphasized in some spinal disorders. Neurological signs and symptoms resulting from cobalamin deficiency most frequently include sensory disturbances, which encompass paresthesia. Research shows that at least 80% of the patients with the accompanying neurological disorders report paresthesia, with significant overlap among those with myelopathy and generalized demyelinating polyneuropathy (Oussalah et al., 2019). The noted correlation between a deficiency in vitamin B12 and neurological symptoms serves to emphasize the necessity of rigorous diagnostic testing in patients who present with paresthesia and numbness, especially in settings in which nutritional deficiencies are prevalent. Further, the manifestations of these sensations impact more than just patient comfort, dramatically influencing patient quality of life and functionality. Chronic numbness and paresthesia may cause psychological distress and impairment in daily functioning, particularly in executing physical activity. Symptomatic control is usually attained with a multidisciplinary approach comprising physical therapy, nutritional supplementation, and, in advanced cases, surgery. Management of the underlying etiology of numbness and paresthesia, especially when related to nerve pathology from spinal disease, is important. Reversal of deficits such as vitamin B12 deficiency can lead to major recovery of neurological function, indicating the value of intense treatment strategies tailored to the specific patient's requirements (Mansueto et al., 2012) (Figure 6.11).

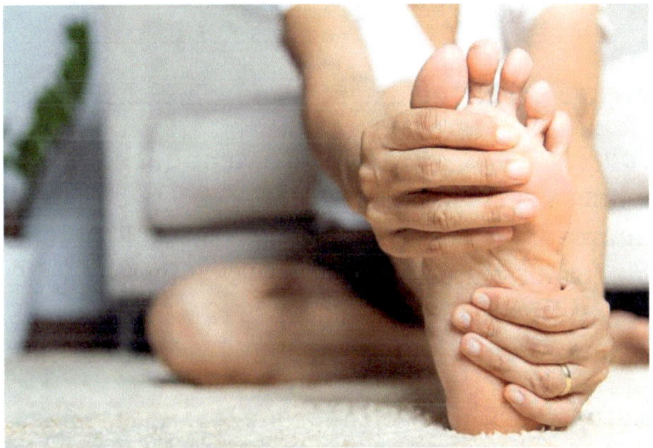

Figure 6.11. Numbness and tingling.

Source: https://www.northshore.org/globalassets/healthy-you/blog/2022/numbness-tingling-pain.jpg.

6.4.3. Mobility Issues

Mobility issues become a significant concern for spinal disorder patients as the loss of movement hampers the ability to do everyday activities and impacts the quality of life of an individual. Pain and restricted movement are caused by several diseases involving herniated disks, scoliosis, and spinal stenosis. The relationship between spinal well-being and mobility is intricate; if the spine is compromised, physical function is not the only aspect impacted but also psychological well-being. Actually, disability due to back pain has reached epidemic proportions in industrialized countries and there exists a pressing need for effective management. Support for self-care must be given priority since patients would probably require reassurance to return to physical activity and work without bed rest for more than 48 hours. The identification of mobility issues in spinal disorders makes it possible an integrative treatment model that recognizes the fact that healing is both a physical and psychosocial process. Studies also emphasize that mobility complications in spinal disorders need to be addressed actively. For instance, complications arising from surgery can significantly hamper patient recovery and mobility rehabilitation. Systematic evaluation of neuromuscular scoliosis patients revealed that surgeries often led to a high rate of complications, and nearly 30% of the patients experienced adverse effects that would exacerbate mobility impairments (Turturro et al., 2017). The above findings emphasize the necessity of careful preoperative planning and comprehensive patient education on potential risks. Secondarily, improvement in the policy of postoperative care and the skill of surgery will avoid these complications and consequently lead to better outcomes in terms of mobility. This calls for clinicians to monitor closely the potential interaction between surgical technique and late mobility problems in patients suffering from spinal disorders. Other than surgical complications, there are psychosocial factors that play an important role in influencing mobility outcomes in spinal disorder patients. Chronic pain and associated psychological distress can severely impair patients' physical activity capacity, thus perpetuating the cycle of immobility. In line with evidence, negative psychosocial factors can worsen physical symptoms, rendering the process of recovery challenging (Lee et al., 2021). The holistic approach, thus, to both psychological and physical aspects of mobility impairment is imperative for successful rehabilitation. This might involve cognitive behavioral therapy, pain management strategies, and support groups to enable patients in their recovery process. The comprehension of the different aspects of spinal disorders enables the health providers to design comprehensive management plans that address mobility and well-being. Ultimately, creating a forward-thinking, patient-centered approach to mobility challenges can lead to better health outcomes for individuals who live with spinal disorders.

6.5. Diagnosis of Spinal Disorders

Diagnosis of spinal disorders is an intricate process that integrates clinical assessment with advanced imaging modalities. The initial step in the process is a careful history and physical examination by the clinician to ascertain symptoms such as pain, weakness, and restriction of motion. This clinical foundation is essential because it provides the necessary framework for the precise location of the spine involved and the nature of the symptoms produced by the patient. Subsequently, imaging procedures such as X-rays, MRI, and CT scans are employed to visualize structural abnormalities of the spine, including herniated discs, spinal stenosis, or fractures. Prompt and accurate diagnosis of these disorders is instrumental in determining the proper treatment regimen and improving patient outcomes, substantiating the crucial role of integrative diagnostic processes in spinal therapy. Advancements in technology through imaging have significantly enhanced the accuracy of diagnosing disorders of the spine. Techniques such as MRI not only capture the intricate image of the spinal cord and surrounding soft tissues but also allow for the assessment of compression and inflammation of the nerve roots. These tools assist the clinician in making a more accurate diagnosis, which is a vital component in devising personalized treatment plans. Moreover, quantitative data and computer-based diagnosis are being incorporated more and more in the evaluation of spinal disorders. For instance, artificial intelligence applications used for imaging interpretation can lead to more precise patient outcome predictions following surgical treatment, particularly with operations like posterior spinal fusion.

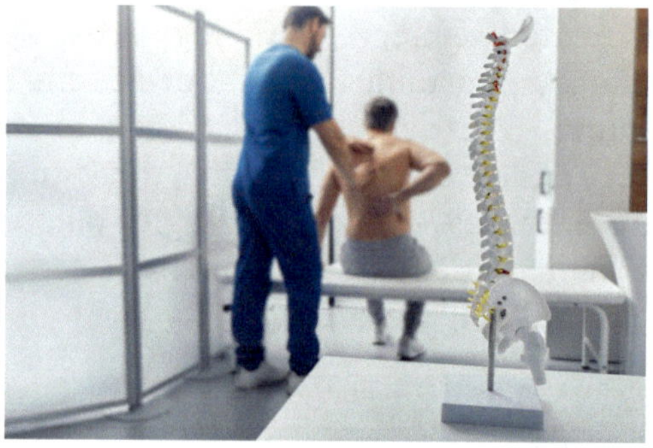

Figure 6.12. The diagnosis of spinal disorders.

Source: https://external-content.duckduckgo.com/iu/?u=https%3A%2F%2Fana-neurosurgery.com%2Fwp-content%2F upload s%2Fshutterstock_2288089461-1024x676.jpg&f=1&nofb=1&ipt=bce4addeac94368719faba3e52b6d6f40eb8b4f41ff2cbb09250dd6ecc418179.

Here, algorithms consider numerous variables, including age, sex, and some clinical symptoms, contributing to a general understanding of the disorder and its optimal management (Babaee et al., 2017). Beyond imaging and clinical examinations, interdisciplinary team function is crucial in diagnosing spinal disorders. Doctors such as neurologists, orthopedists, and physiatrists generally work together in order to formulate an overall understanding of a patient's condition. This multidisciplinary strategy ensures all parameters of the patient's health are considered, leading to more advanced diagnosis. Patient-reported outcome measures and preferences are also being increasingly incorporated into diagnosis because they can give insight into symptom intensity and general quality of life. In conditions like Mucopolysaccharidosis IVA, where spinal involvement is common, individualized management guidelines are essential in optimizing care (Akyol et al., 2019). This patient-focused and collaborative process not only enhances diagnostic accuracy but also promotes enhanced clinical outcomes and patient satisfaction with spinal disorder care (Figure 6.12).

6.5.1. Physical Examination

In the assessment of spinal disorders, physical examination plays a crucial first step in determining causation and planning further management. Detailed history is the first step in a full physical examination, questioning the patient's pain, weakness, or sensory change symptoms regarding their onset, duration, and nature. Clinicians use a formal approach to measure spinal range of motion, palpation of paravertebral muscle for spasm or tenderness, and assessment of neurological function on strength testing and reflexes. By thorough examination, healthcare practitioners can detect red flags like motor impairment or bladder dysfunction requiring referral to a specialist or advanced imaging evaluation. Where uncomplicated back pain is the issue, there is good evidence that the majority of patients will not show significant pathology, and hence targeted conservative management strategies can be used as guidelines suggest, stressing the importance of facilitating clients' return to normal activity (Lee et al., 2021). Second, physical examination enables clinicians to differentiate among various disorders of the spine, such as herniated discs, degenerative disc disease, and stenosis of the spinal canal. Using certain tests, e.g., straight leg raises or flexion testing, clinicians can contribute to the determination of the etiology of radicular pain from nerve root irritation or compression. The key is to correlate the physical examination findings with the patients' history and reported symptoms and create an individualized management plan. Physical therapy, manipulation, or, if necessary, pharmacological therapy for pain relief may be included in such a plan. Early and accurate diagnosis of the disorder through meticulous examination is a significant element in halting the progression of symptoms and limiting disability, finally aiming to advance long-term functional outcomes for the patient population (Lee et al., 2021). Moreover, the use of the physical examination is also pertinent to the formulation of appropriate rehabilitative management and guiding multimodal treatment of patients with chronic spinal disorders. In complex disease cases like Mucopolysaccharidosis VI, for which spinal complications can occur, an interdisciplinary team of health professionals, from physical therapists to occupational therapists, can work with the diagnostic data obtained from the physical examination. The specific findings on musculoskeletal state, flexibility, and motor function as an integrated whole can influence sophisticated management strategies, both operative and nonoperative. This integration is critical in optimizing patient quality of life, as some conditions that necessitate continuous appraisal and tailored interventions occasionally require constant monitoring and support systems to address not just physical but also psychosocial concerns.

6.5.2. Imaging Techniques

Imaging modalities play a pivotal role in the diagnosis and management of spinal disorders, as they provide medical practitioners with the ability to view and examine complex anatomical structures of the spine. Traditional modalities, such as X-rays and computed tomography (CT), are commonly utilized due to their availability and ability to visualize bone pathology, but will fall short in viewing soft tissue and neural alterations in spinal disorders. The limitations of conventional imaging have spurred interest in advanced imaging techniques, such as magnetic resonance imaging (MRI). MRI excels in its capacity to provide detailed images of soft tissues, including intervertebral discs, nerve roots, and the spinal cord. As our understanding of spinal disorders evolves, so too must our imaging methods, paving the way for innovations that may lead to more effective treatment strategies and improved patient outcomes. Emergent imaging modalities promise much in the illumination of the complex interactions of the biological factors involved in causing spinal disorders. An example would be the integration of fat and water imaging on MRI, which has been shown to more clearly depict degenerative changes and is useful for distinguishing symptomatic from asymptomatic findings. These newer techniques are significant in that traditional imaging results have a tendency to reveal several non-specific findings, which can be seen in asymptomatic patients, thus making it hard to understand the clinical significance of such results (Elliot et al., 2018). The incorporation of these sophisticated imaging methods into routine clinical practice is significant, since they can increase diagnostic sensitivity and serve to guide certain therapeutic approaches customized to the patient's requirements. Additionally, emerging imaging devices, such as PET, are uncovering the mechanisms of neuroinflammation in many of the spinal conditions. In these diseases like multiple sclerosis, TSPO-selective radioligand PET imaging has emerged as a valuable tool in the detection of neuroinflammatory processes within the spinal cord that are not accessible with routine imaging techniques (Abourbeh et al., 2012). This visualization of neuroinflammation, in addition to presenting more information regarding the disease process, signifies the trend toward more individualized, targeted medicine. Through the combination of these new imaging technologies, clinicians can gain a more mechanistic insight into spinal disorders and, ultimately, improved treatment options with enhanced patient outcomes for spinal health (Figure 6.13).

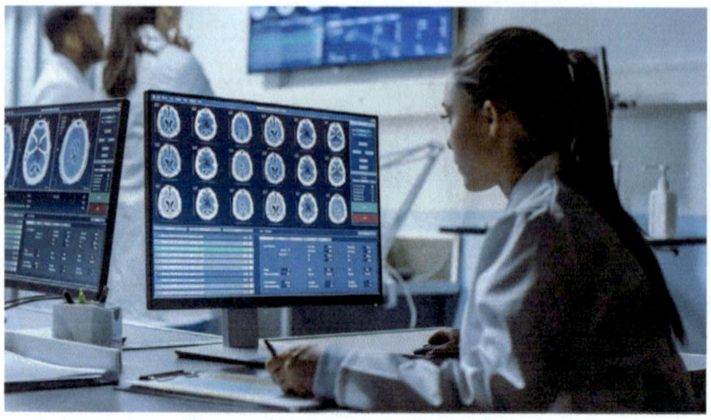

Figure 6.13. Imaging techniques play a pivotal role in the diagnosis and management of spinal disorders.

Source: https://external-content.duckduckgo.com/iu/?u=https%3A%2F%2Fwww.healthcarebusinesstoday.com%2Fwp-content%2Fuploads%2F2020%2F07%2Fimage1.jpg&f=1&nofb=1&ipt=a7fab21f04430aa6503f9ccf34e74f81d2bbfaa7eab25c61b1787a55909985f4.

6.5.3. Neurological Assessments

Neurological examinations play a central role in the comprehensive assessment of spinal disorder patients since they provide useful information on the structure and function of the nervous system. These examinations uncover the mysteries of neurological function, such as motor and sensory pathways, that can be impaired by spinal cord compression or nerve impingement. Through systematic evaluation of reflexes, muscular strength, and sensory modalities, clinicians are able to ascertain the specific neurological deficits resulting from disorders such as herniated disc or spinal stenosis. Accurate identification of the nature of these deficits is crucial in developing effective treatment plans and interventions in order to ultimately enhance patient outcomes. Apart from that, a thorough neurological examination becomes a point of reference for observing the evolution in the patient's condition over time and performing timely therapeutic adjustments as and when necessary. For spinal disorders, various standard neurological examination techniques have been developed to gauge the function of both the central and peripheral nervous systems. These include comprehensive examinations such as the Glasgow Coma Scale to check for consciousness and specific tests such as the pinprick or light touch tests to check sensory function. In addition, imaging modalities such as MRI and CT scans usually occur in concert to get visual confirmation of structural derangements such as extruded discs or bony lesions that have a tendency to exacerbate neurological impairment. Such assessments are not only diagnostic baseline but also necessary for the guidance of surgical treatment and rehabilitative efforts if indicated. This multi-fold approach integrates clinical findings with imaging diagnosis, thereby enabling a more successful treatment of the spinal disorders' complexities. Due to the heterogeneous impact of spinal disorders on neurological function, an interdisciplinary approach to management and assessment is required. This involves collaboration not just between orthopedic specialists and neurologists but also among physiotherapists, occupational therapists, as well as other medical practitioners involved in attending to patients. As illustrated in guidelines for diseases like Moquino A syndrome, sharing similar challenges of skeletal and neurological presentation, a team-based approach is essential to provide improved management of such patients' requirements (Akyol et al., 2019; Hendriksz et al., 2015). This collaboration enhances the accuracy of neurological testing and increases treatment possibilities by combining knowledge from several fields. Ultimately, these synergies enhance improved clinical outcomes, exemplifying the importance of complicated and sophisticated neurological examinations in the broader context of spinal disorder care (Figure 6.14).

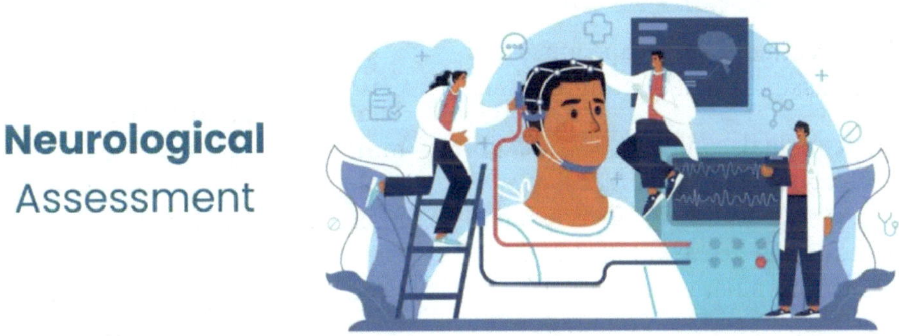

Figure 6.14. Neurological assessments play a critical role in the comprehensive evaluation of patients with spinal disorders.

Source: https://www.medicoverhospitals.in/images/articles/neurological-assessment-begumpet.webp.

6.6. Treatment Options for Spinal Disorders

The environment for treatment of spinal disorders encompasses an array of modalities, all customized to address the particular nature and severity of the condition. Numerous patients are treated initially with conservative management by way of physical therapy, pain control, and the use of orthotic equipment. These treatments have a likelihood to adjust symptoms, increase mobility, and restore functionality without invoking immediate demand for invasive intervention. Physical therapy, in particular, has been shown to enhance strength, flexibility, and coordination, all of which significantly reduce pain and enhance quality of life. The efficacy of these conservative methods underscores the worth of a comprehensive treatment plan that addresses the specific needs of specific patients and clinical presentation. Conservative measures being inadequate in symptom reduction, aggressive treatment methods can be utilized. Surgery, from minimally invasive to complex spinal surgery, may be necessary to repair anatomical conditions such as a herniated disc, spinal stenosis, and deformity. These surgeries are to fix inherent structural defects, remove nerve compression, or stabilize the spine.

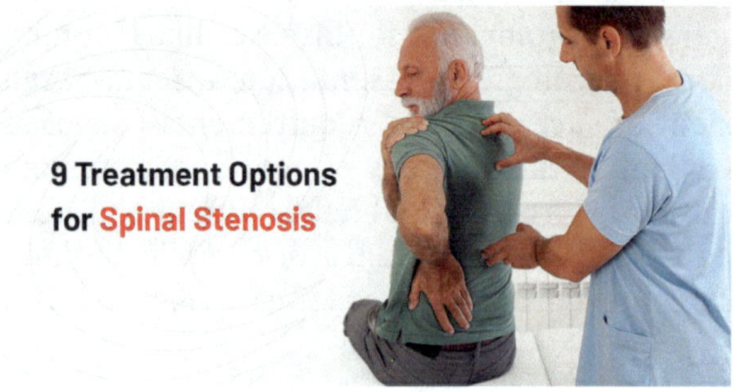

Figure 6.15. The treatment landscape for spinal disorders encompasses a variety of modalities.

Source: https://external-content.duckduckgo.com/iu/?u=https%3A%2F%2Fwww.sciatica.com%2Fwp-content%2Fuploads%2F2023%2F05%2F01-9-treatment-options-for-spinal-stenosis-5446ac6f.jpeg&f=1&nofb=1&ipt=ca433da962ad70ee70e76ad0eb6b59131f1e36433158a1be95c5aa0f82312c5e.

The decision to proceed with surgery is typically made after several considerations, such as the overall health of the patient, the degree of neurological impairment, and the dangers that the surgery can pose. Further, enhanced surgery techniques and equipment keep enhancing the outcomes of the patient, with remarkable diminishment in the period of recovery and post-surgery outcomes. New treatments for spinal disorders also include new therapies such as gene therapy and regenerative medicine, which are exciting fields for spinal care. Research into such modalities as stem cell therapy and tissue engineering is in progress to repair damaged spinal structures and stimulate healing at the cellular level. These new approaches hold promise for the solution of historically entrenched difficulties inherent in chronic spinal disorders, as well as for overall function and quality of life in so-affected individuals. As the topic continues to advance, ongoing evaluation and refinement of treatment protocols are needed, which function to justify the call for evidence-based practices in the betterment of care. With the intricacies of spinal disorders, multidisciplinary treatment that involves various forms of therapy can significantly enhance patient outcome and satisfaction in accordance with the overall objective of improving the quality of life of those suffering from these complex conditions (DeLong et al., 2008; Akyol et al., 2019) (Figure 6.15).

6.6.1. Non-Surgical Treatments

The range of non-operative spinal disorder management has widened significantly, and patients are offered a diverse range of management options in the quest to eliminate pain and restore function. Physical therapy stands head and shoulders above the rest, employing targeted exercise to enhance strength, flexibility, and posture. Targeting core stabilization and sound body mechanics, physical therapy not only reduces pain but also averts subsequent injury. In addition to helping to decrease pain and encourage healing, modalities such as electrical stimulation and ultrasound are used to further accomplish these goals. This combination therapy enables a holistic recovery process, with individualized treatment planning required in order to address unique patient needs, ultimately leading to improved mobility and quality of life. Pharmacological therapy is also a critical element of non-operative spinal disorder treatment. Nonsteroidal anti-inflammatory drugs (NSAIDs) are usually prescribed to reduce inflammation and pain that accompany most spinal conditions. In patients who have more severe or chronic pain, physicians can consider prescribing more potent analgesics or adjunctive treatment such as muscle relaxants or anticonvulsants. A combination of these pharmacotherapy modalities as part of a comprehensive management plan is ideal to produce optimum outcomes in patients. But adequate care must be taken towards probable side effects and harm associated with long-term drug intake.

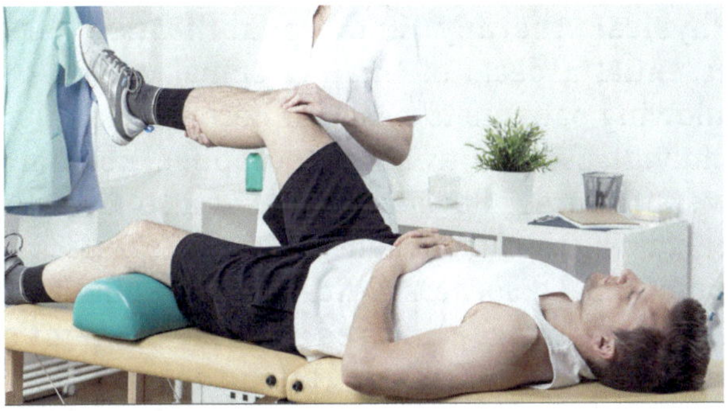

Figure 6.16. The landscape of non-surgical treatments for spinal disorders has expanded significantly.

Source: https://www.laudclinic.com/wp-content/uploads/2020/05/Physiotherapy-banner-1.jpg.

This demands constant monitoring and evaluation of the health condition of the patient to be able to provide maximum as well as risk-free therapy regimen. In addition, newer modalities of treatment are being developed in the field of non-surgical treatment of spinal disorders. One of these is the use of regenerative medicine modalities, including platelet-rich plasma (PRP) injection and stem cell therapy, to capitalize on the body's own repair processes to promote healing of tissue. Science indicates that such interventions have promise for being helpful in patients with disc degeneration or other spinal irregularities, although further study is required to ascertain their long-term safety and efficacy. In addition, complementary therapies such as acupuncture and chiropractic treatments have gained popularity, providing patients with further means of managing pain and promoting spinal health. Through the adoption of these diverse non-surgical interventions, healthcare professionals are able to create comprehensive treatment programs that treat the physiological and psychological dimensions of spinal conditions alongside motivating patient empowerment and engagement in the recovery process (Figure 6.16).

6.6.2. Surgical Interventions

Surgical interventions are most critical in treating many spinal conditions, particularly when conservative treatment fails to alleviate disabling symptoms. They become the treatment of choice for conditions such as herniated disc, spinal stenosis, and degenerative disc disease. The goal of such operations tends to aim at decompressing the spinal cord or nerve, stabilizing the spine, or repairing spinal deformity. Most of the surgical treatments include discectomy, laminectomy, or spinal fusion, depending on the pathology and the condition of individual patients. Surgery is a useful way to relieve pain and improve function, although it encompasses a serious estimation of risks and benefits over expected postoperative complications. The outcome of the surgery is based on the overall condition of the patients, the complexity of the disorder, and adherence to postoperative rehabilitation procedures. Moreover, the evolution of surgical techniques, including minimally invasive surgery, has revolutionized spinal surgery practice. Minimally invasive spinal surgery (MISS) applies smaller cuts and sophisticated instrumentation that reduces tissue trauma, decreases scarring, and promotes quicker recovery times. Techniques like endoscopic discectomy and percutaneous fusion are examples of this evolution. These technologies not only attempt to maintain spinal stability but also enhance recovery patterns for patients. However, success with these techniques depends significantly on the preoperative imaging and assessment. Furthermore, clinical trials and studies still go on in advancing these methods, examining long-term outcomes and quality of life after surgery. These developments hold a promising future for spinal surgery, with more emphasis on patient welfare and improved recovery profiles.

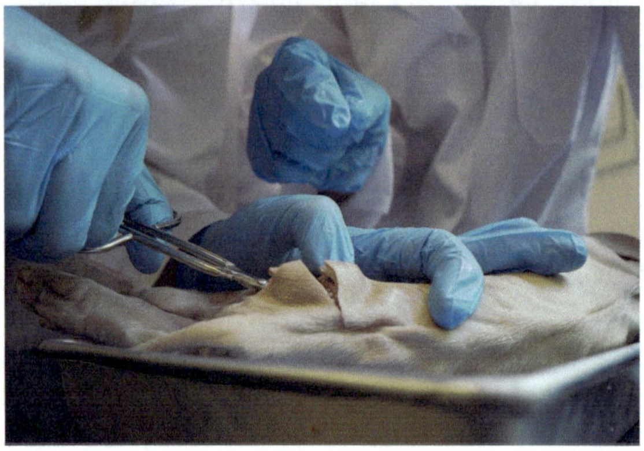

Figure 6.17. Surgical interventions play a critical role in the management of various spinal disorders.

Source: https://external-content.duckduckgo.com/iu/?u=https%3A%2F%2Fblog.explo.org%2Fhubfs%2Fyale%2Facademics%2Fslideshows%2F20170629_103615%2F6-29_Surgical_Interventions_-_12_of_20.jpg&f=1&nofb=1&ipt=f33a05c94c3af9feae9e2e3d3a0f7ffe8b69a7e1cd8f8894134de1a36c4a0324.

Finally, multidisciplinary participation in the surgical planning of spinal disorders indicates how complex spinal disorder treatment is. Consultation with orthopedic surgeons, neurosurgeons, physiatrists, and pain management professionals ensures proper and holistic care, both surgical and nonsurgical. Consultation among these professionals ensures an individualized treatment protocol that enhances surgical outcomes and patient satisfaction. The recent publication of evidence-based guidelines, e.g., management of disorders such as Mucopolysaccharidosis (MPS) IVA and MPS VI, is reflective of the necessity for consensus-building in approaching surgery. These guidelines not only optimize management strategies but also provide a blueprint for surveillance and follow-up. With the application of these collaborative frameworks, healthcare practitioners can better deal with the complexities of spinal pathologies, eventually leading to more optimal and tailored therapeutic interventions (Akyol et al., 2019) (Figure 6.17).

6.6.3. Rehabilitation and Physical Therapy

Physical therapy and rehabilitation are essential aspects of treating spinal disorders, allowing patients to heal and become healthier individuals. The treatments applied not only work towards alleviating pain but also towards enhancing the functionality of patients suffering from spinal disorders. Efficacious rehabilitation treatments are tailored to the patient's individual requirements, taking into account factors such as the sequence of severity, patient age, and comorbid illness. Most importantly, interventions focus on the restoration of physical activity early on as a treatment modality, in accordance with prevailing trends against prolonged bed rest. Through self-care and encouraging engagement in daily activities, rehabilitation programs attempt to empower patients to become active participants in their own recovery process, which is instrumental in psychological health and physical well-being. Comprehensive rehabilitation usually entails a multidisciplinary process that includes a variety of therapeutic interventions aimed at addressing the complex needs of patients with spinal disorders. Physiotherapy is also at the core of such treatment protocols, and the evidence suggests a beneficial effect on patient outcomes in spinal pain and associated conditions. As has been highlighted in literature, the role of physiotherapy extends beyond resolving immediate pain; it also involves the development of strength, flexibility, and endurance through targeted exercise regimens. Besides, psychological and behavioral aspects are increasingly playing a significant role in managing the psychosocial factors that can aggregate spinal pain, so that increased resilience and self-management are possible. The harmony between physical and mental health is the most important factor to enable successful rehabilitation, pointing to the need for an integrated treatment plan that supports sustained recovery (Howard-Wilsher et al., 2016). Secondly, the economic implications of physical therapy and rehabilitation are significant and must be carefully planned for by healthcare policymakers. Cost-effectiveness studies indicate that the majority of rehabilitation interventions are highly effective, improving individual health outcomes in addition to lowering overall health spending because of their preventive nature. For instance, systematic reviews have pointed out that several rehabilitation interventions, including physiotherapy, not only improve the quality of life in spinal disorder patients but also result in cost savings when they are applied to the fullest. The possibility of rehabilitation in decreasing the ever-rising economic burden of chronic pain conditions highlights its importance in contemporary healthcare systems. Such conclusions call for more investigation into providing good rehabilitation services, especially in resource-challenged regions, to ensure that every individual with spinal disorders accesses the necessary rehabilitation services (Howard-Wilsher et al., 2016).

SUMMARY

The systematic study of spinal disease has illuminated the complex interaction among anatomical shape, physiological function, and clinical picture in spinal disorders. As this study closes, diseases such as herniated disc, spinal stenosis, and idiopathic scoliosis illustrate the potential for massive morbidity due to spinal architectural abnormalities. Understanding of the complex mechanisms controlling spinal health, including those of biomechanics and neurology, is crucial to the understanding of these diseases. Finally, clinical evidence underscores the importance of early diagnosis with current imaging techniques, particularly MRI, to successful management. The new advances not only provide for the possibility of early treatment but also maximize the effectiveness of conservative care, being extremely useful in avoiding the aggravation of such conditions. Therefore, current research into spinal pathology and its treatment remains crucial to improved patient treatment and quality of life. In managing spinal disorders, treatment strategies need to be tailored to suit the specific presentation and needs of each patient. Evidence-based practice, coupled with the principles of patient-centered care, have been shown to be useful in the provision of maximal therapeutic gain. As noted in the literature, conservative therapy in the form of physical therapy and pharmacotherapy frequently offers much relief with minimal attendant risks, as with surgical procedures. Furthermore, novel interventions such as steroid treatment of conditions like spontaneous intracranial hypotension offer new avenues to relief and emphasize the need for ongoing research into pharmacological interventions (Russo et al., 2018). Thus, the bringing together of clinical evidence, patient information, and interdisciplinarity is paramount in the guidance and management protocols that can effectively treat the multifactorial nature of spinal disorders. The ultimate outcome of this study is that the care of spinal disorders requires a multifaceted approach that integrates current scientific reality with clinical expertise and patient attitudes. Consensus-based expert guideline development, for instance, for Mucopolysaccharidosis IVA, enhances care for complex conditions that impact spinal health and associated systems (Akyol et al., 2019). These paradigms assist healthcare providers in using standardized management approaches with some latitude for adaptability to fit the particular patient profile. Additionally, ongoing education and research are essential to uncover new information regarding spinal disorders, ultimately closing knowledge and treatment gaps. This combined system not only attempts to alleviate symptoms but also hopes to enhance the general quality of life for those who have suffered from spinal disorders, where innovation in diagnostic and care methods is crucial.

A deep insight into spinal disorders reveals significant findings regarding their impact on patient health and quality of life. Among the significant ones is the evaluation of symptomatic adult spinal deformity (SASD), which explains the relationship between the severity of spinal deformities and health-related quality of life. Recent studies have indicated that patients with SASD have significantly lower physical component summary (PCS) scores than the general U.S. population, with studies finding a PCS for SASD patients of 40.9 versus 50 in the general population. This imbalance points to the disabling nature of spinal disorders and requires greater awareness among health practitioners regarding the nature and severity of spinal deformities that are associated with disability, thus ensuring that diagnosis and treatment are made more effective (Bess et al., 2016). To the discourse on spinal disorders is added recent therapeutic innovation, particularly where genetic disorders like spinal muscular atrophy (SMA) are involved. The introduction of nusinersen, an antisense oligonucleotide, is a significant advancement in the therapeutic paradigm. Designed for intrathecal administration, nusinersen reprograms the splicing of survival motor neuron 2 premessenger RNA to enhance the synthesis of the survival motor neuron protein, which is crucial to motor neuron function. Clinical trials proved to be promising, with significant improvement in motor function and survival, although they have not been able to achieve the developmental milestones of the same age (Meylemans & De Bleecker, 2019). This emphasizes the need for ongoing research and development via innovation of successful treatments for spinal disorders. Lastly, the synopsis of the major points on spinal disorders emphasizes the need for an integrated approach towards understanding and managing these disorders. The relationship of the resulting physical disability of spinal deformity with psychological impact on the patient cannot be overemphasized. Also, the recent onset of targeted therapies like nusinersen reveals the rapidly shifting paradigm of management in this area, which can be a cause of renewed optimism in the patients of genetic muscular disorders. Therefore, more clinical trials and research are necessary in order to more clearly explain the complexities of spinal pathologies and develop wide-ranging strategies that enhance patient outcomes and quality of life (Bess et al., 2016; Meylemans & De Bleecker, 2019).

CLOSER LOOK

PHYSICAL THERAPY

Physical therapy is a healthcare profession focused on improving movement, reducing pain, restoring function, and preventing disability. It plays a vital role in the rehabilitation of individuals affected by injury, illness, surgery, or chronic conditions. Physical therapists use evidence-based techniques to help patients regain strength, flexibility, balance, and coordination, enabling them to return to daily activities and improve their quality of life. Physical therapy involves a comprehensive assessment of posture, movement patterns, muscle strength, joint mobility, and functional ability. Based on this evaluation, personalized treatment plans are designed. Common interventions include therapeutic exercises, manual therapy, stretching, electrotherapy, heat and cold therapy, and posture correction. Specialized programs are also developed for sports rehabilitation, neurological conditions, cardiopulmonary disorders, pediatric care, and geriatric rehabilitation. In orthopedic cases, physical therapy is essential for recovery after fractures, joint replacements, sprains, and musculoskeletal injuries. It helps reduce pain, prevent stiffness, improve circulation, and promote tissue healing. In neurological rehabilitation, physical therapy supports patients with stroke, spinal cord injuries, and Parkinson's disease by enhancing mobility and independence. Preventive care is another important aspect, focusing on injury prevention, ergonomic education, and fitness training. Overall, physical therapy provides a holistic, patient-centered approach that supports recovery, enhances physical function, and promotes long-term health and well-being.

REFERENCES

1. Abourbeh, G., Thézé, B., Maroy, R., Dubois, A., Brulon, V., Fontyn, Y., Dollé, F., Tavitian, B., & Boisgard, R. (2012). Imaging microglial/macrophage activation in spinal cords of experimental autoimmune encephalomyelitis rats by positron emission tomography using the mitochondrial 18 kDa translocator protein radioligand [^{18}F]DPA-714. *The Journal of neuroscience : the official journal of the Society for Neuroscience, 32*(17), 5728–5736. https://doi.org/10.1523/JNEUROSCI.2900-11.2012(accessed on 26th June 2025).
2. McClurg D, Walker K, Aitchison P, et al. Abdominal Massage for the Relief of Constipation in People with Parkinson's: A Qualitative Study. *Parkinsons Dis.* 2016;2016:4842090. doi:10.1155/2016/4842090(accessed on 26th June 2025).
3. Bess, S., Line, B., Fu, K. M., McCarthy, I., Lafage, V., Schwab, F., Shaffrey, C., Ames, C., Akbarnia, B., Jo, H., Kelly, M., Burton, D., Hart, R., Klineberg, E., Kebaish, K., Hostin, R., Mundis, G., Mummaneni, P., Smith, J. S., & International Spine Study Group (2016). The Health Impact of Symptomatic Adult Spinal Deformity: Comparison of Deformity Types to United States Population Norms and Chronic Diseases. *Spine, 41*(3), 224–233. https://doi.org/10.1097/BRS.0000000000001202(accessed on 26th June 2025).
4. Akyol, M. U., Alden, T. D., Amartino, H., Ashworth, J., Belani, K., Berger, K. I., Borgo, A., Braunlin, E., Eto, Y., Gold, J. I., Jester, A., Jones, S. A., Karsli, C., Mackenzie, W., Marinho, D. R., McFadyen, A., McGill, J., Mitchell, J. J., Muenzer, J., Okuyama, T., ... MPS Consensus Programme Co-Chairs (2019). Recommendations for the management of MPS IVA: systematic evidence- and consensus-based guidance. *Orphanet journal of rare diseases, 14*(1), 137. https://doi.org/10.1186/s13023-019-1074-9(accessed on 26th June 2025).
5. Pahl, M. A., Brislin, B., Boden, S., Hilibrand, A. S., Vaccaro, A., Hanscom, B., & Albert, T. J. (2006). The impact of four common lumbar spine diagnoses upon overall health status. *The spine journal : official journal of the North American Spine Society, 6*(2), 125–130. https://doi.org/10.1016/j.spinee.2005.04.014(accessed on 26th June 2025).
6. Russo C, Buono V, Fenza G, Zandolino A, Serino A, Manto A. Spontaneous intracranial hypotension: two steroid-responsive cases. *Pol J Radiol.* 2018;83:e229-e233. Published 2018 May 22. doi:10.5114/pjr.2018.76380(accessed on 26th June 2025).
7. Yalin Zheng, M. S. Nixon and R. Allen, "Automatic lumbar vertebrae segmentation in fluoroscopic images via optimised concurrent Hough transform," *2001 Conference Proceedings of the 23rd Annual International Conference of the IEEE Engineering in Medicine and Biology Society*, Istanbul, Turkey, 2001, pp. 2653-2656, doi: 10.1109/IEMBS.2001.1017328.(accessed on 26th June 2025).
8. Chou, D., Mummaneni, P., Anand, N., Nunley, P., La Marca, F., Fu, K. M., Fessler, R., Park, P., Wang, M., Than, K., Nguyen, S., Uribe, J., Zavatsky, J., Deviren, V., Kanter, A., Okonkwo, D., Eastlack, R., Mundis, G., & International Spine Study Group (2018). Treatment of the Fractional Curve of Adult Scoliosis With Circumferential Minimally Invasive Surgery Versus Traditional, Open Surgery: An Analysis of Surgical Outcomes. *Global spine journal, 8*(8), 827–833. https://doi.org/10.1177/2192568218775069(accessed on 26th June 2025).
9. Babaee, M., Soleimani, P., Zali, A., Mohseni Kabir, N., & Chizari, M. (2017). A Predictive Model for Assessment of Successful Outcome in Posterior Spinal Fusion Surgery. *International*

Clinical Neuroscience Journal (ICNJ), 4(4), 143-151. Advance online publication. https://doi.org/10.15171/icnj.2017.05(accessed on 26th June 2025).

10. Benea, V., Georgescu, S. R., Mitran, C. I., et al. (2016). The current treatment of erectile dysfunction. https://core.ac.uk/download/144552982.pdf (accessed on 26th June 2025).
11. Hendriksz, C. J., Berger, K. I., Giugliani, R., Harmatz, P., Kampmann, C., Mackenzie, W. G., Raiman, J., Villarreal, M. S., & Savarirayan, R. (2015). International guidelines for the management and treatment of Morquio A syndrome. *American journal of medical genetics. Part A, 167A*(1), 11–25. https://doi.org/10.1002/ajmg.a.36833(accessed on 26th June 2025).
12. Boardman, F. K. (2014). Experiential knowledge of disability, impairment and illness: The reproductive decisions of families genetically at risk. https://core.ac.uk/download/16664970.pdf (accessed on 26th June 2025).
13. Morris, C., Bowers, R., Ross, K., Stevens, P., & Phillips, D. (2011). Orthotic management of cerebral palsy: recommendations from a consensus conference. *NeuroRehabilitation, 28*(1), 37–46. https://doi.org/10.3233/NRE-2011-0630(accessed on 26th June 2025).
14. Keddie, S., Jaunmuktane, Z., Brandner, S., Shah, S., Maddison, P., Rees, J. H., Hanna, M. G., Lunn, M. P. T., Reilly, M. M., Rossor, A. M., & Carr, A. S. (2018). A diagnostic conundrum. *Practical neurology, 18*(2), 137–142. https://doi.org/10.1136/practneurol-2017-001801 (accessed on 26th June 2025).
15. Burnand, B., Larequi-Lauber, T., Porchet, F., et al. (1998). Indications à la laminectomie: Adéquation et nécessité. https://core.ac.uk/download/77170853.pdf (accessed on 26th June 2025).
16. Poltawski, L., Watson, T. & Byrne, G., (2008). Physiotherapists' perceptions of problematic musculoskeletal soft tissue disorders. International Journal of Therapy and Rehabilitation 2008 15:10, 437-444. (accessed on 26th June 2025).
17. Turturro, F., Montanaro, A., Calderaro, C., Labianca, L., Di Sanzo, V., & Ferretti, A. (2017). Rate of complications due to neuromuscular scoliosis spine surgery in a 30-years consecutive series. *European spine journal : official publication of the European Spine Society, the European Spinal Deformity Society, and the European Section of the Cervical Spine Research Society, 26*(Suppl 4), 539–545. https://doi.org/10.1007/s00586-017-5034-6(accessed on 26th June 2025).
18. Camilleri, M. (1999). Functional bowel disease: A challenging frontier in gastroenterology. https://core.ac.uk/download/46601769.pdf (accessed on 26th June 2025).
19. Mansueto, P., Di Stefano, L., D'Alcamo, A., & Carroccio, A. (2012). Multiple sclerosis-like neurological manifestations in a coeliac patient: nothing is as it seems. *BMJ case reports, 2012*, bcr2012006392. https://doi.org/10.1136/bcr-2012-006392(accessed on 26th June 2025).
20. Elliott, J. M., Hancock, M. J., Crawford, R. J., Smith, A. C., & Walton, D. M. (2018). Advancing imaging technologies for patients with spinal pain: with a focus on whiplash injury. *The spine journal : official journal of the North American Spine Society, 18*(8), 1489–1497. https://doi.org/10.1016/j.spinee.2017.06.015(accessed on 26th June 2025).
21. Lee SW, Nguyen D, Mack D, Aguila E, Thomas M, Doddy K. Conservative Management of Low Back Pain. *HCA Healthc J Med.* 2021;2(5):319-328. Published 2021 Oct 29. doi:10.36518/2689-0216.1261(accessed on 26th June 2025).

22. Travlos, V., Downs, J., Wilson, A., Hince, D., & Patman, S. (2019). Mental wellbeing in non-ambulant youth with neuromuscular disorders: What makes the difference?. *Neuromuscular disorders : NMD, 29*(1), 48–58. https://doi.org/10.1016/j.nmd.2018.08.013(accessed on 26th June 2025).

23. Estrine, J., & DeLisle, L. (2006). Stress: Putting the brain back into medicine. https://core.ac.uk/download/71356692.pdf (accessed on 26th June 2025).

24. Howard-Wilsher, S., Irvine, L., Fan, H., Shakespeare, T., Suhrcke, M., Horton, S., Poland, F., Hooper, L., & Song, F. (2016). Systematic overview of economic evaluations of health-related rehabilitation. *Disability and health journal, 9*(1), 11–25. https://doi.org/10.1016/j.dhjo.2015.08.009(accessed on 26th June 2025).

25. Oussalah, A., Julien, M., Levy, J., Hajjar, O., Franczak, C., Stephan, C., Laugel, E., Wandzel, M., Filhine-Tresarrieu, P., Green, R., & Guéant, J. L. (2019). Global Burden Related to Nitrous Oxide Exposure in Medical and Recreational Settings: A Systematic Review and Individual Patient Data Meta-Analysis. *Journal of clinical medicine, 8*(4), 551. https://doi.org/10.3390/jcm8040551 (accessed on 26th June 2025).

26. Stricsek, G., Gillick, J., Rymarczuk, G., & Harrop, J. S. (2018). Managing the Complex Patient with Degenerative Cervical Myelopathy: How to Handle the Aging Spine, the Obese Patient, and Individuals with Medical Comorbidities. *Neurosurgery clinics of North America, 29*(1), 177–184. https://doi.org/10.1016/j.nec.2017.09.014(accessed on 26th June 2025).

27. Abbati, G. *et al.* (2017). MRI-Based Surgical Planning for Lumbar Spinal Stenosis. In: Descoteaux, M., Maier-Hein, L., Franz, A., Jannin, P., Collins, D., Duchesne, S. (eds) Medical Image Computing and Computer Assisted Intervention – MICCAI 2017. MICCAI 2017. Lecture Notes in Computer Science(), vol 10435. Springer, Cham. https://doi.org/10.1007/978-3-319-66179-7_14(accessed on 26th June 2025).

28. Jeffries, M. (2016). Management of rapid eye movement sleep behavior disorder in patients with Parkinson's disease. https://open.bu.edu/bitstream/2144/19178/1/Jeffries_bu_0017N_12300.pdf (accessed on 26th June 2025).

29. Larauche, M., Mulak, A., & Taché, Y. (2011). Stress-related alterations of visceral sensation: Animal models for irritable bowel syndrome study. https://core.ac.uk/download/323080393.pdf (accessed on 26th June 2025).

30. DeLong, M. R., Gazzaniga, M. S., Marder, E., & Wichmann, T. (2008). 2008 progress report on brain research. https://core.ac.uk/download/71349141.pdf (accessed on 26th June 2025).

31. Meylemans, A., & De Bleecker, J. (2019). Current evidence for treatment with nusinersen for spinal muscular atrophy: a systematic review. *Acta neurologica Belgica, 119*(4), 523–533. https://doi.org/10.1007/s13760-019-01199-z(accessed on 26th June 2025).

32. Sivhugwana, Innocentia (2022). Factors related with the functional outcome of patients who sustained tibial plateau fractures. Dissertation (MSc (Physiotherapy))--University of Pretoria, 2022. https://core.ac.uk/download/565849089.pdf

33. Walker, B. F. (1993). Disc disease: A summary and review. https://core.ac.uk/download/11242068.pdf (accessed on 26th June 2025).

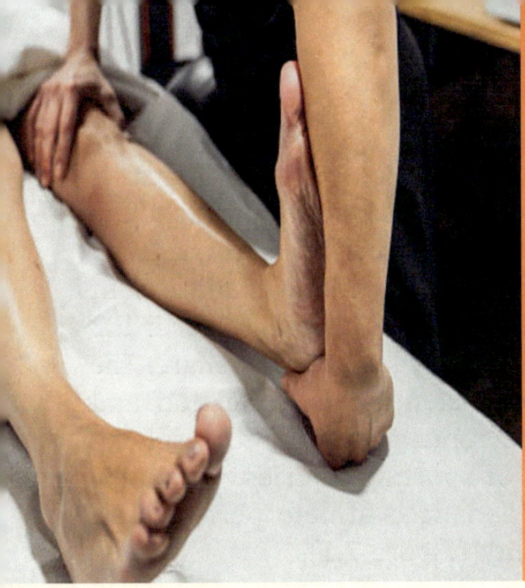

Chapter 7

SPORTS INJURY ASSESSMENT AND DIAGNOSIS

Contents

Introduction 201

7.1. Types of Sports Injuries 204

7.2. Mechanisms of Injury 207

7.3. Initial Assessment Techniques 211

7.4. Diagnostic Tools and Technologies 214

7.5. Role of Medical Professionals 217

7.6. Treatment Protocols 221

Summary 225

References 228

Introduction

In the world of sports, injury evaluation and diagnosis have become an essential part of athlete performance and healthcare. As the competitive landscape evolves, the need for rigorous methods in evaluating sports injuries grows. Training intensity, fatigue in athletes, and environmental conditions are all contributors to sports injuries. The practitioner can utilize these factors to create proper methods to prevent injury and recovery. This pre-emptive process not only safeguards the health of athletes but also optimizes their training programs. Incorporated into this process is the application of interdisciplinary approaches that combine knowledge from medicine, nutrition, and psychology to facilitate integrated care of the athlete, and therefore address not only the physical manifestations but also the underlying psychosocial origins of impaired performance. The three-dimensional character of sports injury demands a high-level understanding of its etiologies and the prevailing importance of reliable assessment tools. Research suggests clinical testing principles must inform methodologies to support precise diagnosis and good rehabilitation practice. A paradigm shift to the implementation of high-tech biomechanical assessments can significantly enhance the quality of assessment by sports health professionals. New technology, such as optical gait analysis systems, highlights cutting-edge developments in the area. The technologies reduce measurement error and maximize the accuracy of data capture in clinical practice.

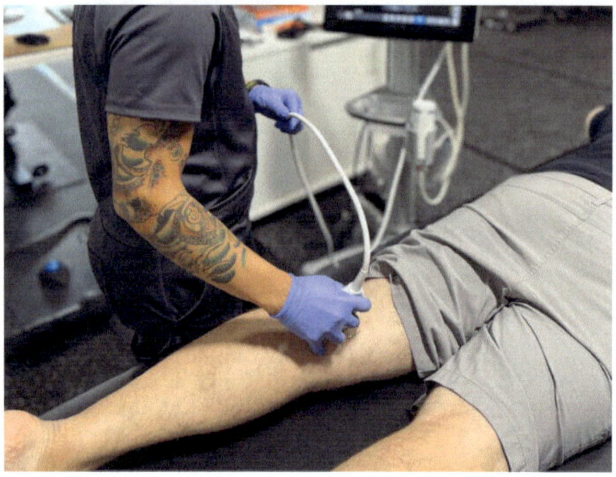

Figure 7.1. Sports injury evaluation.

Source: https://yourphysiciancoach.com/wp-content/uploads/2024/02/sportsinjuryevaluation1-e1709663335988.jpg.

Practitioners can thus make evidence-informed decisions, hence making individual athlete-specific interventions. Coupling new data interpretation methods with existing knowledge is also crucial in managing various injury presentations appropriately. Aiding in individualized interventions and outcome prediction are both essential when building efficient rehabilitation programs. Despite how much there has been advancement, current clinical gait analysis methods remain lacking in a broad theoretical framework for the mechanics of human walking. This lack necessitates ongoing research and model generation to simulate diverse interventions, optimizing the potential to achieve unique athletes' idiosyncratic biomechanical portraits resulting from injury. Also, development of the evidence base via subsequent clinical trials will validate the efficacy of injury management practices to enable clinicians to perform the best practice necessary for athlete welfare. The interaction with scientific investigation and clinical practice remains central to resolving the intricacies of sporting injuries, ultimately translating to enhanced athlete performance and sustainability (Figure 7.1).

Definition of Sports Injuries

It requires a thorough understanding of their multi-spectrum nature, which comprises various types and degrees. Sports injuries may be categorized primarily as acute and chronic injuries. Acute injuries, which occur suddenly while playing sports or exercising, are known as acute injuries, usually arising from trauma in terms of sprain, fracture, or concussion. On the contrary, chronic injuries are due to slow development and tend to include repetitive stress on some parts of the body, creating conditions such as tendonitis or stress fractures. Such a multifaceted injury involves a strenuous evaluation and diagnosis process because the implications of recovery and the athlete's long-term well-being, based on the type and degree of the injury, could be significantly different. The consequences of sports injuries extend beyond the physical and reach the athletes at a psychological, social, and economic level. For instance, athletes can experience emotional pain due to enforced time off, which can affect their psychological health and desire to play competitively once more. Furthermore, the economic expense of medical treatment and rehabilitation may be overwhelming for both the athletes and their families. Preventive measures, such as correct training techniques and use of equipment, are essential in restricting the number of injuries. Knowledge of the potential risks and the best ways of prevention can drastically reduce the impact of injury in sporting environments, further highlighting the relevance of ongoing education and research into sports safety procedures. Of all the types of sports injuries, concussions are problematic since they have insidious and transitory symptoms that can mask the existence of severe pathology. Mild traumatic brain injury (mTBI), which is also referred to as a concussion, results from a blow to the head, either directly or indirectly, leading to changes in brain function. Unfortunately, no universally recognized diagnostic criterion for mTBI exists, making precise evaluation difficult, with a risk of misdiagnosis and vulnerability to further injury. The latest innovative eye-movement measures hold promising avenues for the identification of impairments with concussions, which will have standardized diagnostic criteria established. As research unfolds in this field, it will be important to continue refining the methodologies for evaluation to support enhancing athlete safety and providing valuable input for effective management interventions within the context of sports injury assessment and diagnosis (Sage, 2018; Stuart et al., 2020).

Importance of Assessment and Diagnosis

In the world of sports injury diagnosis and evaluation, the ability to conduct thorough evaluations is of the utmost importance in treatment outcomes and the return to optimal function of athletes. Accurate assessment methods provide for critical information concerning the nature and severity of the injury, on which appropriate rehabilitation procedures must be directed. Since most injuries are caused by overworking and sudden movements, knowledge of the specific mechanisms for such injuries, including muscle ruptures in the hamstrings during sprinting at high speeds, enables practitioners to formulate specific recovery programs. Using modalities like MRI and ultrasound, clinicians can ascertain the exact location and level of damage, thereby giving individualized care to athletes that corresponds to their injury patterns. Ultimately, a good assessment process encourages well-informed decision-making, allowing maximum recovery time and increasing athletes' readiness to safely resume competitive sport (Marrero et al., 2025). Furthermore, the diagnosis is not only a means to the determination of the injury but also a stepping stone to prevention. A good assessment and diagnosis protocol uncovers patterns of injury to construct proactive measures, reducing risks. This is particularly important in young sportspeople, who are increasingly at risk of sports injury. Research has demonstrated that collision and high-impact sports have a propensity to raise the risk of injury in adolescents and need to be assessed thoroughly in order to inform risk management policies. Understanding the specific vulnerabilities that are attached to various sports enables coaches and health professionals to implement special training regimens and injury prevention measures. These advanced measures not only enhance safety but also contribute to the growth of sports in the long term and provide sustainable performance (Ryabcev et al., 2024). Ultimately, the general importance of diagnosis and assessment can be perceived through its contribution to customizing the best rehabilitation strategies. Following the initial trauma, tailored rehabilitation processes are dependent on proper diagnostic data. For instance, identification of sites where muscle ruptures happen in the hamstrings will directly influence the choice of therapeutic modalities employed in rehabilitation. Further, the incorporation of physical rehabilitation techniques enhances healing so that athletes can regain function at an improved rate. Rehabilitation science verifies the requirement for assessment that clarifies injury mechanisms and ensuing recovery patterns on the basis of incorporation of methods like physiotherapy and therapeutic exercises. As attested by studies indicating the higher efficacy of organized rehabilitation facilities in young sport athletes, the role of constant monitoring throughout the entire chain of recovery cannot be overemphasized (Ryabcev et al., 2024) (Figure 7.2).

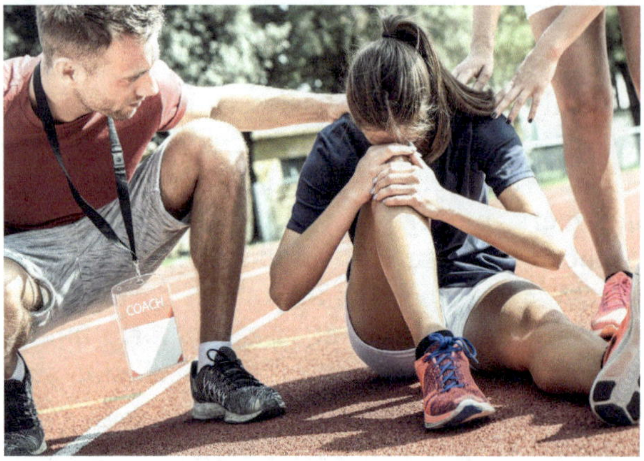

Figure 7.2. The importance of early treatment of sports injuries.

Source: https://www.pbmchealth.org/application/files/4015/7468/3679/Peconic_Bay_Medical_Center_The_Importance_of_Early_Treatment_of_Sports_Injuries_IMAGE1.jpeg.

7.1. Types of Sports Injuries

In sports, injuries also come in various forms, depending on the physical demands and individual movement of a specific activity. Acute injuries are among the most prevalent types of sports injury, occurring suddenly during an activity, such as sprains, strains, fractures, and concussions. Being hit directly or falling is most likely to cause these injuries, where the symptoms are immediately apparent and demand a timely evaluation and diagnosis. As an example, the anterior cruciate ligament (ACL) sprains and tears commonly encountered during basketball and soccer matches, such as sudden changes in direction, may have significant long-term effects if left unattended immediately. An understanding of the mechanisms behind these acute sports injuries is important in order to formulate proper prevention programs and provide appropriate medical intervention in a timely manner to negate their effects on athletes' performance and health. Chronic injuries, on the other hand, result from long-term cumulative stress and are typically associated with poor conditioning or poor technique. Stress fractures and tendonitis are textbook examples of this kind, as they result from continuous overuse with insufficient recovery time. Endurance athletes such as runners and cyclists are most susceptible to this kind of injury, which can accumulate gradually with minimal warning and typically does not go unnoticed until it significantly affects performance. Detailed assessments, i.e., physical examinations and imaging studies, are necessary for proper chronic injury diagnoses. Preventive measures, e.g., strength training, flexibility training, and correct training regimens, are critical to reducing chronic injury incidence, ultimately enabling athletes to maintain their competitive edge while keeping downtime to a minimum. Diagnosis and treatment of these different types of injuries need a complicated insight into the particular demands made on different parts of the body during sports. Sports-specific injury examinations are crucial for formulating rehabilitation and recovery programs to suit the particular needs of each sports player. Other developments, such as virtual triage clinics, have also arisen as cutting-edge solutions towards enhancing the referral process for treating sports injuries. For instance, a study on knee injuries illustrated the significance of sporting injuries on the overall injury burden, where 41.2% of the cases were a result of sporting activity. Early diagnosis after thorough examination provides the patient with the appropriate treatment, either surgical or conservative, thereby enhancing recovery rates and preventing further complications. Effective management is not merely based on injury type knowledge but also on applying evidence-based practices that translate into optimal athletic performance and overall health (Figure 7.3).

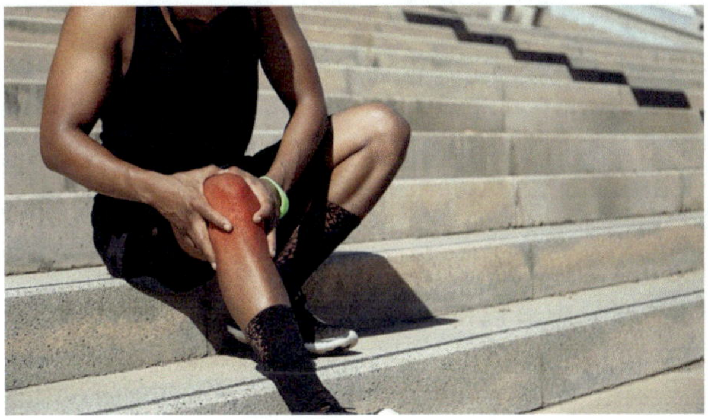

Figure 7.3. ACL injury.

Source: https://mandayahospitalgroup.com/wp-content/uploads/2024/04/cedera-acl.jpg.

7.1.1. Acute Injuries

Abrupt onset and instant effects of acute sporting injuries make them a common problem amongst sportspersons of all ages and stages of competence. Acute sports injuries are commonly caused by abrupt high-impact collisions, abrupt directional changes, or falls and lead to injury of soft tissues, bones, or joints. Examples include sprains, fractures, and strains, which need prompt assessment and treatment to prevent adverse outcomes. Accurate diagnosis is essential in acute injury care, as it directs treatment protocols and healing therapies. Moreover, an understanding of the etiology of such injuries, i.e., overexertion or technical error, can significantly enhance prevention. With appropriate care of athletes in an appropriate and timely fashion, sports practitioners can contribute to optimal performance states along with preventing possible complications throughout the sporting year. In sports injury assessment, the role of newer imaging modalities has increased significantly in the diagnosis of acute injuries. Magnetic Resonance Imaging (MRI), in particular, has been invaluable in unveiling the intricacy of injuries such as those of the anterior cruciate ligament (ACL). Literature points out the need to recognize not only the ACL tear but also some associated injuries, such as meniscus tears and bone contusions. The range of MRI findings in children demonstrates the need for a graduated diagnostic approach with respect to age-related anatomical considerations. It identifies a significant difference between trauma in children and adults; while the adult will tend to manifest more overt complications, the child is prone to display covert but clinically relevant signs that make the diagnosis more difficult.

Whiplash Associated Disorder

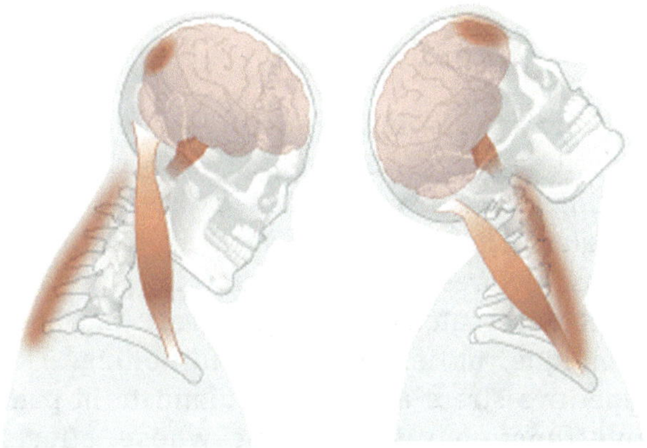

Figure 7.4. Whiplash-associated disorder (WAD).

Source: https://ptclinic.com/medlibrary/images/v2/wad.gif.

Correct interpretation of these imaging results can greatly assist health practitioners in creating tailored rehabilitation plans and tracking the patient's recovery process, thus getting back to optimal performance levels. The setting in which acute injuries occur also greatly affects their diagnosis and treatment. Research within the field of Whiplash Associated Disorders (WAD) illustrates that the environment—whether a road traffic accident or a sports setting—may influence clinician opinion and diagnosis outcome. Experienced physiotherapists have been inconsistent in their classifications of diagnosis based on the situation of injury, suggesting potential bias in assessment strategies. The inconsistency suggests the need for a consistent diagnostic protocol and guidelines with the goal of simplifying sports injury assessment. Through the resolution of the inconsistencies that arise in different contexts, sports health professionals can sharpen their diagnostic accuracy and treatment impact, hence improving the overall care of sportspeople. Identification of these context-dependent factors is vital in designing integrated injury management protocols for improving effective recovery and minimizing the risk of complications from long-term acute injury (Figure 7.4).

7.1.2. Chronic Injuries

Chronic sports injuries typically occur as repetitive strain or overuse, and they are distinguished from sudden causative acute injuries. These injuries, such as tendinitis, stress fractures, and bursitis, develop gradually, often exacerbated by inadequate rest, improper technique, or inadequate conditioning. The repetitive stress effects can culminate in pain and functional impairment whose effects can significantly detract from an athlete's performance. Proper assessment of chronic injury is necessary since misdiagnosis leads to inefficient interventions and extended recovery periods. Sophisticated imaging devices, such as MRI, become significant in the accurate determination of the cause of pain and inflammation, enabling clinicians to craft detailed rehabilitation programs to facilitate athletes' return to play. When addressing chronic injuries, an extensive comprehension of the anatomical structures involved is of significance. The deltoid ligament, for instance, is also a crucial stabilizer of the ankle and is often blamed for chronic instability when it's damaged. Chronic strain of this ligament can develop due to mishandling of acute sprains, yielding long-term effects on an athlete's mobility and overall sporting capability. Symptoms may involve persistent pain, inflammation, and ankle bouts of giving way, all crippling performance. As emerging studies have brought forth, accurate diagnosis is important, and while MRI is the gold standard for imaging, diagnostic MSK ultrasound is a suitable alternative, and the additional benefit of real-time assessment and more interaction with the rehabilitation process. This dual nature of assessment modalities presents improved clinical results in the guise of individually tailored interventions. New therapy for chronic sports medicine injury increasingly encompasses emerging methods such as neuromodulation. This treatment, which modulates nerve function to provide pain relief and promote healing, has been effective in reducing recovery times and improving overall functioning. Neuromodulation can safely reverse the underlying mechanisms of pain and potentially alleviate the reliance on traditional pharmacologic treatments. Patients with chronic pain or non-optimal recovery from injury might benefit significantly from these interventions, especially if traditional measures failed. Yet, as recent literature has proposed, neuromodulation's long-term efficacy and clinical utility need to be continually explored. Comprehending these dynamic treatments in depth, coupled with a solid evaluation framework, will further enable medical practitioners to provide optimal patient outcomes for chronic sports injuries and promote an enhanced quality of life among athletes.

7.1.3. Common Examples of Sports Injuries

Sports injuries are prevalent in nearly every physical endeavor, the most common of which are sprains, strains, and fractures. Sprains, where ligaments are stretched or torn, tend to afflict athletes engaged in high-impact activities such as basketball or soccer. These injuries tend to be accompanied by swelling, bruising, and limited motion; hence prompt assessment is valuable for effective treatment. Strains, on the other hand, are overstretching or tearing of tendons or muscles, usually as a result of sudden physical movement. Fractures, or bone breaks, are highly common in contact sports like rugby or football, wherein athletes are susceptible to impact. A good understanding of such injuries makes their assessment possible and guides athletes toward effective interventions and rehabilitation. Another notable category of sports injuries is more severe conditions, such as anterior cruciate ligament (ACL) injury, which is also popularly known for the high incidence rate in sports involving sudden stops or changes of direction. ACL tears are particularly common in athletes who play sports like soccer, basketball, and skiing, where players subject their knees to severe stress.

The effects of an ACL tear extend beyond immediate pain and inflammation and often necessitate surgery and prolonged rehabilitation. Interestingly, studies indicate that digital health apps may support patients during rehabilitation because they provide vital education on recovery and treatment options (Schmidt et al., 2024). Through this innovative method, sportspersons remain active participants in the healing process even when face-to-face physiotherapy is not always available. In addition to ligament sprains, overuse injuries are a significant issue for athletes. Tendonitis, bursitis, and stress fractures are all the result of repetitive strain and chronic abuse in terms of time, most commonly found in running, swimming, and tennis. Overuse injuries progress slowly, with symptoms of pain, swelling, and diminished strength, which makes them challenging to diagnose and treat. Overlooking these overuse injuries can lead to chronic conditions that bench athletes for months. With the realization of the importance of prevention, medical experts identify correct training techniques and recovery periods as the solution to not having such injuries. Furthermore, being adequately grounded in injury prevention significantly decreases the likelihood of overuse injuries, resulting in better overall performance and lifespan in sports for athletes.

7.2. Mechanisms of Injury

In understanding the injury mechanisms in sports, it is important to understand how individual anatomical structures and biomechanical forces are involved in the injury risk. Complicated interactions of forces like tension, compression, and shear perform critical functions in a variety of sporting scenarios. For instance, in sports involving abrupt direction changes—e.g., soccer or basketball—players tend to experience high stresses in critical structures such as the anterior cruciate ligament (ACL). Furthermore, assessment of these injuries has become increasingly advanced to encompass expert visual assessments, such as studies like the development of the ACL Injury Risk Estimation Quiz (ACL-IQ) for the prediction of injury risk factors through expert observation. These advancements highlight the importance of including biomechanics within practical clinical methods for the best possible prevention of risk from ACL injury in sport (Petushek et al., 2015). In addition to mechanical forces, biological injury responses also have a significant contribution to injury mechanisms, particularly in concussions. Sports concussions, with their multicausal etiology, not only involve direct impacts but also rotational accelerations that have the potential for causing multifaceted pathophysiologic changes in the brain. Recent research using blood biomarkers has elucidated these mechanisms, illustrating the manner in which protein levels like glial fibrillary acidic protein (GFAP) and ubiquitin C-terminal hydrolase-L1 (UCH-L1) can function as objective indicators of concussion severity and recovery. This biological understanding enhances the capacity to diagnose and diagnose concussions through a combination of clinical assessment and biomarker research, thereby resulting in better management of the injury among sporting personalities (McCrea et al., 2020).

In addition, the combination of biomechanical examination with biomarker research has far-reaching significance for the prevention and rehabilitation of injury in sports. Through explanation and quantification of the correlation between mechanical stress and biological response, clinicians are able to develop personalized programs for intervention. These might involve exercises to strengthen vulnerable muscle groups, maximize biomechanics, and ultimately reduce the risk of injury. The implication is that a better understanding of mechanisms of injury enhances diagnostic capability but also yields insight into effective treatment approaches for athletes. Therefore, ongoing research on mechanical and biological factors is essential in informing sports injury assessment processes, thereby allowing athletes to obtain optimal care (Figure 7.5).

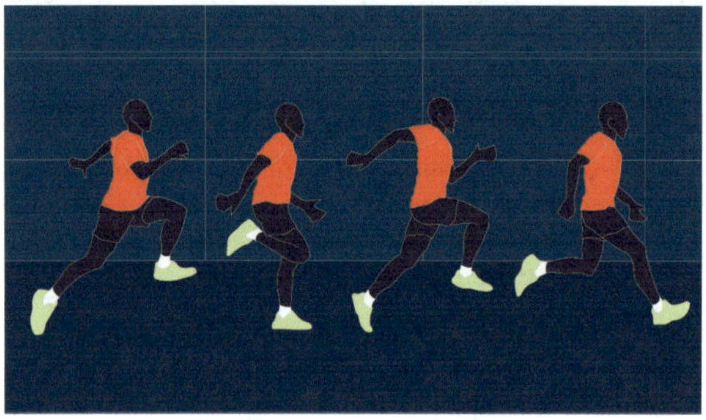

Figure 7.5. Optimizing sprint technique to reduce hamstring injury risk.

Source: https://www.sportsmith.co/wp-content/uploads/2023/12/Hamstring_Injury.jpg.

7.2.1. Impact Injuries

The prevalence of impact injuries in contact sports necessitates elaborate investigation of their evaluation and diagnosis, particularly in terms of their long-term effects. Impact injuries range from the concussion to a severe neurotrauma, with great importance on athletes' physical and mental health. Awareness of these injuries has increased manifold, placing a commitment to understanding the mechanisms of them and their effects. Research has established that recurring head injuries, prevalent among sportspeople like football and boxers, can result in long-term illnesses like Chronic Traumatic Encephalopathy (CTE). CTE is particularly concerning as it is only diagnosable post-mortem, leaving a huge challenge for physicians in today's era to intervene and provide treatment for potential dangers. With ongoing research, the research must move beyond elite sports participants to include young participants, thereby increasing the information on impact injuries within different populations (Sage, 2018). The complexities of diagnosing impact injuries are also amplified by the multiplicity of symptoms experienced by athletes. The injuries can either be acute in nature, as with concussions, or long-term conditions built over time, referred to as cumulative neurotrauma. This complicates it to be certain of making a diagnosis since the majority of the athletes will not report or might blame the symptoms on fatigue or performance. The early diagnosis is important since severe, untreated impact injuries may lead to permanent cognitive disability or physical disability. There have been evaluation protocols that have been created to assist in diagnosing such injuries, which include symptom checklists and cognitive assessment tools. However, reliance on self-reports from athletes can include biases, hence requiring objective measures that can measure the real size of an athlete's condition fairly accurately, especially in conditions like CTE that require more advanced assessment (Sage, 2018). As opposed to neurotrauma, lower limb injuries like Medial Tibial Stress Syndrome (MTSS) pose other problems in sports injury diagnosis and evaluation. Though MTSS is a common ailment in athletes, the uncertain etiology of this condition makes it challenging to prevent and treat. Research is now focused on the transition from reactive treatment to preventive intervention. This involves the identification of risk factors, early symptom recognition at the onset, and tailored training programs aimed at preventing stress on the lower limbs. A wide range of treatment strategies is available—everything from old-fashioned rest and rehab methods to new and more technological forms of therapy. In the end, knowledge of the nature of impact injuries such as MTSS and prevention can greatly enhance athletic safety and performance. More research is critically needed to continue to hone these approaches and make them adaptable to the ever-changing environment of sports injuries (Figure 7.6).

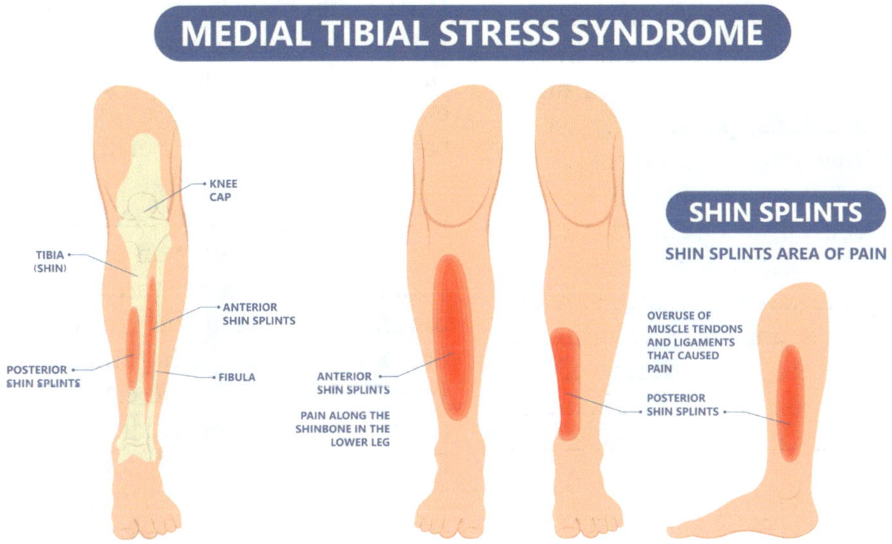

Figure 7.6. Medial tibial stress syndrome.

Source: https://static.wixstatic.com/media/e1bfa1_0a57d33c098a4c86aed237df218f3d97~mv2.jpeg/v1/fill/w_1000,h_629,al_c,q_85,usm_0.66_1.00_0.01/e1bfa1_0a57d33c098a4c86aed237df218f3d97~mv2.jpeg.

7.2.2. Overuse Injuries

Overuse injuries are a significant problem within sport, specifically within sports individuals who subject themselves to repetitive movements over extended periods of time. Unlike acute injury, which is abruptly incurred from trauma, overuse injuries develop gradually as a result of successive stress to muscle, tendon, and bone. The gradual nature of onset of overuse injury renders it tricky to diagnose, particularly as symptoms may initially be so subtle and progress gradually in severity. Players usually ignore the initial signs of pain, assuming that they can work through it, which can lead to more severe conditions. In that case, preventive measures, such as proper training regimens, proper resting periods, and the addition of cross-training, play a significant role in lowering the risk of such injury, which allows players longevity and productivity in sports. Research has outlined the importance of efficient assessment tools in the identification and management of overuse injuries. For example, utilization of the Oslo Sports Trauma Research Center Overuse Injury Questionnaire (OSTRC-O2) modified for different populations allows for culturally sensitive assessment of college athlete overuse injuries. As emphasized in a recent research, high return rates and satisfactory internal consistency of these questionnaires reflect their validity and reliability in monitoring sporting health and overuse injuries among various population groups. By using such standard assessment devices, practitioners are able to gain information regarding the prevalence, site, and severity of overuse injuries. This data not only aids in early diagnosis but also directs individualized interventions to maximize recovery and optimize function with a lower risk of re-injury. In the case of local muscle injuries, assessment of overuse conditions is even more critical. The hamstrings, for instance, are susceptible to injury in high-demand athletic activities, particularly when exposed to repetitive stress. As discussed in recent literature, hamstring strains both occur during and result from sprinting and stretching, and recovery patterns also differ based on the nature of the injury. Diagnostic imaging methods, such as MRI and ultrasound, are pivotal to the evaluation of the nature and severity of the injuries, with details on the involvement of connective tissue and anatomical localization of the injury. Therefore, understanding the mechanism of overuse injury, in conjunction with appropriate diagnostic interventions, allows healthcare practitioners to implement evidence-based rehabilitation programs with emphasis on return to sport in a progressive manner, ultimately enhancing the health and performance of the athlete as highlighted in Marrero et al. (2025).

7.2.3. Environmental Factors Contributing to Injuries

Understanding the environmental etiology of sports injuries is important to effective injury evaluation and prevention planning. Numerous extrinsic factors, such as the surface upon which one is playing, weather conditions, and equipment, have the potential to influence athlete safety. For instance, uneven or poorly conditioned playing fields may lead to ankle sprains or loss of footing and resulting falls in sports involving sharp direction changes or sudden decelerations. Additionally, unfavorable weather, i.e., rain or heat, can impede the performance of an athlete and increase the risk of injury in the form of heat stress or dehydration. Thus, the quantification of such environmental factors at the time of injury occurrence aids in comprehending the situation that leads to injuries and facilitates the formulation of safer environments for sports.

Most importantly, certain sports possess specific environmental conditions that create their profiles of injury. Weightlifting sports, for example, have specific environmental hazards, considering that the weights in question can present a higher threat of harm in terms of poor safety planning. Literature is such that activities like strongman and Highland Games entail excessive injury rates due to the intense physical stress and the risk of environmental damage while competing and training (Keogh & Winwood, 2017). These exercises occasionally require being performed in certain training and facility conditions, which, if not well-maintained, tend to amplify risks of injury. Knowing how environmental factors interact with injury rates in different sports helps to economize risk assessment procedures and inform best practices of training and competition environments. In addition, athlete density and level of competition can dictate injury rates. In team sports, close playing surfaces generate more contact injuries via collision, and competitive environments tend to push participants beyond their safety limits, and hence be more prone to injury. Stress on specific injuries, such as Medial Tibial Stress Syndrome (MTSS), illustrates the need for a better understanding of the same; MTSS is often linked with poor training conditions and poor warm-up strategies (Yamasaki, 2019). Thus, the integration of environmental assessments into the injury diagnosis guarantees a multi-disciplinary approach to the prevention of injury, with a focus on creating appropriate physical environments where athletes can minimize the risk of injury and enhance performance overall.

7.3. Initial Assessment Techniques

The major methods of examination used in sport injury diagnosis play a vital role in establishing the degree and type of an injury. The approaches typically start with a comprehensive history-taking process whereby the clinician obtains details of the patient's symptoms, mechanism of injury, and medical history. This process is very important because it provides a basis for understanding the context surrounding the occurrence of the injury. Moreover, a clinical examination is then performed, wherein the area of problem is observed and palpated to identify signs of swelling, bruising, or tenderness. This comprehensive approach, combining objective and subjective findings, becomes a grounding platform for future interventions and rehabilitation strategies. As highlighted in recent consensus sessions among experts, standardized assessment methods ensure that every clinician employs the same protocol in making accurate diagnoses and consistent findings, e.g., with inguinal disruption, previously referred to as sportsman's hernia (Sheen et al., 2013). Following a primary history and physical examination, special tests can then be used to further determine the nature and degree of the injury. These tests may include functional tests that measure the athlete's motion range, strength, and stability. For instance, in cases of suspected injuries to the joints, clinicians can employ stress tests to establish the integrity of the ligaments and adjacent tissues. Imaging techniques such as ultrasound or MRI may also be prescribed, particularly in cases where internal structures are suspected to be compromised. These imaging modalities provide useful information that allows practitioners to visualize injuries not visible with clinical examination alone. The integration of these preliminary assessment tools not only guides the accurate diagnosis of sport injury but also therapeutic decision-making. Employing a multidisciplinary approach, as supported by recent studies, also enhances treatment effectiveness through tailoring intervention to the unique athlete requirements (Sage, 2018). Lastly, the efficiency of initial assessment strategies relies on the clinical competence of the clinician and adherence to established protocols.

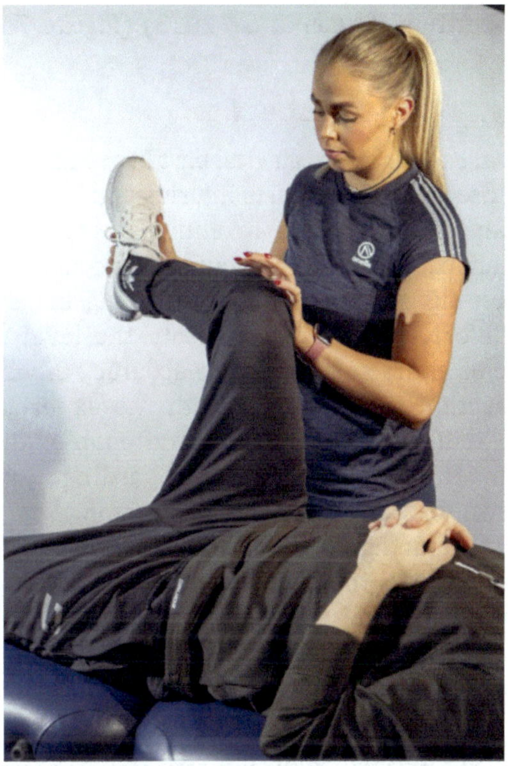

Figure 7.7. Injury assessment and diagnosis Aisling Flynn, athletic therapy.

Source: https://www.aislingflynnathletictherapy.ie/wp-content/uploads/2024/04/injury-assessment-and-diagnosis-aisling-flynn-athletic-therapy_8-jpg.webp.

The need for ongoing education and training of practitioners cannot be stressed enough, as outdated procedures can result in misdiagnosis or inappropriate treatment schemes. Additionally, the creation of effective communication between the clinician and athlete during the assessment process results in trust and encourages rehabilitation protocol compliance. Sharing a common discussion of treatment options can empower the athletes and enhance their rehabilitation process. As continued advancements in the development of sports injury are researched, the enhancement of initial evaluation techniques will be a powerful force in decreasing risks and optimizing long-term results for athletes at every level of competition (Sheen et al., 2013) (Figure 7.7).

7.3.1. Visual Inspection

Visual examination is a vital part of the diagnosis and assessment of sports injuries and is utilized as an initial process in clinical assessment. Clinicians use visual examination to ascertain visible signs of injury, such as swelling, bruising, or deformity, that may indicate the level and type of injury sustained. The accuracy of visual inspection largely varies with the experience and ability of the clinicians and enables them to make sound judgments regarding timely treatment and follow-up inspection. Various sports, particularly high-impact sports like American football, entail certain challenges that need to be taken into account in visual inspection. A proper diagnosis at the initial phase can prove to be a long way in improving the efficacy of treatment and establishing the recovery duration of the athletes. Hence, detailed visual assessment is a critical component of multimodal management of sports injuries. Beyond its use in initial assessment, visual assessment provides for ongoing observation over the recovery process. Throughout rehabilitation progression, practitioners have progressively employed visual assessment for monitoring changes in the appearance of the injury, such as resolution of swelling and range of motion. Ongoing monitoring allows early recognition of possible complications, which can guide alterations to the treatment plan if needed. More advanced technologies, such as real-time imaging and automatic recognition of complications by wound detection machines, are increasingly being used as supplements to routine visual inspection and provide more objective data for practitioners. Most significantly, within the context of acute injury, these improvements are able to offer support in visualizing changes not immediately apparent to the naked eye. Use of such technology can augment the clinician's skill to observe recovery and enable return to athletic function in a safe manner. The practice of visual inspection is ultimately predicated upon an understanding of the mechanisms involved across the spectrum of injuries, thus aiding diagnosis and management. Through examination of specific patterns of injury and their clinical consequences, clinicians can develop targeted individualized rehabilitation programs for the distinct rehabilitation needs of each athlete. The ability to conduct a precise visual assessment not only improves the diagnostic capability of the clinician but also encourages effective communication with athletes regarding the injury and recovery pattern. With advances made in the discipline of sports medicine, the function of visual examination, accompanied by emerging diagnostic modalities, cannot be stressed enough, since integration of old methods with new technologies eventually enhances patient care and optimizes athletic performance. Through continued emphasis on education in visual assessment techniques, medical professionals can optimize diagnostic effectiveness and aid overall wellness and functioning of the athletes.

7.3.2. Palpation Methods

In the clinical evaluation and diagnosis of sports injury, palpation is a key method by which clinicians are able to determine a particular type of injury and appropriately plan treatment. Palpation is a manual examination in which pressure is applied with the fingertips over various structures of the body, like bones, joints, and soft tissues. Depending upon palpation, clinicians can detect abnormal clinical signs such as swelling, pain on pressure, and heat representing internal damage. Through systematic assessment of these physical parameters, clinicians can form an informed clinical opinion on the injury severity and nature. In addition, palpation augments clinicians' knowledge of athletes' status, which allows for targeted interventions to assist recovery as well as enhance performance. Consequently, the incorporation of palpation techniques into daily assessment solidifies the diagnostic protocol in sports medicine. Although effective, the palpation technique also often supplements other diagnostic modalities for use in assisting the evaluation of injury. Palpation, studies have determined, is more accurate when utilized with imaging modalities such as ultrasound and MRI. For example, a recent prospective study highlighted the major advantage of ultrasound in the diagnosis of anterior talofibular ligament (ATFL) tears, with a total sensitivity of 87.5%, and even higher in patients who presented after four days of trauma (Abdulqader et al., 2025). This indicates that while palpation provides us with important qualitative information, incorporating imaging modalities enhances the diagnostic process so that it is complete. Moreover, reliance on palpation alone may lead to misdiagnosis or late detection of complicated injuries, thus reinforcing the necessity for a multi-dimensional approach in the evaluation of sports injuries. In conclusion, palpation methods continue to be a central component in the process of assessing sports injuries. Their utility in the detection of physical signs of injury is advantageous, but users need to know their limitations when used in isolation. Ongoing evolution of testing techniques demands that sports medicine professionals continue to refine their palpation ability and simultaneously apply advances in imaging technology to provide the best patient outcomes. As depicted in study evidence for various conditions, such as the research on sport-related minor traumatic brain injuries, no method is an absolute gold standard; evidence of how evolving and combining old-fashioned examination techniques with newer technologies plays a key role (Haste et al., 2025). This blended system not only ensures accurate diagnosis but also facilitates effective treatment planning attuned to the unique needs of each athlete (Figure 7.8).

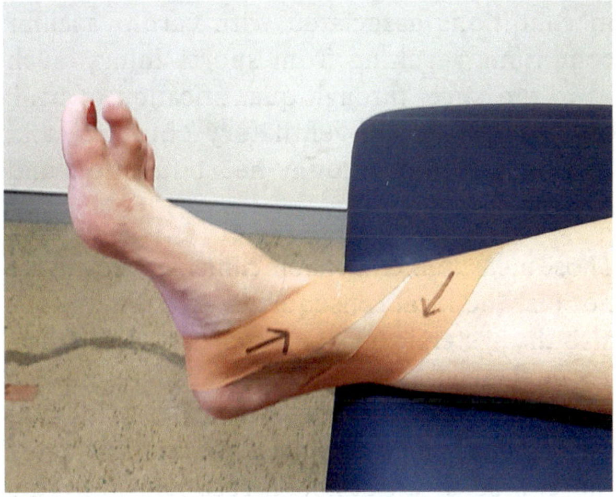

Figure 7.8. Sustentaculum tali palpation.

Source: https://www.sportsinjurybulletin.com/AcuCustom/Sitename/DAM/092/9209-sinus_fig3.jpg.

7.3.3. Functional Testing

Functional testing is a critical component of sport injury evaluation and diagnosis, allowing clinicians to test the capacity of an athlete to perform certain bodily movements following an injury. Functional testing usually entails the application of a set of tests related to the injured area, determining the range of motion, strength, and coordination. By accurately measuring such parameters, functional tests indicate how severe the injury is and give a baseline for rehabilitation to target. The King-Devick (KD) test and other assessments of performance are frequently applied, although they are subject to variability in sensitivity, underlining the need for a global strategy for injury measurement. In the absence of such gold-standard measures in this discipline, the necessity of combining multiple testing protocols is utmost to enable appropriate diagnosis and planning for rehabilitation (Haste et al., 2025). In addition to more traditional tests, newer and more technologically sophisticated ones, such as cardiopulmonary exercise testing (CPET), further enhance functional testing for sport injury assessment. CPET is most relevant in conditions associated with cardiovascular conditions resulting from sports injury, such as to the knee, through quantification of peak oxygen uptake and ventilatory efficiency and also taking into account heart function and capacity for exercise.

Those measurements enable clinicians to evaluate not just the local consequence of an injury but also the systemic effect on sports performance. Through accurate analysis of cardiopulmonary information and damage, medical practitioners can build a more advanced understanding of the course of an athlete's recuperation. This sophisticated understanding then goes on to impact rehabilitation regimes, encouraging highly person-centered interventions that cater to athletes' distinctive functional needs and performance goals (Segreti et al., 2024). Functional testing methods become essential not only in the treatment of acute injuries but also in informing long-term athletic training programs. Under repeated testing, progress and rehabilitation efficacy over time can be tracked, and clinicians are able to make informed adjustments to treatment protocols that meet the best interests of athletes. With return to competition justified, functional tests are able to verify readiness and potential for future performance, and safe and effective return to sports. This dynamic testing minimizes the risk of re-injury by uncovering any remaining deficiencies or imbalances that could have been missed during initial rehabilitation. Functional testing is, hence, an important instrument throughout the whole sports injury management continuum, enabling recovery as well as longevity of sporting careers for athletes (Haste et al., 2025) (Figure 7.9).

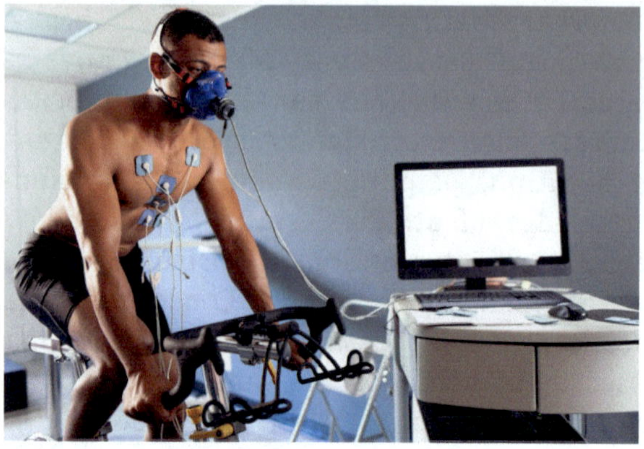

Figure 7.9. Cardiopulmonary exercise test.

Source: https://external-content.duckduckgo.com/iu/?u=https%3A%2F%2Fworkwellfoundation.org%2Fwp-content%2Fuploads%2F2023%2F02%2Fimage3.jpg&f=1&nofb=1&ipt=90b74450601c7a39b41a33cac3825e59e9f05d9294befe00c453b533e9d0ca4c.

7.4. Diagnostic Tools and Technologies

The advent of modern diagnostic machines and technologies has revolutionized the diagnosis and assessment of sports injuries. Classical methods such as patient history and physical examination are now supplemented—and sometimes even replaced—by advanced methods providing more precise and objective results. Technologies like magnetic resonance imaging (MRI) and computed tomography (CT) scans have become essential while assessing the severity of injury, particularly in complex injury cases, including the musculoskeletal system. Also, the use of portable diagnostic machines further enhances in-field assessments to aid timely medical decisions regarding player safety and treatment. As such, the development of diagnostic machines not only increases the accuracy of injury detection but also promotes proactive intervention of athlete well-being, leading ultimately to enhanced sports injury rehabilitation outcomes. For sports-related mild traumatic brain injury (SR-mTBI), the development of diagnostic technology is essential to ensure effective monitoring and evaluation. A systematic review highlighted various instruments used for SR-mTBI evaluation on the day of injury. Despite testing 46 approaches, researchers found no single gold standard for diagnosis. King-Devick (KD) testing was also a widely used method; however, its sensitivity had important variability in between studies, and the area under the curve (AUC) varied from 0.51 to 0.92.

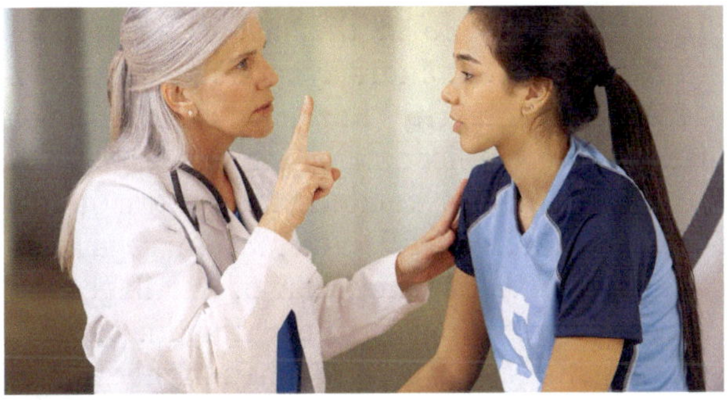

Figure 7.10. Physician evaluating a student athlete's head injury.

Source: https://www.brainscope.com/hs-fs/hubfs/physician-evaluating-student-athlete-head-injury.jpeg?width=1213&name=physician-evaluating-student-athlete-head-injury.jpeg.

The findings emphasize the need for standardized diagnostic methods that integrate a number of tools to evaluate SR-mTBI in a more stable and consistent fashion. By incorporating contemporary techniques, clinicians are able to maximize diagnostic accuracy, thus elevating athlete safety, treatment algorithms, and long-term health outcomes as indicated by the evidence in the study (Haste et al., 2025). For musculoskeletal trauma, i.e., lateral ankle sprain, diagnostic ultrasound has been highly regarded as an advanced tool for investigation. This technology offers real-time imaging that is not only cost-effective but also provides complete insight into soft tissue injury, including the calcaneofibular ligament (CFL) and the anterior talofibular ligament (ATFL). With musculoskeletal diagnostic ultrasound application, practitioners can more clearly visualize injuries, which allows proper diagnosis and tailored treatment planning to be facilitated. The article points to standardization of ultrasound examination techniques as a means of enhancing diagnostic accuracy and patient outcomes. With medicine becoming increasingly reliant on such technologies, the application of diagnostic ultrasound to the diagnosis of sports injuries will expand, and more efficient and thorough management of athlete health will follow (Manske et al., 2024) (Figure 7.10).

7.4.1. Imaging Techniques (X-rays, MRIs)

Imaging techniques play a key role in sports injury evaluation and diagnosis, providing valuable information to support management and treatment planning for the injury. X-rays are typically the first imaging technique employed, particularly in cases where there is suspicion of fracture or dislocation. The technique entails the application of ionizing radiation to generate images of bone structures for clinicians to identify abnormalities such as fractures, malalignments, or disruptions of the joint. While helpful in diagnosing acute injury, X-rays do not do well at visualizing soft tissue injury, like in sports injuries. An understanding of the strengths and weaknesses of X-ray imaging is essential so that healthcare providers can make informed decisions about what to do next in diagnosis, so that athletes can receive appropriate attention in a timely fashion as per clinical guidelines (Yuen et al., 2019). When compared to X-rays, Magnetic Resonance Imaging (MRI) provides a clear image of the hard and soft tissues and is therefore particularly valuable in diagnosing complex sports injuries. MRI uses powerful magnets and radio waves to create clear images of soft tissues such as muscles, ligaments, tendons, and cartilage. This capacity to identify early conditions like tears, strains, and overuse injuries that are not visible on X-ray imaging can be pivotal in the treatment of athletes. In one study assessing foot lesions, MRI proved highly valuable in providing good preoperative assessments of a variety of soft tissue injuries (Hs et al., 2017). Thus, clinicians prefer to use MRI when committed athletes present persistent pain or performance limitations that do not respond to initial treatment, thereby providing an opportunity for a specific rehabilitation process. Employment of advanced imaging technologies, including X-rays and MRIs, enhances the general diagnostic process in sports injury assessment. Clinicians must be capable of determining which imaging modality is most appropriate based on the clinical presentation of the patient and the suspected type of injury. An effective sports injury evaluation algorithm typically begins with X-rays to rule out fractures and proceeds to an MRI if soft tissue injuries are suspected. These imaging techniques not only help with diagnosis but also help with effective communication between the medical team and sportsmen for easy explanation of the injury and its significance. Therefore, a good understanding of imaging modalities is essential to maximize the treatment and rehabilitation of injured sportsmen, thereby leading to improved recovery outcomes in sports medicine (Yuen et al., 2019)

7.4.2. Ultrasound in Injury Assessment

Point-of-care ultrasound (POCUS) incorporation in sports injury assessment is a valuable advance in sports medicine. POCUS provides real-time imaging, with immediate feedback provided to the clinician while the injury is being evaluated. The portability of the equipment enhances accessibility, enabling its use at more than one location, such as sideline assessment during a game. This is a valuable function in the acute injury setting where immediate decision-making is needed to optimize management for the athlete. Compared to traditional imaging techniques such as X-ray and MRI, POCUS not only costs less but also reduces patient radiation exposure, thus gaining popularity in practice in sporting settings. Consequently, the application of POCUS enhances the pace and accuracy of musculoskeletal injury diagnosis, thus leading to improved management options as well as enhanced athlete rehabilitation pathways (Koziak et al., 2025). Ultrasound imaging has proved to be very effective in the diagnosis and follow-up of different sports injuries, especially those affecting soft tissue, including muscles, tendons, and ligaments. Research has revealed that POCUS plays a major role in the fast evaluation of injuries because it offers dynamic visualization of structural integrity (Koziak et al., 2025). For instance, its application in the assessment of the knee joint has demonstrated ultrasound's ability to offer useful information regarding conditions like degeneration of cartilage and associated pathologies. In the domain of knee injuries, studies have established high levels of correlation between ultrasound findings and established clinical assessment parameters like the Visual Analogue Scale (VAS) and the Western Ontario and McMaster Universities Osteoarthritis Index (WOMAC). These correlations validate ultrasound as a precise instrument in clinical practice, lending credibility to its validity in sports medicine practice. Ultrasound is not just a diagnostic instrument; it has an essential function in guiding therapeutic intervention and monitoring recovery, too. By monitoring injury status change over time, clinicians can assess treatment regimens' effectiveness and make informed changes by real-time feedback. This interactive cycle of feedback is particularly precious in sports, where the return-to-play policy is based on an athlete's functional status and recovery progress. The growing evidence supporting ultrasound in assessing sports injury speaks to its promise of optimizing management protocols, establishing a culture of evidence-based practice. With the field of science continuing to evolve, further research on standardizing ultrasound protocols and extending operator training will undoubtedly allow ultrasounds to position themselves as a crucial aspect of the extensive examination and diagnosis of sports injuries (Koziak et al., 2025) (Figure 7.11).

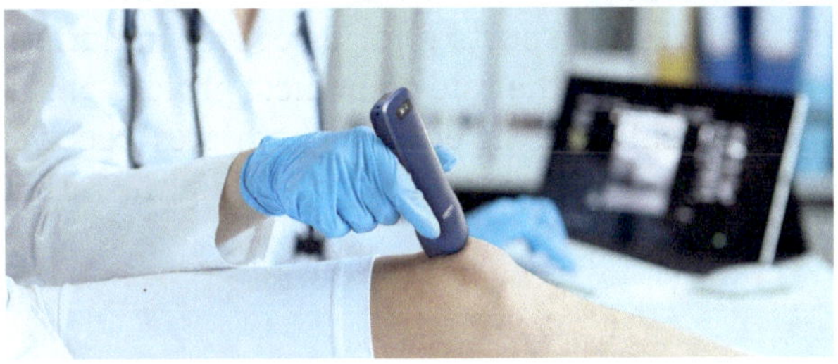

Figure 7.11. Integration of point-of-care ultrasound (POCUS) in sports injury assessment.

Source: https://external-content.duckduckgo.com/iu/?u=https%3A%2F%2Fimg.medicalexpo.com%2Fimages_me%2Fprojects%2Fimages-g%2Fhow-does-pocus-point-of-care-ultrasound-work-43432-17986645.jpg&f=1&nofb=1&ipt=d6ec1b24ac3111ee4dfed91c0948dd213f3480aff36c288036c4f08a7ecf70ad.

7.4.3. Role of Diagnostic Software

With the advent of diagnostic software, sports injury assessment has become much simpler and more effective with faster and more accurate diagnoses. Injury assessment was commonly done through subjective assessments by physicians. Diagnostic software, however, employs complex algorithms and machine learning techniques to process humongous amounts of data, enabling a more objective assessment of injuries. With the help of predictive analytics, these systems are capable of detecting patterns and risk factors for a variety of sports injuries and thereby determine measures of prevention. A shift from a reactive to proactive model benefits not just athlete safety but also returns on performance, hence diagnostic software becomes an invaluable resource for modern sports medicine (Musat et al., 2024). Maybe the single largest effect diagnostic software has had on the assessment of sports injuries is in analyzing imaging results more accurately. For instance, software driven by deep learning can interpret MRI scans for diagnosing anterior cruciate ligament (ACL) tears—high-impact sports-related injuries. In such cases, application of machine learning models like Inception-v3 facilitates efficient classification and identification of accurate injuries, thus proving useful for clinicians to formulate a correct treatment strategy. The precision and scale of evaluation offered by such resources help in providing timely and adequate treatment to the athletes, reducing recovery times, and preventing further complications (Senthilkumar et al., 2024). Also, the role of diagnostic software extends beyond initial assessment through its ability to facilitate ongoing monitoring and rehabilitation. Diagnostic software paired with wearable technology can track an athlete's performance data in real time, including details about their physical condition and potential overuse injuries. By continuously tracking movement patterns, biomechanical stressors, and muscle fatigue, these systems provide medical practitioners with the information needed to alter training programs and rehabilitation regimens. This integration of diagnostic software promotes a combined approach to the care of athletes, with a guarantee that improved performance will not compromise safety. Generally, this integration of technology into sports medicine through diagnostic software reflects a shift towards tailored and data-based athlete health management (Musat et al., 2024).

7.5. Role of Medical Professionals

Medical staff play a vital role in the assessment and diagnosis of sports injuries, owing to their advanced technical skills and proficiency in anatomy, physiology, and biomechanics. Their expertise is important in assessing the severity and nature of injury, so that proper interventions are conducted. This is particularly the case with anterior cruciate ligament injuries, where visual assessment can be complemented by other advanced evaluation methods. Evidence indicates that skilled movement analysis, for instance, can confidently estimate the risk of ACL damage in sports participants through a useful approach, reducing what previously was founded on extensive biomechanical testing (Petushek et al., 2015). With measures like the ACL Injury Risk Estimation Quiz (ACL-IQ), healthcare professionals can enlighten themselves considerably about an athlete's risk profiles and ultimately enhance prevention and optimize individualized interventions according to an athlete's specific needs. Additionally, concussion management underscores the significant responsibility of doctors in evaluating sports injuries. Owing to the complexities and variability that accompany concussive injuries, precise diagnosis and management protocols need to be established to ensure the safety of athletes. Doctors are responsible for applying a combination of traditional evaluation methods and newer technologies, such as ocular-motor testing and neuroimaging, to properly detect and diagnose concussions. Current clinical management guidelines emphasize the symptom-guided course, in which improvement is generally initiated by the resolution of symptoms prior to returning to play. The proactive nature of this complexity necessitates professionals to be familiar with concussion management intricacies and advocate for an athlete's well-being through the recovery period (Gardner, 2017). Finally, collaborative efforts of medical personnel extend well beyond diagnosis and assessment; they are also key in educating athletes, coaches, and parents about risk and prevention of injury. By exchanging information on proper training techniques, warm-up processes, and the importance of early symptom recognition, medical personnel can directly ensure safer playing surfaces. This learning component is key to building a culture of safety in sport because it empowers all involved with the ability to prioritize injury prevention. Moreover, the research and development that continuously look for new methods of measuring injuries allow medical staff to stay innovative in sports medicine, continually refining their practice and assisting with creating better outcomes for athletes. As sports injuries evolve in nature and complexity, the role of medical professionals will remain vital in ensuring athletes receive comprehensive care and support (Figure 7.12).

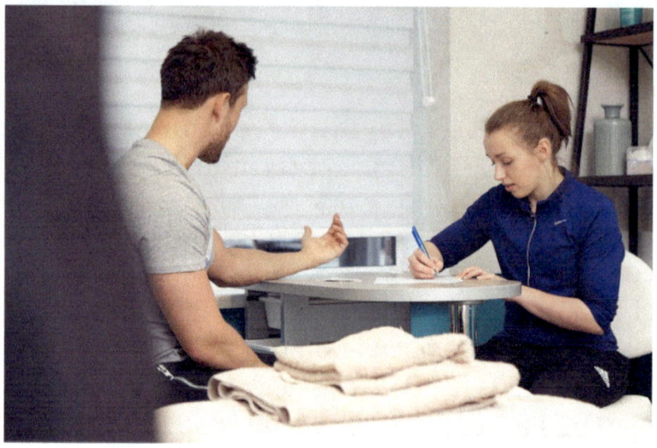

Figure 7.12. Injury assessment and treatment.

Source: https://resolveandrestore.co.uk/wp-content/uploads/2023/01/Injury-Assessment.jpg.

7.5.1. Sports Physicians

Sports physicians are at the core of diagnosis and assessment of sports injuries due to their special training in the particular health issues of athletes. They are trained in the combination of orthopedics, rehabilitation, and exercise physiology and use this training to make the right diagnosis and develop personalized treatment plans. Their primary focus of work is not only rehabilitation but also ensuring the safe return of athletes to competition. Involvement of sports doctors enhances the management of sports injury since studies have shown that athletes assessed by medical professionals have greater adherence to return-to-play (RTP) advice. Specifically, a concussion study among high school sportspeople highlighted that athletes were most appropriately served by a group of physicians and athletic trainers, highlighting the key contribution of medical professionals in ensuring appropriate recovery routes (Sivhugwana, 2021). Apart from diagnostic purposes, sports physicians use sophisticated means of evaluation to identify and minimize injury risks. For instance, the application of visual examination protocols allows skilled practitioners to review athletes' movements, thus better predicting potential injury risks compared to traditional biomechanical analysis. This procedure, outlined in the ACL Injury Risk Estimation Quiz (ACL-IQ), has established that certified professionals with a degree in exercise science can reliably recognize ACL injury risk by observation. Compared to conventional, resource-wasting techniques, this cost-cutting measurement can lead to timely interventions that can decrease injury rates in athletes (Petushek et al., 2015). Furthermore, the portability of such methods highlights that sports doctors are not merely caretakers but are indeed stakeholders in the development of injury prevention measures. Furthermore, sports doctors play a pivotal role in educating athletes and coaching staff on injury prevention and management methods. By providing evidence-based guidelines and keeping lines of communication open, they can help implement best practices within training, conditioning, and recuperation regimes. This training aspect is crucial, particularly in team sports with multiple stakeholders. Bringing together sports doctors, coaches, and players in joint work fosters a sensitization culture towards injury and the healing process. Thus, such collaboration not only optimizes the performance and health of players but also builds a long-term sense of injury prevention and management culture for competitive sports (Sivhugwana, 2021). Therefore, the diverse function of sports physicians includes evaluation, risk control, and education that form a substantial contribution to the total well-being of athletes.

7.5.2. Physical Therapists

The role of the physical therapist in diagnosing and evaluating sports injuries is fundamental to effective management and rehabilitation. Physical therapists are trained to perform a comprehensive assessment that not only addresses the physical aspects of injuries but also movement patterns that underlie and may contribute to injuries. This is especially relevant as abnormal movement patterns have been associated with lower extremity injuries and thus require the application of accurate assessment tools to recognize particular dysfunctions. These assessments enable physical therapists to create a baseline of an athlete's status of injury, which informs the construction of individualized rehabilitation programs. In addition, therapists can incorporate screening criteria to identify risk factors, eventually focusing on preventive measures that can prevent the recurrence of future injuries in athletic involvement. As research progresses in the understanding of sports injury, physical therapists are increasingly mandated to incorporate both conventional and advanced treatment methods. For instance, the treatment of widespread conditions such as Medial Tibial Stress Syndrome (MTSS) reveals the need for novel techniques. Traditional treatments generally focus on maximizing flexibility and strength, but recent research emphasizes the value of prevention since it is discovered that the measures taken in advance are considerably superior to post-injury reactive measures. Physical therapists ensure the long-term health of an athlete by focusing on prevention along with reducing overall healthcare costs associated with recurrent injury. This realignment of focus encourages exploration of new treatment approaches and enhances sporting performance by enabling the athlete to compete without limitation. Physical therapists are also at the forefront of interdisciplinary sports injury management. Communication with the other medical practitioners, including the athletic trainer, physician, and coach, is essential for integration of all aspects of an athlete's case. Physical therapists often serve as the first evaluators and can provide information regarding musculoskeletal status and resultant performance effects. Their assessment, which has demonstrated excellent reliability and validity, can be applied to assist with eligibility decisions and return-to-participation. Given that almost 90% of visual assessments are consistent with quantitative measurements of movement, physical therapists are best placed to help rehabilitate athletes back to sport in a safe manner while minimizing the likelihood of reinjury (Harris-Hayes et al., 2014). In developing an evidence-based practice, such practitioners can ensure that athletes receive the most appropriate treatment during their recovery journey (Figure 7.13).

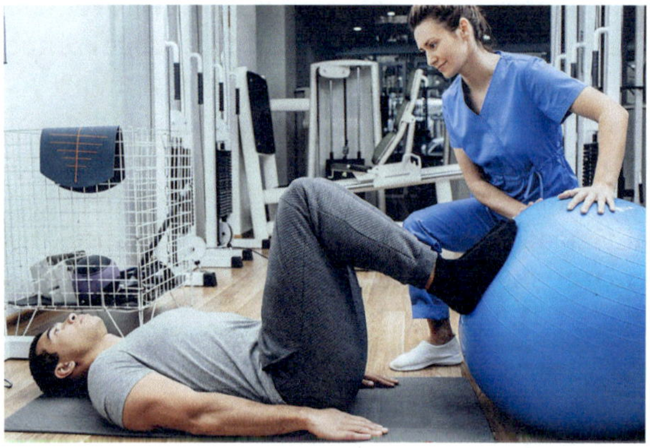

Figure 7.13. Role of physical therapists in sports injury assessment and diagnosis.

Source: https://sportydoctor.com/wp-content/uploads/Sports-Physical-Therapy2.jpg.

7.5.3. Athletic Trainers

Athletic trainers are an integral part of the evaluation and diagnosis of sports injuries because they are the first line of defense for the injured athlete. Athletic trainers are educated and have the skill set to evaluate most forms of athletic trauma, from acute injury like sprain, strain, and fracture to chronic illness like tendonitis or overuse syndromes. The athletic trainer's skill also encompasses interpreting the findings of the assessment and then planning intervention measures that will be taken immediately. One of the most important aspects of their job is using advanced diagnostic techniques to identify various kinds of injuries so that athletes are offered appropriate and timely treatment, which will ultimately enhance their recovery rates and result in a safe return to play. The integration of new technologies into sports training is changing the landscape of injury diagnosis and treatment. One such case is the advent of three-dimensional (3D) printing, which has enabled the creation of patient-specific anatomical models that enhance training and treatment protocols. The models enable better hands-on learning for athletic trainers, as they can simulate various injuries and practice assessment and management skills in a simulated setting. However, current limitations raise challenges, such as the insensitivity of commonly used polymer materials to be detected under standard X-ray imaging, which remains a valuable tool in clinical assessment (Piatt et al., 2024). Overcoming the limitations by developing radiopaque materials has the potential to revolutionize practice and make athletic trainers better prepared for real-world clinical scenarios. Overuse injuries are most prevalent in repetitive motion sports, demonstrating the critical role that athletic trainers have in monitoring and sustaining athletes' physical condition. For example, overuse injuries like swimmer's shoulder and patellofemoral pain syndrome are found widely among elite swimmers through intense training programs, demonstrating the importance of earlier intervention and diagnosis (Zhao et al., 2024). Athletic trainers play an important role in the identification of these injuries, preventive interventions, and the development of rehabilitation programs specific to overuse injuries. Their integrated practice includes monitoring training loads, teaching athletes about the risk of injury, and encouraging proper recovery habits as a means of countering the impact of overuse injuries. By making preventative efforts the focal point and establishing a culture of awareness, athletic trainers not only enhance athletes' performance but also their overall health and well-being significantly as well.

7.6. Treatment Protocols

Within the context of sports injury diagnosis and assessment, the establishment of efficient treatment methods is central to achieving optimal patient outcomes. For example, the rehabilitation of multifilament knee injuries (MLKIs) has experienced great progress, depending to a large extent on the adoption of a streamlined method for diagnosis and intervention. There has been an emerging international agreement focusing on the necessity of a general classification system that distinguishes mechanisms of injury and assesses non-ligamentous structures involved to facilitate a uniform understanding among clinicians. The agreement required surgical treatment as the initial option, especially for young patients, based on the reality that early and complete surgical intervention can lead to improved recovery. This methodical process not only maximizes clinical communication but also enhances the delivery of care across different settings of medical practice so that patients are given the best treatment protocols for taking care of their specific injuries, as evidenced by the high interclass agreement of specialists within the discipline (Murray et al., 2024). Moreover, concussion management has been an urgent matter in sports medicine that demands the application of aggressive treatment protocols. Most recent recommendations place a focus on the earlier diagnosis and initiation of appropriate management steps to prevent long-term consequences of concussion and mild traumatic brain injury (mTBI). The guidelines are primarily focused on cognitive and physical recovery evaluation and outlining the necessity of graduated reconditioning towards athletic return. However, it is clear that there is a strong deficiency of master therapeutic intervention recommendations, which might hinder productive recovery processes. In addition, it has not been successful to utilize a one-size-fits-all mechanism because the responses are widely different in individual patients.

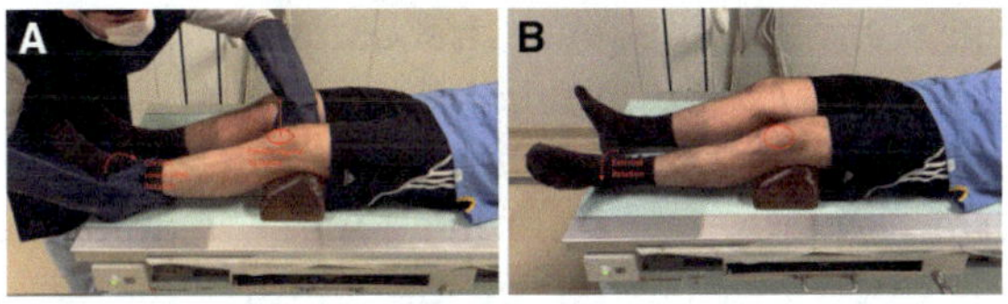

Figure 7.14. Management of multifilament knee injuries (MLKIs).

Source: https://cdn.ncbi.nlm.nih.gov/pmc/blobs/a6d6/7768114/7cd93b4eec3d/gr3.jpg.

As such, continued efforts to further create treatment protocols with both diagnosis and individualized therapeutic interventions are essential to enhancing clinical outcomes among athletes suffering from concussions (Luigi et al., 2023). Application of evidence-based treatment protocols in various sports injuries is an essential innovation in the quality of care for athletes. Multidisciplinary working, as in the MLKIs concord, encourages an injury management approach that encompasses rehabilitation protocols beyond immediate treatment to encompass extended rehabilitation procedures. The provision of established communication channels between healthcare experts, athletes, and coaches is equally vital, ensuring information regarding recommended protocols and rehabilitation time frames is imparted to all. Multidisciplinary working reduces risks that are emergent from too early a return to play, which may potentially lower re-injury levels. With ongoing research in sports injury management, further improvement of treatment protocols based on empirical evidence will remain central. This adaptive model will support the dynamic order of sports and athlete health, allowing ongoing participation and maximum performance (Luigi et al., 2023; Murray et al., 2024) (Figure 7.14).

7.6.1. Immediate Care and First Aid

The initial response of first aid and direct care provided to the athlete following a sporting injury is essential to his or her health and the best recovery. Adequate first aid procedures not only address the immediate physical needs of the injured individual but also avoid the long-term formation of complications. For instance, a proper evaluation of the injury leads to immediate actions such as ceasing bleeding, immobilizing injured areas, and alleviating pain. This is especially true in collision sports where an injury to a limb may involve extensive trauma. Coaching, training, and educating athletes about basic first aid techniques can render sports safer and reduce the likelihood of dire consequences. Consequently, immediate care models not only respond to the body complexity of an injury but also foster a conducive climate that reinforces the importance of athletes' health and safety in sport. In situations where trauma may have long-term effects, such as concussion, strategies to deal with it immediately become even more critical. Experience has shown that proper evaluation and concussion treatment can influence recovery mechanisms and the prevention of resulting chronic disorders like Chronic Traumatic Encephalopathy (CTE) due to cumulative brain damage in contact sports (Sage, 2018). Identifying symptoms such as confusion, dizziness, or unconsciousness by coaches and trainers is the most important because they are likely to be the first to realize if something is amiss. With prompt observation and adequate first aid treatment, the required care can be provided, which will allow them to make informed judgments regarding continued sporting activity. Thus, immediate care is more than first-response practice alone; it is the precursor to injury management that is focused on both short-term comfort and longer-term health outcomes. Beyond the immediate phase of injury management, the integration of clinical prediction rules (CPRs) into immediate care practice can enhance the assessment process for sports injury (Knox et al., 2017). They are designed to facilitate clinical judgment and decision-making and provide guidance that aids in the identification of interventions needed. Examples are CPRs for specific injuries, like those that require imaging following an ankle sprain, that assist first responders in making rapid and effective evidence-based decisions. They are critical in the immediate setting since the capability to quickly assess can restrict the risk of increasing the severity of an injury. Consequently, education and training in CPRs must be integrated into the course of study for sports medicine programs, equipping next-generation professionals with the know-how needed to optimize immediate treatment and first aid during sporting events. Overall strategy emphasis is placed on ensuring appropriate initial responses in the scenario of sports injury diagnosis and assessment.

7.6.2. Rehabilitation Strategies

Rehabilitation planning is essential for injured athletes since it enables the return of function and performance with little risk of subsequent re-injury. The rehabilitation program, once tailored to the individual athlete, should be based on an in-depth evaluation of the particular injury of the individual athlete, as well as an assessment of the severity and the injury mechanisms. For instance, syndesmotic sprains, or high ankle sprains, necessitate a multi-modal rehabilitation process many times involving immobilization and exercises. Rehabilitation is started in the initial phases with anti-inflammatory measures to decrease inflammation and swelling, moving to range of motion and strengthening exercises. This progression is essential to enable the safe return of athletes to intense activity, thus making the rehabilitation plan dynamic and responsive to the athlete's rehabilitation status, consequently enabling reintegration to sports activity (Szukics et al., 2025). Furthermore, rehabilitation strategies can be greatly aided by the use of individualized approaches based on the individual's unique injury profile and rehabilitation needs. Evidence indicates that the aggregation of athlete data, including histories of previous injury and exercise habits, can be utilized to guide personalized rehabilitation strategies. By applying methods such as random forest models, clinicians can more accurately establish sport injury risk and subsequently design personalized rehabilitation interventions. Biomechanical analysis of data to consider a player's joint stability and muscle strength also enhances individualization. Hence, not only do these personalized rehabilitation plans treat return to health from injury, but also maximize overall athletic function and pleasure, uncovering the significance of personalization in rehabilitation strategies (Cao et al., 2025). Finally, an indispensable aspect of successful rehabilitation strategies is ongoing assessment and adjustment throughout the course of recovery. The repeated surveillance of the athletes' progress through ongoing assessments plays a simple role in altering rehabilitation interventions as a response. Clinical professionals can utilize objective examinations to assess functional abilities and track any psychosocial concerns that can influence the recovery process of the sportsmen. Through an open communication culture, sportsmen can express concern and preference, which in turn contributes to better adherence to rehabilitation programs and ultimately more effective outcomes. This athlete-centered and responsive approach not only aids physical recovery but also mental toughness and confidence, so that the athletes are physically and mentally equipped to return to their sport at peak performance (Cao et al., 2025; Szukics et al., 2025).

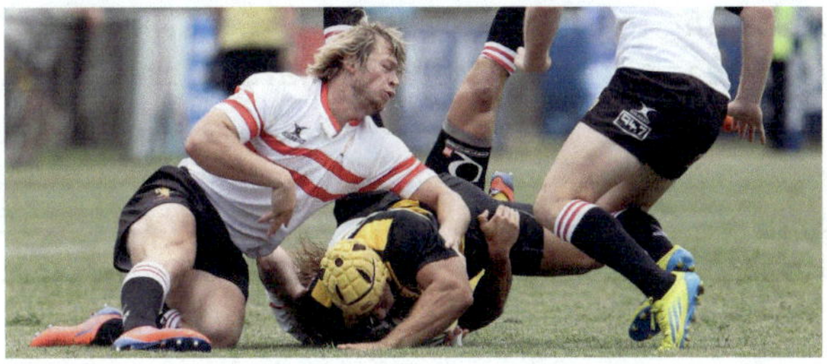

Figure 7.15. Shoulder separations in sports.

Source: https://hartfordsportsorthopedics.com/wp-content/uploads/2020/09/Shoulder-Separations-in-Sports.jpg.

7.6.3. Return-to-Play Criteria

Return-to-play (RTP) protocols are a significant tool of sports injury diagnosis and assessment, particularly for concussion. They aim to ascertain a player's safety and preparedness for competitive competition after a head injury. An effective RTP program typically involves multiple phases, beginning with a complete medical evaluation and symptom survey to establish baseline cognitive and physical performance. Following an initial assessment, the sportsperson may go through a stepwise process of exertion in the form of light physical exercise, sport-specific drills, and heightened practice sessions. The final stage provokes the sportsperson into regaining their former baseline without symptom recurrence, thereby lowering the risk of further injury and promoting long-term health. The application of RTP criteria is particularly relevant in light of growing concern regarding long-term effects of concussions, such as Chronic Traumatic Encephalopathy (CTE). Increased awareness has driven much investigation of the relationship between contact sports, repetitive head impacts, and neurocognitive outcomes and, by extension, the need for stringent RTP guidelines. As noted in a recent study, RTP determinations should not only be founded on alleviating existing symptoms but also on the athlete's broader trend of recovery and potential risks involved in returning to play too rapidly. The conflict is between needing to play and having the responsibility to safeguard athlete safety, particularly in adolescent athletes, whose brains may be uniquely vulnerable to the long-term effects of unrecognized head trauma. Further, the incorporation of evidence-based practices in RTP criterion development can greatly enhance decision-making among sports professionals. As research continues to examine the interconnections of repetitive head trauma and diseases like CTE, it is certain that standardized RTP guidelines must accordingly adjust. These standards would include neurocognitive testing and extensive evaluations to appropriately assess an athlete's recovery. Adoption of these principles assists in the development of a culture in which the welfare of athletes is valued over the pressures of competition. With the weight of the accumulating evidence, including what has been learned from studies on the long-term cognitive effects of contact sports, both coaches and medical staff need to collaborate to develop functional RTP strategies that safeguard athletes, educate communities, and support safer sporting participation as a whole (Sage, 2018; Rodaset al., 2019).

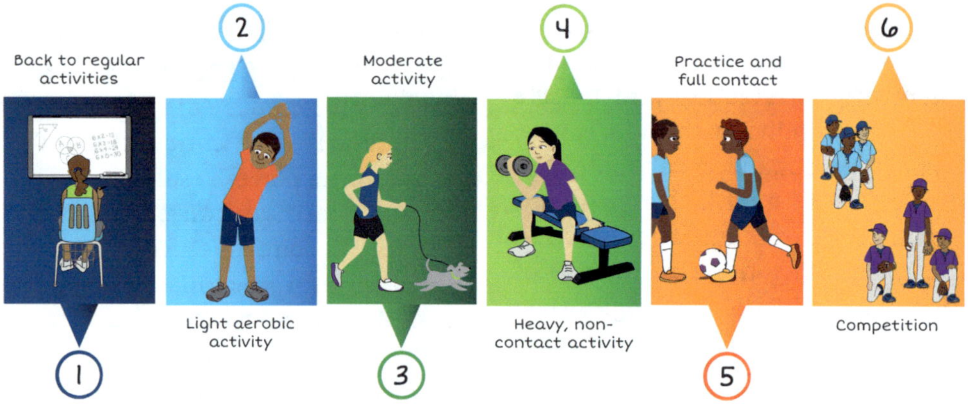

Figure 7.16. The return-to-play (RTP) criteria represent a crucial aspect of sports.

Source: https://www.cdc.gov/heads-up/media/images/2024/07/HU_RTP-Graphic_V2_1643.png?_=31024.

SUMMARY

Diagnosis and assessment of sports injuries are fundamental components of the athletic healthcare model. By systematic evaluation and interdisciplinary design, clinicians can properly identify the severity and type of injury, making informed diagnoses that guide the direction of treatment intervention. This is not merely a question of identifying physical impairment but also regarding psychological impacts of injury that have a significant bearing on a student-athlete's overall performance and recovery course. The convergence of physical rehabilitation and emotional resilience calls for the embracing of a holistic approach that targets both physical and psychological well-being during recovery. Secondly, technology has transformed assessment in sports medicine through more accurate and timely diagnosis. By employing technologies such as imaging modalities, wearables, and data analysis, clinicians can leverage detailed knowledge of an athlete's physiological response and use these findings in personalized rehabilitation programs. Much as these innovations enhance diagnosis effectiveness and pace, they also require ongoing learning by professionals so that they are conversant with new methods. Thus, culture development for ongoing learning among medical professionals is essential in guaranteeing high-quality standards in sports injury evaluation and diagnosis. Finally, effective management of sports injuries relies on cooperation between medical professionals, coaches, and players themselves.

Mutual understanding of assessment protocols can give more informed decisions in training plans, prevention procedures against injuries, and rehabilitation programs. Here, interdisciplinary communication integration is paramount, which ensures cohesion among all involved in their rehabilitation objectives and performance enhancement. As development of the sports environment continues, there will be a recognition of the need for structured assessments and adaptive treatment approaches that will be key to minimizing injury impact and improving athlete longevity and performance in his or her discipline. Effective sports injury diagnosis and evaluation are founded upon the integration of multidisciplinary approaches, such as in the case of inguinal disruption or Sportsman's groin. Experts in a consensus conference emphasized interdisciplinary practice, including input from radiologists, physiotherapists, and surgeons. By using the collaborative methods, there is better comprehension of the injury, along with the fine details that define the condition. The contract articulated that 'inguinal disruption' be the term adopted instead of outdated words like Sportsman's hernia, symbolizing better diagnosis. Abnormal tension around the inguinal ligament detection matters in guiding therapeutic interventions from physiotherapy to operations for purposes of tension relief and strengthening of the area, thereby enhancing athletes' recovery and future performance outcomes (Sheen et al., 2013). Among the weight-training sports, awareness of injury epidemiology is a pivotal factor towards enhancement of performance and safety. Structured analysis of injury incidence between various weight-training activities offers a variety of risks, typically largely influenced by age, sex, and competitive status. As noted observationally, evidence indicates that bodybuilding has the lowest rate of injury, while strongman and Highland Games rates of injury are higher at up to 7.5 injuries per 1,000 hours. These findings underscore the significance of targeted injury protection measures, particularly among high-risk sports. While the study environment varies in intensity, with various studies employing retrospective designs, overall patterns indicate noteworthy anatomical regions vulnerable to injury, i.e., the shoulder, the knee, and the lower back, in guiding coaches and athletes during their preparation and training schedule (Keogh & Winwood, 2017). Lastly, the intersection of injury evaluation methods and findings of epidemiological studies indicates the multifaceted nature of sports injuries and the need for evidence-based methods. Multidimensional consensus on such syndromes as inguinal disruption is an archetype of the kind of interdisciplinary diagnosis that can effectively treat sports injuries. Meanwhile, rewriting the injury dynamics in weight-training sports with improved study designs will have a lasting impact on athletes' safety and well-being. Closing the gap between evidence at the bedside and everyday practice is of utmost importance to maximize injury prevention and management measures. Overall, these results advocate a proactive, informed approach to sports injury assessment and diagnosis to ultimately enhance athlete performance while minimizing the risks of injury through evidence-based practice.

CLOSER LOOK

ACUTE INJURIES

Acute injuries are sudden physical injuries that occur unexpectedly, often as a result of accidents, falls, sports activities, or direct trauma. They typically develop quickly and are characterized by immediate pain, swelling, bruising, and loss of function. Common examples include sprains, strains, fractures, dislocations, cuts, and contusions. Acute injuries can affect muscles, bones, joints, ligaments, and soft tissues, and their severity can range from mild to life-threatening. Prompt assessment and early treatment are essential to prevent complications and promote effective healing. Initial management often follows the RICE principle: Rest, Ice, Compression, and Elevation, which helps reduce pain and swelling. In more serious cases, medical intervention such as immobilization, medications, or surgical procedures may be required. Imaging tools like X-rays, CT scans, and MRI help in accurate diagnosis and treatment planning. Rehabilitation through physical therapy plays a crucial role in restoring strength, flexibility, and functional movement after an acute injury. Gradual return-to-activity programs reduce the risk of re-injury and long-term disability. Preventive strategies include proper warm-up, use of protective equipment, safe training techniques, and awareness of environmental hazards. Overall, timely care and structured rehabilitation are key to ensuring full recovery and maintaining long-term musculoskeletal health.

REFERENCES

1. Abdulqader, S., Shakir, N. A., Ahmed, S. A., & Hassan, Q. A. (2025). Ultrasound accuracy in the diagnosis of anterior talofibular ligament acute injury: A single-center study. *Al-Rafidain Journal of Medical Sciences.* https://www.semanticscholar.org/paper/e3fae4bbd1ff19003c0b1d77ace697134911d34d (accessed on 26th June 2025).
2. Petushek, E. J., Cokely, E. T., Ward, P., Durocher, J. J., Wallace, S. J., & Myer, G. D. (2015). Injury Risk Estimation Expertise: Assessing the ACL Injury Risk Estimation Quiz. *The American journal of sports medicine, 43*(7), 1640–1647. https://doi.org/10.1177/0363546515580791 (accessed on 26th June 2025).
3. Alsaeed, J. K., Salman, S. S., Alsuwat, K. J., Aldoseri, A. A., Mustafa, S. A., Alzahrani, R. A., Alasmari, A. M., et al. (2024). Prevalence and awareness of anterior cruciate ligament injuries among full-contact, semi-contact, and non-contact sports athletes in the Kingdom of Bahrain. *Cureus, 16.* https://www.semanticscholar.org/paper/d9ede8f81c001e89c937a4b38df33858d4962844 (accessed on 26th June 2025).
4. Bielak, K., Bańkowski, D., Juda, P., Kłaptoc, P., Łukoś-Karcz, K., Barabasz, K., Pabian, G., et al. (2025). Neuromodulation in sports medicine: New techniques supporting performance, recovery, and chronic injury treatment–A review. *Polish Journal of Sports Medicine.* https://www.semanticscholar.org/paper/05c6fd1463da237e8034867cdeefee21416e1b21 (accessed on 26th June 2025).
5. Rodas G, Bove T, Caparrós T, et al. Ankle Sprain Versus Muscle Strain Injury in Professional Men's Basketball: A 9-Year Prospective Follow-up Study. *Orthop J Sports Med.* 2019;7(6):2325967119849035. Published 2019 Jun 21. doi:10.1177/2325967119849035(accessed on 26th June 2025).
6. McCrea, M., Broglio, S. P., McAllister, T. W., Gill, J., Giza, C. C., Huber, D. L., Harezlak, J., Cameron, K. L., Houston, M. N., McGinty, G., Jackson, J. C., Guskiewicz, K., Mihalik, J., Brooks, M. A., Duma, S., Rowson, S., Nelson, L. D., Pasquina, P., Meier, T. B., CARE Consortium Investigators, ... DiFiori, J. (2020). Association of Blood Biomarkers With Acute Sport-Related Concussion in Collegiate Athletes: Findings From the NCAA and Department of Defense CARE Consortium. *JAMA network open, 3*(1), e1919771. https://doi.org/10.1001/jamanetworkopen.2019.19771(accessed on 26th June 2025).
7. Cao, J., & Chen, H. (2025). Research on sports injury risk assessment and rehabilitation strategy based on big data analysis. *Molecular & Cellular Biomechanics.* https://www.semanticscholar.org/paper/d652fb49d663608b6e6ccc2a8e6a0aedf8dc8034 (accessed on 26th June 2025).
8. Stuart, S., Parrington, L., Martini, D., Peterka, R., Chesnutt, J., & King, L. (2020). The Measurement of Eye Movements in Mild Traumatic Brain Injury: A Structured Review of an Emerging Area. *Frontiers in sports and active living, 2,* 5. https://doi.org/10.3389/fspor.2020.00005(accessed on 26th June 2025).
9. Collins, D., Lewis, N. A., Pedlar, C. R., et al. (2015). Can clinicians and scientists explain and prevent unexplained underperformance syndrome in elite athletes: An interdisciplinary perspective and 2016 update. https://core.ac.uk/download/42137754.pdf (accessed on 26th June 2025).
10. Da Fonseca, G. I. (2024). Effective rehabilitation strategies for muscle injuries in football players. *International Seven Journal of Multidisciplinary.* https://www.semanticscholar.org/

paper/862e4fc83c6b5325cf01681283fd1bbc31c97f35 (accessed on 26th June 2025).

11. Sheen, A. J., Stephenson, B. M., Lloyd, D. M., Robinson, P., Fevre, D., Paajanen, H., de Beaux, A., Kingsnorth, A., Gilmore, O. J., Bennett, D., Maclennan, I., O'Dwyer, P., Sanders, D., & Kurzer, M. (2014). 'Treatment of the sportsman's groin': British Hernia Society's 2014 position statement based on the Manchester Consensus Conference. *British journal of sports medicine, 48*(14), 1079–1087. https://doi.org/10.1136/bjsports-2013-092872(accessed on 26th June 2025).

12. De Luigi, A. D., Bell, K. R., Bramhall, J. P., Choe, M., Dec, K., Finnoff, J., Halstead, M., et al. (2023). Consensus statement: An evidence-based review of exercise, rehabilitation, rest, and return to activity protocols for the treatment of concussion and mild traumatic brain injury. *PM&R, 15*, 1605–1642. https://www.semanticscholar.org/paper/51066b8286ab96c91aa601 5cc30a196fb5e2b5a4 (accessed on 26th June 2025).

13. Clough, A. E., Flynn, J., Home, J. K., Earle, F., & Clough, P. J. (2015). Whiplash: The possible impact of context on diagnosis. *Pain and Rehabilitation, 2015*(38), 4-9. http://www.ingentaconnect.com/content/ppa/pr/2015/00002015/00000038/art00003#expand/collapse (accessed on 26th June 2025).

14. Keogh, J. W., & Winwood, P. W. (2017). The Epidemiology of Injuries Across the Weight-Training Sports. *Sports medicine (Auckland, N.Z.), 47*(3), 479–501. https://doi.org/10.1007/s40279-016-0575-0(accessed on 26th June 2025).

15. Gardner, A. J. (2017). Sports concussion: A clinical overview. https://core.ac.uk/download/322432803.pdf (accessed on 26th June 2025).

16. Jaremko, J. L., Guenther, Z. D., Jans, L. B., & Macmahon, P. J. (2013). Spectrum of injuries associated with paediatric ACL tears: an MRI pictorial review. *Insights into imaging, 4*(3), 273–285. https://doi.org/10.1007/s13244-013-0250-z(accessed on 26th June 2025).

17. Harris-Hayes, M., Steger-May, K., Koh, C., Royer, N. K., Graci, V., & Salsich, G. B. (2014). Classification of lower extremity movement patterns based on visual assessment: reliability and correlation with 2-dimensional video analysis. *Journal of athletic training, 49*(3), 304–310. https://doi.org/10.4085/1062-6050-49.2.21(accessed on 26th June 2025).

18. Haste, P., de Almeida e Bueno, L., Jérusalem, A., & Bergmann, J. H. M. (2025). Performance of current tools used for on-the-day assessment and diagnosis of mild traumatic brain injury in sport: A systematic review. *BMJ Open Sport & Exercise Medicine, 11*. https://www.semanticscholar.org/paper/eff6de952030113bc1f01d55bbf366ebe204f273 (accessed on 26th June 2025).

19. Hayath, T. M., Mercy, S., Sukrutha, S., & Vaishnavi, K. (2024). A novel method on wound identification using machine learning and image processing. *International Journal of Advanced Research in Science, Communication and Technology*. https://www.semanticscholar.org/paper/e58fdbc32e4eb67d701fa0a11d4c6883249f2090 (accessed on 26th June 2025).

20. Hermena, S., Virani, S., Jasim, O., Suttie, A., & Dalgleish, S. (2025). Accelerating care for knee injuries: Impact of a novel acute knee injury virtual triage clinic on timely diagnosis and treatment. *Orthopaedic Proceedings*. https://www.semanticscholar.org/paper/6d331d9b017e48bc64651e2dbfe639a042c78d3b (accessed on 26th June 2025).

21. Hs, D., Kameln, H. A., & Habash, M. Y. (2017). Ultrasonographic assessment of the foot pseudotumor soft tissue lesions. *International Journal of Clinical & Medical Imaging, 04*.

https://www.semanticscholar.org/paper/ec1c9c2fdacc0488a48b1163fb7e7eb1511adc74 (accessed on 26th June 2025).

22. Kazakova, A. V., Chechko, S. M., Golovina, O. N., Katorkina, E. S., Ismatullin, D. D., & Shamshatdinova, A. R. (2025). Clinical case of hematoma of vaginal vestibule. *Medical & Pharmaceutical Journal "Pulse."* https://www.semanticscholar.org/paper/3d743a3e1258e2daadea1d5090e04016a44ffdf2 (accessed on 26th June 2025).

23. Knox, G. M., Snodgrass, S. J., Stanton, T. R., Kelly, D. H., Vicenzino, B., Wand, B. M., & Rivett, D. A. (2017). Physiotherapy students' perceptions and experiences of clinical prediction rules. *Physiotherapy, 103*(3), 296–303. https://doi.org/10.1016/j.physio.2016.04.001(accessed on 26th June 2025).

24. Koziak, W., Dudek, S., Makieła, M., Bętkowska, A., Kornacka, A., Dudek, W., Szostak, K., et al. (2025). The application of point-of-care ultrasound in sports medicine: A narrative review. *Quality in Sport.* https://www.semanticscholar.org/paper/c517440cb493bca3fa64412d0aa221420686c749 (accessed on 26th June 2025).

25. Lu, Y., Chiu, J., Chen, A. C., Hsu, K. Y., Chan, Y. S., Zhang, E. C., & Sheu, H. (2025). Chinese translation and validation of the Oslo Sports Trauma Research Center questionnaires on overuse injuries and health problems. *Orthopedic Journal of Sports Medicine, 13.* https://www.semanticscholar.org/paper/64f4b257ee96b4f87967f345032e4ac7a1d484f1 (accessed on 26th June 2025).

26. Manske, R., Wolfe, C., Page, P., & Voight, M. L. (2024). Enhancing the diagnosis of lateral ankle sprains: The role of MSK diagnostic ultrasound in evaluating ATFL and CFL. *International Journal of Sports Physical Therapy, 19*, 245–249. https://www.semanticscholar.org/paper/0627671172d772d624f53b8b93e677d8ccc14b38 (accessed on 26th June 2025).

27. Manske, R., Wolfe, C., Page, P., & Voight, M. L. (2025). Diagnostic musculoskeletal ultrasound in the evaluation of the deltoid ligament of the ankle. *International Journal of Sports Physical Therapy, 20*, 641–647. https://www.semanticscholar.org/paper/d3fba7ed2b579c510763f66dfc675945b7d3c470 (accessed on 26th June 2025).

28. Marrero, A. M., Mazza, L. A., Cedola, N., Neville, M. F., Trueba, R. H., Napoli, A., Pascual, T. A., et al. (2025). MRI and US in hamstring sports injury assessment: Anatomy, imaging findings, and mechanisms of injury. *Radiographic, 45*(5), e240061. https://www.semanticscholar.org/paper/2a0bd38052555ba3de3616be77bc7fec93328f84 (accessed on 26th June 2025).

29. Murray, I. R., Makaram, N. S., Geeslin, A. G., Chahla, J., Moatshe, G., Crossley, K. M., Kew, M., et al. (2024). Multiligament knee injury (MLKI): An expert consensus statement on nomenclature, diagnosis, treatment and rehabilitation. *British Journal of Sports Medicine, 58*, 1385–1400. https://www.semanticscholar.org/paper/2da910c7329be2483c92d6b19ddf6f3609d4c404 (accessed on 26th June 2025).

30. Musat, C., Mereuță, C., Nechita, A., Tutunaru, D., Voipan, A., Voipan, D., Mereuta, E., et al. (2024). Diagnostic applications of AI in sports: A comprehensive review of injury risk prediction methods. *Diagnostics, 14.* https://www.semanticscholar.org/paper/77f8ec6321be2c25c11b9a4d9dccc414ff875e6c (accessed on 26th June 2025).

31. Sivhugwana, Innocentia (2022). Factors related with the functional outcome of patients who sustained tibial plateau fractures. Dissertation (MSc (Physiotherapy))--University of Pretoria, 2022. https://core.ac.uk/download/565849089.pdf

32. Piatt, S., Tiari, S., Mihaly, H., & Chen, L. (2024). Preparation of a 3-D printable radiopaque composite using zirconium oxide composite. *Volume 4: Biomedical and Biotechnology Engineering*. https://www.semanticscholar.org/paper/5d1e8e4a31d4367c405d067401f32e8bdaf37ef3 (accessed on 26th June 2025).

33. Reardon, C. L., Hainline, B., Miller Aron, C., Baron, D., Baum, A., Bindra, A., Budgett, R., et al. (2019). Mental health in elite athletes: International Olympic Committee consensus statement (2019). *British Journal of Sports Medicine, 53*, 667–699. https://doi.org/10.1136/bjsports-2019-100715 (accessed on 26th June 2025).

34. Ryabcev, S., Zhmurova, T., & Ryabceva, O. (2024). The effectiveness of the use of physical rehabilitation means for sports injury in the post-immobilization period. *Issues of Establishing the Severity of Harm Caused to Human Health as a Result of Exposure to a Biological Factor*. https://www.semanticscholar.org/paper/ff768c48e05db47fae719c056cf24f5cfd3b42e9 (accessed on 26th June 2025).

35. Sage, M. (2018). Neurocognitive findings in adults who played youth football. https://open.bu.edu/bitstream/2144/33032/5/Sage_bu_0017N_14075.pdf (accessed on 26th June 2025).

36. Schmidt, S., Krahl, D., Podszun, J., Knecht, S., Zimmerer, A., Sobau, C., Ellermann, A., et al. (2024). Combining a digital health application with standard care significantly enhances rehabilitation outcomes for ACL surgery patients. *Knee Surgery, Sports Traumatology, Arthroscopy: Official Journal of the ESSKA*. https://www.semanticscholar.org/paper/c8c54849580bbba2085aacc5702a5413fcb9443b (accessed on 26th June 2025).

37. Segreti, A., Fossati, C., Mulè, M. T., Fanale, V., Crispino, S. P., Coletti, F., Parisi, F., et al. (2024). Assessment of cardiopulmonary capacity in deconditioned athletes because of knee injury. *The Journal of Sports Medicine and Physical Fitness, 64*(7), 615–623. https://www.semanticscholar.org/paper/8fa9d3d475aeeaca9167f2206559860e468d9939 (accessed on 26th June 2025).

38. Senthilkumar, K. T., Sekhar, S. S., Kumar, B., Sujithra, L. R., Vinoj, J., & Nithya, R. (2024). Experimental assessment between dissimilar techniques and methodologies to sports knee injury using magnetic resonance imaging. *South Eastern European Journal of Public Health*. https://www.semanticscholar.org/paper/40a9c1543fb37505f256fa247a21f408c6bfb22b (accessed on 26th June 2025).

39. Steffel, J., Collins, R., Antz, M., Cornu, P., Desteghe, L., Hæusler, K. G., Oldgren, J., et al. (2021). 2021 European Heart Rhythm Association practical guide on the use of non-vitamin K antagonist oral anticoagulants in patients with atrial fibrillation. *EP Europace, 23*, 1612–1676. https://doi.org/10.1093/europace/euab065 (accessed on 26th June 2025).

40. Szukics, P. F., Murray, D. P., Robaina, J., Potter, T., Vargas, L. A., Chapman, C., & Yagnik, G. P. (2025). Sideline management of syndesmotic injuries in the athlete: Evaluation, management, and return to play. *Video Journal of Sports Medicine, 5*. https://www.semanticscholar.org/paper/fb4a8284b99e741aa665360b12b1f18d28386a57 (accessed on 26th June 2025).

41. Tang, L. (2025). A study of the effectiveness of ultrasound imaging in the early detection of cartilage degeneration in the knee joint of athletes. *Molecular & Cellular Biomechanics*. https://www.semanticscholar.org/paper/68bee30f26d4a730c8265ef54a22b38ecc1747c5 (accessed on 26th June 2025).

42. Tenforde, A. S., Borgstrom, H., DeLuca, S., McCormack, M., Singh, M., Soo Hoo, J., & Yun, P. H. (2022). Best practices for extracorporeal shockwave therapy in musculoskeletal medicine:

Clinical application and training consideration. *PM&R, 14*, 611–619. https://doi.org/10.1002/pmrj.12790 (accessed on 26th June 2025).

43. Yamasaki, S. (2019). A review of the treatment and prevention options for medial tibial stress syndrome. https://core.ac.uk/download/213464302.pdf (accessed on 26th June 2025).

44. Zhao, M., Chen, Y., & Sun, L. (2024). The prevalence and management of overuse injuries among adolescent swimmers in China. *Studies in Sports Science and Physical Education*. https://www.semanticscholar.org/paper/bfcdbb32d68c24dbba87feb354699c35e30143d9 (accessed on 26th June 2025).

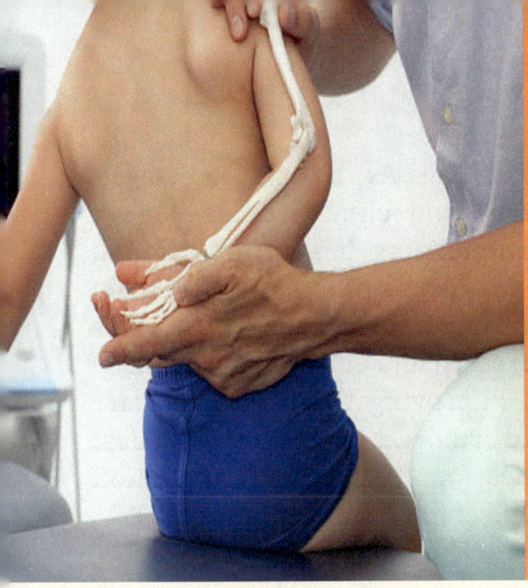

Chapter 8 PEDIATRIC ORTHOPEDICS

Contents

Introduction ... 233
8.1. Developmental Anatomy and Physiology ... 237
8.2. Common Pediatric Orthopedic Conditions ... 241
8.3. Diagnostic Approaches ... 244
8.4. Treatment Modalities ... 248
8.5. Challenges in Pediatric Orthopedics ... 252
8.6. Advances in Pediatric Orthopedic Research ... 255
Summary ... 260
References ... 263

Introduction

Pediatric orthopedics is a field of specialist medicine concerned with the diagnosis, treatment, and prevention of disorders of the musculoskeletal system of children. Owing to the unusual physiology and growing nature of children, pediatric orthopedics is different from adult orthopedics. Children are not miniature adults; they possess growing bones and developing musculoskeletal systems, which need specific knowledge of pediatric orthopedic conditions to deliver quality care. Common issues such as congenital malformations, growth cessation, and scoliosis frequently present during the life of a child and need individualized treatment. Detection and management of these conditions at an early stage can significantly influence the future health and quality of life of a child, which makes specialized knowledge in paediatric musculoskeletal health very important. Appreciation of stages of development and growth is one of the main pillars of pediatric orthopedics, which has a direct bearing on treatment modalities. For example, conditions like osteogenesis imperfecta or developmental dysplasia of the hip require proper attention to be accorded to age-appropriate intervention. The health professionals have to balance on a tightrope as far as growth plate behavior is concerned, as inappropriate management can lead to problems like inequality of limb lengths or deformity of a joint over time. Furthermore, psychological and social dimensions of pediatric orthopedic treatment cannot be overlooked. Pediatric patients are often more sensitive to bodily limitations and body image issues; hence, effective communication with both patient and family is essential in facilitating a cooperative therapeutic relationship. Such a process enables synchronizing young patients' physical as well as emotional needs.

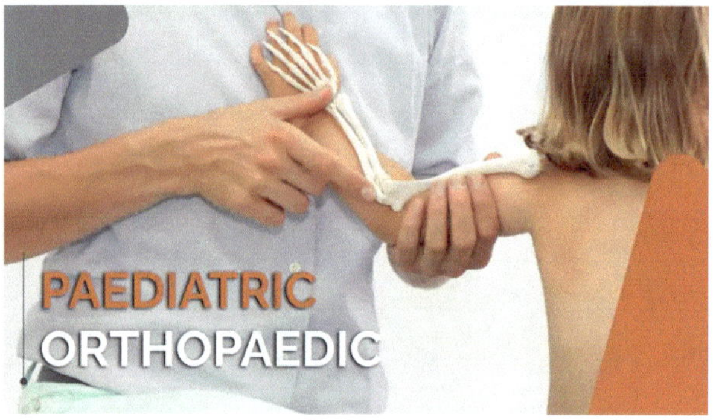

Figure 8.1. Pediatric orthopedics is a specialized branch of medicine focused on the diagnosis.

Source: https://drashwanimaichand.com/blog/wp-content/uploads/2023/11/pediatric-orthopedic-ashwani.webp.

Moreover, advances in technology and surgical procedures in orthopedics for children have revolutionized treatment patterns with greater success for pediatric patients. Minimally invasive methods are increasingly utilized, resulting in reduced periods of recovery and improved postoperative results. Imaging advances, such as the application of MRI and ultrasound, allow for improved diagnosis, and improved implant design specifically anticipates the differences in child anatomy. These advances also open up a need for continued education and training of health professionals. As the science evolves, ongoing research and clinical trials have a key role in rationalizing best practices and ensuring that healthcare practitioners remain current in their competence and expertise. This emphasis on research and education eventually translates into improving the quality of care within pediatric orthopedics, ensuring the best clinical outcomes for a vulnerable population (Loma Linda University, 2002) (Figure 8.1).

Definition and Scope of Pediatric Orthopedics

Pediatric orthopedics is the branch of medicine concerned with the diagnosis, treatment, and management of children's musculoskeletal disorders from infancy to adolescence. The term pediatric orthopedics extends beyond surgery alone; it involves an understanding of growth and development so that treatments support the physical and psychological demands unique to younger patients. Since children's joints and bones are in development, maturity considerations become important factors in the development of successful interventions. The focus on the pediatric-specific aspects of anatomy, physiology, and psychology underscores the importance of this specialty. Thus, pediatric orthopedics not only aims at addressing specific conditions such as scoliosis and congenital deformity but also promotes the healthy growth of children by means of preventive management and rehabilitative care, targeting the more all-encompassing activity of pediatric care (Farre & Rapley, 2017). The field of pediatric orthopedics spans a broad spectrum of diseases that can affect children, ranging from acute trauma to chronic illness. Acute injuries are typically caused by play and sporting activities, and prompt management and treatment are necessary to prevent long-term sequelae. Chronic musculoskeletal disorders, such as limb deformity or developmental dysplasia, require ongoing surveillance and potentially longitudinal management according to the evolving demands of the growing patient. The specialty also interfaces with other interdisciplinary teams that involve physiotherapists, occupational therapists, and pediatricians, making it simple to have an integrated and single approach to care. Moreover, pediatric orthopedics encourages developmental and psychological assessments to appreciate the impact of musculoskeletal disorders on a child's social and emotional well-being (Mustafa, 2015).

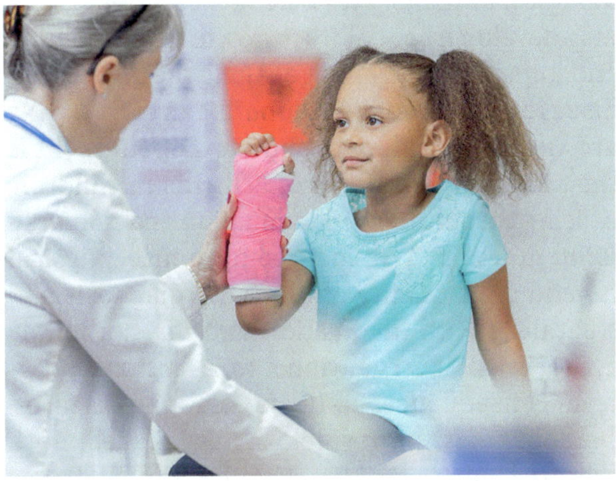

Figure 8.2. Pediatric orthopedics encompasses a specialized branch of medicine focused on the diagnosis.

Source: https://external-content.duckduckgo.com/iu/?u=https%3A%2F%2Fstorage.googleapis.com%2Fjacksonh%2F1%2FPediatric_Orthopedics.jpg&f=1&nofb=1&ipt=6da3019003b71336a7b8ce4f6db15175752033994802fb1cd47e1993442a8d47.

Hence, the specialty is not merely surgical correction but also seeks to optimize overall health outcomes through interprofessional interventions. Moreover, a greater appreciation of the biopsychosocial model of medicine has greatly influenced the practice of pediatric orthopedics. This model centers not just on the physical aspect of injury and conditions but also on the psychological and social effects on pediatric patients. Merging these factors enables pediatric orthopedics practitioners to enhance recovery outcomes better and give a more integrative recovery experience for children. Knowing that children get anxious or afraid of surgical procedures or rehabilitation enhances the quality of care provided. Besides, practitioners also aim to empower the families through learning and the provision of resources so that they can make informed decisions and aid the treatment process. Finally, the pediatric orthopedic practice is progressive and dynamic, heading in more efficient and comprehensive ways towards care that unites physical well-being with psychosocial development (Farre & Rapley, 2017) (Figure 8.2).

Importance of Specialized Care for Children

The worth of specialty care for kids, particularly pediatric orthopedics, simply cannot be overstated. Kids are not mini adults; their developmental, physiologic, and psychological needs vary. Pediatric orthopedic clinicians are specially trained to work with these variations, granting children care commensurate with their development patterns and evolving forms. This was one specialized intervention that was vital, especially for conditions such as osteomyelitis, which can significantly impact a child's quality of life and overall development. With the use of age-specific interventions, pediatric orthopedic specialists can better guarantee enhanced long-term health outcomes while avoiding risks associated with complications from general care. In meta epiphyseal osteomyelitis, for instance, there is specialized treatment that is crucial because it not only involves surgical and rehabilitative treatment but also socio-psychological rehabilitation, which is normally overlooked. The intricacies of rehabilitative processes must be channeled towards restoring physical states and psychological outcomes of illness. Evidence in recent years shows that most patients feel that illness alters their life plan considerably, particularly among males with very much higher levels of despair compared to women (Lukianenko, 2017). This calls for a comprehensive treatment practice in unison that combines physical healing with psychological and emotional support. Understanding these points facilitates more holistic rehabilitation practices based on the particular difficulties faced by children. Furthermore, that of habilitation emerges as a supplementary requirement to rehabilitation in the branch of pediatric orthopedics. Habilitation is the process of preventing pathological disorders by ensuring the optimal growth and development of children afflicted with diseases like meta epiphyseal osteomyelitis. This preventive method not only works towards curing existing conditions but also allows children to achieve their maximum potential. Effective pediatric orthopedic care thus involves creating a culture of support that is supportive of long-term resilience and functional autonomy (Lukianenko, 2017). In the end, the emphasis on complex care opens the door to children's ability to live with their physical challenges while maintaining emotional health, highlighting the central role of pediatric specialists in establishing healthier futures for their pediatric patients (Figure 8.3).

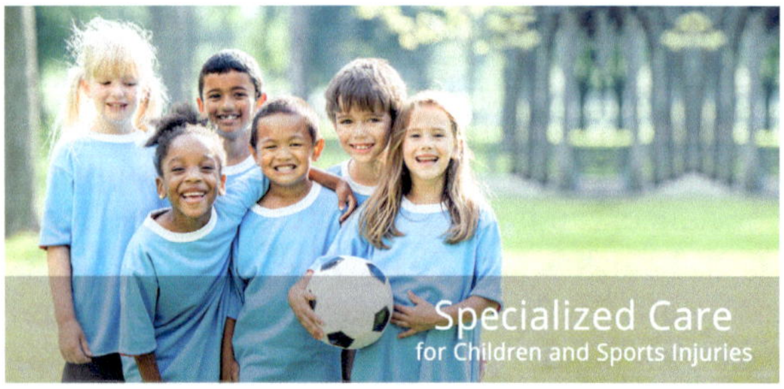

Figure 8.3. The importance of specialized care for children.

Source: https://external-content.duckduckgo.com/iu/?u=https%3A%2F%2Ffootandanklepgh.com%2Fwp-content%2Fuploads%2F2018%2F10%2Fspecialized-care.png&f=1&nofb=1&ipt=ceb44226d1d28a48965dd2ff6f84fe31b6c15a61b7ee23c2b612db30d115d0a5.

Overview of Common Pediatric Musculoskeletal Conditions

The child patient is vulnerable to a variety of musculoskeletal conditions that have a significant impact on their development and growth. The most common among them is osteogenesis imperfecta, which is characterized by brittle bone and recurrent fractures. It is a genetic disease resulting from collagen production defects, lowering the strength and resistance of bones. Patients with osteogenesis imperfecta may develop frequent fractures, limiting mobility and impairing body image. Along the same lines, diseases like juvenile idiopathic arthritis (JIA) are another problem in child orthopedics. JIA is the most frequent form of arthritis in children, causing chronic joint inflammation and impaired joint function that may compromise physical function and quality of life. Early diagnosis and treatment with medication and physiotherapy are critical interventions to avert the long-term consequences of these disabling diseases. Osteogenesis imperfecta and JIA are both critical reminders of the complexity of pediatric musculoskeletal health. Another extremely common condition in pediatric orthopedics is flatfoot, or pes planus. Flatfoot is a foot deformity in which there is a failure of development of the medial bone of the arch of the foot, so that the sole of the foot comes into full contact with the ground. Prevalence of flatfoot in children is a clinical dilemma due to varying beliefs about its clinical significance and management. While an asymptomatic flexible flatfoot often does not require treatment, a symptomatic flatfoot can cause pain and functional impairment for which conservative management strategies, such as activity modification and exercises, are recommended. Moreover, sophisticated biomechanical modeling methods, such as those discussed in Slavens & Harris (2012), are employed to uncover the dynamics of foot mechanics. Such sophisticated methods stress the necessity for interdisciplinarity in pediatric orthopedics in order to develop effective treatment strategies and enhance the success rate of rehabilitative therapy for children with flatfoot. Other conditions, such as scoliosis and Perthes disease, pose peculiar challenges in pediatric orthopedics. Scoliosis, a lateral curvature of the spine, can occur during the adolescent growth spurts and will cause an asymmetry of posture that, when significant, will require monitoring or surgery. Screening programs early in life have been instrumental in the detection of scoliosis, thereby allowing intervention before progressive deterioration sets in and complications occur. Simultaneously, Perthes disease, or avascular necrosis of the femoral head, occurs most frequently in 4- to 10-year-old boys. The illness can produce pain and limited motion of the hip and necessitate a treatment plan with a variety of modalities, including physical therapy and, in some cases, surgery. Both scoliosis and Perthes disease illustrate the heterogeneity of pediatric musculoskeletal disorders, and the necessity for specialist orthopedic intervention to address the particular needs of this vulnerable age group.

8.1. Developmental Anatomy and Physiology

Embryological development plays a central role in pediatric orthopedics since it is the foundation of anatomical structures and their physiological functions. In fetal life, the musculoskeletal system starts developing through primary changes, which begin with the formation of mesodermal structures. These structures differentiate and develop into cartilage and bone, upon which limb development occurs. It is during this period of crisis that congenital deformities, like limb deficiencies or scoliosis, may arise from interference with proceeding developing processes. Awareness of these embryological periods and complications assists medical professionals in diagnosing and designing interventions for children's orthopedic conditions. Notably, the consequences are viewed on examination and management of conditions like flatfoot, as effective treatment regimens can be modified by understanding developmental variation and its physiologic influence during growth phases (Serna, 2015).

Physiologic alterations in childhood also influence the diagnosis and treatment of musculoskeletal disorders. As children grow, the bones and joints undergo dynamic changes as a result of physiological changes in hormones, rates of physical activity, and overall patterns of growth. Bone ossification and maturation occur with the growing bones' mechanical loading, which is essential in shaping conditions treated by pediatric orthopedics, such as osteochondritis dissecans or hip developmental dysplasia. Such conditions are generally treated with an age- and severity-dependent individualized approach comprising a balance between conservative management and surgery.

Understanding the physiological processes of bone growth, i.e., Wolff's Law, assists in predicting what a variety of treatments will accomplish with growth over time and thereby maximize patient outcomes (Kinney, 2007). Understanding how developmental anatomy and physiology are interrelated is vital in overcoming the intricacies of pediatric orthopedic diseases. Professionals must be current with anatomical variations throughout different ages and how these affect treatment. The foundation for an understanding of these differences is rooted in a profound anatomical insight, which has a direct bearing on clinical procedures such as the use of customized orthotics for the treatment of flatfoot. Because many pediatric patients have flat feet, measuring the efficacy of these interventions relies heavily on the anatomical and physiological insight gained from understanding the development process. As research evolves, experts are in a better position to correctly dictate management practices to ensure they adhere to the established developmental standards (Serna, 2015) (Figure 8.4).

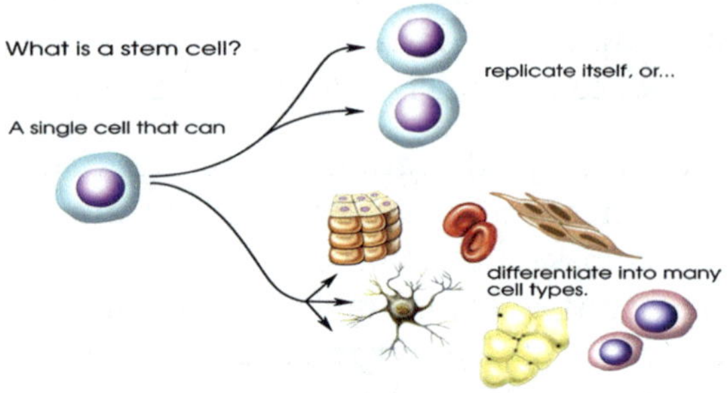

Figure 8.4. Embryological development is integral to understanding pediatric orthopedics.

Source: https://external-content.duckduckgo.com/iu/?u=https%3A%2F%2Fimage.slidesharecdn.com%2Fdevelopmentanatomyandphysiologyofhaematopoiesishematological-copy-170730173129%2F75%2FDevelopment-anatomy-and-physiology-of-haematopoiesis-hematological-copy-4-2048.jpg&f=1&nofb=1&ipt=27e3f058418458ce764a915bdf895f8b435fd0481d954b55f6b7719473942ee0.

8.1.1. Growth Patterns in Children

Patterns of childhood growth are intertwined with their own bone development, and this plays an important part in pediatric orthopedics. Growth occurs through the initial widening of the growth plates, or epiphyseal plates, which are found at the distal end of long bones. They are made of cartilage and are the site of longitudinal growth of bones. The elasticity of growth plates in children renders them susceptible to injury, i.e., fracture. An intimate understanding of growth patterns helps physicians to anticipate potential complications caused by such injuries. Significance of recognition of different patterns of physeal injury is highest as improper treatment has long-term effects like angular deformity or growth arrest, hence highlighting early treatment and precise observation during maturation phases among the pediatric population (Sabharwal & Sabharwal, 2018). Additionally, growth patterns in children can be affected by several factors, such as genetics, diet, and general health status. Appropriate eating habits are highly important during growth years, as macro and micronutrient deficiencies can lead to stunted growth and bone development. For example, calcium and vitamin D are essential for bone strength, whereas protein is important for overall development. Along with nutritional factors, exercise also matters; physically active children tend to have superior bone strength and density compared to inactive children. By recognizing such factors, pediatric orthopedic practitioners can tailor interventions to optimize the outcome of growth.

Early treatment and detection of any growth abnormalities are important, especially for patients with growth plate injury, as this can significantly alter their long-term physical growth pattern (Aber, 2016). Knowledge of the typical growth patterns and variants in specific pediatric populations is essential for planning effective treatment in orthopedics. Dysmorphic growth patterns may be indicative of intrinsic medical conditions or injuries that need to be treated. For instance, kids with osteogenesis imperfecta experience less than normal growth in the case of bone fragility. Conversely, awareness of normal growth patterns makes it easier for early detection of such conditions. Further, implementing injury severity scores for pediatric populations can help clinicians make more informed decisions about treatment modalities, particularly where limb amputation or reconstructive surgery is the option. The development of pediatric-specific guidelines can address particular dilemmas in assessment and management of growth-related injuries, thereby enhancing the process of decision-making among parents and clinicians (Aber, 2016; Sabharwal & Sabharwal, 2018) (Figure 8.5).

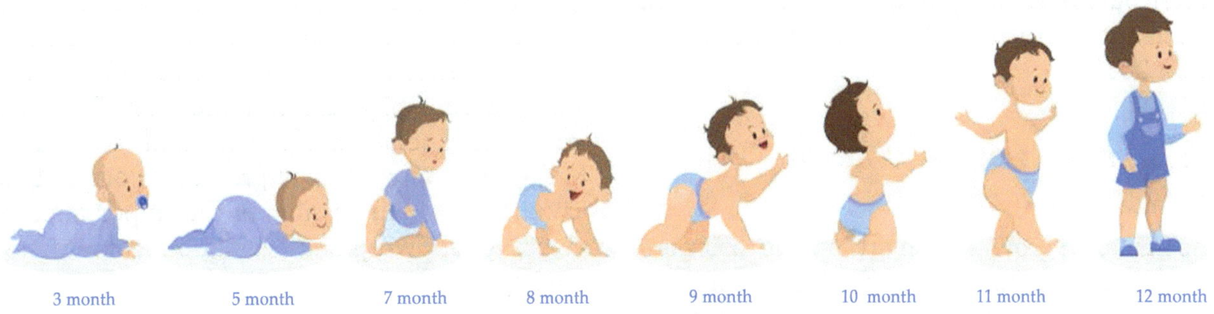

Figure 8.5. The growth patterns in children.

Source: https://external-content.duckduckgo.com/iu/?u=https%3A%2F%2Fi.pinimg.com%2Foriginals%2F46%2F93%2Fd5%2F4693d5ce7be4601932c06c3f40302f17.png&f=1&nofb=1&ipt=709fbb44ca43ec0c96a43c559f43d8211c19b74fbf42208a583d406b4eb1eff1.

8.1.2. Differences Between Pediatric and Adult Musculoskeletal Systems

The musculoskeletal anatomy of children and adults is very different, with significant implications for pediatric orthopedics. The skeleton of the child contains a greater proportion of cartilage, required for growth and development. The cartilage is less rigid than the more rigid, ossified bone that an adult will possess, so the bones in children are more resistant to certain fractures but more susceptible to damage of the growth plates. Juvenile skeletal tissues undergo continuous remodeling based on mechanical stress and trauma, allowing for recovery from injury that would have more ominous consequences in the adult. Treatment of children by pediatric orthopedics thus often maintains a secondary focus on promoting growth, using techniques that are quite distinct from those used in adults. Understanding these differences is of prime importance in designing appropriately individualized treatment protocols to maximize the recovery and long-term musculoskeletal health of children. Another fascinating difference occurs in the healing process typical of the pediatric musculoskeletal system. Children heal faster than adults due to an active growth phase and increased metabolic rates. The open growth plates are a challenge in that an injury in these areas can lead to limb length discrepancies or angular deformities if neglected. Also, traumatization of children's bones usually leads to a greenstick fracture, an incomplete fracture that doesn't lead to total disruption of the bone structure. This is contrary to the more complete and more complicated fractures commonly seen in adults. Therefore, the treatments need to be adjusted not just by the nature of the injury but also by the age and growth status of the patients, highlighting the relevance of specialized expertise in pediatric orthopedics. In addition, the psychological considerations for the management of musculoskeletal injuries in children are quite different from those of adults. Younger patients tend to have increased anxiety surrounding medical procedures, as this varies with their developmental level and inadequate understanding of healthcare principles. Parent roles assume significance in such cases, particularly in being able to make informed choices about treatment plans. Studies suggest that parents tend to struggle with low health literacy, affecting their capacity to cope with healthcare choices for their children. Developing injury severity scores tailored to pediatric use, i.e., a modified Predictive Salvage Index (PSI), would do a great deal to refine decision aids for parents and medical professionals. Application of the same scoring in pediatric orthopedic practice boosts better communication, thereby leading to better outcomes and parental satisfaction with treatment protocols (Slavens & Harris, 2012; Aber, 2016).

8.1.3. Impact of Growth on Orthopedic Conditions

The impact of growth upon orthopedic disorders is of particular significance in the field of pediatric orthopedics, where the dynamic process of developing musculoskeletal tissues coincides with unique challenges. In development, the bones and muscles of children are rapidly changing, not just in form but in function as well. This growth may influence the onset and severity of certain orthopedic disorders, for example, limb deformity or scoliosis. Specifically, adolescents are able to exhibit signs of disorders such as Adolescent Idiopathic Scoliosis (AIS), whose spinal curvature may be exacerbated by growth spurts. Notably, research has demonstrated that pre-operative patients with AIS exhibit different degrees of pain and anxiety when compared to brace patients, and such may have long-lasting implications on their emotional and physical health (Wihak, 2016). It is hence necessary to know how growth influences orthopedic conditions so that intervention options in children are maximized, so that physical correction, along with psychological support, is given. Besides scoliosis, growth influences other conditions such as Morquio A syndrome, which is also a concern due to its musculoskeletal impact. The metabolic disease is capable of producing orthopedic manifestations of enormous magnitude, especially as the patients age and continue to grow in size. Lower and upper extremity deformities are common in children with Morquio A syndrome, and such developments can significantly impact their quality of life. Therefore, early diagnosis becomes highly crucial for effective management of these conditions. A combined approach of orthopedic experts, along with the development of complete treatment guidelines, will further improve the control of extremity-associated complications (White et al., 2014). These interventions will require individualization to meet the unique growth patterns of children involved and not only correct physical complications but also promote social integration and emotional well-being. The effect of growth on orthopedic conditions again highlights the importance of ongoing follow-up and evaluation from infancy through adolescence.

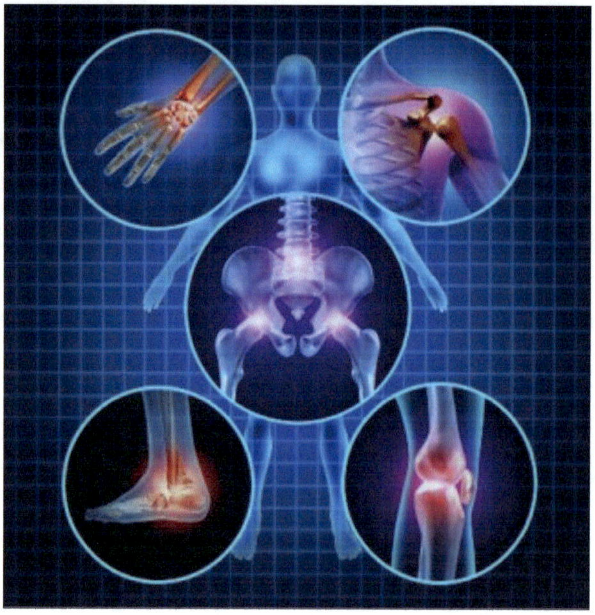

Figure 8.6. The impact of growth on orthopedic conditions.

Source: https://external-content.duckduckgo.com/iu/?u=https%3A%2F%2Fwww.leximed.com.au%2Fwp-content%2Fuploads%2F2020%2F02%2FPicture1.jpg&f=1&nofb=1&ipt=be2ee3f9904d59c53a81a8be3d688b50ff933402de5a7abfb08c74df2ebfb019.

As children go through various stages of development, orthopedic professionals must remain watchful for signs of impending disorders or deterioration of existing conditions. For instance, the adolescent growth spurt not only increases the risk for scoliosis and related conditions but can also serve to amplify symptoms of prior conditions, necessitating early intervention. Parents and caregivers are also significant by being actively involved in follow-up management and observing changes in their child's physical function or symptoms. Integration of growth considerations in the treatment plan not only guarantees effective treatment of pediatric orthopedic conditions but emphasizes the holistic strategy required for achieving optimal long-term outcomes in such patients, a notion completely indispensable in any successful pediatric orthopedic program (Figure 8.6).

8.2. Common Pediatric Orthopedic Conditions

Pediatric orthopedics involves a wide range of disorders that can affect the musculoskeletal system in children, particularly while they are still developing. These disorders range from congenital deformities, fractures, and deformities. Congenital deformities, for instance, clubfoot and developmental dysplasia of the hip, arise during fetal development and could require immediate management after birth. Treatment and early detection are essential to improve long-term results and allow normal growth patterns. Fractures, although common in active children, are particularly challenging to manage because of the varying processes of healing in children compared to adults. The treatments applied to treat such fractures not only need to address the physical but also take into consideration the psychosocial effects on the activity and well-being of a child, since neglecting the latter may result in chronic problems in later life. Of the extensive list of conditions treated in pediatric orthopedics, one that is especially significant is the management of osteomyelitis. Osteomyelitis, an infection of the bone most commonly from bacterial infection, can be a serious complication if left untreated. In particular, in children, meta epiphyseal osteomyelitis is challenging to diagnose and treat because it is not nearly as evident in its presentation and also can have long-term implications on development and growth. Unfortunately, rehabilitation measures for the illness minimize important socio-psychological rehabilitation processes. Research reveals that a high proportion of the affected patients cite interruptions of life planning due to illness, which highlights the psychological burden it places on children and families, particularly in males who view their treatment as more detrimental to their future plans (Lukianenko, 2017). Intensive rehabilitation, therefore, must include physical healing as well as psychological counseling to allow for complete recuperation. Also emphasized is the growing field of pediatric orthopedics involving diseases like scoliosis and benign tumors like osteochondromas. Scoliosis, with its abnormal spinal curvature, may present during periods of rapid growth, and intensive monitoring and treatment must be provided to avoid such long-term sequelae as impaired respiratory function or chronic pain. There are various available treatments, from bracing to surgical correction, depending on the severity of the curve and the child's growth potential. Similarly, benign tumors generally have to be managed with a multimodal approach, based on management and surveillance, so that they do not interfere with the normal musculoskeletal development of the child. Technical improvements in imaging and clinical methods, such as gait analysis, are essential to expanding the knowledge about these conditions, so that tests and treatments can be tailored to meet the particular requirements of every child and obtain the best outcomes (Baker, 2006).

8.2.1. Congenital Deformities (e.g., Clubfoot, Hip Dysplasia)

The spectrum of congenital deformities encompasses a spectrum of musculoskeletal disorders, two of the most frequent being clubfoot and hip dysplasia in pediatric orthopedics. Congenital talipes equinovarus, also known as clubfoot, is characterized by a disordered position of the foot that, if left untreated, may lead to serious loss of function. Traditionally, treatment approaches have ranged from non-operative conservative procedures, like serial casting, to operative methods. Present developments have positioned the Ponseti technique as the gold standard for the treatment of idiopathic clubfoot. Nonetheless, despite its effectiveness, there is a high rate of recurrence, with studies indicating that non-adherence to the brace has a considerable influence on outcomes (Goyal et al., 2023). Understanding these nuances is vital for pediatric orthopedic clinicians who wish to optimize the treatment given to children with this ailment. The other great challenge in pediatric orthopedics, in addition to clubfoot, is hip dysplasia. Developmental dysplasia of the hip (DDH) is a disorder in which the joint of the hip does not properly develop in infants and young toddlers, and not diagnosing and treating early leads to long-term ramifications. The severity of the condition can range from mild to severe, from subluxation to complete hip dislocation. Early detection through routine screening and imaging is essential for effective intervention. Bracing procedures, such as the Pavlik harness, are the primary treatment modalities that work to reduce the hip joint and maintain proper alignment during critical developmental stages. Variability according to treatment substantiates the requirement for individualized management strategies, emphasizing the utility of multidisciplinary care that includes surgical, orthotic, and rehabilitative treatment. Congenital deformity in the form of clubfoot and hip dysplasia has significant implications for the physical health of involved children, as well as their psychological adaptation and social adjustment. Families also tend to encounter emotional and logistical issues associated with caring for such conditions, thus requiring a holistic approach that specifically addresses both the medical and psychosocial aspects. Studies have shown that children with congenital deformities have higher levels of anxiety and loneliness, making supportive interventions critical. In addition, the need for patient education cannot be overstressed; informing families about treatment options, desired outcomes, and potential complications provides a framework in which treatment adherence is supported and effective care is guaranteed. Integrating these factors into the larger pediatric orthopedic care provides health practitioners with the ability to offer greater support to families and promote overall quality of life for children dealing with these birth abnormalities (Figure 8.7).

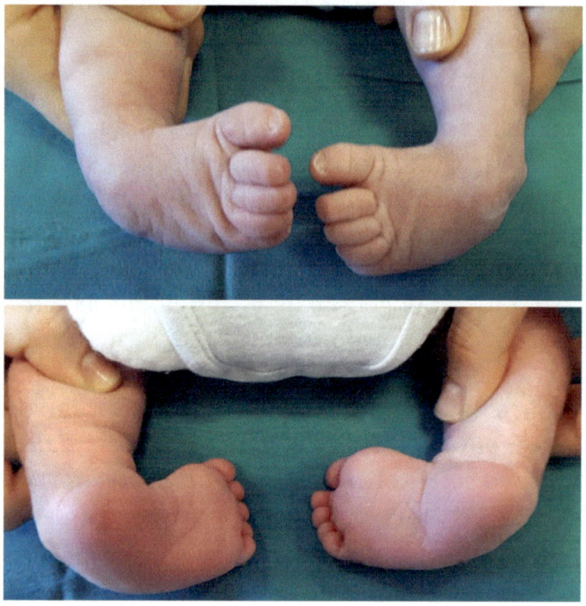

Figure 8.7. Congenital deformities.

Source: https://media.springernature.com/lw1200/springer-static/image/art%3A10.1186%2Fs13052-020-00842-3/MediaObjects/13052_2020_842_Fig1_HTML.png.

8.2.2. Acquired Conditions (e.g., Fractures, Scoliosis)

Acquired conditions of pediatric orthopedics encompass a wide range of musculoskeletal conditions that have a significant influence on the growth and development of a child. Of these, fractures are particularly prevalent because children are so active and liable to falling and sports injuries. Child fractures are generally different from adult fractures in terms of healing and treatment, since the bones of children are developing. These fractures tend to be challenging in management and evaluation for optimal stability and alignment, since their improper treatment can result in long-standing functional impairment or deformity. Additionally, in children, healing occurs with the inclusion of a more hypertrophic callus formation, which could prove challenging to control early mobility and rehabilitation. Understanding the variations in pediatric fractures is necessary so that clinicians are able to provide the optimal best in care for an uneventful recovery course in children. Scoliosis emerges as a second significant acquired disorder of pediatric orthopedics, presenting as unilateral curvature of the spine. Idiopathic scoliosis is the most researched, but the acquired ones can occur for a multitude of reasons, such as neuromuscular disease, injury, or infection. Acquired curvatures must be subjected to a comprehensive clinical assessment in order to diagnose etiology and appropriate intervention methods. Traditional modalities of treatment usually involve bracing and surgery, particularly if the curvature is swiftly progressive. Recent advances in intervention strategies, including the Magnetically-controlled growing rod (MCGR), are, however, a departure from the control of early-onset scoliosis. This technology, besides progressive correction of spinal deformities, reduces the need for repetitive invasive surgery and therefore shortens recovery times, improving the quality of life in such children (Stokes et al., 2014). Treatment of acquired conditions like fractures and scoliosis in children demands multidisciplinary care, taking physiological growth as well as psychosocial considerations into account. Among the most important factors in treating such conditions is minimizing ionizing radiation exposure, especially if serial imaging for follow-up of treatment response is necessary. The emerging role of noninvasive imaging modalities, such as ultrasound, presents a promising alternative for imaging and validating the treatment effect in a risk-free manner compared to radiographic imaging (Horn et al., 2021). With advancing pediatric orthopedics, the use of new technologies will be essential to maximize outcomes in patients and general safety. On the whole, a close understanding of acquired conditions in children, along with better treatment and imaging strategies, is crucial for maximizing healthy growth and addressing sequelae appropriately in the long term (Figure 8.8).

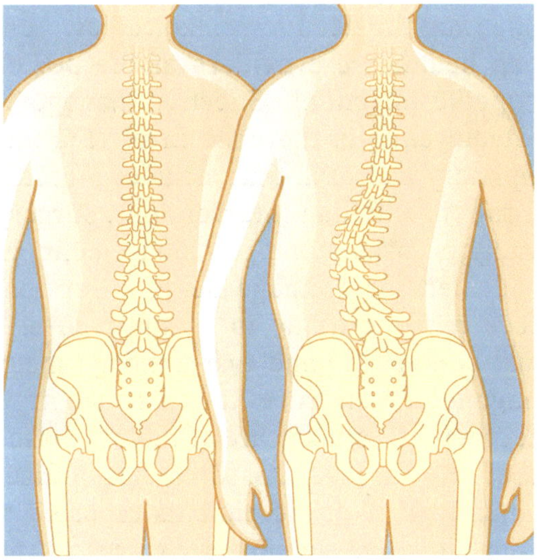

Figure 8.8. Acquired conditions in pediatric orthopedics.

Source: https://external-content.duckduckgo.com/iu/?u=https%3A%2F%2Fweillcornellbrainandspine.org%2Fsites%2Fdefault%2Ffiles%2Fscoliosis-normal-v-curve-lg.jpg&f=1&nofb=1&ipt=5ce056fa225d7d2b9510d73073ddd18a511ad136776ff06c9d4cc1d2557dcf28.

8.2.3. Inflammatory and Infectious Conditions (e.g., Osteomyelitis)

The pediatric population is particularly susceptible to countless inflammatory and infectious conditions, primarily osteomyelitis.

Osteomyelitis, or inflammation of the bone, usually results from bacterial infections, the most common being *Staphylococcus aureus*. In children, such infections are prone to occur after trauma, during surgery, or secondary to hematogenous spread from the remote sites of infection. The clinical presentation of osteomyelitis is extremely varied and manifests as fever, pain, and swelling over the sites involved, which can present in such a way that will lead the physician to misdiagnose if not well assessed. Proper and prompt diagnosis is essential for effective management, as delayed treatment will be followed by long-term disability and chronic pain, thereby highlighting the need for enhanced awareness among healthcare providers of the pediatric orthopedic infections. Effective management of osteomyelitis in the child involves a multidisciplinary approach that includes medical as well as rehabilitation interventions. Surgery is typically a cornerstone of management, with debridement or drainage being an option to remove necrotic tissue to enable recovery. It should be kept in mind that although medical management can cure the disease, it can sometimes fail to take care of the psychosocial side of the disease. Research has indicated that nearly 15% of the patients reported that osteomyelitis has significantly disrupted their life plans, and this is particularly so among male patients (Lukianenko, 2017). Therefore, besides physical rehabilitation, psychological and social impacts of the disease must be tackled as a vital component of comprehensive care, such that the involved children are provided with adequate care during the course of their recovery. Rehabilitation of children with osteomyelitis also has to go beyond the cure of the body, such as through counseling and psychological care, as well as social reintegration. Implementing a holistic approach that incorporates therapeutic interventions and counseling can significantly enhance rehabilitation in general. Interestingly, one study pointed out the need to engage with the socio-psychological factors, citing that most of the patients reported their capacity to achieve life aspirations was diminished through the condition, thus emphasizing the need for proper habilitation systems specific to this population (Lukianenko, 2017). By combining medical and surgical care with psychosocial rehabilitation, clinicians are able to create a more supportive environment conducive to recovery, ultimately improving quality of life and enabling better long-term outcomes for children with osteomyelitis and similar illnesses.

8.3. Diagnostic Approaches

Successful diagnostic approaches in pediatric orthopedics are responsible for accurate assessment and intervention treatment. One of the principal methods is clinical gait analysis and an important tool to determine the biomechanics of a child's locomotion. State-of-the-art optical systems offering retro-reflective marker tracking further enhance the accuracy of these examinations. These systems have advanced to the point where measurement of anthropometric data and the movement of soft tissue over underlying bones is the main challenge. Also, integrating computational techniques is particularly appealing because it may enable clinicians to address these challenges in real-time, hence improving the quality of gait evaluation in pediatric patients in general. These advances underscore the importance of advanced diagnostic methods in enabling proper diagnosis of musculoskeletal disorders in children (Baker, 2006). Interpretation of findings from gait analysis is also important in informing clinical decisions regarding intervention strategies. Lacking a validated grand theory of the way individuals exhibit certain patterns of ambulation, physicians must resort to individual mechanical explanations that will not necessarily provide them with an accurate portrait of the patient's condition.

Consequently, a new paradigm is evolving that focuses on what individual muscles do and how they contribute to the process of moving. This development involves the development of subject-specific models incorporating three-dimensional imaging of the musculoskeletal anatomy of a child and kinematic and kinetic data.

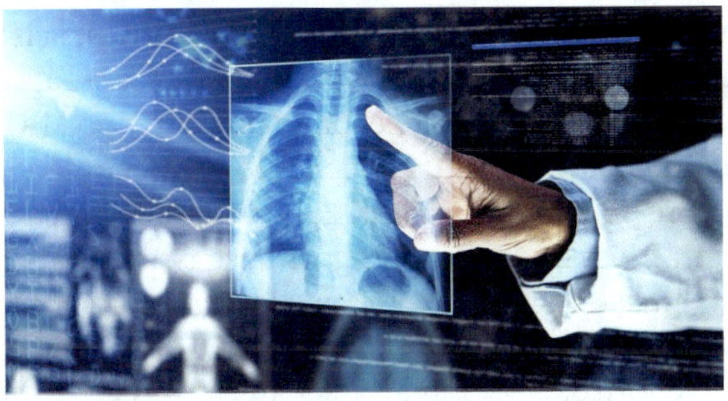

Figure 8.9. The effective diagnostic approaches are pivotal for accurate assessment and treatment intervention.

Source: https://external-content.duckduckgo.com/iu/?u=https%3A%2F%2Fd2jx2rerrg6sh3.cloudfront.net%2Fimages%2Fnews%2FImageForNews_778067_17139484923881440.jpg&f=1&nofb=1&ipt=3435069d21304bd06930c81782282303cc22388ddddc7767e433727c1d90647.

The use of such precise models can help to facilitate an increased level of understanding of the pattern of movement and pathology, allowing the clinician to adjust interventions more suitably and improve the outcome for patients in pediatric orthopedics (Baker, 2006). Lastly, estimation of the likely effectiveness of alternative treatment interventions depends on rigorous clinical trials and computational simulation of interventions. Practice is hampered by the absence of evidence-based information that can guide clinicians regarding the choice of the appropriate treatment courses. The study of simulation models of walking mechanisms in children with musculoskeletal issues offers a promising potential for predicting the outcomes of various interventions. Ultimately, the validation and refinement of these models could close existing knowledge gaps and lead to more informed clinical decision-making. As developmental advancements continue within pediatric orthopedics, the growing attention on these diagnostic methods is critical to ensuring the advancement of practice and research, such that care not only functions effectively but is cost-effective as well (Figure 8.9).

8.3.1. Clinical Evaluation and History Taking

The history taking and clinical evaluation process is of utmost significance in pediatric orthopedics, as is the creation of the foundation for an effective understanding of the patients condition. Children are particularly problematic due to their developmental status, which affects communication and understanding. Communication with the child as well as with his/her parents is important, as it provides a very comprehensive series of facts about the history of the child, including any previous musculoskeletal trauma and family orthopedic disorder patterns. The ability of the clinician in questioning using open-ended questions can take us a great distance toward enhancing the quality of gathered data, while facts like the site of pain, duration, and any aggravating or relieving factors are documented with care. Such an extensive background enables the practitioner to develop a more accurate clinical picture and tailor follow-up evaluation, thereby improving the general management approach in pediatric orthopedics. While taking history, specific attention should be paid to developmental milestones and concerns in growth patterns since these are critical components in the diagnosis of pediatric orthopedic conditions. For instance, a slow rate of progression toward motor skills could be an indicator of underlying musculoskeletal disorders that require investigation. By paying attention to a rational sequence of viewing growth lines and developmental histories, clinicians receive vital information regarding conditions such as osteogenesis imperfecta or hip dysplasia. This focus on developmental context not only allows for easier identification of specific orthopedic issues but also aligns with evidence-based medicine principles. Through the incorporation of evidence from relevant studies, clinicians can enhance patient outcomes and decision-making processes clinically. This transition from results interpretation to data collection is an unbroken process of investigation crucial in pediatric orthopedics that creates a trajectory for efficient management strategies. Finally, the combination of clinical examination and history taking with modern diagnostic equipment creates a synergistic effect that enhances pediatric orthopedic patient care. Using imaging tests and other assessment techniques together with well-documented histories can determine the type and extent of musculoskeletal problems. It thus supports evidence-based communication among the care team, which facilitates joint treatment planning. Furthermore, adopting evidence-based guidelines derived from a systematic review of the extant literature, e.g., for the management of shoulder surgery, can make the clinical pathway rational. These standards can be the yardsticks of best practice, improving the delivery of care quality and the maximization of resource utilization. The painstaking approach to the process of clinical evaluation and history taking, thus, does not serve merely as prerequisites; they are actually integral to the entire pathway of care in pediatric orthopedics, yielding improved clinical outcomes in children (Oliva et al., 2015; Sivhugwana, 2021).

8.3.2. Imaging Techniques (e.g., X-rays, MRI)

In pediatric orthopedics, imaging modalities are the most critical diagnostic devices for precise diagnosis and treatment of musculoskeletal conditions in children. Traditional imaging, such as X-rays, is extremely useful for bone shape and alignment and is therefore useful for diagnosing fractures, congenital malformations, and developmental dysplasia. They are simple and non-invasive, which enables them to have quick evaluations that can have a major impact on treatment. But while X-rays are useful for imaging bony structures, they are less good at assessing soft tissue. Thus, increased sophistication in imaging is necessary to have a better insight into a child's orthopedic condition so that the clinician can make precise diagnoses and craft interventions with increased specificity. Magnetic Resonance Imaging (MRI) has become a central technology in pediatric orthopedics, providing unprecedented definition in the imaging of soft tissues, such as muscles, ligaments, and cartilage. Its non-ionizing properties make it especially valuable for children, who are more susceptible to the impact of radiation. MRIs can accurately detect problems like osteochondritis dissecans, benign tumors, and muscle ruptures, thus widening the diagnostic arsenal at the disposal of pediatric orthopedic specialists. Further, advances in MRI technology, such as increased resolution and faster scanning times, have rendered it more applicable to clinical practice. The evidence is increasingly showing that the integration of MRI findings with clinical assessment can lead to better-informed treatment, which eventually leads to optimized patient outcomes and clinical efficacy in pediatric orthopedics. The future of pediatric orthopedic imaging is directed towards the creation of techniques to enhance the diagnostic capability and therapeutic effect. Imaging advances, including three-dimensional (3D) imaging, may enable the direct visualization of joint and bone anatomy, essentially closing the existing gap between standard imaging and the need for precise anatomical information. As defined in recent literature, the integration of functional tests and advanced imaging can provide further insight into motion mechanics, treatment outcomes, and eventual prognoses in children (Baker, 2006). Finally, predictive modeling from imaging data can assist clinicians with virtually simulating interventions and thereby allowing them to choose the most appropriate treatment modalities (Oliva et al., 2015). This imaging advance not only enhances clinical practice but is capable of revolutionizing the way pediatric orthopedic conditions are diagnosed and treated (Figure 8.10).

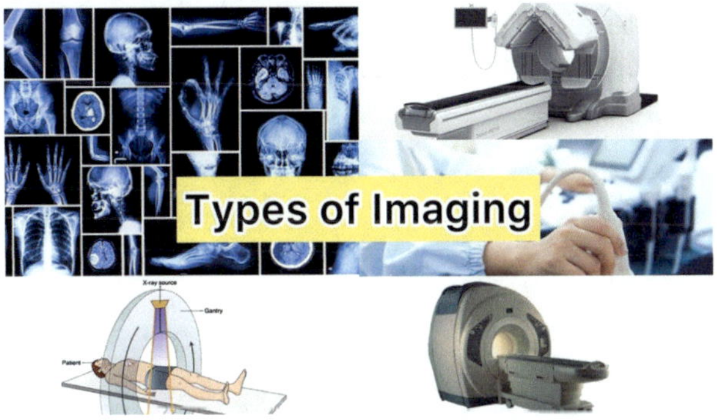

Figure 8.10. In the field of pediatric orthopedics, imaging techniques play a crucial role in the accurate diagnosis.

Source: https://external-content.duckduckgo.com/iu/?u=https%3A%2F%2Fi.ytimg.com%2Fvi%2Fv-bVEJ1IyUw%2Fmaxresdefault.jpg&f=1&nofb=1&ipt=f4eb2534aa6d16ae87c8fe71f0f72d1fa02ed880d0cefcbe8662fdd0f788553b.

8.3.3. Role of Physical Examination in Diagnosis

A thorough physical examination forms the core of pediatric orthopedics, forming the first step in the diagnosis of musculoskeletal conditions. The signs presenting in children are likely to be nonspecific or vague and inclined to make diagnosis difficult. Hence, the clinicians must be able to perform a meticulous physical examination and detect discrepancies in movement, strength, and alignment that may be suggestive of underlying pathology. Results such as disturbances in gait, joint range of motions, and pain symptoms can all provide vital information that guides follow-up evaluation and treatment plans. Additionally, treatment for issues such as flatfoot often depends on the outcomes of physical examination, where symptomatic and asymptomatic presentation are distinguished by the clinician to create an effective management plan, which again verifies the role of detailed physical examination in making accurate diagnoses (Oliva et al., 2015). Furthermore, the intricate relationship between a child's physical capability and his or her developmental milestones emphasizes the importance of physical examination in pediatric orthopedics. As children grow up, their musculoskeletal systems drastically alter, and age-adjusted evaluation becomes necessary. When performing physical exams, medical professionals can evaluate a child's strength, coordination, and flexibility, which play a significant role in determining potential developmental delay or abnormality. A successful physical examination enables the practitioner to distinguish between normal developmental variations of orthopedics and those necessitating intervention. It is particularly crucial in differentiating benign from more serious conditions that may necessitate surgical intervention. In this respect, practitioners also rely on evidence-based guidelines to inform decisions about the form and extent of intervention and treatments (Oliva et al., 2015), thereby ensuring that children's individual development requirements are adequately met. In addition to diagnosing conditions, physical examination plays a crucial role in follow-up and evaluating the effectiveness of ongoing treatments in pediatric orthopedics. Regular examinations allow medical practitioners to observe a child's progress and change treatment plans when necessary. For example, in the treatment of flatfoot, frequent monitoring of changes in symptoms and physical examination may guide the process of deciding between conservative and surgical intervention. The dynamic nature of a child's growth ensures that circumstances for management may alter, and therefore, a responsive management approach is required. By incorporating results of physical examinations systematically into the decision-making process, orthopedic professionals can ensure maximally optimized care specially designed to the child's pattern of growth and unique orthopedic needs. This responsiveness ultimately maximizes the overall effectiveness of treatment outcomes for pediatric orthopedics (Serna, 2015).

8.4. Treatment Modalities

Treatment options in pediatric orthopedics vary greatly and are directed to overcome the unique musculoskeletal issues posed by growing children. Conservative treatment remains a cornerstone for treating many disorders, particularly fractures.

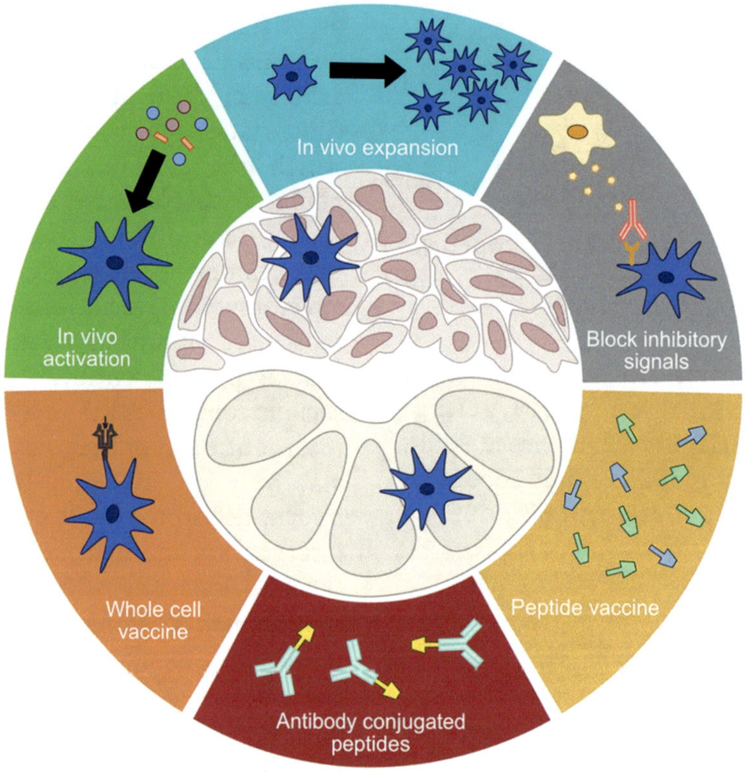

Figure 8.11. The treatment modalities encompass a range of approaches tailored to address the unique musculoskeletal challenges.

Source: https://external-content.duckduckgo.com/iu/?u=https%3A%2F%2Fwww.researchgate.net%2Fpublication%2F341543685%2Ffigure%2Ffig2%2FAS%3A893610618781696%401590064782292%2FTreatment-modalities-targeting-DCs-A-number-of-current-treatment-modalities-aim-to.png&f=1&nofb=1&ipt=3e2a49a51b5ce9d85364d465f77017ec17675aaaedd6c66ff02a684445cc8594.

An excellent example is managing femur fractures of preschool children through conservative care in the form of spica cast immobilization or skin traction. It emphasizes the stability and immobilization in order to achieve healing. More intrusive techniques, such as intramedullary nailing with a flexible rod, have been found to be effective for older children, as demonstrated by a study in which nine preschool children underwent this procedure with positive results. The length of hospital stay averaged four days, which implies a comparatively rapid recovery process within the field of pediatric medicine (Ridder et al., 2008). These conflicting methods emphasize the importance of personalized therapy plans that consider the developmental stage of the child. In the scenario of benign bone tumors, i.e., simple bone cysts, therapeutic modalities have evolved to a great extent to provide techniques for minimal invasiveness to ensure optimum therapy. One such important approach is by employing minimally invasive techniques, such as percutaneous curettage with titanium elastic nailing (TENS) and allogenic bone grafting. This method comes in handy in the treatment of diseases like pathological fractures secondary to a simple bone cyst, as demonstrated in a case where a 14-year-old boy was managed. Minimally invasive surgery decreases trauma, minimizes recovery, and enables a speedy return to function. Postoperatively, fracture healing and complete filling of the cyst cavity with the allograft were observed in the boy (Lakhwani, 2013). These advances emphasize the necessity for the selection of treatment modalities in equipoise between effectiveness and patient-related parameters. Moreover, the selection of treatment modalities in pediatric orthopedics extends beyond surgical and non-surgical types to include physical therapy and rehabilitation methods. These ancillary therapies are very useful in maximizing recovery and improving long-term functional outcomes. Following surgical procedures, therapies adjusted to the child's needs, such as strength training and flexibility exercises, can promote best healing and ensure future injury prevention. There is evidence indicating that prompt intervention with physical therapy plays a very important role in motor development and independence of pediatric patients. For this reason, incorporating multidisciplinary methods that merge surgical interventions, rehabilitative treatment, and follow-up monitoring becomes vital in pediatric orthopedics. This integrated care model underscores the dynamic interplay between various treatment modalities to enable the overall wellness of child patients (Figure 8.11).

8.4.1. Non-Surgical Interventions (e.g., Physical Therapy, Bracing)

Similarly, non-surgical modalities such as bracing and physical therapy are equally crucial in the management of pediatric orthopedic conditions, particularly in AIS. While surgery may most commonly appear to be imminent for severe deformities, the first line of action typically involves less forceful interventions that aim to halt further curvature of the spine. Physical therapy is a primary intervention, focusing on the strength of the spinal musculature and enabling postural control. These treatments can significantly enhance the quality of life in children with AIS by allowing them to manage their condition without resorting to surgery at once. By establishing a firm foundation of physical function and body sense, physical therapy can enable young patients to take charge of their treatment process, contributing to improved global outcomes. Bracing, another essential non-operative treatment, is customized to avoid exacerbation of spinal curvatures in growing adolescents. Several studies indicate that bracing can significantly lower the risk of progression of the curve, especially when the spinal curvature ranges from 20° to 40° (Negrini et al., 2015). The success of bracing relies on adherence, since the frequency and consistency with which the brace is worn correlate directly with successful outcomes. However, the psychological impact of bracing should not be ignored; teenagers often have problems with self-concept and social acceptance while wearing such appliances. Strengthening supportive structures, like counseling and group work, may be effective in lessening such experiences and ensuring treatment compliance. By such collective measures, bracing remains a focal point in the conservative management of scoliosis and other such diseases. In addition, overall treatment of pediatric orthopedic conditions centers on interdisciplinary practice, including bracing and physical therapy. When evaluating how effective these interventions are, research shows that they are able to impact not just the physical aspects of one's condition but also psychological well-being and family dynamics (Wihak, 2016). When fears related to treatment are alleviated, families are better able to adapt to their child's orthopedic condition. The nuances of choosing between operative and non-operative methods emphasize the importance of collaboration among orthopedic surgeons, physical therapists, patients, and families. Ultimately, the investment in non-operative care not only corrects the deforming nature of conditions such as AIS but also creates resistance and resilience in young patients to the extent that they can maintain active lifestyles and emotional well-being despite advancing age (Figure 8.12).

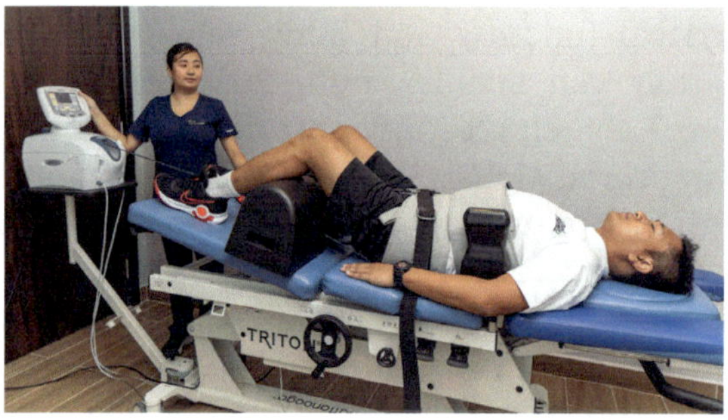

Figure 8.12. Non-surgical interventions such as physical therapy and bracing.

Source: https://external-content.duckduckgo.com/iu/?u=https%3A%2F%2Ffranklinchiropracticdubai.com%2Fwp-content%2Fuploads%2F2022%2F08%2Fd0400b48a2a79d8775e7ff8381786c54-xxlarge-1.jpeg&f=1&nofb=1&ipt=5dc97086240630ee7f6aa03693a9b335132db3fa8cafaa5d9daaf66821992c0b.

8.4.2. Surgical Options and Considerations

In pediatric orthopedics, surgical treatments are commonly adapted to accommodate the specific anatomical and physiological characteristics of children. A critical consideration in pediatric orthopedic operations is growth disturbance since the child's skeletal structure is maturing. Surgeons need to assess carefully the timing of surgery since surgical intervention done too early or too late may result in complications such as limb deformities or joint dysfunction. Additionally, the surgical procedure of preference must be taken into account for the child's activity level as well as the anticipated future level of sports participation. Later surgical techniques, such as minimally invasive procedures, have become increasingly popular due to shorter recovery times and the reduced risk of complications, allowing quicker return to daily activity and sport (Baker, 2006). Advancements in surgical materials and techniques have dramatically expanded the success of pediatric orthopedic surgery. As an example, the use of living donor hamstring tendon (LDHT) grafts from the parent to reconstruct the anterior cruciate ligament (ACL) has gained popularity due to its acceptable mid-term results. It is reported that evidence shows it provides usable graft survival rates simultaneously while decreasing the risk for donor site morbidity when compared to traditional autograft procedures (Cooper et al., 2018). As children experience higher incidence rates of recurrent ACL injury, the LDHT technique may be a viable alternative that holds out for equally good outcomes. However, longer-term studies will be required to establish these findings and monitor the potential consequences as the child grows up. When arriving at decisions regarding surgical intervention, clinicians should seek shared decision-making with families. Factors such as the growth stage of the child, the severity of the orthopedic issue, and postoperative anticipated rehabilitation all require open debate. By providing comprehensive information, health workers can enable parents and caregivers to understand the benefits and limitations of various surgical options. Additionally, by using a multidisciplinary practice involving occupational therapists and physiotherapists, postoperative rehabilitation can be optimized, with enhanced functional results in children. Effective surgical treatment in pediatric orthopedics is hence multi-faceted, focused not just on the technical success of the surgery but also on the collaborative care and support of the child and family throughout the treatment process (Baker, 2006).

8.4.3. Post-Operative Care and Rehabilitation

Post-operative rehabilitation and treatment are critical components of pediatric orthopedics, with significant effects on recovery and late function. After surgical interventions, children typically experience rehabilitative and psychological adaptation. Adequate post-operative care typically includes pain management, vigilance for potential complications such as infections, and functional mobility. Rehabilitation protocols in pediatric patients need to be specifically tailored since these children must adapt to the particular developmental requirements of developing bodies. Moreover, the need for family involvement at this time is emphasized, given that parents play pivotal roles in both physical and psychosocial care. Through a child-centered environment, caregivers are able to facilitate resilience and adherence, which remain critical in upholding optimal recovery. Thus, a multi-factor model of post-operative care can facilitate smoother hospital-to-home transitions and significantly improve overall rehabilitation outcomes. Rehabilitation programs in pediatric orthopedics must be customized and dynamic, depending on the specific surgical procedure and the unique needs of the child. Physical therapy is often initiated early in an effort to promote movement and build up involved structures while protecting the operative area from undue stress. Activity can include low-key range-of-motion techniques, balance training, and functional movement geared to the age and degree of cognitive function of the child. Besides that, the integration of play in rehab is particularly beneficial for kids in that it can induce participation and trigger compliance with treatment regimes. Additionally, the psychological aspect of recovery cannot be overlooked; children must cope with activity restrictions and surgical fear.

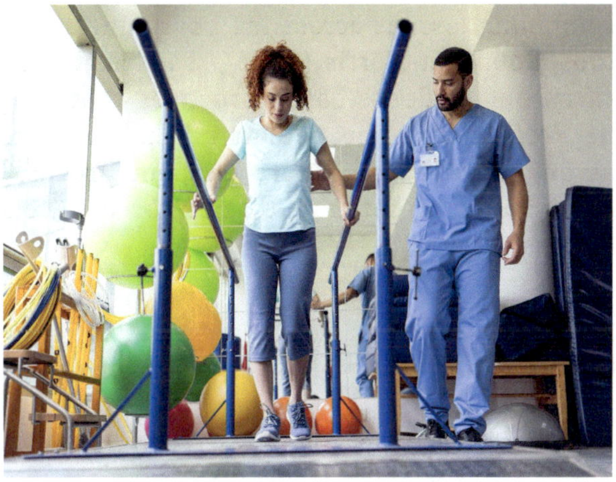

Figure 8.13. Post-operative care and rehabilitation.

Source: https://external-content.duckduckgo.com/iu/?u=https%3A%2F%2Fctspineandortho.com%2Fwp-content%2Fuploads%2F2024%2F03%2FPhysical-Medicine-Rehabilitation.jpg&f=1&nofb=1&ipt=93179688a5219a40f7a50dc514d1557d29903d93a76eec74678357d73a4c57ad.

Rehabilitation workers should therefore incorporate interventions that support emotional well-being as well as physical recovery, eventually fostering an integrated model of recovery. Post-surgical rehabilitation and care can be made even more effective through collaboration between patients, families, and healthcare professionals. Multidisciplinary teams of orthopedic surgeons, psychologists, physical therapists, and occupational therapists can offer extensive care according to the child's specific needs. Regular follow-ups must also be conducted to monitor progress and make changes in rehabilitation programs as needed. Such feedback in such a collaborative setting can help identify barriers to recovery and offer solutions so that children achieve milestones in development. Furthermore, with the increase in life expectancy and the ageing population undergoing orthopedic procedures, as per (Krishna & Pathak, 2020), it casts a light on the need for improved post-operative care protocols that accommodate individual patient issues. By combining lessons across the board, including those found in Morris (2002), it is feasible to carry out evidence-based practices that will be able to redefine pediatric rehabilitation as an improved and more efficient process, culminating in better outcomes for children (Figure 8.13).

8.5. Challenges in Pediatric Orthopedics

Pediatric orthopedics is typified by a myriad of factors that make diagnosis and treatment complex. Heterogeneity in the growth pattern of children is a significant hindrance and can potentially affect the presentation of musculoskeletal disorders. Unlike adults, with well-defined skeletal maturation, children come with disorders that are still developing in relation to their growth. This can lead to misdiagnosis or delayed intervention, since the clinician must be adept at distinguishing between normal variation in development and pathological states. Furthermore, the intricacies of treating fractures in children, where bones are more plastic and responses to healing differ, help to further emphasize the need for specialist expertise in the best management of pediatric orthopedic trauma. These unique considerations require ongoing education and training of practitioners to provide the optimal care particular to this vulnerable population. In addition to the biological complexities, psychological issues are also significant contributors to the issues that are faced in pediatric orthopedics. Children are generally more anxious about medical procedures, which can complicate both the diagnostic process and the treatment process. Panic about pain or uncertain outcomes may cause noncompliance with treatment plans, including follow-throughs as indicated. And even establishing trust and rapport with adolescent patients entails delicate strategies proportional to their stages of growth. Physicians must balance educating children about their illnesses and reassuring them in the interest of minimizing anxiety.

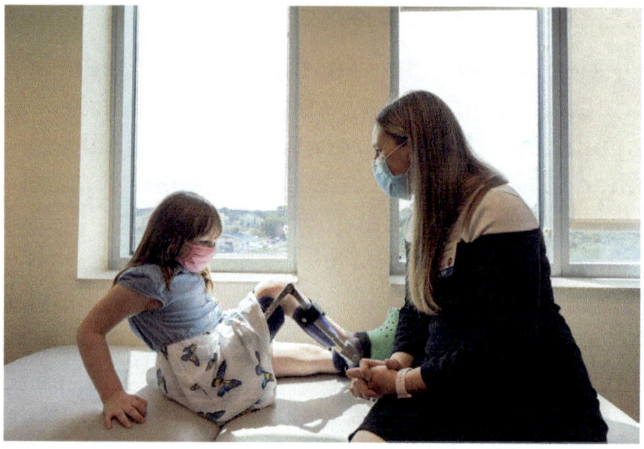

Figure 8.14. The landscape of pediatric orthopedics.

Source: https://external-content.duckduckgo.com/iu/?u=https%3A%2F%2Fufhealth.org%2Fassets%2Fimages%2Fspecialties%2F_1500x1000_crop_center-center_line%2F2462113%2FPediatric-Orthpaedics-facility_JJ103948_2022-07-29-142954_fvjz.jpg&f=1&nofb=1&ipt=af1c73f017f0d40bef9eeca10f3893665662670dc08ac42f2e4fec7407a32486.

This intricate balance is important not only as a means of guaranteeing adherence to treatment protocols but also in facilitating healthy outcomes. Addressing these psychological factors adds yet another layer of complexity to the discipline of pediatric orthopedics, and again underscores the need for a multidisciplinary system of care that includes child life specialists and psychologists. Furthermore, ethical choices occupy a pivotal role in the dilemmas of pediatric orthopedics, particularly when it comes to decision-making for treatment options. The responsibility to ensure patient safety with proper care becomes compromised by concerns about existing treatment costs. Pediatric patients may require innovative solutions that have not been widely studied or proven in medical practices, leaving professionals and families to make difficult choices. Stakeholders in pediatric orthopedics, including manufacturers, regulatory agencies, and clinicians, are presented with these ethical challenges, ensuring that treatment is both safe and effective. It is essential to have complete guidelines and flowing information regarding the dangers and advantages of various forms of treatment so that there can be ethical practice within the field. As pediatric orthopedics develops further, it will be critical to develop solid ethical paradigms to inform practice and assist with evidence-based decision-making among clinicians and families (Stroud et al., 2016; Jones et al., 2019) (Figure 8.14).

8.5.1. Variability in Growth and Development

Variability of growth and development is a critical aspect of pediatric orthopedics, influencing the treatment strategy and overall management plan for the majority of children's musculoskeletal conditions. Knowledge of the physiological dissimilarities between children, such as the disparity as seen with growth spurts and skeletal maturation, needs to be addressed to tailor interventions. For instance, during adolescence, rapid growth changes can lead to conditions like scoliosis, which may require age- and growth-stage-specific treatments. The effect of these growth phases on the success of the treatment cannot be overstated, since early diagnosis and prompt intervention will greatly improve long-term results. Understanding these variabilities allows healthcare professionals to perform appropriate monitoring procedures so that the interventions fall within the child's unique growth and developmental trajectory. Treatment of disorders like Adolescent Idiopathic Scoliosis (AIS) is a quintessential example of the importance of appreciating variability in growth and development. A more recent pre-surgical versus bracing study also identified significant differences in variables such as age, Cobb angle, and psychological stressors associated with different treatment modalities (Wihak, 2016). These differences influence not just the selection of treatment modalities but also the emotional and psychological status of the patient and their family. In particular, pre-surgical families all manifested greater concern about their child's pain and coping with it, which reflects the intricate nature of children with orthopedic conditions. Hence, addressing such psychological aspects alongside physical growth and development becomes essential in ensuring that children with orthopedic issues receive comprehensive care.

Furthermore, in diseases such as Morquio A syndrome, variability in growth and development brings special challenges for treatment. This condition, with a major musculoskeletal presentation, necessitates high levels of specialist care in appreciation of the global presentations of the condition. As demonstrated in more contemporary guidance on the treatment of extremity deformity, prompt diagnosis and specially tailored treatment can lead to improved patient outcomes (White et al., 2014).

Skeletal diversity during Moquino A patients' growth necessitates personalized management, given that conditions affecting the skeleton can differ significantly from one patient to another, hence affecting their overall functionality and quality of life. Through evolving a deep understanding of how growth patterns differ in children, orthopedic practitioners can more effectively deal with the intricacies involved in such hereditary ailments, ultimately to improve intervention and results in pediatric orthopedics.

8.5.2. Psychological Impact of Orthopedic Conditions on Children

The psychological impact of orthopedic disease in children is a strong field of pediatric orthopedics that deserves careful assessment. Iliaffixes such as Adolescent Idiopathic Scoliosis (AIS), besides having an impact on physical well-being, hold an important psychological burden for young patients and their families. It has been suggested that surgical children experience heightened anxiety as well as pain catastrophizing, particularly when facing intense operations such as spinal fusion surgery. Emotional distress at having to wait for surgery may cause helplessness among both children and parents, consequently depriving the child of the ability to deal with the forthcoming medical process. Management of these psychological factors is important to improve overall outcomes and ease recovery in orthopedic patients (Wihak, 2016). Besides, psychological effects are not just limited to preoperative anxiety and include long-term consequences on the quality of life of a child. Operations or chronic illness can lead to stigma and feelings of isolation if the child is unable to participate in normal activities due to pain or because of limitations in mobility. For instance, adolescent patients with bone sarcomas, who are likely to undergo aggressive treatments and extensive lifestyle adjustments, may have challenges with low self-esteem and social adjustment. Those issues underscore the importance of psychosocial support networks, such as psychotherapy and peer groups, that can attenuate the adverse emotional effects and facilitate resilience among child patients. Effective psychological therapy can be capable of eliciting coping mechanisms that enable children to maintain their quality of life regardless of orthopedic complications (Farid, 2023). The inclusion of mental health assessments in treatment plans is also a significant intervention directed at the psychological impact of orthopedic conditions. Scales such as the pediatric Toronto Extremity Salvage Score (pTESS) have been designed to quantify not only the physical, but also the psychological well-being of children with limb surgery. Through these scales, clinicians can assess at-risk patients and modify intervention that moderates both physical rehabilitation and psychology. By including the mental health disciplines within functional assessments, clinicians are better placed to obtain a comprehensive understanding of the child's experience. Not only does this holistic strategy aim to enhance physical outcomes, but also to foster psychological resilience, ultimately to the advantage of children's wellbeing during their orthopedic experiences (Farid, 2023) (Figure 8.15).

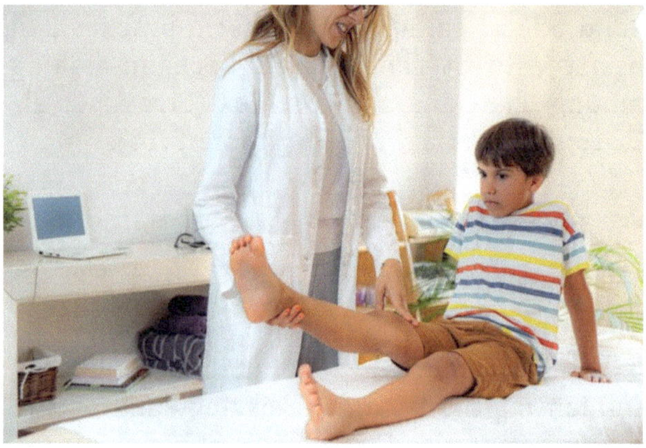

Figure 8.15. The psychological impact of orthopedic conditions on children.

Source: https://external-content.duckduckgo.com/iu/?u=https%3A%2F%2Fbrhealthcare.in%2Fuploads%2Fblogs%2F1715883456_orthopedic_conditions_in_children_early_detection_and_treatment-1.png&f=1&nofb=1&ipt=2cf3c383c35d87ed24d300826db420b2e01680cf9a4470af84e6e2610f6b3e9c.

8.5.3. Access to Specialized Care and Resources

Specialized treatment and availability of resources in pediatric orthopedics are a strong determinant of outcomes and overall quality of life for musculoskeletal disease in children. Prompt access to specialists, such as pediatric orthopedic surgeons and physical therapists, can significantly enhance prognosis with early treatment. Multidisciplinary management of the intricate nature of musculoskeletal issues is usually required, consisting of surgical correction, physical therapy, and follow-up treatment. Denied access to such specialties, children will most likely have delays in diagnosis and treatment that can lead to compounded conditions or lasting harm. As highlighted in many studies on the healthcare of children, systemic barriers of geographic limitations and insufficient insurance coverage continue to bar access to special services, proving the need for targeted interventions for closing these gaps (Sivhugwana, 2021). Furthermore, access to educational information is equally important in the management of pediatric orthopedic conditions. Caregivers and parents should be well-informed on treatment options, rehabilitation protocols, and potential outcomes in order to make proper decisions about their child's care. Education empowers families to make decisions and navigate the health system for appropriate advocacy on behalf of their children and to access proper and timely interventions. Healthcare providers need to emphasize communication and education, using child-oriented materials to present complicated medical data in a readable and comprehensible way. In addition, support networks in the community can provide critical advice and emotional support to families navigating uncharted healthcare systems. With the encouragement of an egalitarian information environment, the healthcare systems can assist patient participation and adherence to treatment regimens, thereby ensuring improved health outcomes as well as the quality of care in pediatric orthopedics (University of Vermont, 1991). As child orthopedics has advanced significantly, disparities continue to prevail concerning access to specialized care among the disadvantaged. Socioeconomic determinants usually dictate the availability of essential services, and low-income families find it extremely challenging to get proper care. Such disparities can add to pre-existing health inequities and result in differential outcomes depending on geographics or socioeconomic status. To overcome these issues, there needs to be a multifaceted strategy involving policy changes that enhance insurance coverage, enhance pediatric specialty clinics' funding, and utilize telemedicine to cover remote populations. In addition, a partnership between academic centers and community organizations can enable increased access to complex care through enhanced outreach programs and services among worthy families. As the field of pediatric orthopedics evolves, equal access must become a pillar of pediatric health, whereby every child gets the opportunity to enjoy outstanding orthopedic care (Sivhugwana, 2021).

8.6. Advances in Pediatric Orthopedic Research

New advances in pediatric orthopedic research have significantly enhanced the understanding and treatment of musculoskeletal disorders in children. In this context, the research of newer surgical techniques has been highly productive. Minimally invasive surgery, with the goal of reducing recovery time and surgical trauma, has been all the rage among pediatric orthopedic surgeons. Not only do they speed up rehabilitation but they also minimize the complications associated with open surgery, such as infection and scarring. Advanced imaging technologies, coupled with robotic operating devices, enable specialists to achieve more precision in surgical procedures, which in turn leads to improved patient outcomes. With scientists refining these methods, the future of pediatric orthopedic surgery looks even brighter with scope for new developments in treatment modalities (Stroud et al., 2016). In addition to surgery advancements, the addition of biological therapies has been a critical component of pediatric orthopedics. For instance, the application of regenerative medicine, such as stem cell therapy, has a huge scope in the treatment of many musculoskeletal disorders. Such therapies aim to capitalize on the body's own repair mechanisms and thus enable recovery in conditions such as osteogenesis imperfecta and juvenile idiopathic arthritis.

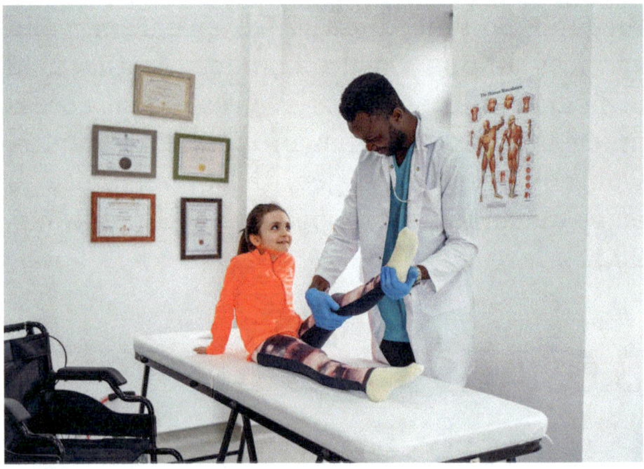

Figure 8.16. Recent advancements in pediatric orthopedic research.

Source: https://external-content.duckduckgo.com/iu/?u=https%3A%2F%2Fmidamericaortho.com%2Ftemplates%2Fyootheme%2Fcache%2FiStock-1306737787-min-8c92d19b.jpeg&f=1&nofb=1&ipt=2e3a2052193451052a7b1f4d228035983173f8579c1494cc56e1336a0f255303.

Research into biologics also intersects with the developing science of gene therapy, promising the possibility of repairing the genetic etiology of orthopedic conditions at the source. With continued research, university and pharmaceutical company partnerships will lead to the development of targeted therapies that meet the needs of pediatric patients in a specifically tailored manner (Sivhugwana, 2021). Furthermore, the role of interdisciplinary research in pediatric orthopedics has increasingly become more critical in dealing with advanced musculoskeletal disorders. Through interdisciplinarity among orthopedists, geneticists, physiotherapists, and others, a greater understanding of the intricate characteristics of such disorders can be obtained. One such example is in the study of the genetic etiology of scoliosis, where efforts have been made through interdisciplinary research to isolate specific markers that can predispose children to spinal deformity. These findings not only direct clinical practice but also enhance patient care through the convenience of earlier detection and intervention methods. The partnership of diverse expertise in such fields is paving the way for novel solutions, ultimately leading to improved quality of life among children when dealing with orthopedic problems (Stroud et al., 2016) (Figure 8.16).

8.6.1. Innovations in Surgical Techniques

The specialty of pediatric orthopedics has witnessed tremendous progress in surgical techniques, with the standard of patient outcomes improving dramatically. Techniques such as minimally invasive surgery (MIS) have gained popularity in recent years, which allow surgeons to manage complex orthopedic pathology in children with minimal trauma to the surrounding tissues. Not only does this yield shorter periods of recovery and less postoperative discomfort, but also less scarring. Through the application of reduced incisions and advanced instrumentation, MIS is attaining precision in procedures such as scoliosis correction and limb alignment. Such technological advancements bring to the forefront the need for modifying surgical methods to suit the personal anatomical and physiological needs of growing pediatric patients and thus foster a culture of constant improvement in surgical therapy (Stroud et al., 2016). Apart from MIS, the application of 3D printing technology in surgery is another thrilling development in pediatric orthopedics.

Surgeons are now able to create patient-specific models and implants, which enhances the process of preoperative planning. Three-dimensional imaging-derived models that are created based on a patient's own anatomy allow for improved visualization of intricate deformity, and therefore, surgical procedures can be optimized to suit individual anatomical variations better. Besides, having customized surgical guides ensures that precision in carrying out complex procedures is possible, leading to enhanced alignment and results, particularly in fracture and joint surgery.

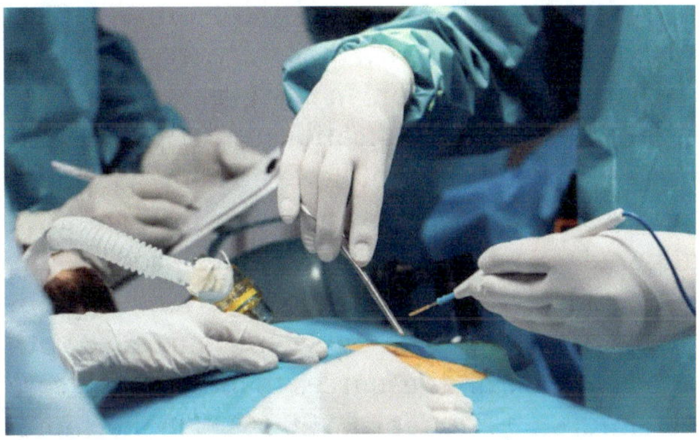

Figure 8.17. The realm of pediatric orthopedics has witnessed remarkable innovations in surgical techniques.

Source: https://drgouravdas.com/wp-content/uploads/2024/10/Innovative-Surgical-Techniques-Used-by-Bhubaneswar-Surgeons-Dr-Gourav-Das-1125x684.webp.

Studies have found that the application of these 3D-printed solutions has already been observed to have vast cost-saving potential, particularly in instances involving complicated cases that require custom implants for children (Tack, 2021). The merging of technology and surgical expertise continues to redefine the practice. Finally, another significant evolution of surgical technique is the use of robotic-assisted surgery in orthopedics for children. Robotic platforms enhance the degrees of freedom and precision of standard surgical instruments, enabling surgeons to better perform difficult procedures. Such technology is of greatest value in the correction of bone deformity or in performing complex joint reconstruction, where precision is paramount. Studies have established that robotic assistance can reduce the incidence of complications and optimize alignment, which is of utmost importance in children because improper alignment can result in long-term disability. The use of robotics in pediatric surgery not only improves procedural processes but also ushers in a new era of orthopedic care that emphasizes safety and efficacy (Stroud et al., 2016). As they continue to evolve, they can shape the future of pediatric orthopedics, eventually enhancing the quality of life of millions of children (Figure 8.17).

8.6.2. Development of New Treatment Protocols

The subspecialty of pediatric orthopedics is experiencing significant development in the development of novel treatment paradigms, driven in large part by the need for improved patient outcomes and the uniqueness of anatomical and physiological variation in children. As advances in medical science continue to unravel the complexities of pediatric musculoskeletal disease, clinicians increasingly are turning to evidence-based medicine to inform their models of care.

The addition of current surgical techniques, including minimally invasive procedures, has proved helpful in reducing recovery and complications. Also, taking up established protocols from adults with respect for variation in children is essential to optimize care. A multidisciplinary team working, including pediatricians, surgeons, and rehabilitation specialists, plays an essential role in refining such treatment protocols to facilitate an integrated approach to managing most orthopedic issues in children. The ongoing quest for new treatment protocols in pediatric orthopedics is also largely driven by the evolution that happens in technology and emerging types of treatment. Advances such as 3D printing facilitate patient-specific guides and implants, which improve surgical precision and outcomes. Developments in regenerative medicine, including the application of stem cells and growth factors, are also being explored to improve healing in complex cases. Development of protocols using these technologies may make for more effective treatments of conditions such as osteogenesis imperfecta and child fractures. With the development of technology, studies targeting the use of these technological advancements in clinical applications are essential. Increased collaboration with industry players and educational institutions fosters an environment in which novel solutions can be expediently tested and executed, enhancing the quality of care provided to younger patients even more.

The development of uniform treatment protocols is also essential for rectifying inequalities of care and ensuring continuity between different healthcare centers. This is particularly relevant in pediatric orthopedics, where variability in treatment technique can lead to different patient experiences and outcomes. Systematic review of the literature, in addition to clinical opinion, can enable the derivation of comprehensive guidelines that address a range of conditions and modes of treatment. Implementation of such guidelines should include consideration not just of clinical efficacy but also of matters such as safety, patient comfort, and ultimate function. In addition, the use of data-driven strategies to measure patient outcomes can reduce the process of refining such protocols with the passage of time. Such an evidence-based strategy is consistent with continued work in the medical sector aimed at enhancing the provision of care through the application of insights drawn from diverse sources, including those presented in Oliva et al. (2015) and Stroud et al. (2016) , towards refining the arena of pediatric orthopedic care.

8.6.3. Future Directions in Pediatric Orthopedic Research

Pediatric orthopedic research in the future will be significantly influenced by advancements in imaging technologies. With the increasing demand for precise diagnostic equipment, three-dimensional (3D) imaging technology has an enormous potential to further improve patient outcomes. According to a systematic review, 3D imaging enhances diagnosis and preoperative planning in complex fractures of limbs, typically due to high-energy trauma. For instance, CT scans enhance diagnostic accuracy by 32% compared to traditional two-dimensional techniques, while MRI has further improved soft tissue evaluation in 28% of cases. More significantly, the application of 3D printing in this regard has been found to be beneficial, with a success rate of 94% in improving postoperative alignment. With these technologies progressing, they will certainly transform the landscape of pediatric orthopedics, equipping surgeons with effective tools and resources to improve the care of children (Vera et al., 2024). Furthermore, the application of robotics in child orthopedic surgery presents another field of research and clinical practice. The creation of robotic-assisted surgical devices initiated a paradigm shift, enabling procedures that require high precision and control. Studies have indicated that such systems not only increase the level of skills among surgeons but also provide scope for minimally invasive operations, thereby reducing recovery times in children. The da Vinci Surgical System is a great case in point of such a technological transformation, with the ability to offer enhanced visualization and articulation in complex procedures. However, robotics is expensive, as adoption is inhibited by the challenges of cost, training requirements, and regulatory barriers. With increasing field, there will also be a requirement for ongoing research to understand the long-term outcome of robotic surgery in pediatric orthopedics, including its potential to act as a solution to surgical autonomy ethical dilemmas (Pushpan & Chinmaya, 2024). Finally, the future of pediatric orthopedic research also must involve research emphasis on personalized medicine and genetics' role in musculoskeletal disorders. The growing field of genomics has the possibility of treatment strategies being tailored individually based on genetic profiles, which maximizes the effectiveness of interventions. Investigations into the genes responsible for conditions such as scoliosis and limb deformities can lead to earlier disease diagnoses and prevention. Machine learning and artificial intelligence can also assist in exploring large data sets for correlations between the outcomes of treatment and genetic factors. By the implementation of these innovations, the pediatric orthopedic field can make its way towards a more empathetic understanding of how to optimize care and redirect health trajectories of musculoskeletal patients in children. Cumulatively, these directions of the future are a positive trend for research that seeks to optimize clinical and quality of care in pediatric orthopedics (Figure 8.18).

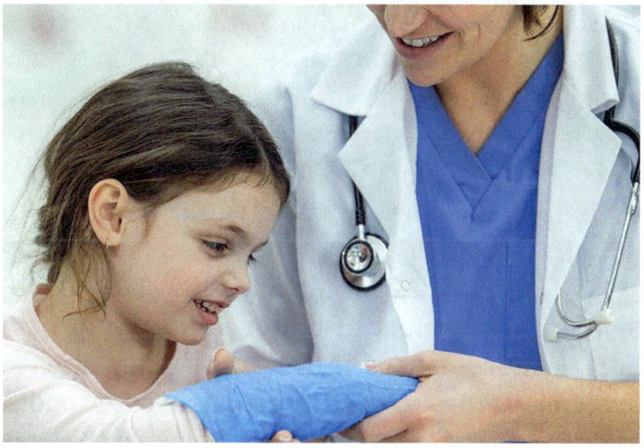

Figure 8.18. Future directions in pediatric orthopedic research.

Source: https://umanitoba.ca/medicine/sites/medicine/files/styles/3x2_900w/public/2023-05/Pediatric-Orthopedic-Surgery-Fellowship-secondaryImage.jpg?itok=bBdSpRDo.

SUMMARY

It is necessary to emphasize the significance of a multidimensional approach to managing musculoskeletal disorders among children. The prevalence of cerebral palsy and other such conditions necessitates not only a clear-cut knowledge of orthopedic intervention but also an understanding of developmental nuances. The literature systematic review conducted, as described in earlier analyses, provides an uncomplicated picture of the evolution of treatment modalities since 1994. By continuously refining treatment protocols and guidelines, health practitioners can optimize outcomes for pediatric patients to the point that interventions are not only efficacious but also specifically tailored to the unique needs presented by various orthopedic conditions, such as those discussed in Morris (2002). This commitment to continuous improvement is essential to the advancement of the overall area of pediatric orthopedics and improved patient outcomes. Furthermore, trends in fracture management surgery, particularly for the humerus, indicate the evolving nature of care in pediatric orthopedics. More evidence has documented a significant rise in the surgical management of proximal humerus fractures, albeit in the consistency of fracture severity over time (Hannonen, 2021). Understanding these trends allows clinicians to make evidence-based treatment choices, which will provide the child with the best possible care available, at least with current evidence and technology. This practice development stresses the importance of both surgical and non-surgical treatments, each having its own merits in accordance with the specific conditions of the injury. With the greater development of pediatric orthopedics, these treatment paradigms must evolve to encompass the latest research and surgical methods. Pediatric orthopedics as a whole stands at a turning point, where evidence-based practice, accompanied by enhanced surgical techniques and technology, will be able to offer a better outcome for the patient. Synthesis of vast amounts of information based on studies like those in this essay is crucial in developing effective treatment regimens. Promoting collaboration among professionals in various disciplines, like rehabilitation and surgery, enables practitioners to deliver holistic care that is consistent with the growth phase of young patients. Lastly, continued progress in this area is not only potentially beneficial for the treatment of existing conditions but also for preventing future orthopedic issues, therefore ensuring better long-term health for children (Morris, 2002; Hannonen, 2021).

Pediatric orthopedics has come a long way in personality, dealing with an array of musculoskeletal disorders that present in children and adolescents. Some of the key issues key to this discipline are the understanding of common conditions like fractures, dislocations, and congenital deformities that often need to be treated uniquely because of the nature of a developing musculoskeletal system. Rotator cuff tears, for instance, although classically discovered in adults, are now increasingly recognized in younger individuals. The management of such injuries is controversial, with many methods being experimented with but without a common consensus on the best procedures, as in the analysis of rotator cuff tear management techniques. Pediatric patients also manifest their healing process differently compared to adults, necessitating the need to have methods that are uniquely designed to address both the functionality and the issue of growth in treatment plans (Oliva et al., 2015). Amongst the usual conditions treated in pediatric orthopedic practice, dislocation of the patella stands out for recurrence risk, especially in dynamic young patients. Post-dislocation treatment is typically conservative or surgical, with more recent data being inclined towards surgical preference for recurrence. Literature that summarizes results indicates that surgically treated patients have a far lower rate of recurrent dislocation, based on the analysis of various trials that compared the efficacy of such treatment. Despite the conflicting success rates, literature acknowledges the need for large studies that would elucidate long-term benefits and relative effectiveness of surgical treatment vs. non-surgical treatment modalities in children (Smith et al., 2015). These findings reflect the ongoing quest in pediatric orthopedics to develop good care paths that maximize outcomes and minimize complications. Furthermore, the challenge of generating evidence-based clinical recommendations in pediatric orthopedics indicates an important area for future research. Heterogeneity of outcomes with treatment and the dangers of operating on children necessitate a robust system for assessment and consensus development among clinicians. For instance, while evidence has determined superiority in certain situations for some operations, total quality of evidence is low and calls have been made for properly designed, multi-center trials that adhere to contemporary research standards. The inclusion of expert agreement on intervention descriptions and patient-specific variables is at the forefront of directing future studies. This emphasis on rigorous research and best practice sharing is central to advancing the field and enhancing the quality of care provided to young patients with musculoskeletal disorders (Smith et al., 2015; Oliva et al., 2015).

CLOSER LOOK

PEDIATRIC ORTHOPEDICS

Pediatric orthopedics is a specialized branch of medicine focused on the diagnosis, treatment, and prevention of musculoskeletal disorders in infants, children, and adolescents. Since children's bones, joints, and muscles are still growing, their orthopedic conditions and treatments differ significantly from those of adults. Early diagnosis and timely intervention are crucial to ensure proper growth and long-term mobility. Common pediatric orthopedic conditions include congenital deformities such as clubfoot, developmental dysplasia of the hip, limb length discrepancies, scoliosis, flat feet, and growth plate injuries. Children are also prone to fractures and sports-related injuries due to high physical activity levels. Diagnosis typically involves physical examination, growth assessment, and imaging techniques like X-rays and ultrasound. Treatment options range from non-surgical approaches such as braces, casts, physiotherapy, and corrective exercises to surgical interventions when necessary. Pediatric orthopedic surgeons carefully consider growth potential while planning treatment to avoid long-term complications. Rehabilitation and follow-up care are essential to monitor development and ensure successful outcomes. Preventive care plays a vital role, including injury prevention education, proper sports training, safe play environments, and early screening programs. Overall, pediatric orthopedics aims to promote healthy musculoskeletal development, restore function, and improve the quality of life for children, enabling them to grow, move, and participate actively in daily and recreational activities.

REFERENCES

1. Aber, R. (2016). Improving health literacy: Parental medical decisions regarding lower extremity amputations. https://core.ac.uk/download/84402968.pdf (accessed on 26th June 2025).
2. Goyal, R. K., Meena, M. K., Agarwal, M., & Sathiyaseelan, N. (2023). Assessing the factors that influence a recurrence of congenital talipes equinovarus in children treated with the Ponseti method . *International Journal of Research in Orthopaedics*, *9*(3), 565–571. https://doi.org/10.18203/issn.2455-4510.IntJResOrthop20231184(accessed on 26th June 2025).
3. Smith, T. O., Gaukroger, A., Metcalfe, A., & Hing, C. B. (2023). Surgical versus non-surgical interventions for treating patellar dislocation. *The Cochrane database of systematic reviews*, *1*(1), CD008106. https://doi.org/10.1002/14651858.CD008106.pub4 (accessed on 26th June 2025).
4. White, K. K., Jester, A., Bache, C. E., Harmatz, P. R., Shediac, R., Thacker, M. M., & Mackenzie, W. G. (2014). Orthopedic management of the extremities in patients with Morquio A syndrome. *Journal of children's orthopaedics*, *8*(4), 295–304. https://doi.org/10.1007/s11832-014-0601-4(accessed on 26th June 2025).
5. Baker, R. J. (2006). Gait analysis methods in rehabilitation. https://core.ac.uk/download/1665518.pdf (accessed on 26th June 2025).
6. Barnes, D., Bedard, T., Cachecho, S., Dahan-Oliel, N., et al. (2019). International multidisciplinary collaboration toward an annotated definition of arthrogryposis multiplex congenita. https://core.ac.uk/download/361285701.pdf (accessed on 26th June 2025).
7. Stroud, C., Dmitriev, I., Kashentseva, E., Bryan, J. N., Curiel, D. T., Rindt, H., Reinero, C., Henry, C. J., Bergman, P. J., Mason, N. J., Gnanandarajah, J. S., Engiles, J. B., Gray, F., Laughlin, D., Gaurnier-Hausser, A., Wallecha, A., Huebner, M., Paterson, Y., O'Connor, D., Treml, L. S., ... Harman, R. J. (2016). A One Health overview, facilitating advances in comparative medicine and translational research. *Clinical and translational medicine*, *5*(Suppl 1), 26. https://doi.org/10.1186/s40169-016-0107-4(accessed on 26th June 2025).
8. Negrini, S., Minozzi, S., Bettany-Saltikov, J., Chockalingam, N., Grivas, T. B., Kotwicki, T., Maruyama, T., Romano, M., & Zaina, F. (2015). Braces for idiopathic scoliosis in adolescents. *The Cochrane database of systematic reviews*, *2015*(6), CD006850. https://doi.org/10.1002/14651858.CD006850.pub3(accessed on 26th June 2025).
9. Oliva F, Piccirilli E, Bossa M, et al. I.S.Mu.L.T - Rotator Cuff Tears Guidelines. *Muscles Ligaments Tendons J.* 2016;5(4):227-263. Published 2016 Feb 13. doi:10.11138/mltj/2015.5.4.227 (accessed on 26th June 2025).
10. Stokes, O. M., O'Donovan, E. J., Samartzis, D., Bow, C. H., Luk, K. D., & Cheung, K. M. (2014). Reducing radiation exposure in early-onset scoliosis surgery patients: novel use of ultrasonography to measure lengthening in magnetically-controlled growing rods. *The spine journal : official journal of the North American Spine Society*, *14*(10), 2397–2404. https://doi.org/10.1016/j.spinee.2014.01.039(accessed on 26th June 2025).
11. Morris C. (2002). A review of the efficacy of lower-limb orthoses used for cerebral palsy. *Developmental medicine and child neurology*, *44*(3), 205–211. https://doi.org/10.1017/s0012162201001943(accessed on 26th June 2025).
12. Horn, J., Rasmussen, H., Bukholm, I. R. K., Røise, O., & Terjesen, T. (2021). Compensation claims in pediatric orthopedics in Norway between 2012 and 2018: a nationwide study of

487 patients. *Acta orthopaedica*, *92*(5), 615–620. https://doi.org/10.1080/17453674.2021.1932922 (accessed on 26th June 2025).

13. Vera, M. D. F., Dávila, D. A. D., Valdés, C. A. J., Zambrano, K. N. M., Chimbo, N. de J. P., & Montero, F. G. S. (2024). 3D imaging techniques for the diagnosis and surgical planning of complex limb fractures: a systematic review. *International Journal of Research in Orthopaedics, 11*(1), 178–185. https://doi.org/10.18203/issn.2455-4510.IntJResOrthop20243418(accessed on 26th June 2025).
14. Cooper, R., Heath, E. L., Pappas, E., Pinczewski, L. A., et al. (2018). 5-year survival of pediatric anterior cruciate ligament reconstruction with living donor hamstring tendon grafts. https://core.ac.uk/download/213607878.pdf (accessed on 26th June 2025).
15. Mortier, D. & De Ridder, K. (2008). Flexible intramedullary nailing in the treatment of diaphyseal fractures of the femur in preschool children. https://core.ac.uk/download/55836013.pdf (accessed on 26th June 2025).
16. Jones, L., Drobe, B., González-Méijome, J. M., Gray, L., Kratzer, T., Newman, S., Nichols, J. J., Ohlendorf, A., Ramdass, S., Santodomingo-Rubido, J., Schmid, K. L., Tan, D., Tan, K. O., Vera-Diaz, F. A., Wong, Y. L., Gifford, K. L., & Resnikoff, S. (2019). IMI - Industry Guidelines and Ethical Considerations for Myopia Control Report. *Investigative ophthalmology & visual science, 60*(3), M161–M183. https://doi.org/10.1167/iovs.18-25963(accessed on 26th June 2025).
17. Farre, A., & Rapley, T. (2017). The New Old (and Old New) Medical Model: Four Decades Navigating the Biomedical and Psychosocial Understandings of Health and Illness. *Healthcare (Basel, Switzerland), 5*(4), 88. https://doi.org/10.3390/healthcare5040088(accessed on 26th June 2025).
18. Farid, N. (2023). Cross cultural adaptation and validation of a self-reporting tool to assess health-related quality of life for Egyptians with extremity bone sarcomas in childhood or adolescence. https://core.ac.uk/download/553327347.pdf (accessed on 26th June 2025).
19. Hannonen, J. (2021). Humerus fractures in children: Treatment trends and surgical techniques. https://core.ac.uk/download/628861958.pdf (accessed on 26th June 2025).
20. Slavens, Brooke A. and Harris, Gerald F., "Biomechanics" (2012). *Biomedical Engineering Faculty Research and Publications*. 21. https://epublications.marquette.edu/bioengin_fac/21(accessed on 26th June 2025).
21. Kinney, A. L. (2007). National scientific facilities and their science impact on non-biomedical research. http://arxiv.org/abs/0705.1797 (accessed on 26th June 2025).
22. Krishna, B., & Pathak, N. (2020). Perioperative management of geriatric patients for orthopedic surgeries. *International Journal of Research in Orthopaedics, 6*(2), 427–434. https://doi.org/10.18203/issn.2455-4510.IntJResOrthop20200749 (accessed on 26th June 2025).
23. Lakhwani, O. P. (2013). Percutaneous method of management of simple bone cyst. https://core.ac.uk/download/pdf/26903648.pdf (accessed on 26th June 2025).
24. Loma Linda University, "2002 - 2003 Bulletin" (2002). School of Allied Health Professions Bulletins. https://scholarsrepository.llu.edu/sahp_bulletin/3 (accessed on 26th June 2025).
25. Lukianenko, D. M. (2017). Substantiation stages of rehabilitation at the patients with meta epiphyseal osteomyelitis. https://core.ac.uk/download/pdf/161864336.pdf (accessed on 26th June 2025).

26. Mustafa, M. S. (2015). A survey on knowledge, attitude & confidence level of disaster management among doctors in Terengganu. https://core.ac.uk/download/154383265.pdf (accessed on 26th June 2025).

27. Pushpan, P., S. P., & Chinmaya, C. (2024). The integration of robotics in surgery: Advancements, challenges, and future prospects. https://core.ac.uk/download/640069977.pdf (accessed on 26th June 2025).

28. Sabharwal, S., & Sabharwal, S. (2018). Growth plate injuries of the lower extremity: Case examples and lessons learned. https://core.ac.uk/download/305124253.pdf (accessed on 26th June 2025).

29. Sivhugwana, Innocentia (2022). Factors related with the functional outcome of patients who sustained tibial plateau fractures. Dissertation (MSc (Physiotherapy))--University of Pretoria, 2022. https://core.ac.uk/download/565849089.pdf

30. Tack, P. (2021). The value of medical 3D printing: Hope versus hype. https://core.ac.uk/download/427574228.pdf (accessed on 26th June 2025).

31. Torres Serna, H. (2015). Bibliographic comparison of the treatments in children with flatfoot. https://core.ac.uk/download/43552910.pdf (accessed on 26th June 2025).

32. University of Vermont. (1991). *University of Vermont, College of Medicine Bulletin*. https://core.ac.uk/download/51066276.pdf (accessed on 26th June 2025).

33. Wihak, A. A. (2016). Preliminary study comparing parent and child functioning by intervention for adolescent idiopathic scoliosis. https://open.bu.edu/bitstream/2144/16112/1/Wihak_bu_0017N_11107.pdf (accessed on 26th June 2025).

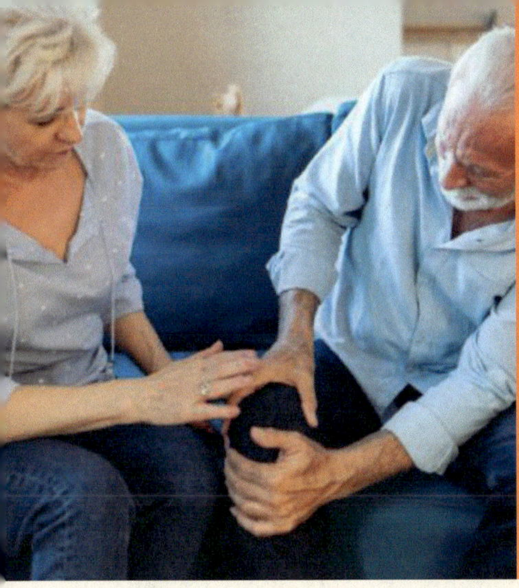

Chapter 9

GERIATRIC ORTHOPEDICS

Contents

Introduction to Geriatric Orthopedics 267
9.1. Common Orthopedic Conditions in the Elderly 271
9.2. Risk Factors for Orthopedic Issues in the Elderly 276
9.3. Diagnostic Approaches in Geriatric Orthopedics 279
9.4. Treatment Options for Geriatric Orthopedic Patients 283
9.5. Challenges in Geriatric Orthopedic Care 287
9.6. Innovations and Advances in Geriatric Orthopedics 290
Summary 295
References 298

Introduction to Geriatric Orthopedics

Geriatric orthopedics has emerged as a critical specialty that treats the individual musculoskeletal problems of elderly persons. The aged population increases with rising age-conditioned orthopedic diseases such as fractures and joint degeneration, and accordingly, the demand for specialty treatment. Geriatric orthopedics is a multidisciplinary discipline that includes expertise from orthopedics, geriatrics, rehabilitation, and nursing to treat the disorders comprehensively. Research has demonstrated the importance of personalized interventions considering both the physiological changes and the comorbidities typical in older patients. Therefore, practitioners are increasingly recognizing the necessity for care systems addressing both mobility and quality of life in the older patient, a shift towards more holistic treatment of orthopedic conditions in the older population. In Malta, the historical context of geriatric care reinforces the cultivation of services most specifically targeted towards this segment. Until 1991, geriatric medicine in the country was largely reserved for long-stay care institutions, such as St. Vincent de Paul Hospital. Specialty services provision in Zammit Clapp Hospital was a core milestone in terms of providing solutions to acute medical problems in elderly patients requiring immediate treatment and rehabilitation, usually referred to St. Luke's Hospital. This shift places a value on specialistic healthcare models that identify not just acute medical problems but also rehabilitation processes essential for elderly patients recovering from orthopedic trauma or surgeries.

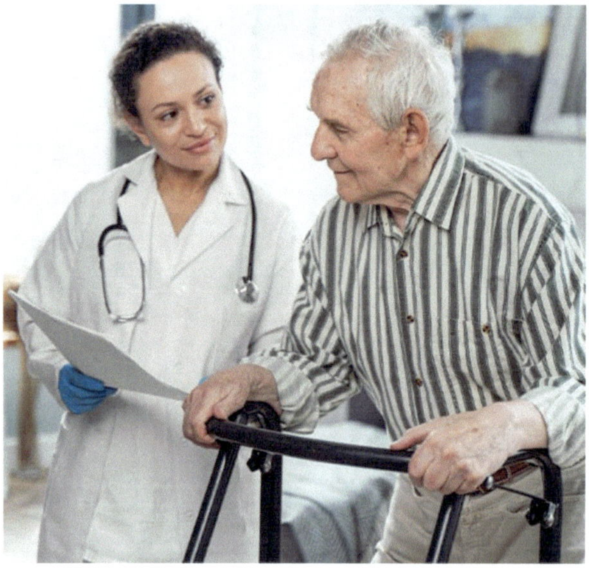

Figure 9.1. The field of geriatric orthopedics.

Source: https://suryahospitals.com/speciality/65648d0fef501Orthopedics---Expertise-Geriatric-Orthopedics_1.jpg.

These developments are significant for the improvement of both the clinical outcomes and overall well-being of elderly individuals. Furthermore, the collaboration among healthcare professionals in geriatric orthopedics enhances the whole treatment of complex cases with elderly patients. Occupational therapy, physiotherapy, and specialist nursing staff work in unison to form a multidisciplinary treatment team, provided that all aspects of a patient's recuperation are addressed. For instance, the integrated interventions of specialties such as occupational therapy and physiotherapy provide the essential support to ensure physical mobility and functional autonomy. Significantly, intervention by orthogeriatric specialist nurses also demonstrates the emerging awareness of nursing contribution in this context, which is increasingly being recognized by clinical settings for their expertise in caring for geriatric patients. This inter-professional partnership not only ensures smooth provision of patient care but also enhances educational opportunities for healthcare workers of geriatric orthopedics, as exemplified through collaboration in the field (Riemen & Hutchison, 2016) (Figure 9.1).

Definition and Scope of Geriatric Orthopedics

Geriatric orthopedics is the orthopedic specialty dealing with the care of musculoskeletal conditions in elderly patients. The specialty's definition is beyond merely simple surgical intervention and encompasses care strategies as a whole tailored to meet the particular physiological and psychosocial needs of the elderly. With advancing age, there are changes that profoundly influence bone density, muscle strength, and balance, which predispose them to fractures and injuries. Thus, geriatric orthopedics is not only interested in surgical intervention such as fracture fixation and replacement arthroplasty but also prevention and rehabilitation measures that enhance quality of life and mobility in elderly patients. This multi-disciplinary venture aims to alleviate the cause of age-related disease, hence ensuring holistic treatment to geriatric patients as per their individual health requirements. Geriatric orthopedics providentially overlaps with the increased incidence of osteoporotic fractures and musculoskeletal conditions in geriatric populations. Treatment and disease prevention are being met within this discipline through pharmacologic and non-pharmacologic interventions. For instance, more recent systematic reviews of literature have proved the efficacy of structured exercise programs, with emphasis on progressive resistance exercise, in preventing falls and consequent fractures among older people following hip fracture surgery. In addition, fracture liaison services with multidisciplinary management have also proved to reduce refracture rates significantly, reflecting the necessity of multidisciplinary models of geriatric orthopedic care (Wilson et al., 2020).

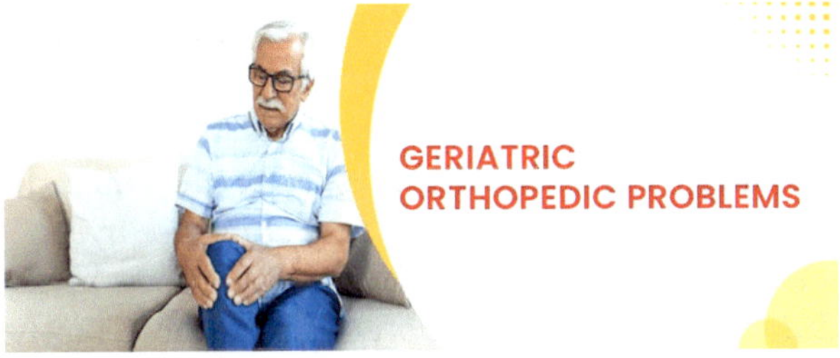

Figure 9.2. Geriatric orthopedics is a specialized branch of orthopedic medicine.

Source: https://external-content.duckduckgo.com/iu/?u=https%3A%2F%2Fi.pinimg.com%2Foriginals%2Fd4%2F47%2F81%2Fd447817ed21ae5d81ecae35783f749d6.png&f=1&nofb=1&ipt=7c2f9496061f6f74bc997e1aaa63e5c1138eb9c8a9acd1d5711620a3e3908b1a.

By tackling comprehensive treatment plans including patient education, exercise, and community support, geriatric orthopedics not only addresses short-term health problems but fosters long-term wellness for its patients. As the field expands, it is more important than ever to establish successful measurement and assessment tools that can further guide clinical practice and research in geriatric orthopedics. One of the critical domains is standing balance assessment, a key competency for mobility and prevention of falls in older populations. From the work of consensus by experts, there has emerged identification of a core set of standard outcomes for measurement of standing balance, utilizing validated instruments such as the Berg Balance Scale and the Mini Balance Evaluation Systems Test (Sibley et al., 2015). These initiatives constitute a significant step towards clinical evaluation standardization, hence increasing the efficacy and reliability of interventions. Last but not least, through the inclusion of evidence-based methods in geriatric orthopedic practice, experts can assist in developing improved patient outcomes, such that the unique problems of older adults are properly addressed in healthcare (Figure 9.2).

Importance of Orthopedic Care in the Elderly

The intricacy of geriatric patients illustrates the great premium of specialist orthopedic service in geriatrics. As the population ages, the prevalence of musculoskeletal illnesses like fractures, arthritis, and osteoporosis rises proportionally. All these share a significant impact on the quality of life by limiting mobility and independence in older persons. Effective orthopedic intervention can alleviate suffering, restore function, and contribute to overall health. For example, surgeries, such as joint replacements, were found to enhance geriatric patients' mobility and satisfaction with life, showing the importance of orthopedics in dealing with their health. Moreover, personalized rehabilitation programs, often initiated in conjunction with surgery, have been found to encourage faster recovery and return to normal activities, pointing to the need for a comprehensive treatment plan in geriatric orthopedics, one that addresses not only physical but also psychosocial healing. Preventive orthopedic care among the elderly is more significant, as care can avert the potential for injury and enhance health outcomes. Falls prevention and promotion of bone health by way of exercise and diet are included in such preventive care. Being a chief determiner of morbidity in older individuals, orthopedic care is not only curative in orientation but also involves measures designed to support the elderly in maintaining their functionality and independence. Physiotherapists and occupational therapists, among other practitioners, play a vital role to play in designing programs tailored to each patient's abilities and needs. Such multidisciplinary programs ensure not only that elderly patients receive necessary surgery or medical intervention but also benefit from worldwide management regimes opposing impending danger before they advance into more complex issues, echoing the preventive nature of orthopedic intervention among elderly populations. Additionally, the complexity of medical comorbidities that often accompany elderly patients necessitates an integrated orthopedic care model to enhance surgical outcomes and avoid complications. Geriatric patients usually present with co-morbidities such as cardiovascular disease, diabetes, and mental impairment that complicate treatment. A multimodal strategy, typically involving experts from various fields, such as orthogeriatric experts, is critical in managing such complexity. Such a collaborative approach is evidenced by effective application of multidisciplinary teams of care with an emphasis on holistic evaluation and tailored intervention programs. Research has established that the effect of such teams is to significantly improve the patients' outcomes, reduce hospital stay, and decrease rates of readmission following orthopedic procedures in the elderly (Cumming et al., 2014; Riemen & Hutchison, 2016). Hence, a comprehensive understanding of both the physiological and psychosocial processes involved with aging is tantamount to optimizing orthopedic care and making it not only essential but imperative in the practice of geriatric medicine.

Overview of Common Conditions Treated

Geriatric orthopedics treats a spectrum of common conditions that have a major effect on the older person's quality of life. The most prevalent condition is osteoarthritis, which is characterized by cartilage and underlying bone degeneration in a joint, producing pain and stiffness that interfere with activities of daily living. Clinical care is usually a combination of non-pharmacological and pharmacological interventions, such as physical therapy, to control pain and improve joint function. Additionally, fractures, particularly hip fractures, are a chronic condition faced by the elderly due to bone density loss. Certain surgical interventions, e.g., hip arthroplasty, may be necessary to restore mobility and independence. The conditions should be recognized as they not only impact individual patients but also add to the burden of healthcare and require a multidisciplinary approach towards orthopedic treatment of the elderly (Lau et al., 2015). Another exceedingly prevalent condition in elderly orthopedics is osteoporosis, which is characterized by the loss of bone mass and density, thus increasing the risk of fracture. Osteoporosis is usually not diagnosed until a fracture is present, and this underscores the importance of preventive screening in the elderly. The treatment regimens are usually lifestyle modification, e.g., dietary change rich in calcium and vitamin D, along with medications designed to slow the loss of bone. Integration of rehabilitation interventions, such as physical therapy, is crucial to muscle strengthening and balance, which contribute to the prevention of falls and fractures. Management of osteoporosis holistically not only includes prevention of fractures but also rehabilitation and maximization of functional outcomes after injury, demonstrating how these treatments are interconnected to maximize quality of life in geriatric patients (Gullà et al., 2013). Also, involvement of joint replacement has become a common mode of treatment increasingly for the elderly suffering from extensive joint degeneration, mainly of the hip and spine. This kind of operation is done for pain relief and restoration of functional mobility when conservative interventions are insufficient. Rehabilitation following an operation is extremely crucial as it involves unique physical training to ensure healing and restore strength. However, the age-related decline and comorbidities in elderly patients necessitate a tailored process of rehabilitation. In this regard, it is essential that a multidisciplinary team comprising occupational therapists, physiotherapists, and surgeons work in harmony to optimize their treatment results. Given the extensive implications for patient autonomy and overall well-being, geriatric orthopedics is as concerned with the surgery as with the entire process of rehabilitation to optimize the outcome in aged patients (Lau et al., 2015) (Figure 9.3).

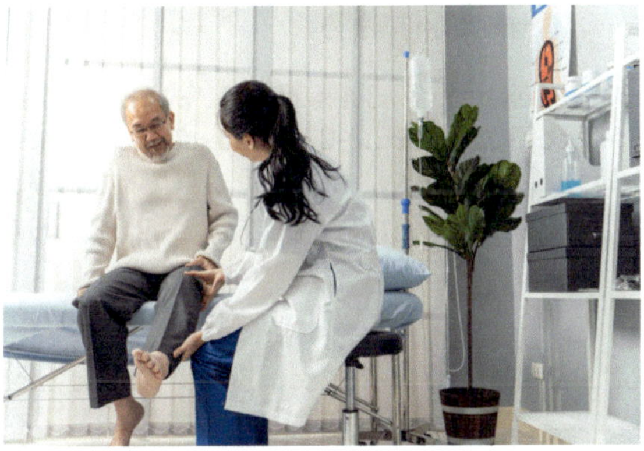

Figure 9.3. In geriatric orthopedics, a variety of common conditions are treated.

Source: https://wp04-media.cdn.ihealthspot.com/wp-content/uploads/sites/115/2023/12/iStock-1401424620-1-768x512.jpg.

9.1. Common Orthopedic Conditions in the Elderly

With an aging population, the prevalence of orthopedic conditions is significantly increased, with resultant debilitation. The most common conditions among older adults include osteoarthritis, osteoporosis, and fractures. Osteoarthritis, which is the loss of cartilage and bone within the joints, can significantly restrict mobility and quality of life. Gradual cartilage loss leads to pain and stiffness, particularly in weight-bearing joints such as the knees and hips. Additionally, osteoporosis causes reduced bone density with possible fractures in patients with a history of falls or who are on drugs that promote further loss of bone. All of these conditions affect physical well-being but also cause declining mental well-being through limitation of social interaction and independence. These older patients are also at higher risk of sustaining fractures due to falls, complicated in many cases by illnesses like osteoporosis. Fractures, especially hip fractures, can lead to severe complications, including longer hospitalization, loss of independence, and increased mortality. Older individuals have multiple comorbidities, which complicate surgical convalescence and rehabilitation. Older patients were, in a cross-sectional study of McGann Hospital, often classified as bed blockers and were found to have high dependency and cognitive impairment with large rehabilitation and discharge problems, evidenced by low Barthel scores (Kumar et al., 2010). This highlights the importance of geriatric assessment and rehabilitation in a community environment as part of comprehensive orthopedic disorder management in order to facilitate recovery and enhance quality of life. Moreover, physical and mental health interaction cannot be overstressed. Mental deterioration, particularly common in the elderly, typically makes orthopedic condition management more difficult. They are prone to not following rehabilitation protocols or being unaware of their postoperative care needs, hence undermining recovery outcomes. The evaluation of patient cognitive abilities at McGann Hospital indicated the universality of low cognitive capacity, hence making their rehabilitation even more complicated (Kumar et al., 2010). Effective interventions, such as intersectoral interventions that integrate medical treatment and community support services, can mitigate the impact of these effects by stimulating both physical recovery and mental activity, aiming ultimately for the improvement in overall quality of life of this high-risk group (Figure 9.4).

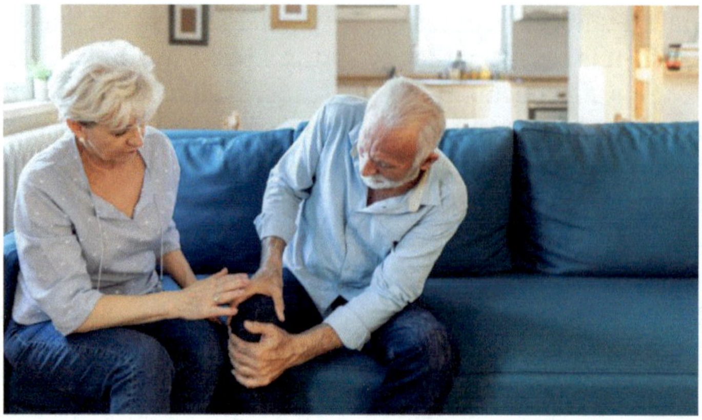

Figure 9.4. The prevalence of orthopedic conditions significantly increases.

Source: https://external-content.duckduckgo.com/iu/?u=https%3A%2F%2Fwww.lifebing.com%2Fwp-content%2Fuploads%2F2023%2F07%2FCommon-Orthopedic-Conditions-Treatment-.jpg&f=1&nofb=1&ipt=372e78159d7d08b448c7bd07691177fa0ffa785ab43a19bca512f161eab62831.

9.1.1. Osteoporosis and Its Implications

The prevalence of osteoporosis in elderly populations has significant implications for individual health as well as public health infrastructures. Osteoporosis is characterized by low bone mass with a high risk of fracture, particularly of the hip, wrist, and spine.

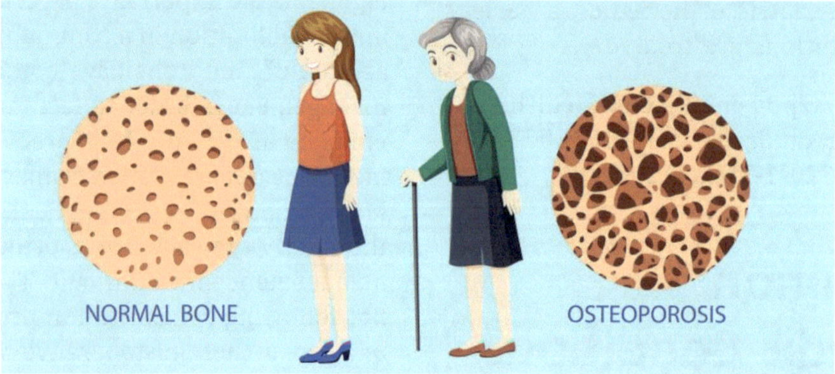

Figure 9.5. The prevalence of osteoporosis in geriatric populations presents significant implications.

Source: https://external-content.duckduckgo.com/iu/?u=https%3A%2F%2Fdenpedia.com%2Fwp-content%2Fuploads%2F2023%2F10%2FiStock-1474048028-e1696567001635-920x398.jpg&f=1&nofb=1&ipt=fa46d38b62d600743a64ce8857a5a44fe8797e7e87e2967c9bc5dd132885411a.

The World Health Organization recognizes osteoporosis as a significant issue due to its association with increased morbidity and mortality among the elderly. Osteoporosis is also a major cause of fractures with resulting debilitating morbidity, including prolonged hospitalization, disability, and diminished quality of life. In this group of people, the economic cost of osteoporosis necessitates urgent attention to prevention. Prevention involves lifestyle modification in the form of increased physical activity and nutritional interventions that are necessary to improve bone health and the prevention of fractures. The latest research suggests that osteoporosis and cognitive impairment in the form of dementia share a common pathological connection. All the research is indicative of the same risk factors and nutritional deficits contributing to both diseases, such as vitamins D and K deficiency and the influence of the APOE4 allele on fracture susceptibility (Downey et al., 2017). This common attribute has significant implications for orthopedic geriatrics since the physical and cognitive complexity of managing osteoporosis sufferers needs to be considered by professionals. More investigation into the interplay between these two conditions needs to be undertaken, with particular reference to reversing malnutrition and enhancing the levels of vitamins in susceptible individuals. Without sophisticated awareness of such correlations, treatment planning may neglect important considerations of patient management with the potential to exacerbate both skeletal and cerebral decline. Furthermore, the implementation of successful falls and fractures prevention measures has become a public health priority. The synergistic collaboration of bodies such as the European Union Geriatric Medicine Society and the International Osteoporosis Foundation has emphasized the necessity for multidisciplinary approaches in terms of bringing fall prevention together with fracture liaison services (Blain et al., 2016). The strategies are implemented not only to manage existing osteoporotic conditions but also to decrease the incidence of falls and subsequent fractures among the older population proactively. By integrating evaluation and management protocols into various healthcare environments, geriatric orthopedic providers can significantly minimize the individual and social burden of osteoporosis. Finally, the prevention as well as treatment of the physical and cognitive consequences of osteoporosis and falls will enhance the quality of care and health outcomes for older patients (Figure 9.5).

9.1.2. Hip Fractures and Their Management

Amongst the many health issues the elderly are faced with, hip fracture is a significant concern in the subspecialty of geriatric orthopedics. The fractures are typically caused by low-energy trauma, which emphasizes the prevalence of osteoporosis in the elderly. Evidence indicates that osteoporotic hip fractures not only have immediate medical consequences but long-term ones as well, including higher rates of secondary fractures and mortality (Cuschieri et al., 2016). The impacts affect not only individual patients but also put considerable economic burdens on healthcare systems. The estimated cost of these fractures in hospitals and associated healthcare can be exorbitant, proclaiming the need for appropriate management measures (Cuschieri et al., 2016). Therefore, addressing the management of hip fractures is essential in avoiding their multifaceted impacts on geriatric patients as well as healthcare systems. Over the past decade, the establishment and implementation of multidisciplinary geriatric fracture programs (GFP) have become a promising strategy for optimizing outcomes in patients with hip fractures. These programs emphasize an interdisciplinary model of care, attempting to organize the care process from the emergency department (ED) to recovery. Evidence has shown that patients enrolled in GFP had significantly improved results for pain management; ED patients who received *fascia iliaca* compartment blocks and acetaminophen reduced their opioid consumption and total pain levels significantly. Additionally, the first analgesic administration time was delayed, hence enhancing the initial care experience. These advances ensure that a therapeutic process of treatment, which can resolve acute problems, can enhance the quality of life in geriatric patients struggling with the nuances of recovery from hip fractures. Despite improvements in clinical management and pain relief, long-term management of hip fractures in the geriatric patient remains the priority. Evidence suggests that the early implementation of anti-osteoporotic therapy, i.e., bisphosphonates, following surgical treatment can yield immense benefit in the form of lowered re-fracture rates and all-cause mortality (Cuschieri et al., 2016). Accurate coordination of follow-up for patients with the incorporation of these therapeutic regimens is important to prevent future fractures. An ongoing focus on prevention and management could both decrease the social and economic costs of hip fractures and return patients to function and independence. As geriatric orthopedics continues to develop, a dual focus on prevention and short-term post-operative management alongside long-term management will be critical to maximizing outcomes in this vulnerable population (Figure 9.6).

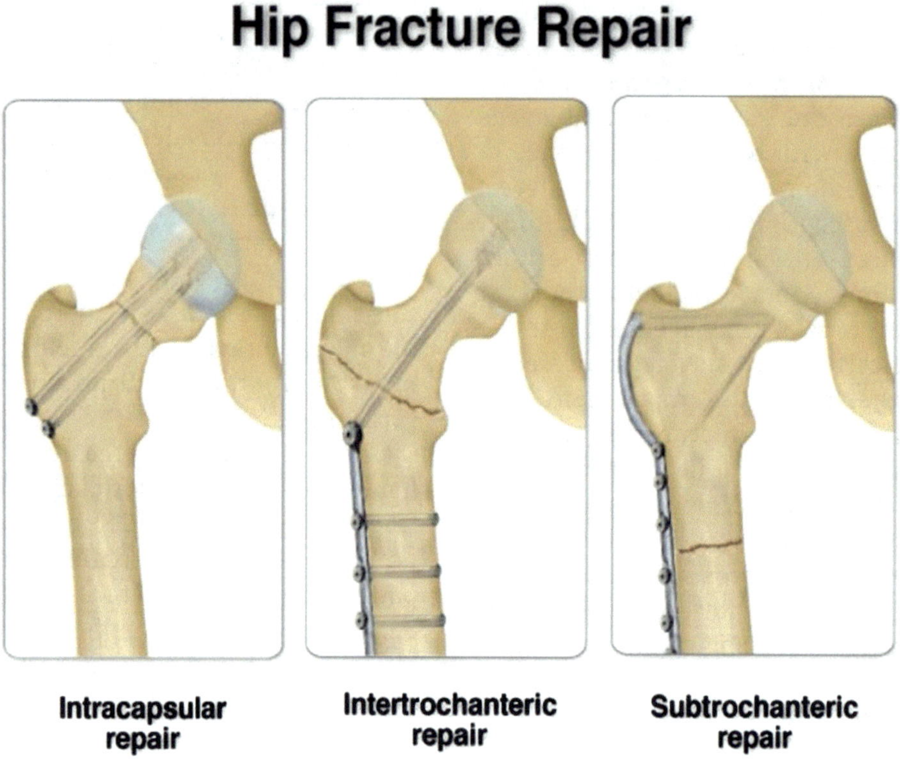

Figure 9.6. Hip fractures and their management.

Source: https://external-content.duckduckgo.com/iu/?u=https%3A%2F%2Fmendmyhip.com%2F_img%2Fhip-intertrochanteric-fracture-repair.jpg&f=1&nofb=1&ipt=59fd7b7abd1272d5131a5d38867eacdd89191bf9e8fd93ff3d7fc995faf24bd2.

9.1.3 Arthritis and Joint Disorders

Arthritis and joint disease constitute a serious issue in geriatric orthopedics. An increase in conditions such as osteoarthritis among aging populations also increases, with consequent debilitating effects on mobility and quality of life among older individuals. Knee osteoarthritis is particularly common, with studies indicating a prevalence of 14% in rural settings and 6% in urban areas in India, pointing towards the commonality of this degenerative joint condition (Sudheer & Jayaprakash, 2017). The clinical relevance of knee osteoarthritis is considerable, typically necessitating interventions of conservative measures such as physical therapy and drugs to more invasive interventions such as joint replacement. Understanding the multifaceted character of arthritis in the elderly is essential for healthcare providers to provide effective, tailor-made treatment modalities addressing physical and also psychosocial requirements of the patients in orthopedic wards. Treatment of arthritis has undergone a revolutionary shift, with improvements in both pharmacologic and non-pharmacologic therapies. As a case in point, intra-articular hyaluronic acid (IAHA) injections are an emerging therapy option for symptom management of knee osteoarthritis. Research confirms that one injection of IAHA can be linked with dramatic pain and functional gain, as evidenced by a clinically important improvement in WOMAC scores among patients (Sudheer & Jayaprakash, 2017). These findings support further exploration of additional new therapies to enhance the quality of life and functional independence among patients. Besides, as geriatric patients tend to have comorbidities, treatment algorithms need to be prescribed in such a way that minimizes side effects and optimizes results. Proper knowledge of treatment modalities for practitioners managing geriatric arthritic patients in the orthopedic field is thus required. Apart from standard surgical and drug treatment, psychological treatment is being noticed more and more for its use in enhancing post-operative results in individuals who undergo joint replacement due to osteoarthritis. Research has shown that the integration of psychological assistance into treatment protocols has beneficial effects, varying by operation type and location, thereby fulfilling the crucial emotional and mental health components of rehabilitation. It is these integrative approaches that underscore the importance of addressing arthritis both as a physiological disorder and as a multifaceted condition involving the complete welfare of an individual. With the development of the field of geriatric orthopedics, the incorporation of psychological considerations into treatment programs will play a key role in establishing comprehensive care that is responsive to the unique needs of the elderly afflicted with arthritis and joint disease (Figure 9.7).

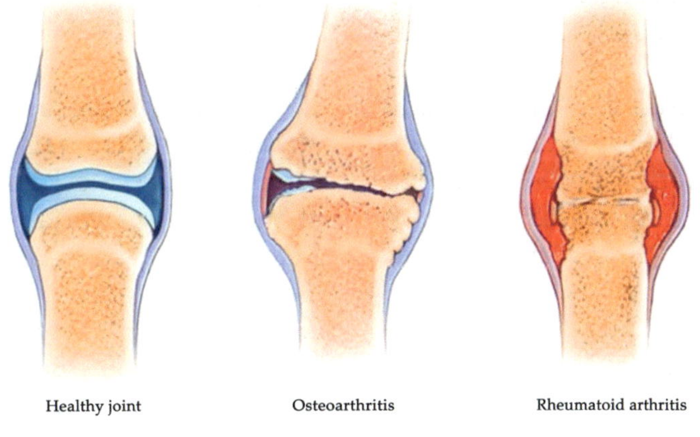

Figure 9.7. Arthritis and joint disorders represent a substantial challenge in geriatric orthopedics.

Source: https://external-content.duckduckgo.com/iu/?u=https%3A%2F%2Fwww.mayoclinic.org%2F-%2Fmedia%2Fkcms%2Fgbs%2Fpatient-consumer%2Fimages%2F2013%2F11%2F15%2F17%2F44%2Fds01122_ds00020_im03689_mcdc7_arthritis_typesthu_jpg.jpg&f=1&nofb=1&ipt=289dbc963ef29db169edd34986b0c01d32107bbd8b6ccd97a6d93ccf5d407b87.

9.2. Risk Factors for Orthopedic Issues in the Elderly

As individuals age, the prevalence of orthopedic disorders increases considerably, often due to a culmination of risk factors, which are particularly common in advanced age. The key stimulus is osteoporosis, when there is decreased bone density and increased fragility. Osteoporotic fractures, and particularly hip fractures, most often follow falls, which become more common in elderly individuals due to impaired balance, coordination, and muscular strength. Physical limitation is only the tip of the iceberg with respect to the impact of these fractures; they often precipitate a cascade of consequent health problems, including increased mortality and substantial costs to the healthcare system. Evidence has shown that re-fracture incidence among older individuals is as high as 11.7% within three years, emphasizing the pressing need for intervention on these simple risk factors along with optimizing follow-up after fracture (Cuschieri et al., 2016). Comorbidities are also another factor of complexity since they tend to go hand-in-hand with aging and may involve diabetes, cardiovascular disease, and cognitive impairment. These conditions aggravate the overall health status of elderly patients and can impair their recovery from orthopedic surgery or treatments. For example, diabetic patients are more likely to experience complications from orthopedic procedures due to poor wound healing and increased risk of infection. In addition, patients with cognitive impairment may be more likely to be nonadherent to rehabilitation programs, thereby inhibiting functional recovery and exacerbating the risk of future falls and fractures. The intricate interaction between the comorbidities and osteoporosis highlights the significance of multifaceted management of the geriatric orthopedic patient with emphasis on personalized tactics that would encompass medical, physical, and social care (Cuschieri et al., 2016). Moreover, social determinants of health play an enormous role in influencing the risk factors of orthopedic disorders in elderly people. Access to healthcare, socioeconomic status, nutrition, and support systems are some of the determinants that have a significant influence on the overall health of aged individuals. For instance, individuals who do not have adequate financial means may be unable to afford necessary drugs, such as bisphosphonates, which have been shown to reduce re-fracture as well as death rates significantly. Research has indicated that early use of anti-osteoporotic medications post-surgery can greatly improve the prognosis in elderly patients. By addressing such social determinants, the healthcare systems can more effectively establish preventive care strategies and intervention schemes to reduce the prevalence of orthopedic issues among the elderly, ultimately enhancing their quality of life and reducing costs associated with repeat fractures and hospitalization.

9.2.1. Age-Related Physiological Changes

The aging process brings with it deep physiological alterations that exert a tremendous impact on musculoskeletal well-being, which is at the heart of geriatric orthopedics studies. Among these alterations, bone densification loss is particularly notable, leading to fractures and osteoporosis becoming more probable in older populations. Bone mineralization loss is largely caused by endocrine imbalances, poor nutrition, and physical inactivity, all of which are common among the elderly. As bone density drops, bones become more susceptible to injury. This makes surgery more complicated. Muscle loss and weakness or sarcopenia, is also another causative factor that exacerbates mobility and diminishes the overall ability to recover from orthopedic surgery. Therefore, there needs to be a more advanced approach in treatment and rehabilitation, with emphasis on individualized intervention that considers special physiological states of geriatric patients. Also, the cardiovascular and respiratory systems undergo changes, making perioperative care in the elderly more challenging. With aging, changes could include decreased cardiac output, increased vascular resistance, and impaired lung function. These would account for a higher incidence of cardiac and respiratory complications during orthopedic surgery. As a result of the aging population, anesthetic considerations must be altered to offset these vulnerabilities. For instance, the selection of anesthetic agents must account for altered pharmacokinetics and pharmacodynamics due to physiological alterations associated with increasing age. Thus, the surgical teams must not only evaluate the orthopedic pathology but also consider the patient's overall health status. This combined strategy is crucial in minimizing risks and optimizing surgical outcomes, like in the example of centenarian patients in the handling of orthopedic procedures (Krishna & Pathak, 2020). Finally, neurophysiological changes also play a critical role in identifying challenges in geriatric orthopedics. Cognitive worsening is prevalent among older patients, resulting in differential responses to anesthesia and pain management. Neuroplasticity with age can alter the perception of pain, and postoperative care is made difficult. Variability demands extreme care in pain management, as the elderly are more susceptible to some of the analgesics and take longer to recover from sedation. Moreover, comorbidities of age commonly make symptom interpretation difficult and impede rehabilitation efforts. Therefore, orthopedic practitioners must perform complete preoperative assessments and close monitoring, with the understanding that the interaction of these age-related physiological alterations significantly contributes to the outcome of patients in geriatric orthopedics (Cumming et al., 2014) (Figure 9.8).

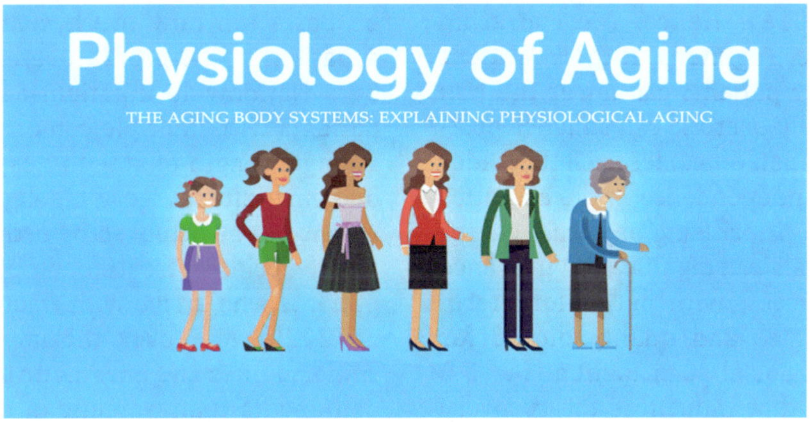

Figure 9.8. The aging process brings about significant physiological changes.

Source: https://external-content.duckduckgo.com/iu/?u=https%3A%2F%2Fnurseslabs.com%2Fwp-content%2Fuploads%2F2016%2F08%2FFeaturedThe-Aging-Body-Systems_-Explaining-Physiological-Aging-768x552.png&f=1&nofb=1&ipt=9865f6d026f47e3ed3f3e6076f7fcd7f91d0649db805dd0aa83b43b4a7f2f961.

9.2.2. Lifestyle Factors and Their Impact

Determinants of lifestyle are particularly significant in the elderly, particularly in geriatric orthopedics. Activity, diet, and social interaction all play their part in determining how musculoskeletal disorders turn out. A good diet with sufficient nutrition, particularly protein and calcium, is also essential for bone health, and this may prevent fractures. Research has established that protein and energy deficits are involved in exacerbating functional outcomes in elderly patients with recovered hip fractures, a factor that underscores the relevance of geriatric nutritional assessment (Blain et al., 2016). Active engagement in physical exercise, including weight-bearing exercises, is also beneficial to bone strength and density, factors vital to preventing falls and consequential injuries. Thus, optimal control of lifestyle factors can enhance recovery profiles and overall well-being in geriatric patients. Exercise plays a two-way role in advancing the welfare of elderly individuals, particularly in the area of orthopedic welfare. Apart from strengthening muscles, exercise also improves equilibrium and coordination, essential for avoiding falls. Falls remain the most common cause of fracture, particularly hip fractures, even in the elderly who may need surgical intervention and lead to prolonged morbidity (Blain et al., 2016). Hence, incorporating tailored exercise regimens into treatment strategies in older patients can lower the risk of falls. Additionally, exercise can enhance post-surgical rehabilitation outcomes such that older patients achieve independence in the activities of daily living. By prioritizing physical activity, health professionals can significantly influence the recovery process, with better long-term functional outcomes and quality of life for older individuals. Social participation is also a basic way of life that influences the recovery and health of older adults as part of geriatric orthopedics. Social interaction and social activity not only maintain emotional and mental well-being but also enhance adherence to regimens of physical training and dietary restriction. Isolation can cause depression and decrease motivation for involvement in rehabilitation exercises, negatively affecting recovery from orthopedic procedures. A study shows that patients with solid social connections are more likely to have increased rates of recovery and better functional capacity following orthopedic intervention (Li et al., 2012). Therefore, the encouragement of social contact and interaction can go a long way in enhancing the rehabilitation process for older patients, affirming the aspect of lifestyle beyond physical health, influencing emotional and psychological well-being in geriatric orthopedics.

9.2.3. Comorbidities and Their Influence on Orthopedic Health

The presence of comorbidities is a prominent factor in the treatment and outcomes of orthopedic health among geriatric patients. With increasing age, the prevalence of chronic conditions such as diabetes, hypertension, and cardiovascular disease also increases, and this can complicate surgery. For instance, while managing hip fractures—particularly those needing hemiarthroplasty or total hip arthroplasty—the co-morbid states should be closely evaluated. Surgical preference may be based on how much comorbidities affect a patient's risk profile overall. It was shown by a Nationwide Inpatient Sample study that patients with multiple comorbidities may have a longer length of stay in hospital and varying outcomes after surgery, highlighting the delicate balance to be achieved by orthopedic surgeons when deciding treatment options for elderly patients who arrive with fractures (Boniello et al., 2020). Moreover, the interaction between comorbidities and anesthetic techniques makes orthopedic management in the elderly even more difficult. All anesthetic techniques are not evidence to produce the same outcome in postoperative mobility—a factor of utmost importance in the recovery of patients who have undergone orthopedic procedure. Although commonly used anesthetic techniques in the guise of general and neuraxial blockades are properly established, the impact on recovery can vary based on the health condition of a person. Studies have pointed out that despite similarities in demographic factors and rates of comorbidity, rates of first mobilization after surgery postoperatively can differ, and may have consequences for subsequent mobility and quality of life (Blain et al., 2016). This highlights the need for individualized anesthetic planning tailored to the precise health profiles of older patients. In addition to anesthetic and surgical considerations, comorbidities also affect rehabilitation planning following orthopedic surgery. Effective rehabilitation in the older patient typically requires an interdisciplinary system that can adjust to varying states of health. Physical therapy may need to be altered based on a patient's cardiovascular status or other chronic disease, impacting recovery time and functional outcome. Comorbid patients may also find it hard to integrate prescribed rehabilitative exercises into their lives due to fatigue or compromise of mobility. As documented in studies, better results in geriatric orthopedics call for understanding the relationship between comorbidities and patients' surgical and recuperation needs, outlining the complexity of individualized patient management in such a population (Blain et al., 2016; Boniello et al., 2020) (Figure 9.9).

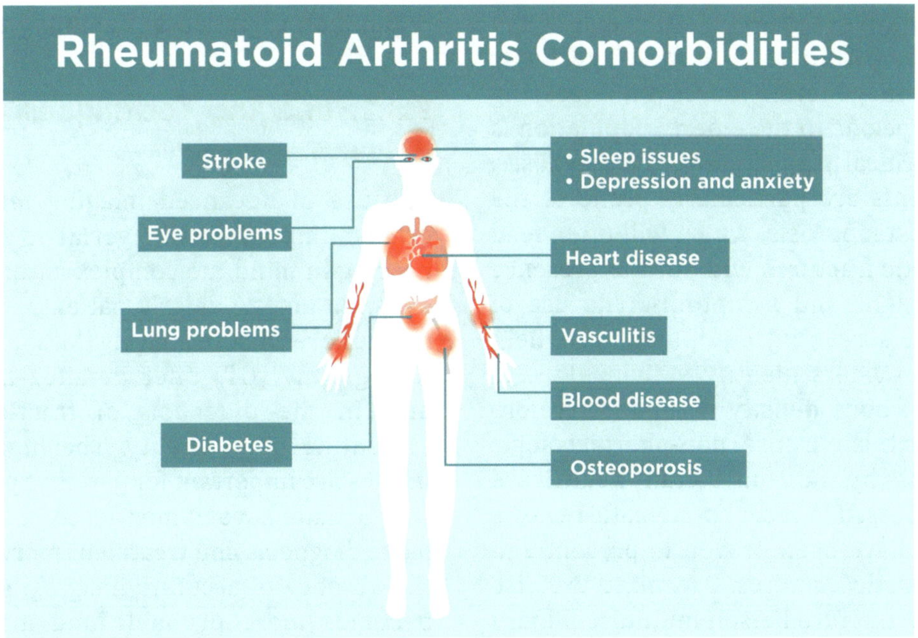

Figure 9.9. The presence of comorbidities significantly influences the management and outcomes of orthopedic health in geriatric patients.

Source: https://external-content.duckduckgo.com/iu/?u=http%3A%2F%2Fcreakyjoints.org%2Fwp-content%2Fuploads%2F0619_Rheumatoid-Arthritis-Comorbidities.jpg&f=1&nofb=1&ipt=f70b833fde04b4b1630c794465419d400520e7f21c6767c5382f400696b87478.

9.3. Diagnostic Approaches in Geriatric Orthopedics

The complexity involved in diagnosing musculoskeletal disorders of the elderly necessitates the incorporation of diverse diagnostic methods in geriatric orthopedics. As elderly patients tend to be accompanied by different comorbidities, traditional methods of diagnosis such as physical examination and radiographic assessment prove to be limiting. A related approach to diagnosis is thus indicated to determine appropriate assessment. High-resolution imaging techniques with MRI and CT offer increased diagnostic resolution by defining intricate bone and soft tissue data. In addition, greater applications of ultrasound in outpatient settings enable real-time assessment of joint and tendon abnormalities and provide useful adjunctive information to conventional modalities. This diagnostic process of integration, therefore, not only improves clinical results but also provides tailored treatment options, thus enhancing patient care within the field of geriatric orthopedics in general. Moreover, assessing risk factors specific to the elderly population is particularly critical in making effective diagnoses. Elderly patients are particularly prone to the disorder of osteoporosis, which will often lead to osteoporotic fractures without the presence of warning signs and symptoms. The use of standardized screening equipment can help healthcare providers identify individuals with a high risk of bone density loss and therefore fractures. For this purpose, non-pharmacologic interventions by non-physician healthcare deliverers, stressed in recent systematic reviews of literature, have been proven to prevent and cure osteoporotic fractures. Organized exercise regimens and fracture liaison multidisciplinary team services have been proven to reduce the incidence of falls and refractures. Hence, identification and remediation of these risk factors are most important in formulating strategic diagnostic and preventive interventions conforming to the individual health patterns of geriatric patients (Wilson et al., 2020). Patient education is also a fast-emerging core component of the diagnostic and management process of geriatric orthopedics. Educating patients regarding their conditions and the bearing of diagnostic outcomes encourages greater participation and adherence to treatment plans. With interdisciplinary teams, non-physician clinicians are able to deliver targeted educational interventions based on the specific needs of individual patients. Targeting evidence-based lifestyle modifications, such as dietary changes and exercise habits, reinforces treatment and prevents further onset of orthopedic conditions. Involving patients in the diagnostic process can also make them more cognizant of the need for follow-up care and promote greater compliance and improved health outcomes. As the specialty of geriatric orthopedics continues to evolve, the intersection of education, testing, and patient activation will undoubtedly shape practice in the management of this diverse and multifaceted population of patients (Cumming et al., 2014).

9.3.1. Imaging Techniques and Their Relevance

The use of advanced imaging methods is of utmost importance in geriatric orthopedics, bearing in mind the complex nature of injuries common among elderly patients. For example, magnetic resonance imaging (MRI) and computed tomography (CT) offer detailed imaging that aids in the diagnosis of fractures and in evaluating bone quality. The high-resolution images are important for geriatric patients since they usually have numerous comorbidities that make diagnosis and treatment more complex. In the absence of accurate imaging, misdiagnosis becomes more probable and may result in ineffective treatment modalities. The value of proper imaging is also highlighted by instance, as in the case of fragility fractures of the acetabulum, where compromised bone quality increases the difficulty of diagnosis (Toro et al., 2022). In the end, the application of these imaging modalities in geriatric orthopedics reaches far beyond simple diagnosis; they allow for optimized treatment plans, which are vital in optimizing patient outcomes. Further enhance the management strategy for the geriatric patient by the use of imaging examinations, since the latter play a crucial role in planning surgical intervention. In orthopedic geriatrics, the choice to operate or otherwise is significantly determined by proper assessment of the nature of a fracture by use of imaging. For example, treatment of acetabular fracture relies partially on imaging to some degree to determine the most suitable action, especially considering the high complication rates for various surgical procedures (Toro et al., 2022). Imaging not only aids in initial diagnosis but also contributes to outcome evaluation after treatment. This cyclical use of imaging and re-examination is vital in demystifying the complexity of surgical procedures and facilitating informed decisions that consider the medical profile of the individual patient and the natural risk of post-operative complications. Early imaging is also crucial for hip fractures, where the urgency for surgery has to be balanced with patient safety.

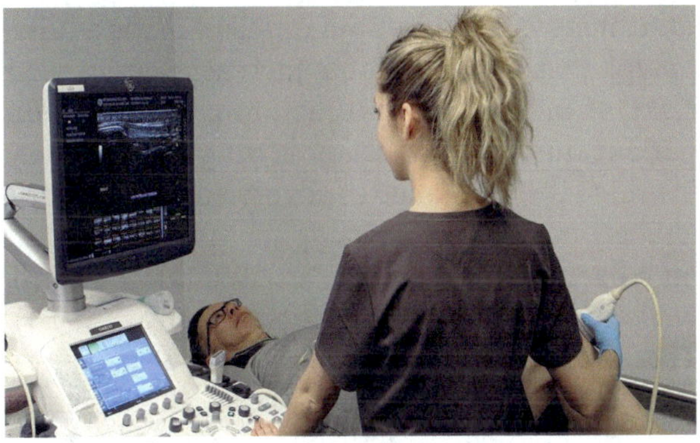

Figure 9.10. Imaging techniques and their relevance.

Source: https://external-content.duckduckgo.com/iu/?u=https%3A%2F%2Fwww.recomind.net%2Fwp-content%2Fuploads%2F2023%2F05%2Fdiagnostic-imaging-systems-875x528.jpg&f=1&nofb=1&ipt=73f594aba59c0d08a8204390e8befe4dc5052459f520f55a4f7163c786a9df0e.

New data indicate that early surgery significantly enhances the result in the elderly patient following fracture, but is at risk for complications due to anticoagulant therapy common among the elderly population. The early use of imaging allows for a better preoperative assessment, which is required to prevent bleeding- and infection-related complications during surgery. The use of imaging modalities not only decides surgical timing but also helps to modulate patient-specific treatment plans based on individual comorbid conditions and overall status. Basically, the use of imaging modalities in geriatric orthopedics is intended to facilitate timely and effective care, with the aim of providing older adults with the best degree of treatment in resolving their orthopedic quandaries (Figure 9.10).

9.3.2. Clinical Assessments and Evaluations

Clinical assessments and evaluations are fundamental components of geriatric orthopedics and the foundation for tailoring successful treatment plans to elderly patients. They are typically extensive histories, physical examinations, and assessments of functional status that are significant in establishing the individualized needs of elderly persons. Targeting such regions as mobility, degree of pain, and comorbidities that exist can help healthcare providers establish a targeted approach to patient treatment. Clinically, evaluations regularly include the utilization of standardized measures aimed at quantifying quality of life, functioning ability, and psychological state, all of which contribute to a better understanding of the intricate nature of an older patient's health status. Critically, this general assessment is similar to the biopsychosocial model that captures the interplay of biological factors, psychological well-being, and social determinants influencing patients' outcomes in geriatric orthopedics (Bornet et al., 2017). Geriatric patient assessment also demands knowledge of the peculiar challenges that they have endured, particularly with regard to accessibility to healthcare services. The majority of older patients have mobility impairments or are residents in isolated areas, thereby greatly impairing their ability to gain access to timely clinical assessment. It is here that telehealth has arrived as an innovative idea, allowing for synchronous real-time interaction between patients and healthcare providers. The method has been found to be successful in expanding access and enabling the performance of assessments in a timely fashion, even from a remote site. Telehealth facilitates not only initial evaluation but also ongoing evaluation and treatment plan revisions, thereby supporting continuity of care. Its integration into geriatric orthopedics is a necessary evolution that underscores the importance of flexibility in delivering care to the ever-changing healthcare needs of older adults (Bywood et al., 2013). Most importantly, the outcomes of clinical assessments significantly influence the formulation of care plans tailored to the specific requirements of geriatric patients. Research has highlighted the strong correlation between functional status, cognition, and quality of life in the elderly. For instance, a study demonstrated that greater functional independence and cognitive health have an important role to play in the overall perceived quality of life in the framework of rehabilitation of geriatric patients. Conversely, comorbidities and depressive symptoms predict poorer outcomes, emphasizing the value of thorough depression assessments and evaluations of comorbidity management as part of clinical assessment. By including these findings in patient assessments, clinicians are able to direct interventions most likely to lead to colossal improvement in overall well-being. Hence, comprehensive clinical evaluation not only guides direct treatment strategies but also guides long-term health trajectories among older adults undergoing orthopedic care (Bornet et al., 2017).

9.3.3. Importance of Patient History in Diagnosis

In orthopedics of the elderly, the importance of obtaining a complete patient history cannot be overstated. Elderly patients have a high number of comorbid conditions that complicate their diagnosis and treatment. A complete patient history helps healthcare practitioners build a better understanding of the patient's overall health, including identifying underlying issues that can mask or mimic orthopedic issues. Preparation of a history of previous injuries, procedures, and current medications is similarly crucial, as this data can directly influence the choice of treatment and potential outcome. For instance, understanding how patients have fared in the past with fractures or joint replacement can guide decisions in the use of further imaging or the appropriateness of surgical options. Accordingly, the taking of a complete patient history is a critical foundation upon which a valid diagnosis and treatment plan can be fashioned. Furthermore, the ability to identify adverse drug reactions based on patient history significantly enhances treatment safety. In populations of older adults, polypharmacy is common, increasing increased risks of medication interaction and impact on patient outcomes. A study highlighted the way in which the incidence of adverse drug reactions (ADRs) was 3.1% in hospital inpatients and an observed association existed for patients with orthopedic treatment (Lobo et al., 2013). Through systematic review of a patient's medication regimen as well as their health history, medical practitioners can effectively reduce these risks. This forward-looking strategy not only helps optimize treatment choices but also facilitates a patient-centered model of care wherein the patient is heard and comprehended regarding his/her medical experience. Finally, what is learned from a patient's history directs real-time clinical decision-making, minimizing complications. In addition, active engagement in open communication with patients regarding their histories promotes a more collaborative healthcare environment. Older patients may have decades of medical history, and allowing them a space to tell their stories is not only beneficial in diagnosis but also empowers patients. The shared strategy also enhances compliance with treatment since patients who feel involved in their care become more dedicated to following medical advice. There is support that detailed patient history-taking can lead to better clinical outcomes as routine protocols in geriatric orthopedics accommodate the multifactorial nature of conditions of old age (Cumming et al., 2014). By centering patient histories, clinicians are better positioned to address efficiently the complexity that comes with geriatric patients, guaranteeing tailored interventions able to significantly improve function and quality of life among this vulnerable group (Figure 9.11).

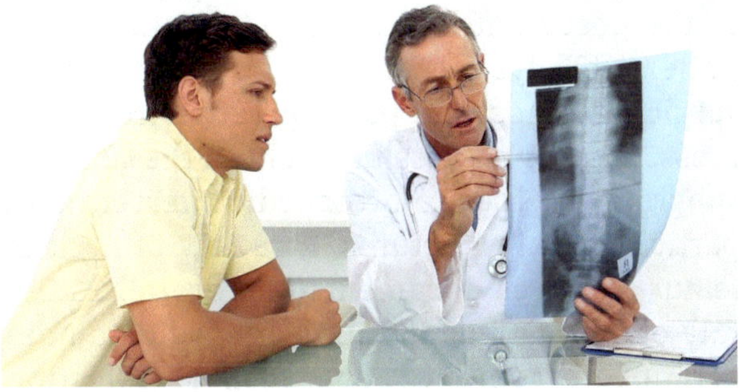

Figure 9.11. The importance of obtaining a comprehensive patient history.

Source: https://external-content.duckduckgo.com/iu/?u=https%3A%2F%2Fthesouthfirst.com%2Fwp-content%2Fuploads%2F2023%2F09%2Fdoctorexplain.jpg&f=1&nofb=1&ipt=d6814864db48f1f5e70dcba5753c8a327265addfd89d21f082b6267919b4ec46.

9.4. Treatment Options for Geriatric Orthopedic Patients

Geriatric orthopedic management is accompanied by unique challenges that involve close scrutiny of the options for treatment. Non-operative treatment is usually the initial line of treatment for fractures that are amenable to conservative treatment. These can be in the form of pain control protocols, physical therapy, and orthopedic bracing and can be intended to facilitate improved mobility and functional outcome with minimal complications. For instance, applying physiotherapy is effective in increasing strength and balance in elderly patients, hence reducing the risk of falls and related injuries. Additionally, relief of pain with medications—i.e., nonsteroidal anti-inflammatory medications (NSAIDs) and acetaminophen—can alleviate pain and improve the quality of patients, hence facilitating the performance of rehabilitation exercises that are very critical to healing (Riemen & Hutchison, 2016). However, in some conditions, surgery may be warranted if conservative management does not work. In the case of odontoid fractures, which occur predominantly in older patients, a multicenter study aimed to measure the degree to which treatment methods affect patient outcomes, with an emphasis on the conflict of decision-making between surgery and non-surgery (Fehlings et al., 2013). While approximately 63.5% of the patients underwent surgical intervention, the study highlighted the complexity of such decisions. The majority of patients with severe comorbidities or advanced age experienced worse outcomes following initial treatment that was non-surgical, and treatment failure was typified by declining mobility and increased complications. Thus, the decision to proceed with surgical treatment should be made following a full assessment of the overall well-being of the patient, fracture type, and comorbidities to maximize benefits and minimize treatment failure rates. Along with traditional treatment regimes, novel strategies and emerging technologies are transforming geriatric orthopedics. Minimally invasive surgical procedures have begun to gain traction in the management of various diseases, with shorter recovery periods, less postoperative discomfort, and fewer complications, which are sine qua non for older patients. Furthermore, more targeted approaches of personalized medicine taking into account the patients' genetic and biochemical profiles are gaining significance so that highly individualized treatment regimens can be designed to improve efficacy and reduce side effects. The convergence of rehabilitation robotics and telemedicine also offers hope in terms of valuable assistance in handling rehabilitation as well as tracking outcomes remotely. With advancing geriatric orthopedics, these advances will likely play significant roles not only in optimizing therapeutic results but also in expanding the purview of useful therapeutic interventions for this vulnerable population (Riemen & Hutchison, 2016) (Figure 9.12).

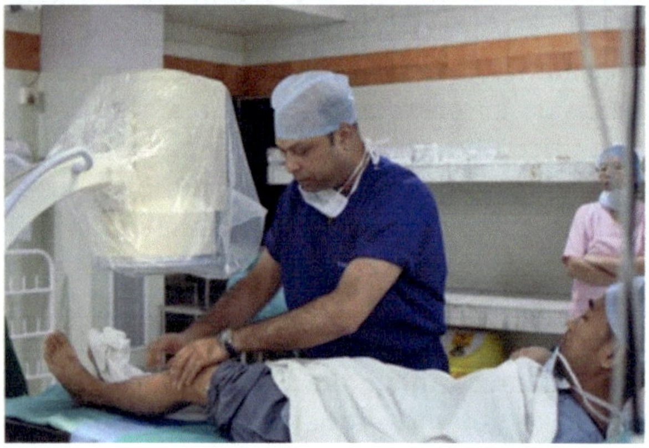

Figure 9.12. Treatment options for geriatric orthopedic patients.

Source: https://external-content.duckduckgo.com/iu/?u=https%3A%2F%2F5.imimg.com%2Fdata5%2FKE%2FFW%2FGLADMIN-67186534%2Fgeriatric-orthopedic-treatment-500x500.png&f=1&nofb=1&ipt=5414793fea6466372ac41509138d8f8b8efcdf2d36163afda44afd9234e6c48b.

9.4.1. Surgical Interventions and Considerations

Geriatric orthopedic operations are typically complex and demand an appreciation of the interaction between physiological and psychological determinants of behavior in elderly patients. As patients get older, they also present with comorbid diseases that challenge surgical recovery. Diabetes, hypertension, and cardiovascular disease are some examples of conditions that must be assessed and managed appropriately preoperatively to prevent anesthetic and surgical repair-related complications. Additionally, the elderly patient may experience greater procedure anxiety due to cognitive impairment or worries of postoperative complications. Implementing individualized care interventions, as cited in the literature, can directly contribute to better health outcomes in this population, such that the surgical approach is tailored specifically to the needs and conditions of the individual patient (Theys et al., 2021). Attention to surgical method and post-operative treatment is essential for successful results in the geriatric subgroup exposed to orthopedic interventions, particularly hip fractures. A review of neck of femur fractures documented an overall 21.8% rate of 90-day readmission largely due to non-orthopedic complications such as infection and cardiovascular disease (Srinivasan et al., 2024). This directs toward the necessity for an orthogeriatric co-management that is a multidisciplinary process, which may consolidate care by integrating surgical and medical treatments specifically tailored to the age group. Systematically addressing the multifactorial etiology of readmission, healthcare providers are able to implement targeted interventions that not only shorten surgical recovery but also ensure the prevention of complications through overall perioperative management. Apart from the surgical operation and early postoperative care, rehabilitation is also a significant predictor of long-term results of geriatric orthopedic surgery. Elderly patients are likely to suffer from severe impairments such as decreased mobility and increased risk of falls during the postoperative period, which can directly affect their quality of life. Therefore, it is crucial to make a rehabilitative plan with strategic physiotherapy and occupational therapy. This is a strategy that promotes patients to regain function and independence, thereby reducing the risk of complications and achieving optimal satisfaction with care. Also, understanding the nuances of pain management in this population is very important, given the risk of adverse drug reactions. Emphasis on a complete rehabilitation plan can ultimately optimize recovery pathways, which supports better health outcomes of geriatric orthopedic procedures (Figure 9.13).

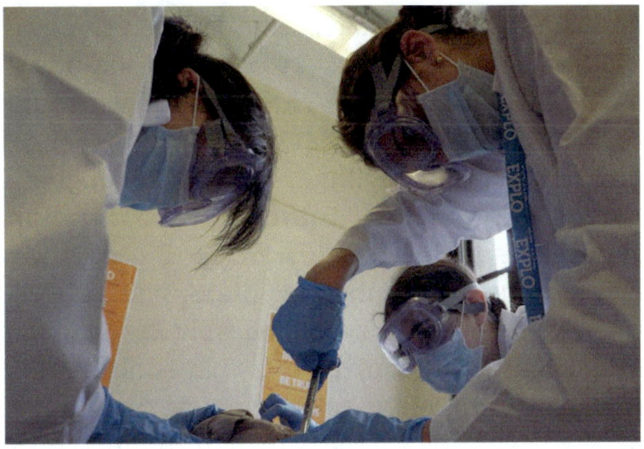

Figure 9.13. Surgical interventions in geriatric orthopedics are often complex.

Source: https://external-content.duckduckgo.com/iu/?u=http%3A%2F%2Fblog.explo.org%2Fhubfs%2Fyale%2Facademics%2Fslideshows%2F20170629_103615%2F6-29_Surgical_Interventions_-_13_of_20.jpg&f=1&nofb=1&ipt=075db27ec04f2b62852098a30c0e228084b5828632c8615940fbb3aaa33f2c29.

9.4.2. Non-Surgical Management Strategies

For orthopedics in geriatrics, non-surgical interventions are also becoming an important part of patient management, particularly with the increasing incidence of musculoskeletal disorders in the elderly. They include a broad spectrum of interventions ranging from pharmacological interventions to physical therapy and lifestyle modification aimed at reducing pain and optimizing functionality. Medications such as analgesics and anti-inflammatory drugs are frequently employed to manage symptoms, but their use should be cautiously weighed, particularly when there is high susceptibility to side effects in the older patient. With these modalities combined, clinicians can formulate a more integrated plan of care tailored to the individual patient's needs, thus reducing the necessity for surgical intervention and associated complications. Another important aspect of non-operative management in geriatric orthopedics is the initiation of rehabilitation protocols. The latter typically consists of physical and occupational therapy, directed towards strength recovery, improvement in mobility, and overall enhancement of the quality of life. Of particular importance are individualized exercise programs directed towards the individual specifics of elderly individuals, such as decreased bone density and loss of muscle mass, which lead directly to fracture hazard and recovery outcomes. Also encompassed is the inclusion of assistive devices and home modification as factors contributing to functional independence. Early intervention with such rehabilitation practices has data showing it significantly decreases the rate of readmission following orthopedic events, and this is evidence supporting an active treatment approach to geriatric patients presenting with musculoskeletal complaints (Srinivasan et al., 2024). Besides, non-surgical management methods also have to include a multi-disciplinary approach with the inclusion of evaluation and modification of underlying states of health. Comorbidities such as cardiovascular disease and diabetes can complicate the recovery of orthopedic pathology, necessitating a combined evaluation of patient health. In this case, interprofessional collaboration among practitioners such as geriatricians, orthopedic specialists, and rehabilitation professionals facilitates multi-modal management of the physical, dietary, and lifestyle aspects of general health. This is highly likely in those with complex individuals, such as centenarians, who are bound to present new challenges during their treatment (Krishna & Pathak, 2020). As geriatric orthopedics continues to evolve, implementing these non-surgical methods will be key to enhancing patients' results while lessening the burden on medical systems.

9.4.3. Rehabilitation and Physical Therapy

The addition of rehabilitation and physical therapy is most crucial in the management of the condition of geriatric patients in the field of orthopedics. Because elderly adults usually reside with musculoskeletal disorders, rehabilitative measures can play a valuable role in their functional capacity and health. Physical therapy is not only directed at the restoration of motion and power following injury or surgery, but also toward the prevention of future complications by educating and activating the patient.

These encompass exercises that intend to improve balance, flexibility, and resistance, which are the main elements for fall risk reduction. Additionally, understanding the psychological aspects of rehabilitation also contributes to challenging elderly individuals to participate actively in their process of rehabilitation, evoking a sense of independence and self-esteem. A central point about geriatric orthopedics is the requirement of interprofessional interaction among health professionals, particularly in the environment of rehabilitation. Physiotherapist, occupational therapist, and nursing staff involvement in team care can permit intense rehabilitation plans tailored to the individual's particular needs. For instance, the application of evidence-based programs that include feedback from various specialists can maximize patient outcomes. Such collaboration is highlighted in a study demonstrating improved recovery times and functional gains when rehabilitation professionals work together (Riemen & Hutchison, 2016). Furthermore, encouraging the culture of teamwork continues to aid both practitioners and patients in general to ensure that the intricate problems encountered by elderly persons during recovery are handled comprehensively and effectively. Powerful evidence confirms the effectiveness of specific rehabilitation treatments in elderly individuals with specific rehabilitation challenges. For example, certain studies have indicated that short-duration high-intensity training programs can offer useful functional benefits in specific patient populations, such as those with cerebral palsy (Blahovec et al., 2012). Translation of these interventions to elderly patients could encourage their mobilization and independence, and thus serve to highlight the value of ongoing research to identify optimal rehabilitation regimens suitable for this group. By investing in evidence-based physical therapy strategies, healthcare providers will be able to enhance results for geriatric orthopedic patients. In total, it is important that rehabilitation be considered at the forefront of the care continuum, thus establishing the groundwork for a more active and stronger aging process (Figure 9.14).

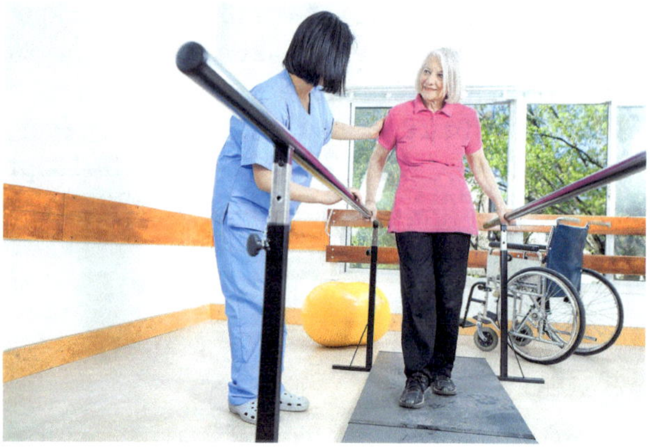

Figure 9.14. The integration of rehabilitation and physical therapy.

Source: https://external-content.duckduckgo.com/iu/?u=https%3A%2F%2Fbethesdahealth.org%2Fwp-content%2Fuploads%2F2018%2F04%2FRehabilitation-clinic-with-elderly-people-and-nurse-626641908_1258x838.jpeg&f=1&nofb=1&ipt=788f11d15c6da6254ee0e496506ab2363001a300b731af386ba6915fcac0c3bd.

9.5. Challenges in Geriatric Orthopedic Care

The intrinsic barriers of geriatric orthopedic care are many and mainly stem from the enormous medical needs of the elderly. Aging is a process of continual decline in physiological function, which most often exaggerates the severity of musculoskeletal pathology. Fractures, and particularly hip fractures, are therefore extremely prevalent and have severe consequences, including loss of independence and extremely high mortality.

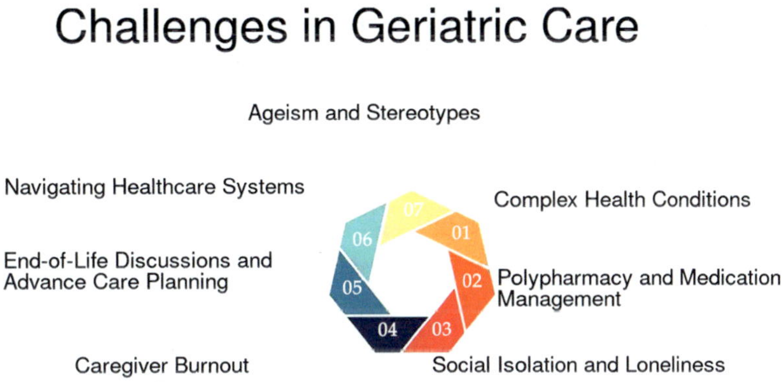

Figure 9.15. The challenges inherent in geriatric orthopedic care.

Source: https://fastercapital.co/i/Geriatric-Care-Best-Practices-Unlocking-Business-Opportunities--Geriatric-Care-Innovations--Challenges-in-Geriatric-Care.webp.

The fact that older people cannot heal effectively from injury also complicates treatment since not only can they have operations, but also long-term rehabilitation. The history of geriatric medicine shows these problems; until 1991, Malta's specialist geriatric medicine was largely confined to long-stay care, showing the lack of immediate, expert treatment for acute medical issues and rehabilitation. This is a reflection of an intrinsic disconnect within the system that remains to threaten the effectiveness and accessibility of orthopedic geriatric care (Fiorini et al., 1998). The other related challenge that accompanies orthopedic issues among the elderly is the psychological aspect. The interaction between physical disability and mental well-being is particularly clear with elderly patients, especially those with severe fractures. Studies have established a significant correlation between patients who have a hip fracture and the mental health of such patients and those of their caregivers. Stress that comes with caring for an elderly person during recovery from a hip fracture may accumulate, and this leads to significant mental pressure on the family members, creating yet another variable contributing to the illness of the patient. These interdependencies complicate care strategies, as a caregiver's mental distress directly impacts the patient's recovery process. The bidirectional impact highlights the need for bio-psychosocial intervention in geriatric patient care, as neglect of the mental health component can contribute to rehabilitation failure. It is therefore crucial to engage patients as well as caregivers to enhance the outcome of geriatric orthopedic care (Bellanti et al., 2016). Besides, financial and resource constraints are significant barriers to the best geriatric orthopedic care. Elderly individuals need more complex services, yet the healthcare system itself is commonly not equipped to handle them. Inefficient hospital resources can lead to overcrowding, delayed surgery, and poor follow-up care, all of which hinder effective and timely treatment. Moreover, differences in insurance coverage and health policies can add disparities to the availability of necessary procedures and rehabilitation programs. These systemic issues not only put an undue burden on healthcare professionals but also significantly negatively affect the quality of life for geriatric patients awaiting treatment. Thus, ameliorating these financial and logistical concerns is essential to guarantee that outcomes for geriatric orthopedic patients are enhanced. Through advocacy for policy change and more resources for specialist care of the elderly, stakeholders may promote progress toward a more equitable system that takes into account the unique needs of this compromised population (Figure 9.15).

9.5.1. Polypharmacy and Its Effects on Treatment

Polypharmacy, or the concurrent administration of two or more drugs, presents challenges to geriatric orthopedics in a way that is different from the general population. Patients in older age groups have multiple co-morbid conditions necessitating complex regimens of therapy. As highlighted in most studies, the prevalence of polypharmacy in the geriatric population can lead to drug-related side effects, hospitalization, and impaired functional status. The elderly patients admitted to orthopedic wards are also being prescribed an average of over three drugs, thus rendering their treatment even more complicated. For instance, as per a recent survey, over 35% of the drugs prescribed were fixed-dose combinations (FDCs), which have the tendency to increase the potential for interaction as well as lower drug adherence because they are hard to administer in one sitting. Hence, specialists should analytically review the entire drug course for each patient in an effort to reduce such risks without compromising therapeutic protocols for diseases such as spondylosis, a disease common among this group (Basheer et al., 2018). In addition to the clinical impact, polypharmacy also has significant impacts on the financial burden on patients as well as healthcare systems. Geriatric patients usually experience high expenditures related to numerous medications, leading to non-adherence based on monetary limitations. The research indicates that poor compliance with prescribed treatments is, at least in part, explained by the pharmacological treatment's high cost arising from polypharmacy. In addition, the restricted use of generics and necessary medicines results in this financial burden. Low-cost solutions can foster compliance and access by elderly individuals, and as such, more rational prescribing must be sought by medical practitioners. By focusing on the usage of basic medication and observing the treatment goals as a whole, then healthcare practitioners can ease the economic strain while improving the therapeutic improvements of elderly patients in orthopedics (Cumming et al., 2014). To address the problems posed by polypharmacy, systematic reviews of medication and individualized management plans are an urgent requirement in geriatric orthopedics. Systematic observation of a patient's medication regimen prevents drug-drug interactions and optimizes therapeutic effects. Implementing procedures such as medication reconciliation and interdepartmental coordination ensures a multidisciplinary care approach. This is particularly relevant in orthopedic clinics where patients are at risk of falls or drug-induced fractures secondary to medication side effects. Education regarding the implications of polypharmacy for both patients and healthcare practitioners is essential. Through establishing a culture of open dialogue and education about possible benefits and risks of medications, healthcare workers have the ability to administer safer and more efficient treatment regimens to older patients in the orthopedic setting (Basheer et al., 2018).

9.5.2. Communication Barriers with Elderly Patients

Communication barriers with older patients are major problems in the practice of geriatric orthopedics, where optimal communication is essential for maximum care. With increasing age, patients can develop various conditions such as hearing loss, cognitive impairment, and sensory deficits that impede their ability to communicate meaningfully. Additionally, healthcare professionals' use of medical jargon becomes an additional barrier. A study with dietitians found that some professionals used non-standardized modes of communication, which could potentially be improved in orthopedic settings where there is the availability of multi-disciplinary teams. Providing clearer, shorter information not only improves understanding but also allows older patients to assist effectively in their care by being able to make informed decisions. Overall, this reinforces better health outcomes, substantiating the role of clear communication in the area of geriatric care (Milte & Miller, 2011). Secondly, the differences in generations and cultures can cause miscommunication between older patients and health workers. Older people typically have backgrounds where respect for a person in authority—like doctors—may stifle open communication. Such tendencies may result in patients' reluctance to speak out in concern or clarification of their treatments, particularly where complex conditions are involved, like in the case of hip fractures. With the highest priority of patient-centered treatment, access to information, and the ability to verbalize questions or concerns, these factors become the focal points; not being able to access these aspects can strip away recovery. More communication strategies, such as utilizing family members during discussion, can allow gap bridging and enable elderly patients to be heard as well as being heard in clinical settings (Ganesh & Sameer, 2024). Finally, incorporating formal communication training for healthcare practitioners can significantly diminish barriers to this type of care. By learning that older patients require specialized methods of communication, practitioners can better address their diverse needs. This kind of training should encompass active listening skills, non-verbal communication skills, and visualization skills to improve verbal communication. Evidence has shown that when practitioners employ tailored approaches, such as medico-terminology breaking down and providing adequate response time, patients receive increased rates of satisfaction and adherence to suggested interventions. This is particularly relevant in geriatric orthopedics, where treatment compliance with rehabilitation protocols is essential in recovery. Lastly, the establishment of a culture of open communication will not only enhance better patient outcomes but also reinforce better clinical outcomes across geriatric orthopedic practice (Milte & Miller, 2011) (Figure 9.16).

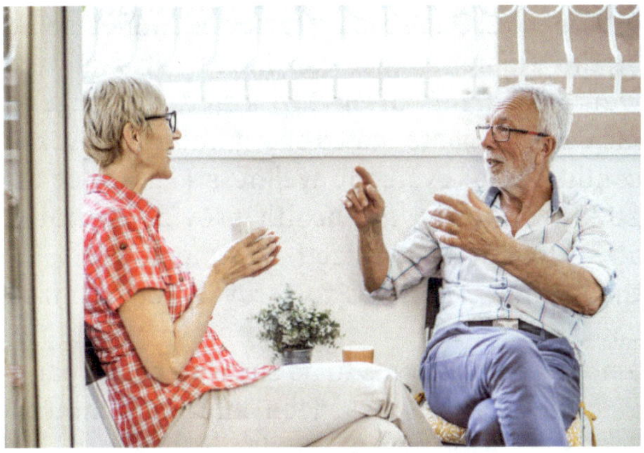

Figure 9.16. Communication barriers with elderly patients are critical challenges in the field of geriatric orthopedics.

Source: https://tiptonplace.com/hubfs/Senior-couple-sitting-and-talk.jpg.

9.5.3. Ethical Considerations in Treatment Decisions

In elderly orthopedics, therapeutic choice often overlaps with patient demographics and social determinants of health issues regarding ethics. Insurance status and race, for instance, can significantly impact treatments and outcomes in older patients with spinal fractures. A critical analysis of data for trauma patients revealed that there was a higher probability for nonwhites to receive definitive treatment using halo orthosis, while white patients received rigid collars (Giles, 2016). These findings question the ethics of equity and accessibility of care and call for healthcare providers to be attuned to recognizing and addressing potential biases that affect clinical decisions. Achieving fair treatment encompasses awareness of the kind of disparities listed above and implementing policies ensuring fairness and justice in treatment processes. Moreover, facilitators and barriers towards recovery following surgical interventions among elderly patients exhibit imperative ethical dimensions of geriatric orthopedics. One scoping review identified some of the elements that can hinder or facilitate weight-bearing after hip fracture surgery, including patients' states of cognition and overall conditions of systemic wellness (Turabi et al., 2023). Ethically, the health providers should advocate for customized treatment plans for these unique barriers to recovery. Customized care enhances the autonomy principle, empowering patients to be engaged participants in care decisions based on informed choices. Also, they bring to light the significance of taking into consideration the general implications of surgical procedures beyond technical success since postoperative experiences have a far-reaching impact on patients' quality of life and long-term outcomes. Finally, the ethical challenges of treatment decisions in geriatric orthopedics are exacerbated by the requirement for informed consent, particularly when working with vulnerable populations. Competence and decision-making capacity may fluctuate in the elderly, particularly those who have cognitive impairment or other illnesses. Clinicians are required to uphold the patient's autonomy against the interest of protecting those who are not necessarily competent to make completely well-informed decisions. This conflict is most extreme in acute care settings where decisions need to be made quickly. Treatment options should be considered in terms of not just patients, but also their families, to ensure a holistic approach to decision-making that takes into account the patient's values and preferences as well as medical advice. The ethical issues at play in treatment decisions thus go far beyond clinical efficacy and into the realm of patient-centered care.

9.6. Innovations and Advances in Geriatric Orthopedics

Current advancements in geriatrics have had a revolutionary impact on the practice of orthopedics, primarily in the form of technology advances that address the unique needs of older patients. Advances in surgery technologies and techniques have made it possible for surgeons to perform minimally invasive surgeries, which reduce recovery times and surgical risk among older patients. The introduction of robots and computer-assisted surgical systems has been pivotal to improving accuracy in joint replacement and fracture fixation surgeries. The systems allow for enhanced preoperative planning and real-time feedback, resulting in improved success rates. Furthermore, the application of telemedicine for pre-operative assessment permits clinicians to assess patients remotely, thereby ensuring that such patients get necessary care with minimal stress or danger, ultimately ensuring better geriatric orthopedic health management practices. Apart from surgery advancements, there has also emerged a growing emphasis on post-surgery rehabilitation within geriatric orthopedics. Research has highlighted the importance of individually tailored rehabilitation programs that address the specific physical needs of older patients recovering from orthopedic procedures. Incorporating physical therapy, occupational therapy, and pain management strategies, these programs seek to enhance functionality and quality of life. Research shows that organized rehabilitation patients are more likely to enhance their autonomy and reduce the risks of falls, which are key challenges among the elderly population. Interventions that enable patient self-management and education for post-operative care are observed to be moving in the direction of a more integrated strategy addressing the physiological as well as psychologic fronts of recovery among geriatric patients.

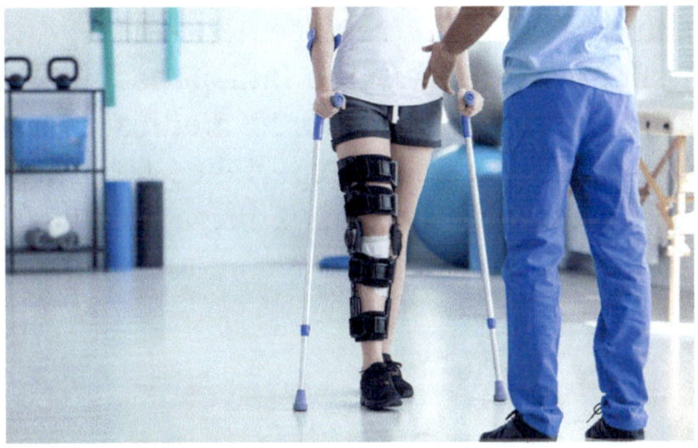

Figure 9.17. Recent advancements in geriatrics have significantly impacted the field of orthopedics.

Source: https://midamortho.com/wp-content/uploads/2023/11/midamortho2.png.

This is most significant because it highlights the importance of individualizing treatment planning based on individual strength and needs, thereby boosting patient satisfaction and health outcomes among geriatric orthopedics. Policy implications are central to sustaining such innovations and making them available within the healthcare system. Evidence-based policy research continues to offer the possibility of strengthening preventive care and care coordination that is especially tailored for the elderly. With the facilitation of patient self-management and palliative care models, stakeholders can better address the multidimensional issues with geriatric orthopedics. The Stern Center's focus on these efforts is indicative of a growing trend towards the alignment of innovative practice with policy action that maximizes outcomes for older adults. Strategic investment in workforce development and support for family caregivers is central to the development of a long-term model of geriatric orthopedic care. As there is a population trend towards an aging population, it will be crucial to place such policies high on the list in keeping with the overall welfare of older patients in orthopedics, ensuring their safety and welfare as they battle age-related orthopedic complications (The Stern Center for Evidence-Based Policy, 2015; Sivhugwana, 2021) (Figure 9.17).

9.6.1. Technological Advancements in Surgical Techniques

During the past decades, advances in surgical technology have revolutionized the field of geriatric orthopedics, enhancing the efficiency of surgery and recovery of patients. A recent example is minimally invasive surgery (MIS), which allows surgeons to perform complex procedures through small incisions. This technique not only reduces postoperative pain but also reduces recovery time, an element that is extremely helpful for elderly patients who recover more slowly from surgery due to related medical concerns. The implementation of video-assisted thoracoscopic surgery, for example, has provided favorable results for those requiring thoracic procedures, demonstrating the ways in which modern techniques are less damaging to the body with the same positive outcomes. Besides, these innovations have enabled the development of sophisticated training simulators that make surgeons more competent so that they can conduct safe and effective procedures for elderly patients requiring orthopedic interventions. Robotic surgery integration is another stellar innovation that has seen increased usage in geriatric orthopedics. Robotic technology provides enhanced precision and accuracy, and surgeons can perform intricate procedures with precision impossible when using traditional methods. This capability is particularly beneficial in joint replacement surgery, where precision is utmost in implant placement and alignment. Therefore, studies have proven that robotic surgery leads to improved outcomes, such as reduced postoperative pain and improved recovery of function. In addition, evidence indicates that older patients experience fewer postoperative complications, which validates the advantage of incorporating technology in surgical procedures. As robotic platforms become more advanced and more widely utilized in orthopedic settings, the future of geriatric surgical care is on the verge of even more innovation. In postoperative care, technology remains at the forefront of assessing and improving patient outcomes. Telemedicine and other strategies are becoming more dominant, providing health professionals with the tools they require to monitor recuperation at a distance. This is particularly beneficial for older patients, who may struggle to reach healthcare centers. Further, using mobile health applications enables patients to indirectly report the severity of pain and recovery to their healthcare providers. To effectively manage postoperative pain—a key variable for modulating the quality of life in old patients undergoing operations such as total knee replacement—integrating formal pain assessment measures such as the Visual Analogue Scale (VAS) is indispensable. With these technological developments combined with enhanced operation procedures, medical systems can enhance the rehabilitation process and present a comprehensive care experience focusing on physical recuperation along with quality of life concerns for the elderly (Ranga Priya et al., 2020; Lalwani & Suvarna, 2021) (Figure 9.18).

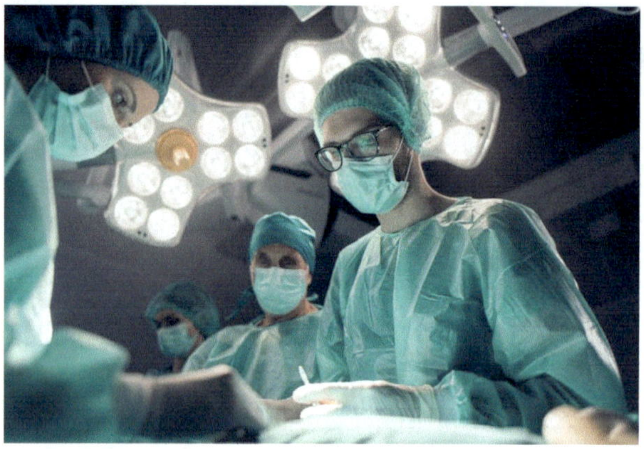

Figure 9.18. The technological advancements in surgical techniques have revolutionized the field of geriatric orthopedics.

Source: https://www.amnhealthcare.com/siteassets/candidate-blog/physician/candidate-blog/locums/locum-tenens-surgery-jobs-min.jpg.

9.6.2. Research on Age-Specific Treatment Protocols

As the population continues to age, age-specific treatment regimens in the field of geriatric orthopedics become increasingly vital. Populations who are older have been determined by studies to respond to injury and treatment differently from younger people. Their bodies slowly respond to the rehabilitation processes, and it is essential to have specialized treatment regimens that emphasize incremental, progressive activity in physical rehabilitation. For example, hip fracture studies—common among the elderly—are insistent on the inclusion of proprioceptive training in the treatment process to combat the inherent difficulties of this age group. Unfortunately, most treatments as of now do not incorporate overt proprioceptive training, and the recovery process does not achieve its full potential. Hence, the creation of age-specific protocols becomes inevitable in order to combat complications and make older patients function normally (Martimbianco et al., 2008). At the same time, it is necessary to study the pharmacological component of therapy in the elderly to create efficient protocols. Elderly patients frequently receive many drugs simultaneously, increasing the risk of ADRs and making treatment more complicated. Current investigations have shown that a significant percentage of hospitalization of elderly patients is caused by ADRs, thus making their orthopedic treatment even more complicated. The polypharmacy issues require healthcare practitioners to develop integrative plans of medication management that are contextually appropriate for older patients who are having orthopedic procedures. By paying attention to the needs and risks of this category of patients, it is possible to enhance the quality of care and limit the dangers associated with regular treatment options (Lobo et al., 2013). Ultimately, encouraging the evidence-based delivery of age-related treatment pathways in geriatric orthopedics will improve outcomes for patients. The shifting profile of orthopedic research demands continuous evaluation and updating of therapeutic approaches, particularly with regard to an aging population. Multidisciplinary management of older patients, with consideration of the developments of pharmacology, rehabilitation, and geriatric medicine, can better meet the multifaceted demands of the elderly. By promoting ongoing research in these areas and progressing toward more individualized treatment schemas, healthcare professionals can serve an essential function in enhancing the functional status and quality of life of elderly patients with orthopedic disorders. These advances will not only increase the clinical results but are also crucial steps toward the redefinition of geriatric orthopedic care in the 21st century.

9.6.3. Role of Telemedicine in Geriatric Care

The telemedicine revolution has changed healthcare delivery, particularly in geriatric medicine, where restricted access is not uncommon. Older people are generally disadvantaged by difficulties in physically attending medical consultations due to mobility issues, chronic conditions, or a lack of transport. Telemedicine overcomes these challenges by providing a virtual consultation platform to allow medical professionals to evaluate and treat patients' health without being physically present. This virtual consultation can be of much use in elderly patients post-surgery, where early follow-up is critical in the healing process. Studies have shown that the deployment of digital health technologies in post-operative care significantly enhances patient engagement and treatment plan adherence, thereby improving overall health outcomes (Zhang et al., 2022). Moving to telehealth not only reduces the physical visit burden but also facilitates a seamless interaction between patients and healthcare providers. In addition, telemedicine enables thorough geriatric assessments, which are essential in order to customize interventions for the distinct needs of older persons. With telehealth platforms, clinicians can perform extensive assessments that cover diverse facets of well-being, such as physical, cognitive, and psychological functioning. This is a holistic method that enables geriatricians to detect possible risks and treat intricate problems better. Additionally, live video consultations also enable doctors to evaluate patients' functional capacity and deliver immediate feedback and ensure adherence to rehabilitation exercises critical for the recovery following orthopedic surgery. Telemedicine interventions not only connect patients with specialists but also support coordinated care from the healthcare team, enhancing the quality of care in geriatric orthopedics as a whole. Thus, telehealth incorporation into paradigms of care for geriatric populations is in alignment with the World Health Organization's ICOPE approach, highlighting its ability to optimize integrated care for older adults (Zhang et al., 2022). While there are considerable advantages of telemedicine, problems still exist in its applicability in all settings, particularly in low-resource settings. The effectiveness of telehealth modalities can be hindered by limited access to technology, poor digital literacy among older patients, and a lack of consistency regarding the willingness of health providers to utilize such modalities. Furthermore, disparities in access to essential health services continue to exist among those living in rural or remote areas, underlining the need for individualized telehealth models that respond to the specific needs of geriatric patients. To meet these challenges, however, requires not only innovative approaches to technology incorporation but ongoing education and support of healthcare providers and patients as well. With the growing older population, ongoing growth in telemedicine can bridge gaps in access to care, ultimately improving health outcomes and quality of life among older adults who have orthopedic challenges (Figure 9.19).

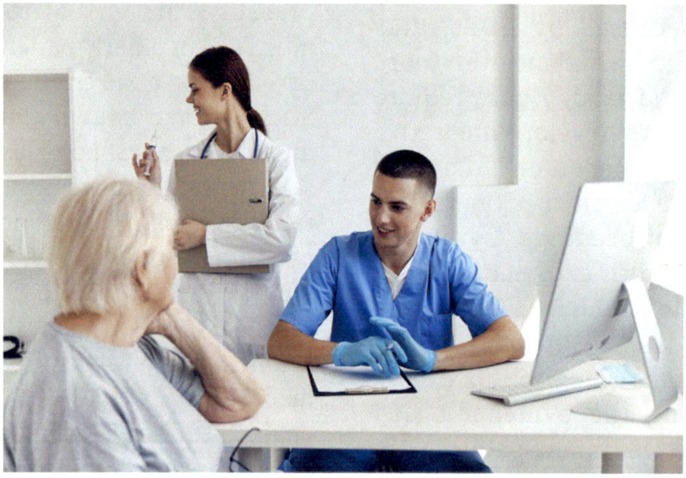

Figure 9.19. Role of telemedicine in geriatric care.

Source: https://staffingly.com/wp-content/uploads/2025/02/telemedicine-in-geriatric-healthcare-scaled.jpg.

SUMMARY

It is obvious that the nuances of this field demand a multifaceted intervention technique in treatment and care. The elderly patient is bound to possess certain problems, including a greater prevalence of comorbidities, lesser physiological reserves, and differences in response to surgery and rehabilitation. As shown in the literature, effective management techniques must include thorough assessments, individualized care planning, and a focus on improving patients' overall quality of life. Such an approach not only aids in treating acute orthopedic conditions but also promotes long-term mobility and independence in elderly patients, hence reducing the risk of future complications or surgeries. Furthermore, inclusion of multidisciplinary teams is also necessary within geriatric orthopedics to offer a comprehensive treatment for patients. Comprehensively high-quality communication and collaboration between orthopedic surgeons, nurses, physical therapists, and social workers provides an avenue for exploring the intricate complications that come with geriatric patients. Studies reveal that suboptimal assessment before interventions may result in negative outcomes such as increased catheterization, which negatively impacts quality of life. Attempting to optimize patient independence by proper assessment, education, and caregiver involvement can significantly enhance patient satisfaction and functional outcomes, as noted by the findings of Abela et al. (1995). Lastly, utilization of valid and reliable measures to quantify individualized care cannot be ignored in geriatric orthopedics. Measures like the Individualized Care Scale (ICS) have been shown to enhance patients' ability to grasp needs and expectations, which can lead to improved care overall. There is evidence to support that when health professionals have precise measures to assess the quality of care, the outcome of patients is dramatically enhanced. Following validation work described in Theys et al. (2021), this will help detect uneven areas for improvement that could be translated to improved nursing practice and patient-focused care for geriatric orthopedics. This global shift in care methods would redefine the therapeutic model for the elderly, being a root-level shift towards individualized, evidence-based geriatric orthopedic care.

Management of older orthopedic patients is a complex array of issues brought out by current research and clinical experience. The most prominent area of concern is managing frail older patients with urgent care requirements for musculoskeletal pathology. Detailed Geriatric Assessments, such as those applied in Leicester, are an all-inclusive approach that addresses not only the immediate medical condition but also functional and social factors that affect the patient's recovery. The model is centered on the synergy of inter-professional collaboration among multidisciplinary teams, including geriatricians, orthopedic surgeons, and nurse practitioners, as part of the attempt to enhance patient outcomes within acute and community care. The new services highlight the need for tailor-made intervention strategies that address the unique needs of the geriatric population while considering the need for effective care coordination at different levels of health services (Conroy et al., 2019). Furthermore, the focus on orthogeriatrics shows particular proof of advances in the treatment of injury specific to the older patient, specifically hip fractures. Hip fracture wards, as a specialist unit, have become a fundamental component in this care pathway, integrating the abilities of anesthetists, orthopedic surgeons, and geriatricians in order to provide maximum treatment outcomes. Specialist units allow more streamlined pathways that maximize recovery and limit complications from surgical procedures. Furthermore, findings in research into odontoid fractures serve to underscore the specific problems in geriatric orthopedics, with very high correlations found between failure of treatment and variables such as age, type of treatment, and sex. Such findings are essential to maximizing clinical guidance and ensuring that the choice of treatment is optimized according to patient-specific profiles (Fehlings et al., 2013). Community-based interventions are equally important in the orthopedic care of the elderly, highlighting the importance of taking care of patients following hospital discharge. Outpatient interventions are integrated to ensure that patients discharged to homes receive adequate follow-up care, with a focus on rehabilitation and recovery. This emphasis on continuity of care continues to be critical to ensuring long-term health results as well as limiting the risk of readmission. By referring to successful local general practitioners and primary care physicians in close consultation, experts are able to create a comprehensive plan that includes not only the physical rehabilitation needs but also the socioeconomic determinants of the patient's readjustment to independent living. The evolving paradigms of geriatric orthopedics reflect increased focus towards fulfilling the varied needs of elderly patients, ultimately towards enhanced quality of life and successful function (Conroy et al., 2019).

CLOSER LOOK

AGE-SPECIFIC TREATMENT PROTOCOLS

Age-specific treatment protocols refer to medical and therapeutic approaches that are carefully tailored to meet the unique physiological, developmental, and functional needs of different age groups. Since children, adults, and older adults differ significantly in terms of growth, metabolism, healing capacity, and activity levels, personalized treatment plans are essential for effective and safe care. In pediatric patients, treatment protocols focus on supporting growth and development while preventing long-term complications. Non-invasive methods such as bracing, physiotherapy, and guided exercises are often preferred, with surgical interventions planned carefully to avoid disturbing growth plates. For adults, treatment aims to restore function, manage pain, and support recovery from injuries or chronic conditions through a combination of medication, physical therapy, and, when necessary, surgery. In older adults, age-specific protocols emphasize pain management, mobility preservation, fall prevention, and management of degenerative conditions such as osteoporosis and osteoarthritis. Treatments are designed to be gentle, considering reduced bone density, slower healing, and the presence of other medical conditions. Rehabilitation focuses on balance training, strength building, and functional independence. Overall, age-specific treatment protocols enhance safety, improve outcomes, and promote holistic care by addressing the distinct physical and functional requirements of each life stage, ensuring optimal recovery and long-term well-being.

REFERENCES

1. Abela, Stephen. "The Outcome of Elderly Patients Following Removal of Indwelling Urinary Catheter," 1995. (accessed on 26th June 2025).

2. Wilson, N., Hurkmans, E., Adams, J., Bakkers, M., Balážová, P., Baxter, M., Blavnsfeldt, A. B., Briot, K., Chiari, C., Cooper, C., Dragoi, R., Gäbler, G., Lems, W., Mosor, E., Pais, S., Simon, C., Studenic, P., Tilley, S., de la Torre, J., & Stamm, T. A. (2020). Prevention and management of osteoporotic fractures by non-physician health professionals: a systematic literature review to inform EULAR points to consider. *RMD open*, *6*(1), e001143. https://doi.org/10.1136/rmdopen-2019-001143 (accessed on 26th June 2025).

3. Conroy S, Brown J, Bell K, Haunton V, Robinson TG, Banerjee J, Martin G, Regen E, Phelps K, O'Kelly K, Kondova D, Williamson I, Wildbur D, Fallmann S,

4. Chen L, Oldridge L, Larkin M, Wilson A, Agarwal S, Bankart J, Subramaniam H, Raghavan R, Panerai R, Clague-Baker N, Chung E, Stahl BC, Chen F, Triboan D, Psychoula I, Northcott A. (2019). East Midlands Research into Ageing Network (EMRAN) Discussion Paper Series. East Midlands Research into Ageing Network (EMRAN) Discussion Paper Series Issue 26 Apr 2019. ISSN 2059-3341.. https://core.ac.uk/download/228199189.pdf (accessed on 26th June 2025).

5. Theys, S., Van Hecke, A., Akkermans, R., & Heinen, M. (2021). The Dutch Individualised Care Scale for patients and nurses - a psychometric validation study. *Scandinavian journal of caring sciences*, *35*(1), 308–318. https://doi.org/10.1111/scs.12853(accessed on 26th June 2025).

6. Turabi, R. Y., Wyatt, D., Guerra, S., O'Connell, M. D. L., Khatun, T., Sageer, S. A., Alhazmi, A., & Sheehan, K. J. (2023). Barriers and facilitators of weight bearing after hip fracture surgery among older adults. A scoping review. *Osteoporosis international : a journal established as result of cooperation between the European Foundation for Osteoporosis and the National Osteoporosis Foundation of the USA*, *34*(7), 1193–1205. https://doi.org/10.1007/s00198-023-06735-5(accessed on 26th June 2025).

7. Blain, H., Masud, T., Dargent-Molina, P., Martin, F. C., Rosendahl, E., van der Velde, N., Bousquet, J., Benetos, A., Cooper, C., Kanis, J. A., Reginster, J. Y., Rizzoli, R., Cortet, B., Barbagallo, M., Dreinhöfer, K. E., Vellas, B., Maggi, S., Strandberg, T., EUGMS Falls and Fracture Interest Group,, International Association of Gerontology and Geriatrics for the European Region (IAGG-ER),, ... International Osteoporosis Foundation (IOF) (2016). A comprehensive fracture prevention strategy in older adults: the European Union Geriatric Medicine Society (EUGMS) statement. *Aging clinical and experimental research*, *28*(4), 797–803. https://doi.org/10.1007/s40520-016-0588-4(accessed on 26th June 2025).

8. Fehlings, M. G., Arun, R., Vaccaro, A. R., Arnold, P. M., Chapman, J. R., & Kopjar, B. (2013). Predictors of treatment outcomes in geriatric patients with odontoid fractures: AOSpine North America multi-centre prospective GOF study. *Spine*, *38*(11), 881–886. https://doi.org/10.1097/BRS.0b013e31828314ee(accessed on 26th June 2025).

9. Toro, G., Braile, A., De Cicco, A., Pezzella, R., Ascione, F., Cecere, A. B., & Schiavone Panni, A. (2022). Fragility Fractures of the Acetabulum: Current Concepts for Improving Patients' Outcomes. *Indian journal of orthopaedics*, *56*(7), 1139–1149. https://doi.org/10.1007/s43465-022-00653-0(accessed on 26th June 2025).

10. Basheer, M., Daud, I., Shaikh, U. S., Sini, K., et al. (2018). Drug utilization pattern in orthopedic outpatient department of a tertiary care hospital in Kerala: A geriatric perspective. https://core.ac.uk/download/539896899.pdf (accessed on 26th June 2025).

11. Bellanti, G., Eleuteri, S., & Falaschi, P. (2016). Hip fracture: Preliminary results supporting significative correlations between the psychological wellbeing of patients and their relative caregivers. https://core.ac.uk/download/98343305.pdf (accessed on 26th June 2025).

12. Blahovec, A., Kuiken, A., Mears, J., Riggins, C., et al. (2012). Immediate effects of high intensity training in children with cerebral palsy GMFCS levels I–III: A pilot study. http://digitalscholarship.unlv.edu/cgi/viewcontent.cgi?article=2323&context=thesesdissertations (accessed on 26th June 2025).

13. Boniello, A. J., Cavanaugh, P., Denehy, K., Kerbel, R., et al. (2020). National trends in total hip arthroplasty for traumatic hip fractures: An analysis of a nationwide all-payer database. https://core.ac.uk/download/288122122.pdf (accessed on 26th June 2025).

14. Bornet, M. A., Monod, S., Pasquier, J., Rochat, T., et al. (2017). Factors associated with quality of life in elderly hospitalized patients undergoing post-acute rehabilitation: A cross-sectional analytical study in Switzerland. https://core.ac.uk/download/132562789.pdf (accessed on 26th June 2025).

15. Downey CL, Young A, Burton EF, et al. Dementia and osteoporosis in a geriatric population: Is there a common link?. *World J Orthop*. 2017;8(5):412-423. Published 2017 May 18. doi:10.5312/wjo.v8.i5.412(accessed on 26th June 2025).

16. Bywood P, Raven M, Butler C. (2013). Telehealth in primary health care settings within Australia and internationally. PHCRIS Policy Issue Review. Adelaide: Primary Health Care Research & Information Service. (accessed on 26th June 2025).

17. Casey, S. D., Hirsch, C. H., Mumma, B. E., Slee, A., et al. (2017). Emergency department pain management following implementation of a geriatric hip fracture program. https://core.ac.uk/download/323071629.pdf (accessed on 26th June 2025).

18. Martimbianco ALC, Polachini LO, Chamlian TR, Masiero D. Effects of proprioception in the rehabilitation process of hip fractures. Acta Ortop Bras. [serial on the Internet]. 2008; 16(2):112-116. Available from URL: http://www.scielo.br/aob. (accessed on 26th June 2025).

19. Li, H. J., Cheng, H. S., Liang, J., Wu, C. C., & Shyu, Y. I. (2013). Functional recovery of older people with hip fracture: does malnutrition make a difference?. *Journal of advanced nursing*, *69*(8), 1691–1703. https://doi.org/10.1111/jan.12027(accessed on 26th June 2025).

20. Cumming, K., Hoyle, G. E., Hutchison, J. D., & Soiza, R. L. (2014). Prevalence, incidence and etiology of hyponatremia in elderly patients with fragility fractures. *PloS one*, *9*(2), e88272. https://doi.org/10.1371/journal.pone.0088272 (accessed on 26th June 2025).

21. Cuschieri, S., Gatt, R., & Grech, S. (2016). Bisphosphonates: A cost benefit analysis patient. https://core.ac.uk/download/46603883.pdf (accessed on 26th June 2025).

22. Srinivasan, P. A., Venugopal, V., Selvarajan, R. M., Dhotare, S., Ganapathy, R., Patel, S., Tariq, M., & Mahmoud, O. (2024). Tackling the challenge of 90-day readmissions in hip fracture management: a retrospective study. *International Journal of Research in Orthopaedics*, *10*(6), 1170–1173. https://doi.org/10.18203/issn.2455-4510.IntJResOrthop20243111(accessed on 26th June 2025).

23. Lobo, M. G., Pinheiro, S. M., Castro, J. G., Momenté, V. G., & Pranchevicius, M. C. (2013). Adverse drug reaction monitoring: support for pharmacovigilance at a tertiary care hospital in Northern Brazil. *BMC pharmacology & toxicology, 14*, 5. https://doi.org/10.1186/2050-6511-14-5(accessed on 26th June 2025).

24. Lau, T. W., Fang, C., & Leung, F. (2016). Assessment of postoperative short-term and long-term mortality risk in Chinese geriatric patients for hip fracture using the Charlson comorbidity score. *Hong Kong medical journal = Xianggang yi xue za zhi, 22*(1), 16–22. https://doi.org/10.12809/hkmj154451(accessed on 26th June 2025).

25. Fiorini, A. (1998). The specialty of geriatric medicine in Malta: At a crossroads. https://core.ac.uk/download/46602151.pdf (accessed on 26th June 2025).

26. Ganesh, A., & Sameer, M. M. (2024). Hip fractures redefined - ERAS protocol's impact: the Indian scenario. *International Journal of Research in Orthopaedics, 10*(6), 1437–1440. https://doi.org/10.18203/issn.2455-4510.IntJResOrthop20243149(accessed on 26th June 2025).

27. Gullà, V., Gabbrielli, F., Lanzafame, P., & Mull, J.P. (2013). Sensorized Garments Developed for Remote Postural and Motor Rehabilitation.(accessed on 26th June 2025).

28. Zhang, J., Yang, M., Ge, Y., Ivers, R., Webster, R., & Tian, M. (2022). The role of digital health for post-surgery care of older patients with hip fracture: A scoping review. *International journal of medical informatics, 160*, 104709. https://doi.org/10.1016/j.ijmedinf.2022.104709(accessed on 26th June 2025).

29. Giles, E. M. (2016). Upper cervical spine fracture at Yale: Factors associated with management and outcomes. https://core.ac.uk/download/232775162.pdf (accessed on 26th June 2025).

30. Riemen AH, Hutchison JD. The multidisciplinary management of hip fractures in older patients. *Orthop Trauma*. 2016;30(2):117-122. doi:10.1016/j.mporth.2016.03.006(accessed on 26th June 2025).

31. Sudheer, U., & Jayaprakash, C. (2017). Clinical outcome of intra-articular hyaluronic acid injection for knee joint osteoarthritis: a prospective interventional study from a tertiary care hospital. *International Journal of Research in Orthopaedics, 3*(3), 595–601. https://doi.org/10.18203/issn.2455-4510.IntJResOrthop20171908(accessed on 26th June 2025).

32. M. Ranga Priya, M. Karthika, Meril Lucy Shibu, B. Kowsalya, & Lini Jacob. (2020). Quality of life in total knee replacement (TKR) patients – A review. *Journal of Applied Pharmaceutical Research, 8*(4), 16-23. https://doi.org/10.18231/j.joapr.2020.v.8.i.4.16.23(accessed on 26th June 2025)

33. Krishna, B., & Pathak, N. (2020). Perioperative management of geriatric patients for orthopedic surgeries. *International Journal of Research in Orthopaedics, 6*(2), 427–434. https://doi.org/10.18203/issn.2455-4510.IntJResOrthop20200749(accessed on 26th June 2025).

34. Kumar, P. N., Parameshwar, S., & Shinge, N. (2010). Bed blockers: A study on the elderly patients in a teaching hospital in India. https://core.ac.uk/download/pdf/87449.pdf (accessed on 26th June 2025).

35. Lalwani, Y., & Suvarna, V. (2021). Global outlook on medical device industry. https://core.ac.uk/download/482241733.pdf (accessed on 26th June 2025).

36. MILTE, R. and MILLER, M. (2011), Dietetic care of hip fracture patients across Australia: Are we doing enough?. Nutrition & Dietetics, 68: 214-220. https://doi.org/10.1111/j.1747-0080.2011.01538.x(accessed on 26th June 2025).

37. The Stern Center for Evidence-Based Policy (2015). Addressing the health needs of an aging America: New opportunities for evidence-based policy solutions. https://core.ac.uk/download/75783019.pdf (accessed on 26th June 2025).

38. Sibley, K. M., Howe, T., Lamb, S. E., Lord, S. R., Maki, B. E., Rose, D. J., Scott, V., Stathokostas, L., Straus, S. E., & Jaglal, S. B. (2015). Recommendations for a core outcome set for measuring standing balance in adult populations: a consensus-based approach. *PloS one, 10*(3), e0120568. https://doi.org/10.1371/journal.pone.0120568(accessed on 26th June 2025).

39. Sivhugwana, Innocentia (2022). Factors related with the functional outcome of patients who sustained tibial plateau fractures. Dissertation (MSc (Physiotherapy))--University of Pretoria, 2022. https://core.ac.uk/download/565849089.pdf

40. Waller, P. G. (2012). Surgical delay for hip fracture clients and the use of Clopidogrel: An integrative review. https://core.ac.uk/download/58824498.pdf (accessed on 26th June 2025).

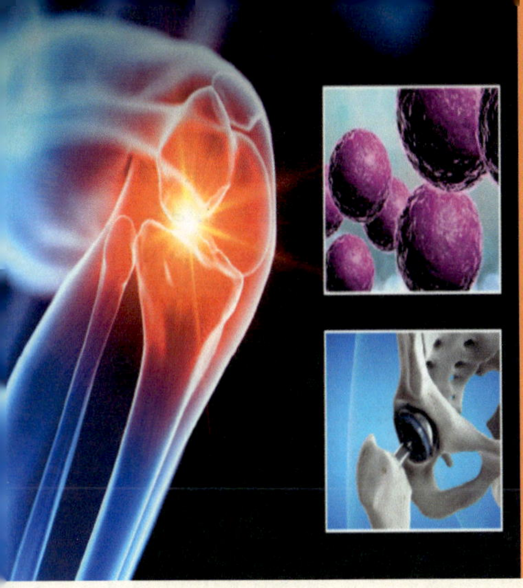

Chapter 10

ORTHOPEDIC INFECTIONS

Contents

Introduction....303
10.1. Types of Orthopedic Infections....306
10.2. Causes and Risk Factors....310
10.3. Symptoms and Diagnosis....314
10.4. Treatment Options....317
10.5. Complications of Orthopedic Infections....321
10.6. Prevention Strategies....324
Summary....328
References....331

Introduction

The development of orthopedic infections is an immediate concern in clinical practice, reaching beyond the surgical and into the nonsurgical setting. Orthopedic infections can be the result of various etiological factors, with SSIs complicating surgical procedures. SSIs constitute approximately 16% of hospital-acquired infections, resulting in severe morbidity, mortality, and added healthcare expenditure. The heterogeneity of SSI management is underscored by the multifactorial etiology of prevention, which demands an evidence-driven and integrated process throughout the continuum of surgery. Involvement in quality improvement projects, such as that found with the One Together collaboration, offers an avenue for healthcare providers to expedite the application of best practices intended to minimize SSI risk, thereby underscoring the importance of solutions that are systemic in nature and cross-practice site individual (Wilson et al., 2015). The heightened sensitivity to the burden resulting from orthopedic infections warrants active control measures based on empirical evidence. Despite significant advances in the pathophysiology of such infections, evidence-based guideline translation into practice is challenging. Challenges such as suboptimal local policies, suboptimal leadership, and a lack of holistic training impede optimal practice adherence to recommended interventions. This gap in implementation often results in a loop of increasing infection rates and adverse patient outcomes, and therefore, it is crucial to ensure greater focus on developing leadership and accountability within healthcare teams. In reaction, attempts at bridging the evidence-practice gap have the power to empower clinicians and optimize patient care in orthopedic settings (Wilson et al., 2015). Also, orthopedic infection complexity justifies personalized treatment regimens.

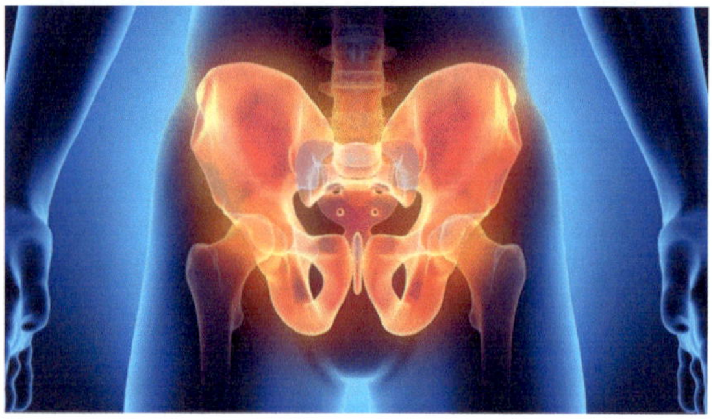

Figure 10.1. The prevalence of orthopedic infections marks a pressing concern in clinical practice.

Source: https://acornprivateclinic.co.uk/wp-content/uploads/2023/03/Untitled-design-13-1-1080x600.png.

Although guidelines are necessary and can be a good reference, they should be sufficiently flexible in managing specific patient demands. Considering the body of healthcare interventions across all disciplines, collaborative practice that leverages insights from medical practitioners and patient advocacy is crucial in maximizing treatment effectiveness. The application of techniques such as modified-Delphi procedures can facilitate concordance among practitioners to formulate individualized management protocols that not only address the clinical presentation of infections but also the psychosocial components of patient care. By prioritizing individualized care algorithms, overall orthopedic infection management practice can be significantly advanced, improving both clinical and patient-reported outcomes (Figure 10.1).

Definition of Orthopedic Infections

Orthopedic infections are a broad category of infections involving the musculoskeletal system, including bones, joints, and the surrounding soft tissues. They may be of diverse origin, from a postoperative infection to an infection due to trauma or hematogenous seeding from a distant infection. They are typically divided into surgical site infections (SSIs), bone infections, and joint infections, each with a distinctive presentation and clinical significance. Surgical site infections – and particularly for orthopedic surgery – are concerning due to the open nature of the surgery site and risk for severe morbidity. For instance, one-year mortality rates following hip hemiarthroplasty can increase as high as 10-40%, and a significant source of such poor outcomes is SSIs (Sprowson et al., 2013). An understanding of the exact definitions of such infections is important so that an accurate diagnosis, successful treatment, and improved patient outcomes are possible. Orthopedic infections are classified on the basis of their onset, which is either acute or chronic. Acute infections usually occur in a short period following trauma or surgery, often with localized inflammation, fever, and systemic disease. Conversely, long-term infections can arise from chronic low-grade infections that last for months or years and have less severe symptoms that complicate their diagnosis. Treatment of such infections is typically complex and can entail surgery, prolonged antibiotic therapy, or both. Research has experienced varied success rates depending on the nature of the infection and condition of the patient, necessitating tailored approaches. For example, multi-center randomized controlled trials of the effectiveness of multiple antibiotic regimens in surgical patients form the basis for evidence-based practices in managing such infections (Schneider et al., 2015). Furthermore, orthopedic infection management is a grave concern due to the complex nature of the musculoskeletal system and the heterogeneity of the pathogenic agents (Sprowson et al., 2013). The most common phenomenon is bacterial infections, where *Staphylococcus aureus* is a common etiology, but it may also be caused by fungi or other microorganisms. The clinical relevance is high since these infections are capable of leading to osteomyelitis, septic arthritis, and amputation in very bad cases. Complications are to be kept to a minimum, and healing promoted through effective surveillance mechanisms and clinical practice by early diagnosis and management.

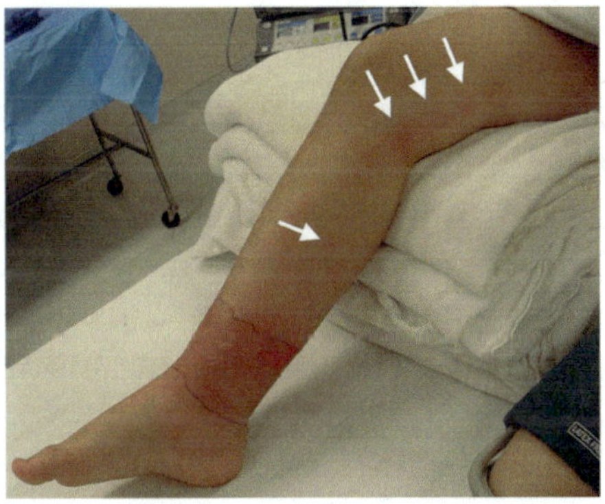

Figure 10.2. The term orthopedic infections.

Source: https://external-content.duckduckgo.com/iu/?u=https%3A%2F%2Fi0.wp.com%2Fmusculoskeletalkey.com%2Fwp-content%2Fuploads%2F2021%2F01%2FC18-FF1-1.gif%3Fw%3D960&f=1&nofb=1&ipt=49c836fa25c25d86e5f598b664b121317ad8fe7c4e19affed1674dde588ab5d1.

Hence, ongoing research on new treatment techniques and prevention is the need of the hour. Research on the definition and implications of orthopedic infection, given the evolving healthcare scenario, will equip healthcare professionals to deliver improved patient care and results in orthopedic surgery (Figure 10.2).

Importance of Understanding Orthopedic Infections

The understanding of orthopedic infections plays a key role in improving patient outcomes and minimizing surgical-related complications. Orthopedic infections, particularly those that are post-surgical, can lead to prolonged hospitalization, increased healthcare expenses, and severe morbidity in patients. Accurate identification and management of such infections are critical not only for the effective management of the infection itself but also for preventing repeated recurrence of such complications. This knowledge entails awareness of the contributing factors for infections, including patient population, comorbidities, and other environmental factors such as environmental change. A case in point is that current research indicates that changes in seasons have wide-ranging implications on periprosthetic joint infection rates and therefore it is critical for healthcare providers to bear this information in mind when examining patients and evaluating risk (Rosas et al., 2017). By doing this, health professionals are able to improve decision-making and improve the quality of care overall. Another element of the value of learning about orthopedic infections is the influence on surgical procedures and protocols. It has been discovered that some season of the year has higher infection rates; thus, knowledge of such trends allows for the formulation of specific preoperative and postoperative care plans. Infection control measures intensified in peak seasons can considerably reduce infections as well as improve surgical outcomes. In addition, understanding orthopedic infection at a deeper level assists practitioners in choosing the right antibiotics and improving patient management techniques, ultimately leading to hospital readmission reduction. Understanding aids the proactive approach among the surgical team, ensuring watchful monitoring as well as intervention. Knowledge of these variables has a significant bearing on the direction of patient care, hence both practicing professionals and those entering the field have to remain current. Additionally, awareness of orthopedic infections has implications beyond individual patient care, extending to encompass public health. Infections can bear on the allocation of healthcare resources, rates of insurance, and even rehabilitation following surgery. Maximum management of these infections will lead to a lower total cost within the healthcare system, since infections not managed adequately can result in costly re-operations and follow-up procedures. The financial burden of orthopedic infection identifies the requirement for specific research and education in this area, to produce evidence-based guidelines that minimize costs but maximize clinical outcomes. Additionally, education of the healthcare providers and patients on prevention and symptoms of orthopedic infections is also imperative. Awareness facilitates patients to actively engage in their care process and adhere to postoperative instructions, resulting in better health and well-being (Stavrakis et al., 2015). The comprehension of orthopedic infections is therefore vital not just for clinical excellence but also towards the creation of an enhanced healthcare system.

10.1. Types of Orthopedic Infections

Orthopedic infections are usually divided first and foremost based on their anatomical site of involvement and pathogenesis, and therefore between superficial and deep infections. Superficial infections, which typically appear at the level of the skin surrounding surgical wounds, typically manifest as erythema, swelling, and pus drainage. These tend to follow surgery and are typically managed by antibiotics or minor surgical interventions. Deep infections, however, penetrate beneath the skin and subcutaneous tissues and extend to the underlying bone and joint machinery. These are far more perilous as they can lead to complications of osteomyelitis or septic arthritis and need more vigorous treatment protocols. Understanding these categories is critical for orthopedic surgeons, as they determine the choice of operation, the requirement for removal of the implant, and management of the patient's condition in general. Orthopedic infections can also be divided according to their cause, both hematogenous and contiguous. Hematogenous infections are carried through the bloodstream to bone and joint tissue, often from a distant infection site or in patients who have a pre-existing systemic condition. Contiguous infections, by contrast, are typically associated with trauma or surgery, whereby the pathogen contaminates the operating field or bone by direct contact with infected hardware. The separation of the two types is of significant treatment implications. For instance, hematogenous infections may be treated with long-term antibiotic therapy aimed at known pathogens, while contiguous infections may need surgical debridement in addition to pharmacological treatment. In addition, some classifications, such as open fractures, can predispose some patients to some pathogens and therefore we need individualized treatment regimens. Moreover, outcomes of orthopedic infections can also be defined significantly by classification systems that could exclude the risk of infection following fractures, especially open fractures. For example, the Gustilo-Anderson classification system remains a critical tool in evaluating open fractures, where its predictive value in fracture-related infections (FRI) has been well established. In studies, Gustilo-Anderson classification was reported to be a more sensitive predictor of FRI compared to Orthopedic Trauma Association-Open Fracture Classification (OTA-OFC), indicating the importance of precise classification in decision-making (Khoury et al., 2024). The implications are important; using the criteria, clinicians can predict such complications as osteomyelitis and adjust their treatment strategies based on this. Therefore, understanding the various categories and types of orthopedic infection enables healthcare professionals to avoid injury and achieve the best outcomes in surgical patients (Figure 10.3).

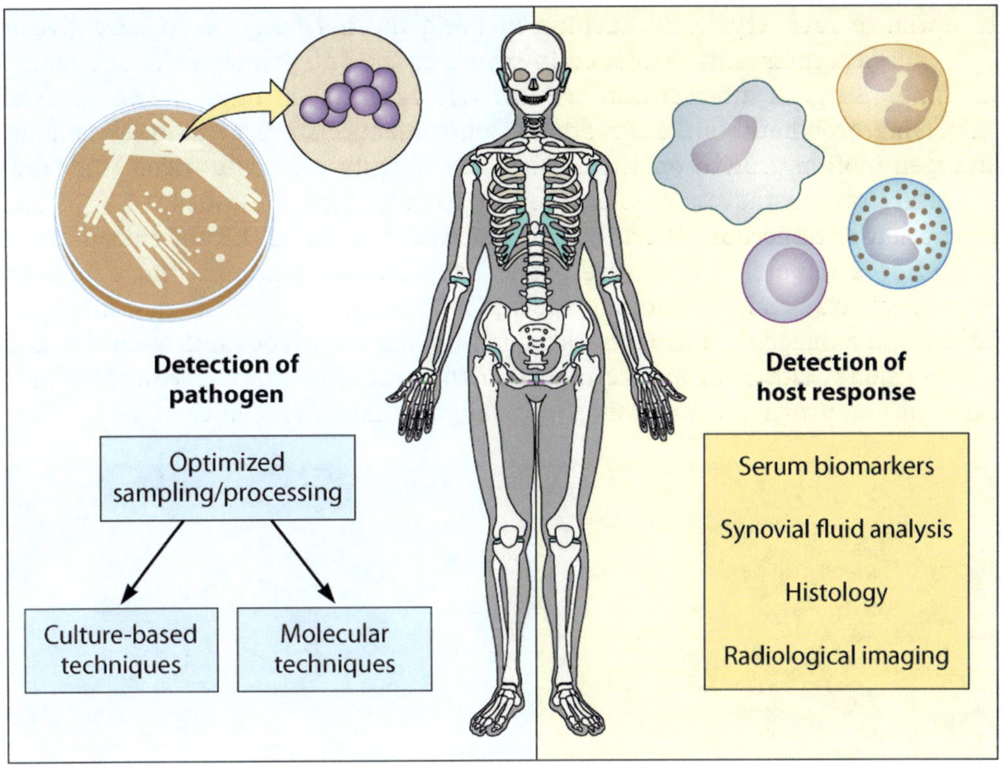

Figure 10.3. Orthopedic infections can be primarily categorized based on their anatomical location and mode of onset.

Source: https://journals.asm.org/cms/10.1128/jcm.02196-21/asset/e95ab353-4ea0-4b40-8148-3c253ee47d05/assets/images/large/jcm.02196-21-f001.jpg.

10.1.1. Osteomyelitis

Osteomyelitis, an infection of the bone leading to inflammation, is a difficult condition in orthopedic medicine. Pathophysiology is multifactorial and most often the result of a compromise of the skin or direct spread from a contiguous infection that permits the introduction of pathogens into bone. In diabetic patients, osteomyelitis is a complication of ulcers of the foot, which may be undetected due to neuropathy, thereby making early detection and treatment challenging. The risk of chronic osteomyelitis explains the need for proper and timely diagnosis since any delay can result in further damage to tissue as well as other complications, including the need for amputation. Explanation of the pathophysiological mechanisms of falling victim to this condition is essential to formulating effective management strategies with a view to restoring bone strength and function in such affected patients. Osteomyelitis management remains controversial among the medical fraternity, mostly due to heterogeneity of clinical presentation as well as health status among patients. Controversy pertains to conservative versus surgical management, particularly diabetic foot osteomyelitis. A study highlighted that a significant proportion of patients, i.e., 63.5%, achieved remission with nonsurgical intervention alone, i.e., antibiotic treatment for an extended duration of 10.8 weeks (Zeun et al., 2016). Specific clinical factors, e.g., pedal pulses, were found to have a significant impact on outcome. Thus, careful assessment and individually formulated treatment plans are essential to optimize recovery while keeping in mind the harmony of conservative modalities and the urgent surgical intervention needed in severe cases. The principles of adequate antibiotic therapy and timely surgical intervention are likewise essential in other forms of osteomyelitis, especially involving prosthetic joints. Prosthetic joint infections are of unique challenge, mainly because pathogen biofilm growth on the surface of implants creates difficulty in eradication. A review of literature reveals that there is a necessity to determine the causative organism in order to direct appropriate antimicrobial therapy, since this will determine the patient's outcome (Fsadni & Fsadni, 2013). It is important to ensure proper coordination among orthopedic surgeons and infectious disease specialists in developing specific management protocols that integrate both the surgical and medical management aspects. Ultimately, being knowledgeable about the complexities of osteomyelitis, along with appropriate management practices, plays a vital role in enhancing patient treatment and prognostic outcomes in orthopedic infection (Figure 10.4).

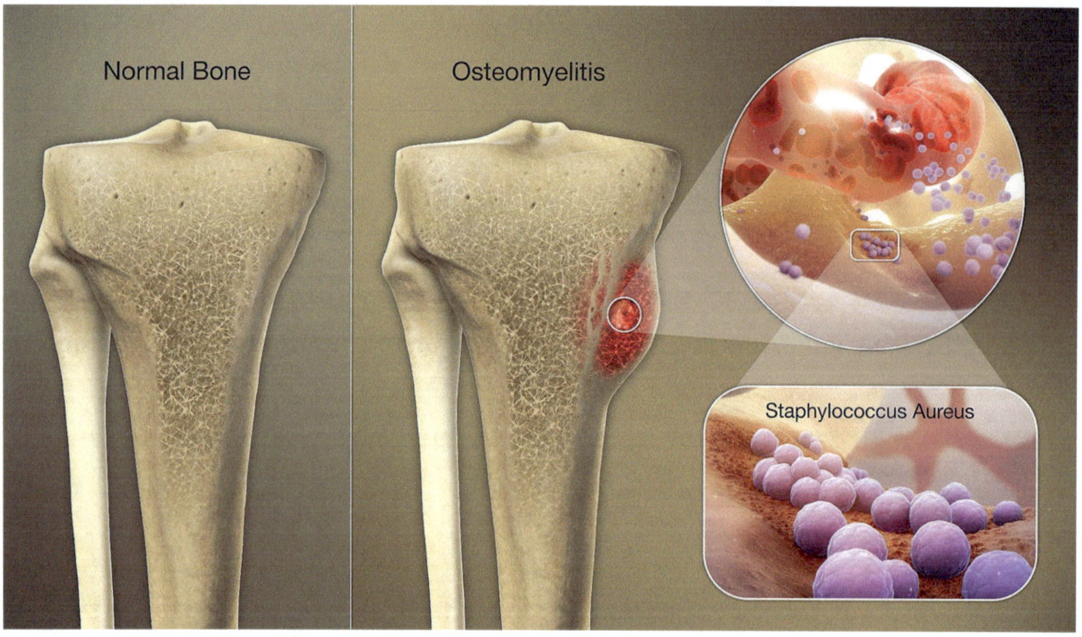

Figure 10.4. Osteomyelitis, an inflammatory condition of the bone caused by infection.

Source: https://geekymedics.com/wp-content/uploads/2024/12/1600px-3D_Medical_Animation_Staphylococcus_Aureus-2.jpg.

10.1.2. Septic Arthritis

Septic arthritis represents a serious complication of infections in orthopedics, and it is chiefly characterized by the joint infection caused by the infectious agent. The condition typically comes with searing pain, swelling, and restriction of mobility, ultimately impairing the integrity of the infected joint. Methicillin-sensitive and methicillin-resistant *Staphylococcus aureus* have been among the most common etiologic microorganisms in the past; yet, an enlarged microbial spectrum that includes Gram-negative bacteria and fungi can also be a causative agent of this devastating condition. Early diagnosis, facilitated through joint aspiration and fluid culture, becomes critical in delineating the microbial etiology. The overall aim in the management of septic arthritis is the eradication of the offending pathogen with simultaneous preservation of joint function. The delay in treatment can increase the risk of joint destruction, again calling for vigilance and efficacy in diagnosing this critical medical dilemma in orthopedic practice. Effective treatment of septic arthritis relies on a combination of antimicrobial therapy and surgical intervention. Initial treatment is most often comprised of the administration of appropriate intravenous antibiotics targeted to the identified pathogen, which is primarily based on cultures drawn from joint fluid. In the more extreme cases, particularly when the formation of an abscess or significant joint destruction occurs, surgery is sometimes required, typically in the form of arthroscopic or open drainage. The type of drainage employed may affect both the rate of recovery and the final result of the joint, as illustrated in research concerning the use of antibiotic spacers in periprosthetic infection. Surprisingly, while both stemmed and stemless antibiotic spacers have shown similar clinical outcomes, the specificity of individual patient cases and severity of infection will guide the decision-making process of the orthopedic surgeons (Padegimas et al., 2017). Integration of the treatment techniques is not just intended to cure the acute infection but also to rehabilitate and restore function, emphasizing the value of comprehensive integrated care. The implications of septic arthritis extend beyond the immediate joint pathology; instead, they involve an overall impact on long-term prognosis, requiring careful follow-up. Possible residual joint dysfunction or risk for subsequent osteoarthritis in the patient after septic arthritis may be due to the initial inflammatory response or architectural compromise within the joint complex. Moreover, the psychological impact of pain and limitation of movement cannot be underestimated after recovery. Longitudinal studies show that a significant percentage of patients can benefit from ongoing rehabilitation in an effort to optimize pre-infection functionality and quality of life levels. Therefore, septic arthritis treatment must tackle not just the removal of infection but an overall rehabilitation plan, so patients can navigate the complex landscape of recovery without undue risk of future joint complications (Kuong et al., 2012) (Figure 10.5).

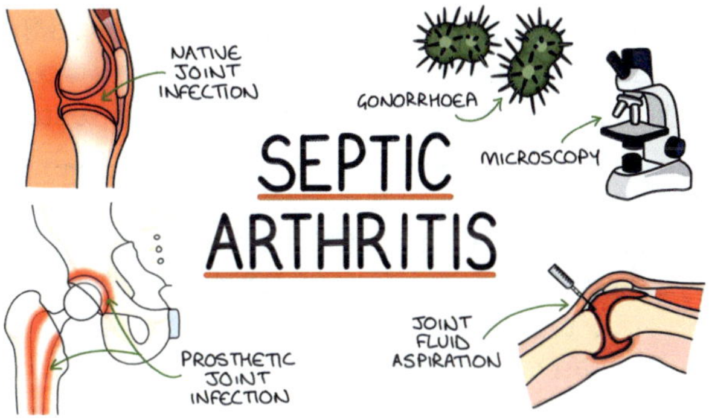

Figure 10.5. Septic arthritis represents a significant complication.

Source: https://i.ytimg.com/vi/ToLPT_FSRwU/maxresdefault.jpg.

10.1.3. Prosthetic Joint Infections

The responsibility of prosthetic joint infections (PJIs) is a challenging issue in orthopedic management, normally the outcome of complex interactions among host, surgical, and microbial factors. With the placement of prosthetic materials in the human body, the risk of infection is increased due to such reasons as biofilm development, which enhances bacteria's ability to attach and colonize surfaces. *Staphylococcus aureus* and *Staphylococcus epidermidis* are usually implicated organisms, and these thrive in such conditions, making diagnosis and treatment challenging. Since infections may occur even under sterile surgical conditions, knowledge of the dynamics of PJIs is essential in order to best optimize preventive protocols and treat existing infections. The institution of local guidelines for identification and proper management of such infection continues to be important in preventing their occurrence and enhancing patient outcomes (Fsadni & Fsadni, 2013). Treatment of prosthetic joint infections needs a multidisciplinary approach, including both surgery and antimicrobial therapy. Prompt detection of the causative organism is critical since proper antimicrobial treatment can influence the outcome significantly. Antibiotics form the cornerstone of the treatment protocol, but their activity can be significantly blunted by biofilm formation on the prosthetic surfaces. Surgical intervention—excision of infected prosthetic material, in most cases—is frequently required for cure, illustrating the fine balance between surgical and antimicrobial treatment of PJIs. Local health policies must prioritize getting surgical teams and infectious disease experts fully trained to enable integration and establish customized protocols that take into account distinctive infection patterns in their patient groups (Smith & Chetter, 2015). Prophylaxis against prosthetic joint infections is still a top priority in orthopedic intervention, and patient optimization before surgery is crucial. Various factors lead to the occurrence of these infections, such as comorbidities, which make patients susceptible to postoperative complications. The preoperative evaluations involving the assessment of patients' general health and modification of risk factors can greatly reduce the risk of PJIs. In addition, continued research into newer technology, such as infection-reducing biological prostheses, holds promising prospects for orthopedic practice. In the integration of preventive components with developments in the surgical technique and materials, the medical field can effectively enhance patient safety and outcomes in terms of prosthetic joint replacement surgery (Fsadni & Fsadni, 2013) (Figure 10.6).

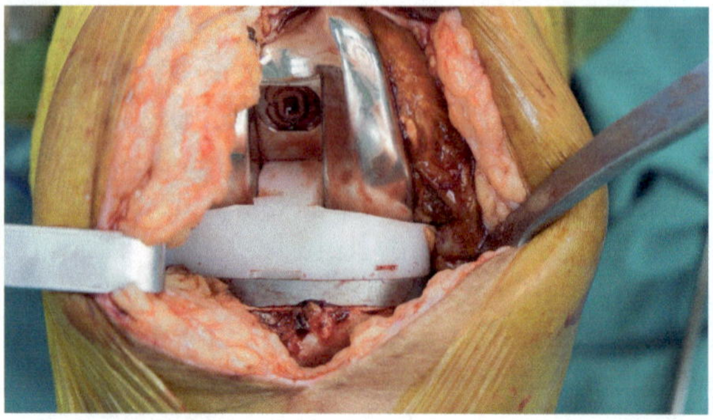

Figure 10.6. The incidence of prosthetic joint infections (PJIs).

Source: https://www.rheumatologyadvisor.com/wp-content/uploads/sites/18/2019/01/arthroplastyofkneesh376986_1449983.jpg.

10.2. Causes and Risk Factors

Orthopedic infections are multifaceted complications resulting from many risk factors, some of which include the nature of surgery performed. Surgery, particularly operative procedures on implantable devices, puts individuals at risk of infection by potential exposure of deep tissues to disease-causing microorganisms. Spinal fusion procedures, for instance, which are often applied in the treatment of idiopathic scoliosis, have been associated with surgical site infections (SSIs) due to pathogens like Propionibacterium acnes. A case-control study highlighted that not only are the occurrences of such infections associated with some pathogens, but also with patient demographics and with surgical complexity. It was identified that acute infection happens shortly after surgery while delayed infection may happen even years after surgery has been conducted, identifying the importance of looking into both the short-term and long-term risk factors in surgical practice (Swarup et al., 2018). Another significant reason for orthopedic infections is factors related to the patient, such as comorbidities, age, and immune status. Patients who are elderly, for example, pose a higher risk of infections due to physiological changes in immune response and wound healing.

A literature review of hip hemiarthroplasty cited alarming rates of post-operative infection at 4.68% in the UK, significantly higher than the less than 1% rate for elective hip procedures (Sprowson et al., 2013). This difference emphasizes the absolute significance of the health status of the patient before surgery in the estimation of infection risk. In addition, diabetes, obesity, and malnutrition also potentially enhance the risk of infection. Because of this, optimization of the health status of potential surgical candidates is most important for minimizing infection rates and associated complications of orthopedic surgery. The use of prophylactic interventions, including antibiotic therapy and asepsis, has been the mainstay in reducing infection risk in orthopedic procedures. While these practices have evolved, the increasing trend for SSIs is generating concern, with extensive studies conducted in search of newer technologies. Present trials evaluating high-dose antibiotic-impregnated cement in hip hemiarthroplasty aim to determine its efficacy in reducing infection rates and enhancing patient outcomes. Outcome of such randomized controlled trials could revolutionize clinical guidance and encourage the adoption of Corrigendum for enhanced infection prevention, particularly among high-risk groups (Sprowson et al., 2013). With ongoing advances by medical professionals in surgical techniques and preventive measures, understanding the etiology and risk factors of orthopedic infections will prove critical in minimizing their occurrence and advancing worldwide patient care.

10.2.1. Bacterial Pathogens

In orthopedic infections, bacterial pathogens emerge as the prime suspect for causing increased morbidity and surgical procedure complications. Infections, particularly following arthroplasty, are a serious issue due to the fine balance required for healing to be effective. Bacterial pathogens such as *Staphylococcus aureus* and *Staphylococcus epidermidis* not only cause increased infection rates but also become critical in necessitating revision surgeries, which then complicate treatment. Studies show infection rates after arthroplasty ranging between 1% and 4%, increasing significantly with revision arthroplasty. Prevention of these complications is significant through the development of novel methods of infection and disinfection so that early therapy can be applied for such pathogens and ultimately improve patient outcomes in orthopedic practice (McDonald et al., 2013). New advances in bactericidal technology, such as high-intensity narrow-spectrum (HINS) light, have shown promising results in minimizing bacterial bioburden in operating rooms. The success of HINS light at specific intensities has been validated through extensive testing, indicating that it can kill orthopedic infection-relevant pathogens without compromise to osteoblast viability. For instance, HINS light exposure at 5 mW/cm2 killed over 98% of *Staphylococcus aureus* and 83% of *Staphylococcus epidermidis*, proving its effectiveness as a potential disinfection tool for orthopedic surgical theatres. Not only does this breakthrough application kill common bacterial pathogens, but it also represents a significant milestone in the diminution of postoperative infection levels, thus the overall success rate of orthopedic procedures (McDonald et al., 2013). To combat the development and dissemination of bacterial pathogens in orthopedic infections, it is imperative to explore novel infection-control strategies founded on biomaterials science. With ever-mounting antibiotic resistance, traditional infection-management techniques are increasingly insufficient. The introduction of nanotechnology in the construction of next-generation biomaterials is an interesting direction towards enhancing infection resistance as well as promoting tissue regeneration. Animal pre-clinical models are essential in the evaluation of the efficacy of new methods of overcoming bacterial infections; however, a knowledge of the limitations of such models is imperative. Results in animals will not always reflect clinical cases, and careful study design with an emphasis on reducing mortality and preventing recurrence of infection is necessary. The application of such new technologies has the potential to improve interventions in the management of orthopedic infections and ultimately improve patient care (Figure 10.7).

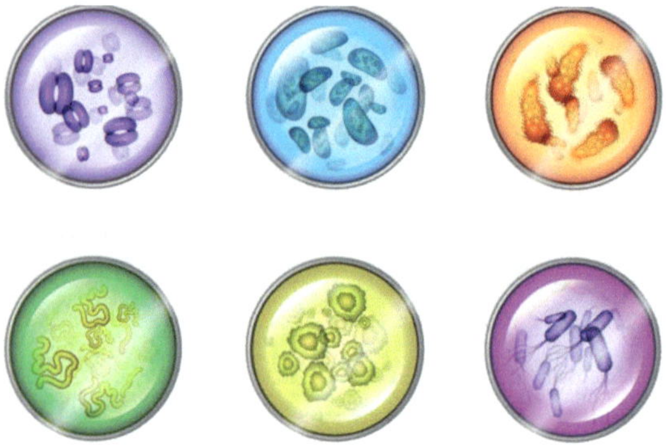

Figure 10.7. The bacterial pathogens emerge as the primary culprits.

Source: https://img.mlo-online.com/files/base/ebm/mlo/image/2022/11/16x9/AdobeStock_224535449.6384d36f46eaa.png?auto=format,compress&fit=max&q=45&w=640&width=640.

10.2.2. Surgical Procedures and Trauma

Surgery, and particularly the management of trauma, has crucial roles to play in orthopedic infection treatment. Trauma patients are often in need of urgent surgical management to facilitate recovery and minimize the risk of complications such as infection. Damage control orthopedics has emerged as a central theme in recent years, particularly in the management of complex injuries from traumatic injury. This is a policy that emphasizes early wound control, immediate fracture reduction, and proper antibiotic prophylaxis, all of which are responsible for preventing infection and ensuring maximum patient outcome. Such surgery, particularly in combat settings, has been proven to be linked with increased rates of recovery as well as reduced mortality, emphasizing the importance of coordinated care strategies in cases of trauma (Ng et al., 2015). The nature of injury in traumatic settings, especially in conflict areas, is especially testing for surgeons. As witnessed during the Libyan civil war, treating serious spinal and limb injuries involves not only technical competence but the ability to improvise under ever-changing conditions and constraints of resource availability. The Gustilo-Anderson system illustrates the severity of injuries, such as Type IIIB/C, which often require extremely complex surgical treatment and rigorous infection management. Creating a multidisciplinary team model has proven useful in the sense that it effectively incorporates the mix of expertise necessary to stabilize complicated cases, thereby enhancing patient outcomes and providing global care. The integration of these strategies demonstrates an extensive understanding of surgical trauma management (Ng et al., 2015). Besides trauma management, infection prevention and treatment remain high on the agenda following surgery. Specifically, in spine surgery, infection of the implant can lead to disastrous complications involving neurological damage and extended disability. New research on animal models for postoperative spine infection illustrates the need for improved methodologies to evaluate infection in terms of a greater range involving parameters such as variability of bacterial strain and long-term outcomes. Extending these models through new methods involving advanced imaging and bioluminescent bacterial strains, researchers aim to refine treatment protocols and prevention. This ongoing study emphasizes the critical interface of surgical treatment, trauma, and infection, ultimately leading to improving patient care and prevention of orthopedic infections.

10.2.3. Patient-Related Factors (e.g., Diabetes, Immunocompromised Status)

Orthopedic infections are strongly influenced by a number of factors related to the patient, particularly comorbid diseases such as diabetes mellitus and immunosuppressive diseases. Diabetic patients are prone to infection due to defects in wound healing, impaired circulation, and impaired immunity.

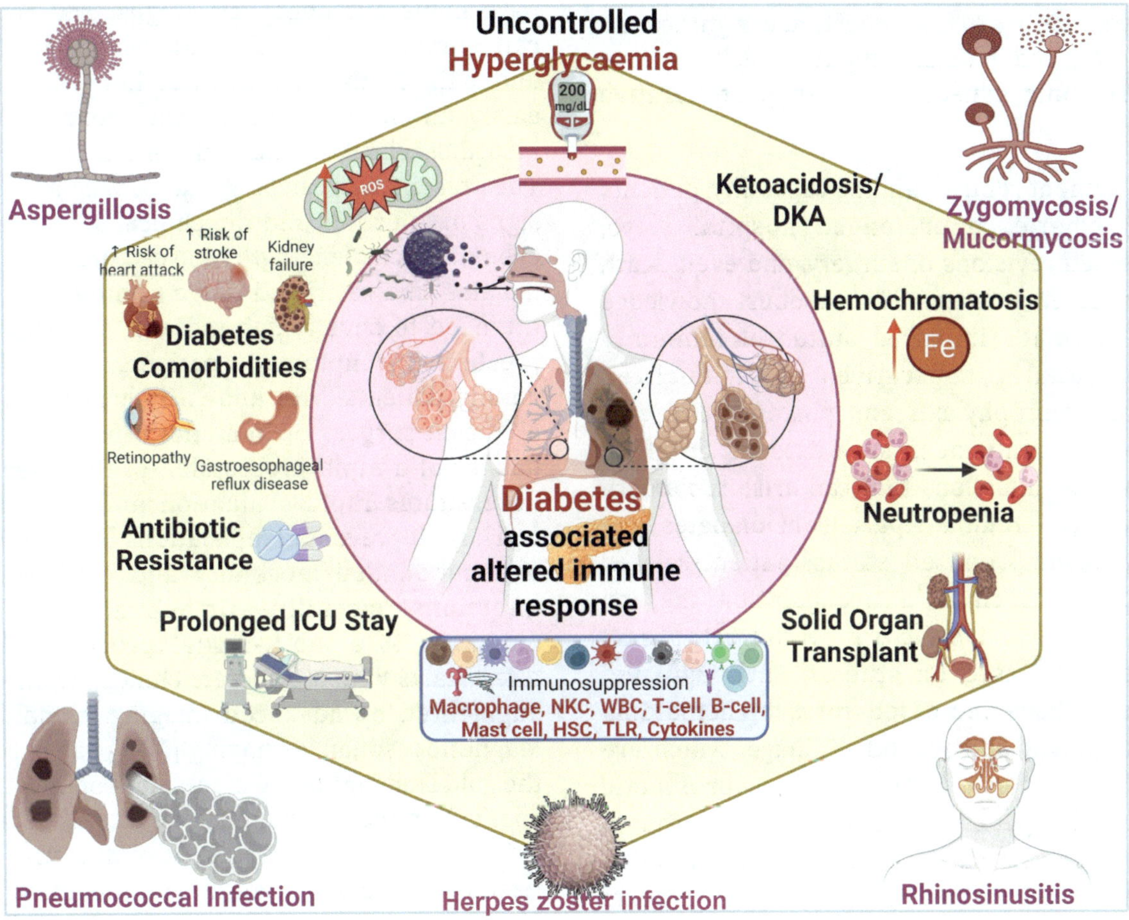

Figure 10.8. Orthopedic infections are significantly influenced by various patient-related factors.

Source: https://pub.mdpi-res.com/biologics/biologics-03-00004/article_deploy/html/images/biologics-03-00004-ag.png?1678264463.

Hyperglycemia can cause dysfunction in neutrophil function and cause an increased risk for bacterial growth, thus rendering these patients extremely vulnerable to infection after surgery. Moreover, studies indicate that diabetics undergoing orthopedic interventions have higher rates of postoperative complications like infections compared to non-diabetic patients. This increased vulnerability necessitates that diabetic patients should be properly assessed before surgery so that preparations are made to minimize such risks and enable quick recovery. The patient's immunocompromised state, whether due to cancer treatment, autoimmune disease, or long-term steroid use, further contributes to the risk of orthopedic infection. The immune system's ability to fight infection is significantly compromised in these patients, which can have catastrophic consequences in postoperative recovery.

Without robust immune capability, patients may experience prolonged hospital stays, increased revisions of surgery, and even death due to severe infection. Thus, a robust knowledge of a patient's impaired status of immunity is essential preoperatively. Individualized antibiotic prophylaxis and postoperative care become paramount in such cases in an effort to prevent infections that can arise secondary to surgical trauma. Apart from diabetes and immunocompromised status, patient-related conditions such as anticoagulation therapy are also causative factors behind orthopedic infections. Based on studies, anticoagulated patients have increased rates of hematoma development and wound drainage, which are established risk factors for periprosthetic infection. Specifically, a study found that a high mean international normalized ratio value of above 1.5 was more prevalent in patients who subsequently developed wound infections and complications following surgery. This underlines the need for careful management of anticoagulation in the perioperative period since wise dosing not only prevents hematoma formation but also is a necessary safety measure precluding later infection, showing the intricate relationship between drug management and patient factors in orthopedic clinical practice (Parvizi et al., 2007; Fang et al., 2017) (Figure 10.8).

10.3. Symptoms and Diagnosis

Recognition of the signs is critical in early diagnosis of orthopedic infections, which can have numerous nonspecific signs. The patient can complain of local tenderness, swelling, and pain at the site of infection, which are easily mimicked by other conditions such as musculoskeletal trauma or degenerative disease. The presentation can be subtle with no apparent signs of infection, and the clinical syndrome is even more challenging. These can include fever, malaise, and restricted range of motion, hence the need to have a high index of suspicion on presenting symptoms in patients, particularly among patients with known risk factors such as recent surgery or immunosuppression. The danger of a rapid progression of the infection necessitates rapid evaluation and diagnostic workup to prevent complications that can lead to compounded morbidity and, with severe infections, mortality. Orthopedic infection diagnosis is a multi-modal process, which often starts with a complete clinical evaluation augmented by advanced imaging modalities. Magnetic resonance imaging (MRI) has become the gold standard in the assessment of infectious spondylitis and other similar conditions because MRI has a superior capacity to image the soft tissue and assess the size of the infection. Moreover, while computed tomography (CT) and nuclear medicine studies can be helpful as well, their utility may be dependent upon the specific clinical context. It is important that clinicians distinguish between infectious processes and other pathological conditions with careful observation of imaging features, as they can be analogous to similar symptoms in other spinal pathologies. Accurate diagnosis relies on a clear understanding of the interdependence between imaging features and clinical presentations, resulting in the right therapeutic interventions to prevent the infection. In fracture-associated infection (FRI), timeliness of recognition and diagnosis continues to be the most important, as the specificity of this disease would pose novel challenges to orthopedic surgeons. FRI is likely to have an insidious and nonspecific presentation, potentially leading to delayed treatment and associated complications of recurrent infection and chronic disability. It is significant to improve clinical outcomes as well as to reduce the huge financial burden caused by these infections on the healthcare system and the public. A systematic approach that combines clinical evaluation with advanced imaging modalities is critical to achieve the highest possible diagnostic accuracy. By giving a deeper understanding of the distinct presentation and diagnostic features of FRI within the broader context of orthopedic infections, practitioners are best able to optimize treatment regimens and ultimately improve patient prognosis (He et al., 2023).

10.3.1. Common Clinical Symptoms

Orthopedic infections can be linked to various clinical signs that are critical for diagnosis and treatment. The most common of these is pain referred to the site of infection, ranging from mild to severe crippling pain. Pain in this case usually correlates with the severity of infection and could increase with movement or pressure at the infected site. In addition, swelling and inflammation are typical findings in the form of erythema or redness over the affected area. These are not only evidence that infection is present but, more importantly, differentiate it from other processes, such as trauma or arthritis. Lastly, systemic signs such as fever and malaise may accompany local findings, indicating a more systemic reaction to infection, which must be watched closely by healthcare providers. Another important symptom of orthopedic infection is purulent drainage, which may occur as the characteristic sign of abscess formation. The quality of this drainage can provide rich information regarding the causative pathogens since different bacterial infections produce exudate of varying qualities. For instance, *Staphylococcus aureus* infections can result in thick, yellow discharge, while other less pathogenic organisms produce a more serous fluid. This clinical presentation requires early intervention, as delayed intervention can result in additional complications, such as necrosis of the surrounding tissue. Further, clinicians must be cautious to distinguish such drainage from other diseases, since infections like necrotizing fasciitis can progress very rapidly and may initially have only a nonspecific presentation (Szilagyi et al., 2023).

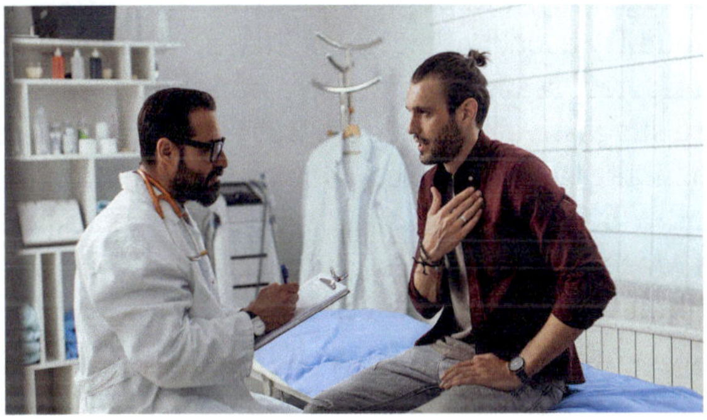

Figure 10.9. Common clinical symptoms.

Source: https://www.cdc.gov/hepatitis-a/media/images/2024/04/hepatitis-a-clinical-signs-symptoms-thumbnail.jpg.

Systemic symptoms like fever, chills, or fatigue can be noticed by patients in certain cases and indicate a more systemic response to the infection. This acute inflammatory reaction can lead to septic arthritis or osteomyelitis, which goes on to influence the overall clinical presentation. These presentations systemically emphasize the requirement of thorough clinical evaluations as they are suggestive of potential complications of orthopedic infections. Identification of such signs can enable early intervention, which is necessary given the fact that untreated orthopedic infections can lead to long-term disability and even mortality. Integration of patient history and physical exam findings with existing imaging modalities may assist in creating a comprehensive treatment plan tailored to the patient-specific presentations, thereby improving outcomes in orthopedic infection management (Dagher et al., 2024) (Figure 10.9).

10.3.2. Diagnostic Imaging Techniques

Diagnostic imaging modalities play a key role in the detection and management of orthopedic infections, significantly enhancing the clinician's ability to make the correct decision. Plain radiography, although often the first imaging modality used, will at times identify nonspecific periosteal reaction or erosive bone changes that are suggestive of infection. But it may be unable to make a distinction between a malignant and a benign process, as with some examples of coccidioidomycosis, wherein lesions had simulated neoplasms on initial X-ray reports. The solution is to add these findings with higher-level modalities such as magnetic resonance imaging (MRI) or computed tomography (CT) scans, which provide greater definition of soft tissue involvement and the process's extent. This general strategy allows for an accurate diagnosis, which prompts early treatment for such complex infections. Additional studies on MRI and CT machines reveal their utility for deeper tissue infection diagnosis and osteomyelitis assessment. MRI is particularly valuable due to increased soft tissue contrast, by means of which inflammatory processes near bone structures can be observed. By detection of abscesses or edema, MRI is more effective in guiding surgery than is routine with current methods. An example was two patients with knee pain, where imaging revealed lytic lesions diagnosed as primary bone tumors that ultimately proved to be extrapulmonary coccidioidomycosis on histology. Such misdiagnoses serve to underscore the importance of incorporating advanced diagnostic imaging techniques in the evaluation of orthopedic infection because they provide critical information that alters the direction of treatment. In conclusion, the use of advanced diagnostic imaging techniques in the evaluation of orthopedic infection cannot be overstated. Each imaging modality provides valuable information that informs clinical decision-making and eventually results in better patient outcomes through timely and proper interventions. Furthermore, it is critical that healthcare professionals understand the uses and differences of these techniques. As demonstrated through examples with the cases of coccidioidomycosis, the utilization of traditional imaging in isolation can lead to misdiagnosis, highlighting the necessity of efficient communication between radiologists and orthopedic surgeons. By sustaining high suspicion and with the help of advanced imaging modalities, clinicians can overcome the obstacles of orthopedic infections and provide accurate diagnoses and implement appropriate treatment in such a complicated case as this (Li et al., 2014; Stavrakis et al., 2015).

10.3.3. Laboratory Tests and Cultures

For orthopedic infections, laboratory testing and cultures play a key role in identifying bacterial pathogens accurately and treating them. Causative organism identification is always important because the information would directly influence the choice of antimicrobial therapy. Laboratory techniques like joint aspirates, blood cultures, and tissue biopsies are used to isolate and identify microbial agents causing infection. The application of such methods allows clinicians to track phenotypic characteristics and conduct further antimicrobial susceptibility testing, which is absolutely necessary for effective treatment planning. As pointed out in the literature, local prevalence studies have the potential to gain an in-depth understanding of the organisms that are most likely to result in prosthetic joint infections and render more specific therapeutic approaches feasible in practice (Fsadni & Fsadni, 2013). Besides, the individual cultures must also be responsive and immediate to adequately manage the nuances of orthopedic infections. Propionibacterium acnes, for instance, has been referred to as a challenging organism to isolate due to its slow growth. Testing within the laboratory must be done for the identification of both acute and delayed infections that may be caused by such pathogens. Acute Propionibacterium acnes infections in a case-control study developed shortly after surgery, with the need for careful observation of postoperative patients for early infection, while delayed infections required more extensive testing (Swarup et al., 2018). Researchers point to the need for strict laboratory protocols in order to aid in the detection and deliver appropriate sensitivity testing for these slow-growing microorganisms that are key causative agents of surgical site infections within orthopedic settings. Lastly, the integration of laboratory tests and culture results with clinical presentations invites an integrative approach in the management of orthopedic infection. With the combination of new diagnostic technologies and old-fashioned methods, providers can refine the accuracy of diagnoses and speed of treatment. Moreover, cross-disciplinary communication between infectious disease specialists and orthopedic surgeons can result in enhanced management guidelines combining surgical treatment with empirical antibiotics. The collaboration not only optimizes patient results but also informs the creation of consensus guidelines. The ongoing research in organism detection and susceptibility patterns will be important in revamping treatment strategies for prosthetic joint infections and other related conditions in orthopedic practice (Fsadni & Fsadni, 2013) (Figure 10.10).

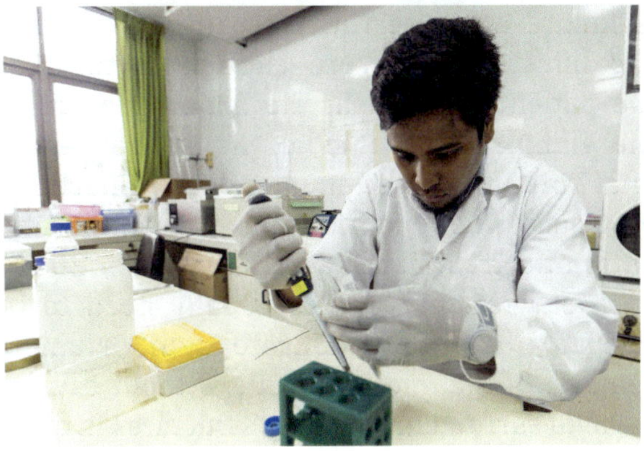

Figure 10.10. Laboratory tests and cultures.

Source: https://www.lalpathlabs.com/blog/wp-content/uploads/2016/09/blood-culuture-test.jpg.

10.4. Treatment Options

Orthopedic infections should be managed multidisciplinarily, involving both pharmacologic and surgical interventions to yield the best patient outcomes. Antibiotic therapy remains an essential component of the treatment, modulated depending on the infecting pathogens, particularly for the management of biofilm-based infections caused by prosthetic implants. It is challenging for bacteria such as *Staphylococcus aureus* and S. epidermidis is their ability to adhere to implant surfaces, thereby forming biofilms, making them resistant to conventional antibiotic therapies (Stavrakis et al., 2015). The complexity necessitates proper microbial identification by cultures and advanced diagnostic imaging techniques, which can guide clinicians on how to select effective treatment modalities. In addition, new developments in antimicrobial coatings and materials for implants promise not only to reduce infections but possibly to prevent them in the first place, implying a preventative approach as much as a reactive one. Surgical treatment might become indicated where there is failure of conservative treatment or when the infection is severe enough to threaten the patient's health. In the majority of cases, the elimination of infected hardware plays a vital role in the treatment of such infections, especially when biofilm formation complicates antibiotic treatment (Stavrakis et al., 2015). Such surgical procedures usually need to be carried out with a delicate equilibrium of removal of the infected tissue without causing harm to surrounding healthy structures in order to maintain the integrity of the infected limb. In addition to debridement and removal of hardware, negative pressure wound therapy is now in vogue to facilitate healing and reduce additional chances of infection. This technology not only helps in wound management, but it also creates a tissue regenerative environment that is very important after debridement. Last but not least, preventive strategies cannot be emphasized strongly enough in the fight against orthopedic infections. Aside from the drug and surgical interventions, enhancing patient health before elective surgery, for instance, comorbidity and nutritional management, can reduce the rate of surgical-site infections significantly (Smith & Chetter, 2015). Furthermore, studies into biological prostheses also advance with the intent of maximizing the body's response to infection and lowering the risks associated with foreign bodies. These developments mirror a movement toward more complete models of treatment that consider the patient's overall health. As our knowledge base in orthopedic infections grows, it is increasingly clear that an interdisciplinary approach will work best in managing this multifaceted and challenging aspect of medical practice.

10.4.1. Antibiotic Therapy

The role of antibiotic therapy in the management of orthopedic infection cannot be overstated. With the prevalence of infection following surgery, and specifically the insertion of orthopedic hardware, appropriate antibiotic therapy is crucial. These patients are at a high risk of surgical site infection, which can significantly prolong recovery, lead to greater morbidity, and necessitate additional surgery. With ongoing progress in the development of antibiotic resistance, certain therapies must be well selected for application in the treatment of infection due to resistant microorganisms by clinicians. Blending different treatment approaches, including new therapies, can maximize the effectiveness of conventional antibiotic regimens in the treatment of severe post-surgical infections (Cascini et al., 2024). Biofilm-forming pathogenicity and specificity complicate the treatment in orthopedic practice. These bacteria, having adhered to implant surfaces, can resist standard antibiotic therapy since they are in an altered physiological state and possess intrinsic mechanisms of resistance. As noted in current studies, the efficacy and function of antibiotics like rifampicin can decline with aging biofilms, leading to chronic infection that defies standard treatment strategies (Youf et al., 2024). Clinicians cannot solely rely on systemic antibiotic therapy but also need to rely on local delivery methods and adjunctive strategies to treat the biofilm infection successfully, hence improving orthopedic treatment patient outcomes. Evidence indicates that employing traditional antibiotic therapy combined with newer treatment modalities may be more effective when treating orthopedic infections. For example, later studies of oxygen-ozone therapy also hold promise for a synergistic action when administered in conjunction with conventional antibiotics, with a proven reduction of infection rates in variously treated patients with orthopedic device-related post-operative wounds (Cascini et al., 2024). This dual therapy may potentially speed up healing and combat the phenomenon of antibiotic resistance for biofilm-related infections. With the evolving trend in antibiotic therapy, there is a need for research and clinical trials to develop evidence-based clinical guidelines with new therapies to optimize infection management in orthopedic surgery in the best possible way and ensure patient safety, along with improving surgical outcomes (Youf et al., 2024) (Figure 10.11).

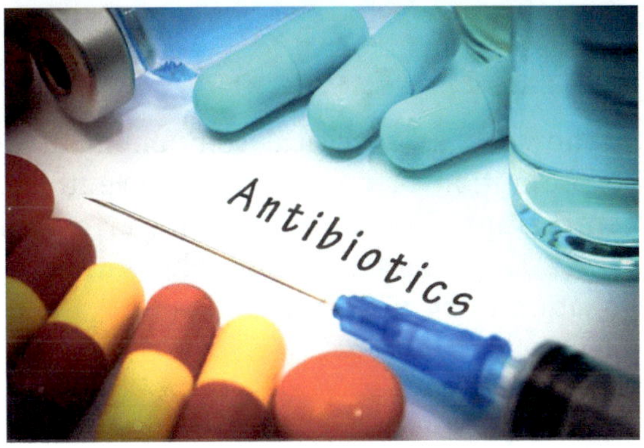

Figure 10.11. The role of antibiotic therapy in the management of orthopedic infections.

Source: https://mumcdnstorage.blob.core.windows.net/cnt/2022/02/Pre-Transplant-Antibiotic-Use-May-Increase-GVHD-Risk.jpg.

10.4.2. Surgical Intervention

The role of surgical intervention in the management of orthopedic infection is critical, particularly when there is failure of conservative therapy to alleviate symptoms or limit infection spread. Surgical maneuvers are likely to involve debridement, whereby the excision of dying and infected tissue initiates healing and facilitates normal function of adjacent sound structures. This technique is especially important in deep surgical site infections (SSIs) after procedures such as hip hemiarthroplasty, whose SSI incidence can raise patient morbidity and mortality rates considerably. For instance, for hip hemiarthroplasty to treat intracapsular fractured neck of femur, the rate of SSI has been estimated to be around 4.68%, a far cry from elective surgery's less than 1% rate, thus conclusively demonstrating the necessity of adequate surgical treatment interventions (Sprowson et al., 2013). In addition to debridement, surgical management can also involve the placement of antibiotic-impregnated material, such as cement, in surgeries. Recent work has considered the use of high-dose antibiotic-impregnated cement in hip hemiarthroplasty to decrease the incidence of post-operative infection. The therapy may offer a double advantage: localized antibiotic treatment and structural support, and so address infection and associated mechanical instability. Outcomes of such interventions remain to be seen, with trials attempting to establish evidence-based recommendations. If successful, these interventions can revolutionize post-operative protocols and lead to improved long-term outcomes for similar patients undergoing these procedures (Sprowson et al., 2013). Detailed information about the microbial community and the orthopedic infection pathogenic organisms is needed to guide surgical interventions. As highlighted in recent publications, there is a clear need for orthopedic and infectious disease specialists to come together to develop a regional consensus for the diagnosis and management of prosthetic joint infection.

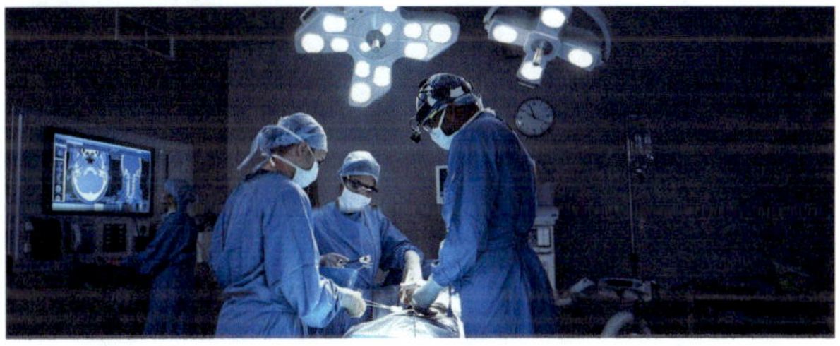

Figure 10.12. The role of surgical intervention in managing orthopedic infections.

Source: https://www.hopkinsmedicine.org/-/media/images/health/2_-treatment/surgical-care/common-surgical-hero.jpg?h=500&iar=0&mh=500&mw=1300&w=1297&hash=FD277EB2AEE62E1B53537767AEE778CE.

The identification of the causative pathogens through effective clinical assessment is key, as this helps clinicians implement appropriate antimicrobial therapy based on the specific infection profile. The synergy of surgical treatment and precise antimicrobial management forms a cornerstone in the management of orthopedic infections, in line with guidelines that emphasize synergistic management in such complex scenarios. The collaboration is not only directed towards managing existing infections but also towards designing preventive strategies to be implemented in clinical practice (Figure 10.12).

10.4.3. Adjunctive Therapies (e.g., Hyperbaric Oxygen Therapy)

Adjunctive treatments have more and more become renowned as a critical component of the treatment of orthopedic infections, particularly in the promotion of healing and prevention of complications. One such treatment is hyperbaric oxygen therapy (HBOT). By administering pure oxygen at pressures greater than ambient conditions, HBOT promotes neovascularization and enhances wound healing rates through improved oxygenation of hypoxic tissue.

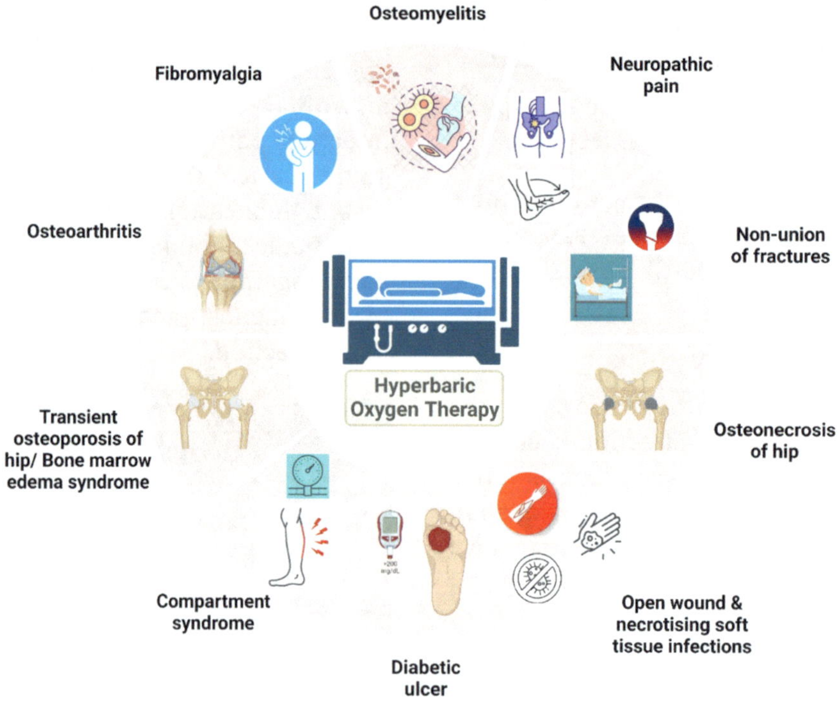

Figure 10.13. Adjunctive therapies have gained increasing recognition in the management of orthopedic infections.

Source: https://media.springernature.com/lw1200/springer-static/image/art%3A10.1007%2Fs43465-023-00837-2/MediaObjects/43465_2023_837_Fig1_HTML.png.

This therapy has been shown to be especially useful in the treatment of chronic, non-healing infected wounds, thereby meeting the pressing need for improved results in orthopedic infection patients that resist conventional treatment. Research has indicated that adjunct therapies like HBOT not only increase healing rates but, further, reduce the incidence of further complications such as amputations or prolonged disability. For instance, studies comparing traditional wound closure to treatments like vacuum-assisted closure (VAC) have evaluated the effectiveness of HBOT. The results show that while VAC is somewhat advantageous in terms of wound closure ease, HBOT can deliver impressive increases in epithelialization and recovery of patients. This combination therapy may be beneficial to patients who have extensive soft tissue injury with an orthopedic infection in that it accesses more than a single mechanism for addressing tissue viability and infection management (Ansari et al., 2022). Further investigation of adjunct treatment shows the necessity of integrating these treatments into standard care pathways for orthopedic infections. Case series and reports exploring the conservative treatment of conditions such as paraspinal compartment syndrome prove the efficacy of HBOT as an adjunctive therapy. It has been revealed that while surgery is the treatment of choice for compartment syndrome, conservative management—e.g., HBOT—has had favorable outcomes in some cases. This emphasizes the requirement of a multidisciplinary approach in addressing complicated infections, necessitating more research in protocols with adjunctive therapy for the optimization of patient outcomes in orthopedic management (LaGreca et al., 2024) (Figure 10.13).

10.5. Complications of Orthopedic Infections

The infections resulting from orthopedic infections have a direct effect on patient outcomes and the efficacy of surgical interventions. Among all the potential complications, the development of surgical site infections (SSIs) is one of the most serious. SSIs can develop in the postoperative environment after procedures such as total hip arthroplasty. The incidence of SSIs in individuals undergoing hip operations is prohibitively high, particularly among high-risk populations. For instance, there is evidence that the rate of SSIs can rise to as high as around 4.68% for hip hemiarthroplasties in the UK compared to less than 1% for elective hip surgery. This extreme contrast emphasizes the need for targeted measures to limit infection hazards among patients who are subjected to such operations, valuing preoperative assessment and infection control to optimize surgical outcomes and reduce their costs. Among the numerous determinants of orthopedic infection complications, seasonal variations have been emphasized by recent investigations. Studies of Medicare data from 2005 through 2014 revealed that winter had the highest rate of periprosthetic infection following total hip arthroplasty, particularly in the Midwest, South, and West United States. These results reinforce the reality that environmental and temporal factors can increase the risk of postoperative infections. Detection of infection rate seasonality patterns and the seasonal variation in risk of surgery can assist clinicians in better patient stratification by risk and potentially optimize the timing of surgery to improve outcomes. Seasonal awareness in clinical practice can facilitate greater patient counseling and proactive prevention of postoperative complications. Treatment of such surgical complications would entail evidence-based interventions, with the use of high-dose antibiotic-impregnated cement in orthopedic surgery being especially worthy of consideration. Research studies have indicated that such interventions were likely to decrease the occurrence of deep SSIs among patients, particularly those who had hip hemiarthroplasties for fractures. By assessing the impact of antibiotic-impregnated materials in the context of a randomized controlled trial, the findings would contribute significantly to clinical practice recommendations in orthopedic surgery. If it is found to be effective, the use of high-dose antibiotics in cement has the potential to significantly decrease the risk of infections, thus enhancing patient morbidity and overall safety of hip surgery. The evidence-based practice will play a vital role in addressing the current challenge of complications linked to orthopedic infections, ultimately proving to be beneficial to both patients and healthcare systems.

10.5.1. Chronic Pain and Disability

The dynamic interplay between disability and chronic pain is complicated and often exacerbated by the presence of concurrent orthopedic infection. Directly, chronic pain can be a product of orthopedic disorders such as arthritis or tendonitis that are common causes of precipitating inflammatory responses leading to chronic aching. These patients are often not only physically but also psychosocially impaired. This dual burden can result in decreased quality of life, with decreased mobility and daily functioning. Moreover, patients have functioning difficulties in carrying out normal day-to-day activities and are more reliant on caregivers and the healthcare system. Evidence shows that the presence of chronic pain strongly corresponds with the inability to perform many activities within both the home and workplace, ultimately increasing their sense of disability and helplessness, calling for the need for intensive management interventions addressing both relief of pain as well as restoration. Consequences of chronic pain extend into more specific domains, such as foot health in patients with rheumatic disease, where optimum care can mean a huge difference to function. As highlighted in more recent studies, suboptimal foot health is prevalent in individuals with chronic disease and this creates complications that further compromise mobility and lead to vicious cycles of disability and pain. Most specifically, the majority of patients have described symptomatic callus and toenail problems that have exacerbated pain in their foot, thereby exacerbating their overall status. A lack of access to podiatric care, despite advice for referral to specialist treatment, explains unmet foot health needs, which can complicate rehabilitation attempts and sustain the formation of further disability. This evidence indicates the importance of whole healthcare approaches where patients are guaranteed to receive comprehensive services that address the scope of their chronic pain and its impact on mobility and daily living, as evidenced in the work of Williams & Bowden 2004). Conservative orthopedic intervention techniques have been useful in managing chronic pain, such as for conditions like rotator cuff syndrome.

Clinical trials of the efficacy of various therapeutic regimens, including Traumeel injections versus corticosteroid injections, provide significant data on the management of chronic musculoskeletal pain. Such approaches not only alleviate pain but also improve the range of motion and functional ability of afflicted patients. With the knowledge of the need for such interventions, medical professionals can better tailor their treatment methods to tackle individual patient demands, thereby enhancing their potential for recovery as well as reducing disability. Information gained through such studies can aid the argument for adopting less invasive methods, towards a transition away from reliance on more aggressive strategies such as surgery, to improve patients' quality of life and overall function, as suggested in Bossche et al. (2015) (Figure 10.14).

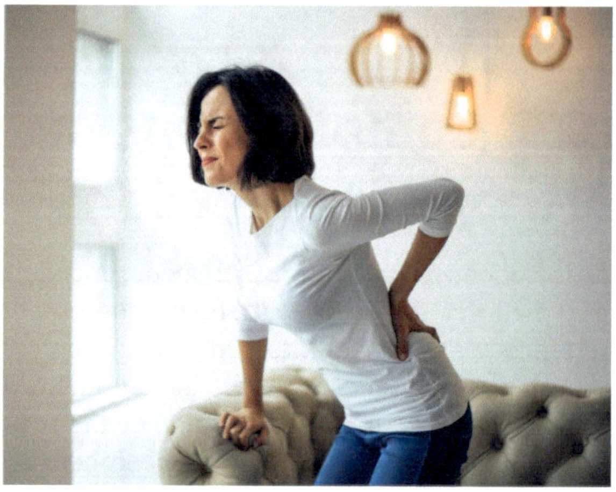

Figure 10.14. The relationship between chronic pain and disability.

Source: https://runningshoehealth.com/wp-content/uploads/2024/05/Is-chronic-pain-a-disability-in-canada_-1024x672.jpg.

10.5.2. Amputation Risks

The urgency to proceed with amputation as a mode of treatment for orthopedic infections often evolves with the severity and chronicity of the infection, underscoring the complexity of managing infectious diseases. For diabetic foot osteomyelitis and other such conditions, conservative treatment has been found to lead to successful outcomes without surgery, with nearly two-thirds of conservatively managed patients becoming afebrile and pain-free within 12 months (Zeun et al., 2016). However, the existence of certain clinical factors, such as the absence of pedal pulses, can prolong the duration of antibiotic therapy required and that risk of amputation, as well as highlight the precarious balance between infection control and limb preservation. This works to highlight the importance of early intervention combined with strict monitoring to prevent the development of an infection that would necessitate surgery and diminish the risks thereof. In addition to the direct physical consequences of amputation, there are also severe psychosocial risks that can influence patients whose limbs are lost due to infection. These would include emotional loss, depression, and anxiety that harm the quality of life and well-being. Studies have identified that patients who undergo transfemoral amputations, especially those with comorbid conditions such as osteoporosis, may be at risk of heightened threats not just for the procedure itself but also for rehabilitation results. As an example, infections following surgery are a barrier to the recovery and rehabilitation processes, which also make psychological adaptation to living with an amputation more complex (Lord, 2016). Hence, taking care of both the medical and emotional needs of amputation becomes essential, underlining the need for multidisciplinary management in patient care. Secondarily, the danger of complications from an amputation due to orthopedic infections cannot be discounted. These include risks such as surgical site infections, difficulty in wound healing, and multiple surgeries, all of which have the potential to significantly alter the recovery course. Poor vascularity and underlying conditions, including diabetes, may be acting to amplify such risks, altering the prognosis of patient management after amputation. As proven in osteomyelitis of the diabetic foot, the location of osteomyelitis is proving to influence the propensity for surgical intervention, as some regions become more dangerous for postoperative complications than others (Zeun et al., 2016). Continuing assessment and attention to unique patient risk factors remain paramount in avoiding these risks, allowing for informed strategic amputation decisions based on a comprehensive understanding of physical health as well as quality of life (Figure 10.15).

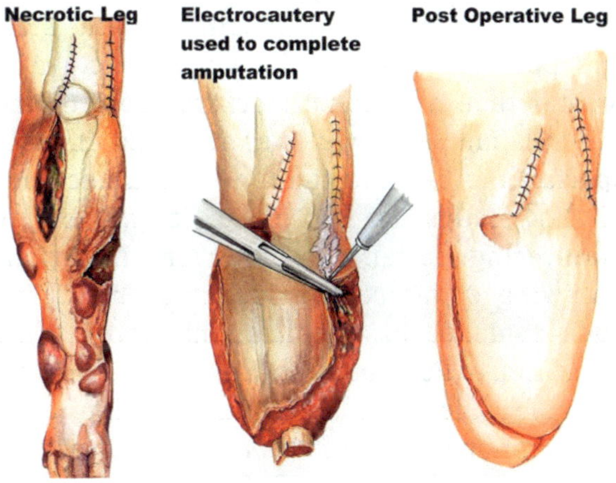

Figure 10.15. The decision to proceed with amputation as a treatment for orthopedic infections.

Source: https://i0.wp.com/diabeticfootonline.com/wp-content/uploads/2015/04/amputation.jpg?w=736&ssl=1.

10.5.3. Systemic Infections and Sepsis

The relationship between orthopedic infections and sepsis is a critical subject of clinical interest. Sepsis, which is a potentially lethal organ dysfunction secondary to an uncontrolled host response to infection, may be due to localized infection sources like those of the musculoskeletal system. The severity of sepsis is often graded based on criteria that evaluate the systemic inflammatory response syndrome (SIRS) as well as the presence of infecting pathogens. Most noteworthy is the early detection and intervention, as delayed intervention can elevate the risk of morbidity and mortality. It could also be challenging to distinguish sepsis from SIRS, with the need for reliable biomarkers in the acute care setting of orthopedics. Recent studies have explored the use of biomarkers for the early detection of sepsis cases, with a focus on the usefulness of procalcitonin (PCT) in distinguishing between SIRS and sepsis. Research has discovered that PCT levels are strongly correlated with the degree of severity in a patient's clinical state and possess sensitivity and specificity rates greater than traditional markers like CRP and pro-inflammatory cytokines IL-6 and IL-8. Of special interest, the timeliness and accuracy of diagnostics by PCT make it valuable in monitoring patients with severe infections following orthopedic procedures or trauma. Such evidence has implications favoring the utilization of PCT as a routine diagnostic adjunct in orthopedic clinics for better enabling early intervention strategies and maximizing patient outcomes (BalcI et al., 2002). Management of systemic diseases such as sepsis in orthopedic patients calls for a multidisciplinary approach. The infections may be of operative origin, secondary to immobilization, or even medical in origin and require collaborative input from orthopedic surgeons, intensivists, and infectious disease specialists. Management success may not only include prompt antibiotic therapy but also aggressive supportive care to maintain organ function. The complexity of such cases demands close monitoring of clinical parameters along with sophisticated diagnostic modalities to enable timely interventions. As advanced care progresses, a more precise comprehension of the pathogenetic processes of sepsis and systemic infections will be essential in developing specific therapeutic interventions that optimize recovery and minimize complications in patients with orthopedic conditions (Fang et al., 2017).

10.6. Prevention Strategies

Implementation of optimal prevention practices is vital in reducing the incidence of orthopedic infections, particularly surgical site infections (SSIs). Multifactorial etiology of infections necessitates a whole-person approach to addressing host, environmental, and pathogen factors. Optimization of patient measures is central to this, including optimal preoperative assessment to identify and overcome risk factors like obesity, diabetes, and smoking. Optimized recovery protocols can also be instituted with a focus on physical conditioning and nutritional status to help reduce postoperative risk of complications. It has been proven that optimizing these factors in patients can significantly reduce infection rates, thereby contributing towards improved surgical outcomes and patient satisfaction. In addition to patient optimization, careful preparation of the operating room environment must be done to prevent SSI. This includes maintaining scrupulously sterile methods during the operation and employing adequate antimicrobial prophylaxis. Appropriately applied surgical drapes, barriers, and meticulous skin antisepsis can reduce microbial contamination considerably. Additionally, prosthetic material care should be taken with care because, in most situations, the availability of implants hinders infection outcomes. Recent evidence demonstrates that the etiological organisms of SSI typically are *Staphylococcus aureus*, which persists in biofilms. Therefore, preventive interventions ought to be extended to the selection and use of materials during surgery, since these determine the risk of infection as well as the health outcomes of the patient, calling for adherence to set standards and procedures (Smith & Chetter, 2015). Postoperative care is also important in preventing orthopedic infection. Adequate monitoring for early symptoms of infection, in addition to patient education regarding wound care, can aid in the identification of potential complications prior to them being severe. Operative teams need to encourage open discussion with patients in order to inform them of symptoms such as more pain, swelling, or drainage so that there can be early intervention. Furthermore, utilization of follow-up care strategies through consistent assessment and possible interventions such as irrigation and debridement in case of inflammation is easily able to manage possible infections once they arise. It is important to continue researching these prevention techniques, particularly as the mechanisms used in surgical site infection prevention continue to progress, with greater attention being directed towards the importance of having a standardized protocol based on the individual surgical scenario (Swarup et al., 2018).

10.6.1. Preoperative Measures

Preoperative measures play a vital role in averting the risk of orthopedic infections, particularly surgical site infection (SSI). Firm practices begin with diligent patient selection for recognizing individuals who are most likely to be at higher risk for infection. Risk factors such as diabetes, obesity, and a smoking background have been shown to compromise immune function and heal poorly. By controlling these modifiable risk factors before surgery, healthcare providers can decrease the occurrence of SSIs greatly. For instance, tight glycemic control in diabetic individuals before undergoing surgery is required because elevated blood glucose levels are associated with an increased rate of infection. Furthermore, smoking cessation programs need to be implemented since smoking has an adverse effect on wound healing and tissue oxygenation, ultimately slowing the recovery process and making infection a greater risk (Atesok et al., 2020). Apart from patient selection, achieving the best health through preoperative assessments has a major impact on outcome. Preoperative tests and examinations screen for any existing medical conditions that would predispose to infection. This process may involve widespread blood testing, imaging procedures, and referral to specialists where necessary. The use of a system for screening and elimination of nasal carriers of *Staphylococcus aureus*, such as methicillin-resistant strains, reduces the incidence of postoperative infections even more (Smith & Chetter, 2015). The use of prophylactic antibiotics, scheduled appropriately to be given when surgical procedures begin, has also been shown to appreciably lower the rate of SSIs. They not only contribute to patient safety but also enhance healthcare resource utilization by reducing the need for revision surgery and its costs. Patient education is also an important component of preoperative practices in preventing orthopedic infections. Appropriate explanation of how complying with preoperative guidance is important can empower the patient to take charge of their health. Ensuring patients are properly educated on the effects of their lifestyle habits is a key function in ensuring compliance with mandatory health modifications. For example, education interventions can highlight the necessity of proper nutrition, fluid intake, and avoidance of tobacco and alcohol, all of which can enhance overall surgical outcomes. Further, providing guidance on post-surgery infection control and wound treatment raises the sustained initiative towards infection prevention in the post-operative phase. With the incorporation of these preoperative measures, clinicians establish a solid foundation for infection rate minimization and patient outcome improvement in orthopedic procedures (Smith & Chetter, 2015; Atesok et al., 2020) (Figure 10.16).

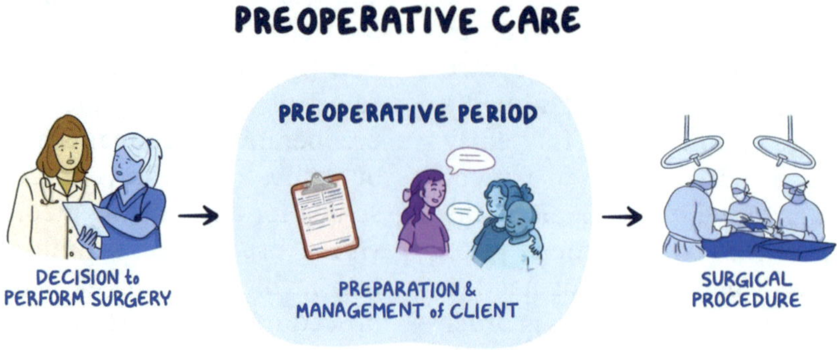

Figure 10.16. Preoperative measures play a crucial role in mitigating the risk of orthopedic infections.

Source: https://d16qt3wv6xm098.cloudfront.net/7u_7UhwdRqOF0Aosh9NcEsG0T-OWhpKE/_.jpg.

10.6.2. Postoperative Care

Postoperative care is one of the main areas in treating patients who have been treated with orthopedic surgeries, particularly in avoiding infections. The recovery phase is correlated with a heightened risk of complications since the body has to heal while it is exposed to the invasive alterations caused by the surgery. Adept postoperative care protocols are significant in minimizing the infection risk, one that can have critical implications for recovery times and patient outcomes overall. Some of the most important aspects of postoperative management are checking for infection at the surgical sites, managing the administration of antibiotics, and pain control. Additionally, close observation throughout this time can lead to the detection of any complications early on, which, if treated on time, may prevent major complications such as unplanned reoperation or prolonged hospital stay, further justifying the importance of an effective postoperative protocol. Incidence of postoperative infections may be influenced by various factors, one of which is the season of the year in which the operation is performed. Analysis of Medicare claims in a retrospective study revealed that periprosthetic joint infection rates were highest for winter months, suggesting environmental factors have a significant influence on patient outcomes. Specifically, the seasonality of infection rates highlights the need for adaptive postoperative care modalities sensitive to the environment dominating each season. For instance, heightened vigilance in the winter may involve infection control practices and patient education on the presentation of postoperative infections. Through an understanding of these seasonal variations, medical practitioners can use differential interventions to optimize care and, perhaps, lower the levels of postoperative infections, thus improving patients' recovery patterns (Rosas et al., 2017). In addition, for surgical procedures such as those involving neuromuscular scoliosis, the postoperative care process should be suitably comprehensive in order to address the heightened levels of complications characteristic of such complicated procedures. Statistical processing has given proof that certain surgical methods can lead to varying rates of complications, illustrating the necessity for matching postoperative management to the patient's specific surgical condition. As a large percentage of complications occur as a result of postoperative problems, specific knowledge of probable adverse outcomes is necessary for designing prevention tactics. This is underscored by the call for individualized postoperative care protocols that not only screen for infection but also change with the individual needs posed by certain surgical procedures. Hence, advocating a preventative outlook through informed care can considerably improve patient outcomes and reduce the carga das complications in orthopedic surgery (Turturro et al., 2017).

10.6.3. Patient Education and Awareness

The importance of patient education and awareness in orthopedic infections cannot be overstressed. Education makes patients responsible and involved in their treatment, resulting in better health outcomes. Patient awareness about the risk factors surrounding orthopedic surgery allows them to be better equipped to recognize early signs of infection, such as swelling, redness, and fever. This proactive approach enables early intervention, which is critical because undrained infections can lead to severe complications like prolonged hospital stay and reoperation. Education regarding compliance with postoperative protocol—wound care, for example, and taking all prescribed courses of antibiotics—also greatly enhances the likelihood of successful outcomes. Overall, encouraging awareness and critical information among patients encourages a partnership of care that is central to the prevention of the development of orthopedic infections. Beyond the direct delivery of education, the application of systematic methods toward patient awareness can prove very valuable. For instance, multi-component interventions combining education with behavior change strategies have proved effective in various healthcare settings. These interventions can include patient and caregiver workshops, educational pamphlets, and visual aids to describe the symptoms and hazards of orthopedic infections. With the employment of various communication modalities, health professionals are able to address various levels of health literacy among patients so that important information can be conveyed and understood. Moreover, a questioning-promoting culture can enhance participation and cooperation with therapy. This is in accordance with current evidence indicating that increased awareness of potential complications, such as infections, leads to a more vigilant patient population and consequently lower incidence rates of adverse outcomes (Rawson et al., 2017). Of utmost significance is the role of healthcare workers in ensuring patient education is not downplayed. The effectiveness of training programs relies on the commitment of medical professionals to placing priorities into action and involving themselves in cooperative decision-making. Staff courses for better communication skills and teaching patients can equip healthcare professionals with the skills required to communicate critical information. In a study, it was found that perioperative staff often lacked uniform knowledge regarding infection prevention practices, and there was an urgent need for increased training (Godfrey et al., 2013). By ensuring that such people are well-educated on orthopedic infections, they can act as patient educators, thus setting a situation where educated patients are able to make informed decisions based on their health goals. Ultimately, a balanced strategy that incorporates systemic education, effective communication, and patient engagement results in reducing orthopedic infections as well as enhancing patient safety as a whole (Figure 10.17).

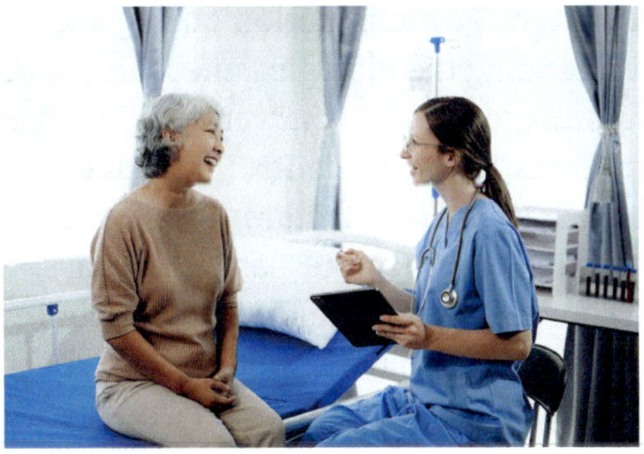

Figure 10.17. The significance of patient education and awareness.

Source: https://flearningstudio.com/wp-content/uploads/2024/12/how-to-improve-patient-education.jpg.

SUMMARY

Generally, orthopedic infections are a complex problem that demands a complex approach to prevention, diagnosis, and treatment. The evidence suggests seasonal patterns play an overwhelming role in the incidence of periprosthetic infections, with winter having exceptionally high rates in various parts of the United States (Rosas et al., 2017). This observation highlights the necessity of making risk assessment tools responsive to temporal concerns, such that healthcare workers can more appropriately implement preventive measures. Additionally, this seasonality would enable enhanced scheduling of surgery and postoperative care, ultimately resulting in enhanced patient outcomes by mitigating infection risks based on time. The development of antibiotic-impregnated surgical implants is a great way to combat orthopedic infection effectively. Progress in local antibiotic delivery systems, for example, the use of vancomycin and tigecycline on biocompatible coatings, has indicated dramatic decreases in bacterial colonization and osteomyelitis and implant loosening prevention (Stavrakis et al., 2019). Such evidence suggests the feasibility of single-stage surgeries with improved efficiency of treatments and patient recovery times. By adopting such technology into practice, surgeons can more effectively manage the intrinsic risks of infection associated with orthopedic implants. Last but not least, the ongoing development of research into orthopedic infections indicates a future that is marked by enhanced patient safety and surgical outcomes. An understanding of the multifactorial etiology of these infections, consisting of host factors, microbial resistance patterns, and environmental influences, allows clinicians to adopt an expanded approach. There is a requirement for further investigation into both the technological and biological borders of orthopedic practice to further reduce infection risks. As more information becomes available, the potential for further therapeutic interventions and outcomes within orthopedic care becomes increasingly attainable, further supporting evidence-based practice in its fight against these prevalent conditions.

In the debate of the multifaceted subject of orthopedic infections, it is imperative to highlight points of significance that encompass the pathophysiology, diagnostic challenge, and therapeutic protocols of these conditions. The etiologic causes of orthopedic infections are varied, ranging from bacterial contamination during surgery to hematogenous seeding from another septic source. Understanding the biological mechanism behind these infections is essential for the development of successful therapeutic interventions. Furthermore, the development of antibiotic-resistant pathogens complicates infection control, demanding ongoing studies and alteration of treatment protocols. Recognition of these factors provides the foundation upon which effective clinical pathways can be established. Over the past few years, the need for standardized diagnostic criteria has come to the forefront, particularly in the context of fracture-related infections (FRI). The difficulty of FRI diagnosis is underscored by the absence of widely accepted guidelines, and this can lead to variability in patient outcomes and treatment. In response to this dilemma, the AO Foundation and the European Bone and Joint Infection Society collaborated to propose a consensus definition for FRI to facilitate standardization of diagnostic protocols and optimize patient outcomes. This platform emphasizes convergence between clinical examinations and imaging and laboratory tests, in line with an all-encompassing assessment method that adapts to the specific needs of individual patients (Govaert et al., 2019). Creation of these standards is crucial, not only to enhance the efficacy of treatment but also to promote uniformity in research and clinical care. Treatment of orthopedic infection is itself complex and involves a multifactorial regimen of controlling surgical intervention, antibiotic therapy, and ongoing monitoring practices. Management of FRI in particular necessitates an intense understanding of microbiology and modification of treatment regimens based on the specific pathogens present. Consensus guidelines stress the necessity to obtain microbiological specimens from infection sites in order to guide relevant antibiotic choices, an essential step in averting the failure rate of treatment (Halvorsen et al., 2022). Further, novel approaches in molecular biology and histopathologic research are enhancing diagnostic specificity and maximizing therapeutic outcomes. As our perception of orthopedic infection changes, it is very important to lay great emphasis on research studies with an eye towards refining diagnostic and treatment modalities such that the quality of care to infected patients is improved.

CLOSER LOOK

POSTOPERATIVE CARE

Postoperative care refers to the comprehensive medical and nursing management provided to patients after surgery to ensure safe recovery, prevent complications, and promote healing. It begins immediately after the procedure and continues until the patient has regained adequate function and strength. Effective postoperative care plays a crucial role in reducing pain, minimizing infection risk, and restoring normal physiological functions. Key components include monitoring vital signs, managing pain, maintaining wound hygiene, and preventing complications such as infections, blood clots, and respiratory problems. Proper medication administration, fluid management, and nutritional support are essential to enhance recovery and tissue repair. Early mobilization and physiotherapy help improve circulation, reduce stiffness, and prevent muscle weakness, particularly after orthopedic and abdominal surgeries. Patient education is an important aspect of postoperative care. Clear instructions on wound care, medication use, physical activity, and follow-up visits help patients actively participate in their recovery. Emotional support and reassurance also contribute to reduced anxiety and better healing outcomes. Individualized care plans are developed based on the type of surgery, patient health status, and recovery goals. With advancements in surgical techniques and rehabilitation strategies, postoperative care has become more efficient and patient-centered. Overall, comprehensive postoperative care ensures faster recovery, reduces hospital stay, improves patient comfort, and supports a safe return to daily activities and long-term well-being.

REFERENCES

1. Padegimas, E. M., Narzikul, A., Lawrence, C., Hendy, B. A., Abboud, J. A., Ramsey, M. L., Williams, G. R., & Namdari, S. (2017). Antibiotic Spacers in Shoulder Arthroplasty: Comparison of Stemmed and Stemless Implants. *Clinics in orthopedic surgery*, *9*(4), 489–496. https://doi.org/10.4055/cios.2017.9.4.489(accessed on 26th June 2025).
2. McDonald, R. S., Gupta, S., Maclean, M., Ramakrishnan, P., Anderson, J. G., MacGregor, S. J., Meek, R. M., & Grant, M. H. (2013). 405 nm Light exposure of osteoblasts and inactivation of bacterial isolates from arthroplasty patients: potential for new disinfection applications?. *European cells & materials*, *25*, 204–214. https://doi.org/10.22203/ecm.v025a15(accessed on 26th June 2025).
3. Ansari, T. A., Arora, S., Barik, S., Meena, R. K., et al. (2022). Comparison of topical oxygen with vacuum assisted closure in wound healing in a low resource setting. https://core.ac.uk/download/544240271.pdf (accessed on 26th June 2025).
4. Atesok, K., Gokaslan, Z. L., Heffernan, M. J., Papavassiliou, E., et al. (2020). Current strategies in prevention of postoperative infections in spine surgery. https://core.ac.uk/download/299811520.pdf (accessed on 26th June 2025).
5. LaGreca M, Badragheh A, Jones N, Falconiero T, Danshaw B. Conservative Management of a Rare Clinical Phenomenon: Paraspinal Compartment Syndrome - A Review of Existing Literature. *J Orthop Case Rep*. 2024;14(12):229-236. doi:10.13107/jocr.2024.v14.i12.5082(accessed on 26th June 2025).
6. Balcı, C., Gürses, E., Kaptanoğlu, B., Sungurtekin, H., et al. (2002). Usefulness of procalcitonin for diagnosis of sepsis in the intensive care unit. https://core.ac.uk/download/pdf/3244068.pdf (accessed on 26th June 2025).
7. Stavrakis, A. I., Loftin, A. H., Lord, E. L., Hu, Y., Manegold, J. E., Dworsky, E. M., Scaduto, A. A., & Bernthal, N. M. (2015). Current Animal Models of Postoperative Spine Infection and Potential Future Advances. *Frontiers in medicine*, *2*, 34. https://doi.org/10.3389/fmed.2015.00034(accessed on 26th June 2025).
8. Stavrakis, A. I., Zhu, S., Loftin, A. H., Weixian, X., Niska, J., Hegde, V., Segura, T., & Bernthal, N. M. (2019). Controlled Release of Vancomycin and Tigecycline from an Orthopaedic Implant Coating Prevents *Staphylococcus aureus* Infection in an Open Fracture Animal Model. *BioMed research international*, *2019*, 1638508. https://doi.org/10.1155/2019/1638508(accessed on 26th June 2025).
9. Swarup, I., Gruskay, J., Price, M., Yang, J., Blanco, J., Perlman, S., & Widmann, R. (2018). *Propionibacterium acnes* infections in patients with idiopathic scoliosis: a case-control study and review of the literature. *Journal of children's orthopaedics*, *12*(2), 173–180. https://doi.org/10.1302/1863-2548.12.170212c (accessed on 26th June 2025).
10. Ng, C., Mifsud, M., Borg, J. N., & Mizzi, C. (2015). The Libyan civil conflict: selected case series of orthopaedic trauma managed in Malta in 2014. *Scandinavian journal of trauma, resuscitation and emergency medicine*, *23*, 103. https://doi.org/10.1186/s13049-015-0183-2(accessed on 26th June 2025).
11. Williams, A. E. & Bowden, A. P (2004). Meeting the challenge for foot health in rheumatic diseases. https://core.ac.uk/download/1662145.pdf (accessed on 26th June 2025).

12. Rosas, S., Ong, A. C., Buller, L. T., Sabeh, K. G., Law, T. Y., Roche, M. W., & Hernandez, V. H. (2017). Season of the year influences infection rates following total hip arthroplasty. *World journal of orthopedics, 8*(12), 895–901. https://doi.org/10.5312/wjo.v8.i12.895(accessed on 26th June 2025).

13. Busscher, H. J., Frijlink, H. W., Grainger, D. W., Hinrichs, W. L. J., et al. (2020). Accepting higher morbidity in exchange for sacrificing fewer animals in studies developing novel infection-control strategies. https://core.ac.uk/download/288122146.pdf (accessed on 26th June 2025).

14. Turturro, F., Montanaro, A., Calderaro, C., Labianca, L., Di Sanzo, V., & Ferretti, A. (2017). Rate of complications due to neuromuscular scoliosis spine surgery in a 30-years consecutive series. *European spine journal : official publication of the European Spine Society, the European Spinal Deformity Society, and the European Section of the Cervical Spine Research Society, 26*(Suppl 4), 539–545. https://doi.org/10.1007/s00586-017-5034-6(accessed on 26th June 2025).

15. Li, Y. C., Stavrakis, G., Hanrahan, C. J., Jones, K. B., & Randall, R. L. (2014). Coccidiomycosis infection of the patella mimicking a neoplasm - two case reports. *BMC medical imaging, 14*, 8. https://doi.org/10.1186/1471-2342-14-8Stavrakis(accessed on 26th June 2025).

16. Cascini, F., Franzini, M., Andreoli, A., Manzotti, A., Cadeddu, C., Quaranta, G., Gentili, A., et al. (2024). Use of oxygen-ozone therapy to improve the effectiveness of antibiotic treatment on infected arthroplasty: Protocol for a superiority, open-label, multicenter, randomized, parallel trial. *BMJ Open, 14.* https://www.semanticscholar.org/paper/f158b1aa6222a43c51dda816e21c06e47e787d78 (accessed on 26th June 2025).

17. Rawson TM, Moore LS, Tivey AM, et al. Behaviour change interventions to influence antimicrobial prescribing: a cross-sectional analysis of reports from UK state-of-the-art scientific conferences. *Antimicrob Resist Infect Control.* 2017;6:11. Published 2017 Jan 13. doi:10.1186/s13756-017-0170-7(accessed on 26th June 2025).

18. Smith, G. & Chetter, I. (2015). Infection in prosthetic material. Surgery - Oxford International Edition, Volume 33, Issue 11, 559 – 564 https://core.ac.uk/download/151157240.pdf (accessed on 26th June 2025).

19. Kuong, E. E., To, M., Yuen, M. H., Choi, A. K., Fong, C. M., & Chow, W. (2012). Pitfalls in diagnosing septic arthritis in Hong Kong children: ten years' experience. *Hong Kong medical journal = Xianggang yi xue za zhi, 18*(6), 482–487.(accessed on 26th June 2025).

20. Dagher, T., Dwyer, E., Baker, H. P., Kalidoss, S., & Strelzow, J. A. (2024). "Dr. AI will see you now": How do ChatGPT-4 treatment recommendations align with orthopedic clinical practice guidelines? *Clinical Orthopedics and Related Research, 482*, 2098–2106. https://www.semanticscholar.org/paper/70d1805367e053588ad237d6e3d7aaf08b4e42b9 (accessed on 26th June 2025).

21. Godfrey, M., Smith, J., Green, J., Cheater, F., Inouye, S. K., & Young, J. B. (2013). Developing and implementing an integrated delirium prevention system of care: a theory driven, participatory research study. *BMC health services research, 13*, 341. https://doi.org/10.1186/1472-6963-13-341(accessed on 26th June 2025).

22. Fang, C. X., Lau, T. W., Leung, F. K. L., To, M. K. T., et al. (2017). Infection after fracture osteosynthesis–Part I: Pathogenesis, diagnosis and classification. https://core.ac.uk/download/95556649.pdf (accessed on 26th June 2025).

23. Fsadni, C., & Fsadni, P. (2013). Prosthetic joint infections. https://core.ac.uk/download/46602347.pdf (accessed on 26th June 2025).

24. Wilson J, Topley K, Stott D, Neachell J, Gallagher R. The OneTogether collaborative approach to reduce the risk of surgical site infection: identifying the challenges to assuring best practice. *J Infect Prev*. 2015;16(3):118-125. doi:10.1177/1757177414564204(accessed on 26th June 2025).

25. Parvizi, J., Ghanem, E., Joshi, A., Sharkey, P. F., Hozack, W. J., & Rothman, R. H. (2007). Does "excessive" anticoagulation predispose to periprosthetic infection?. *The Journal of arthroplasty*, *22*(6 Suppl 2), 24–28. https://doi.org/10.1016/j.arth.2007.03.007(accessed on 26th June 2025).

26. Signore A, Glaudemans AW, Galli F, Rouzet F. Imaging infection and inflammation. *Biomed Res Int*. 2015;2015:615150. doi:10.1155/2015/615150(accessed on 26th June 2025).

27. Zeun, P., Gooday, C., Nunney, I., & Dhatariya, K. (2016). Predictors of Outcomes in Diabetic Foot Osteomyelitis Treated Initially With Conservative (Nonsurgical) Medical Management: A Retrospective Study. *The international journal of lower extremity wounds*, *15*(1), 19–25. https://doi.org/10.1177/1534734615596892(accessed on 26th June 2025).

28. Govaert, G. A. M., Kuehl, R., Atkins, B. L., Trampuž, A., Morgenstern, M., Obremskey, W. T., Verhofstad, M. H. J., et al. (2019). Diagnosing fracture-related infection: Current concepts and recommendations. *Journal of Orthopedic Trauma, 34*, 8–17. https://doi.org/10.1097/bot.0000000000001614 (accessed on 26th June 2025).

29. Halvachizadeh, S., Dreifuss, M., Rauer, T., Kaiser, A., Ubmann, D., Pape, H. C., & Allemann, F. (2025). Does the AO/OTA fracture classification dictate the anesthesia modality for the surgical management of unstable distal radius fractures? A retrospective cohort study in 127 patients managed by general vs. regional anesthesia. *Patient Safety in Surgery, 19*. https://www.semanticscholar.org/paper/46782955c682b9ba7102e37fe9a79a6ee48f208e (accessed on 26th June 2025).

30. Halvorsen, S., Mehilli, J., Cassese, S., Hall, T. S., Abdelhamid, M., Barbato, E., De Hert, S., et al. (2022). 2022 ESC Guidelines on cardiovascular assessment and management of patients undergoing non-cardiac surgery. *European Heart Journal, 43*, 3826–3924. https://doi.org/10.1093/eurheartj/ehac270 (accessed on 26th June 2025).

31. Khoury, P. H., Hazra, N., DeMartino, A., Birungi-Huff, K., Slobogean, G., O'Toole, R. V., & O'Hara, N. N. (2024). Is the Orthopedic Trauma Association-Open Fracture Classification better than the Gustilo-Anderson Classification at predicting fracture-related infections in the tibia? *Journal of Orthopedic Trauma, 38*, 655–660. https://www.semanticscholar.org/paper/9ad500f30f9f32f6467a268005c272c3f9793e29 (accessed on 26th June 2025).

32. Lord, S. J. (2016). Osseo integrated total hip replacement connected to a lower limb prosthesis: A proof-of-concept study with three cases. https://core.ac.uk/download/61305091.pdf (accessed on 26th June 2025).

33. Schneider, P., Heels-Ansdell, D., Thabane, L., Ghert, M., & PARITY Investigators (2021). Prophylactic Antibiotic Regimens In Tumor Surgery (PARITY): a multi-center randomized controlled study comparing alternative antibiotic regimens in patients undergoing tumor resections with endoprosthetic replacements-a statistical analysis plan. *Trials, 22*(1), 223. https://doi.org/10.1186/s13063-021-05147-2(accessed on 26th June 2025).

34. Simpson, H. E., Yu, T., & Jiang, N. (2023). Current concepts of fracture-related infection. *International Journal of Clinical Practice, 2023.* https://www.semanticscholar.org/paper/926f9e3ec0d47046884975d31673bcea860b3a65 (accessed on 26th June 2025).

35. Sprowson, A. P., Jensen, C. D., Gupta, S., Parsons, N., Murty, A. N., Jones, S. M., Inman, D., & Reed, M. R. (2013). The effect of high dose antibiotic impregnated cement on rate of surgical site infection after hip hemiarthroplasty for fractured neck of femur: a protocol for a double-blind quasi randomised controlled trial. *BMC musculoskeletal disorders, 14*, 356. https://doi.org/10.1186/1471-2474-14-356(accessed on 26th June 2025).

36. Szilagyi, J., Kuester, V., & Reznicek, J. (2023). Pediatric necrotizing fasciitis. *Journal of the Pediatric Orthopedic Society of North America, 5.* https://www.semanticscholar.org/paper/27a48f9994862948451fcd44847f0bb0bfc0cfe1 (accessed on 26th June 2025).

37. Vanden Bossche, L., & Vanderstraeten, G. (2015). A multi-center, double-blind, randomized, placebo-controlled trial protocol to assess Traumeel injection vs dexamethasone injection in rotator cuff syndrome: the TRAumeel in ROtator cuff syndrome (TRARO) study protocol. *BMC musculoskeletal disorders, 16*(1), 8. https://doi.org/10.1186/s12891-015-0471-z(accessed on 26th June 2025).

38. Xu, Z., Zhu, W., Zhou, S., Yang, Z., Xiang, L., Zhang, J., & Liu, K. (2025). Diagnostic imaging confusion in infectious spondylitis. *Journal of Orthopedic Surgery and Research, 20.* https://www.semanticscholar.org/paper/33fb613d12a4c0dda4f82df5e998b4c1e934f586 (accessed on 26th June 2025).

39. Youf, R., Schewior, R., Mannala, G., Zhao, Y., Alt, V., & Riool, M. (2024). *Galleria mellonella* larvae: A promising animal model to study biofilm maturation in orthopedic infections. *Orthopedic Proceedings.* https://www.semanticscholar.org/paper/04070047566b730ec2fbcc6b3eae9a9087c3e5d8 (accessed on 26th June 2025).

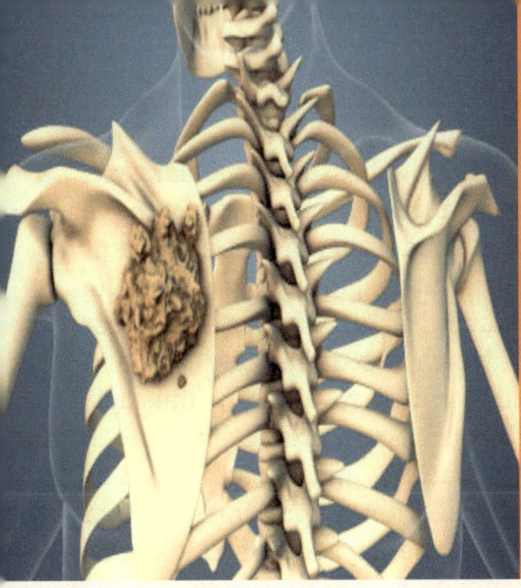

Chapter 11

TUMORS OF BONES AND SOFT TISSUES

Contents

Introduction....335
11.1. Types of Bone Tumors....338
11.2. Types of Soft Tissue Tumors....341
11.3. Symptoms and Diagnosis....345
11.4. Treatment Options for Bone Tumors....348
11.5. Treatment Options for Soft Tissue Tumors....352
11.6. Prognosis and Outcomes....356
Summary....361
References....364

Introduction

The oncology discipline has come a long way in the diagnosis and treatment of a variety of cancers, including bone and soft tissue tumors. While less common than carcinomas, these neoplasms present unique difficulties in their diagnosis, treatment, and control. Sarcomas, the most frequent tumor of the bone and soft tissue tumors, are derived from mesenchymal cells and may present in any part of the body. Extensive studies are necessary because these tumors have diverse biological behaviors, differences in response to conventional therapy, and some prognostic factors. As a result of the difficulties in their molecular and histopathological characteristics, new diagnostic methods such as FAP-PET imaging have the potential to advance detection and treatment algorithms for sarcoma patients, as suggested by results from a recent observational trial that was a harbinger of the growing role of targeted imaging methods (Siegel et al., 2021). The rising incidence of bone and soft tissue tumors reported by the American Cancer Society warrants urgent attention to this neglected area of oncology.

The last few years have seen cancer cases estimated to rise, based on estimates in 2021 revealing nearly 1.9 million new cancer cases in the United States alone (Siegel et al., 2021). While general trends of cancer mortality have declined due to earlier diagnosis and improved therapy, the unique character of sarcomas, including the common late diagnosis and multifaceted therapeutic regimens, underscores the need for increased education and exposure in practitioners. Increased awareness of the pathology and clinical significance of these tumors will lead to earlier diagnosis and better outcomes and quality of life in patients with these neoplasms. Furthermore, technological progress and growth in imaging technology, like the increasing application of FAP inhibitors in PET scanning, represent a significant landmark in our ability to monitor tumor activity and guide therapeutic approaches. The application of FAP-PET is proven to have major benefits, e.g., good positive predictive values and sensitivity, eventually impacting clinical management and patient outcome. As the evidence of this study on FAPI-PET indicates, these new technologies give scientists and physicians a clearer understanding of tumoral activity as well as more ability to personalize treatment regimens according to patient-specific needs (Siegel et al., 2021). Continuing research and financing in this branch of study are needed to improve diagnostic accuracy and treatment outcome, thereby addressing the current need for upgrading the tumor management of soft tissues and bones.

Definition of Tumors

In oncology, a tumor is defined as an abnormal growth of tissue that results when cells grow uncontrollably. This aspect of uncontrolled cellular growth distinguishes tumors from normal tissues, which operate strict regulatory mechanisms to restrict growth and apoptosis. Cancers are all tumors, but not all tumors are cancers; tumors are benign or malignant in nature. Benign tumors do not invade surrounding tissue or metastasize, whereas malignant tumors invade and can move throughout the body. Identifying this important difference is crucial in diagnosing and treating bone and soft tissue disease. Of special interest are bone tumors, which arise from bone cells, and soft tissue tumors, which result from muscles, fat, nerves, or fibrous tissues, presenting various histopathological features and clinical courses, underscoring the need for proper classification to direct appropriate therapy. The high incidence of tumors arising in bones and soft tissues emphasizes their clinical significance, as such tumors would constitute serious morbidity. While some tumors appear as primary tumors, others are secondary tumors because of metastasis of cancer in distant organs. The etiology in such tumors may be multifactorial in nature, including genetic factors, environmental factors, and other associated risk factors. With advancing technology, the role of nanotechnology in tumor diagnosis as well as treatment holds much promise. Specifically, nanomedicine offers targeted drug delivery systems that maximize the efficacy of existing therapies while minimizing the side effects of conventional treatments. The prospects of nanomedicine as a game-changer in the treatment of bone and soft tissue tumors are evident as it facilitates personalized and targeted interventions tailored to each patient's needs (Patra et al., 2018). expertise in the definition and categorization of tumors will likewise develop on the basis of new evidence and the evolving nature of cancer biology. As each new diagnosis and treatment method emerges, such frameworks will need to be capable of keeping pace with the developing knowledge of tumor pathophysiology and response to therapy. New studies of the molecular mechanism of tumors are likely to have a significant role in establishing such frameworks guiding practice in the clinical setting. Besides, interdisciplinary research will also enhance our knowledge of the complexities of tumor biology and thus lead to new prevention, diagnosis, and therapeutic strategies. Consequently, tumor definitions' ongoing construction—as elaborated in a number of assessment studies—will be central to driving more precise and patient-oriented models of cancer care (Tonetti et al., 2018) (Figure 11.1).

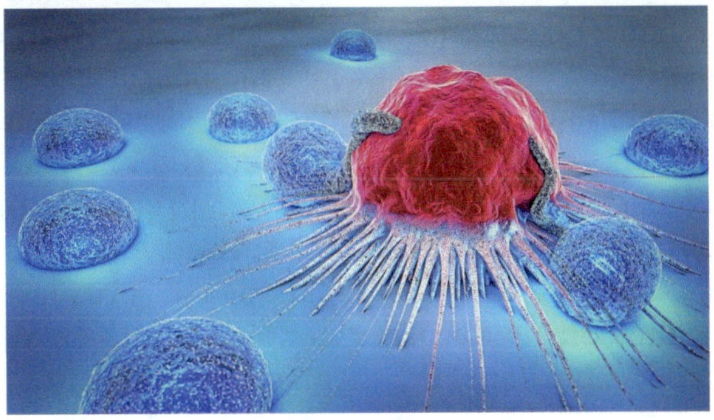

Figure 11.1 A tumor is defined as an abnormal mass of tissue.

Source: https://pacificcross.com.vn/wp-content/uploads/2021/07/khoi-u.jpg.

Importance of Studying Bone and Soft Tissue Tumors

Bone and soft tissue tumor research is critical not just for the development of medical science but also for improving patient care. Understanding the heterogeneity of tumors in terms of pathology, genetic makeup, and clinical behavior helps achieve more accurate diagnosis and tailored treatment strategies. The very crux of this science is knowing the behavior of the tumors, which can be highly variable between patients. By examining the genetic and molecular origins of tumors, scientists can design targeted therapies that enhance the efficiency of treatments and reduce side effects. For instance, recent research in nanomedicine has shown that nanotechnology holds enormous potential to target therapeutic agents more precisely to the location of the tumor and thereby enhance the effectiveness of current treatments while reducing toxicity to healthy tissues (Patra et al., 2018). These innovations address the urgency of tumor biology and the ever-changing nature of cancer management. Furthermore, studies on bone and soft tissue tumors provide information on the epidemiology and risk factors of these cancers. Through the discovery of genetic predisposition, environmental exposures, and lifestyle components that cause tumors, scientists can better plan for prevention methods and early detection schemes. This aspect is particularly vital for at-risk populations, potentially reducing the incidence of aggressive forms of cancer by the application of preventive interventions. Further, clinician practice across a range of patient populations provides an opportunity to obtain data that informs health policy and distribution of resources to maximize efforts in public health aimed at reducing disparities in cancer care. As a result, the study of these tumors not only adds to understanding their fundamental biology but also enables communities with improved health outcomes and increased awareness, consistent with broader public health goals.

The returns on bone and soft tissue tumor research also extend into the realm of precision medicine, revolutionizing practice in oncology at its core. With the advent of new treatment modalities and diagnostic tests, oncologists increasingly require integrating minute details about tumor types, biomarkers, and patient characteristics into decision-making tasks. Through this integration, treatment plans are allowed to be customized to align therapies with the individualized tumor profile, which can lead to improved survival rates and quality of life for the patient. Additionally, with significant findings emerging in cancer studies, they drive the formulation of clinical guidelines and standards of care required in enabling the transmission of the most updated evidence-based care to patients in time. As fast-paced as the field is, research in bone and soft tissue tumors remains core in driving innovation and therapeutic outcomes for affected individuals (Tonetti et al., 2018).

11.1. Types of Bone Tumors

In the scenario of bone tumors, there are many different classifications that all have particular characteristics and clinical relevance. Primary bone tumors can be broadly categorized as benign or malignant. Benign tumors, such as osteochondromas and enchondromas, are not invasive by nature and are usually asymptomatic unless they become painful or uncomfortable, depending on their location. Conversely, primary malignant bone cancers like osteosarcomas and Ewing sarcomas are malignant with the potential to metastasize to distant organs from their original location. Differentiating between the two is important in deciding whether or not the treatment approach would be observation alone in the case of benign tumors, whereas malignant tumors would require a widespread oncologic intervention that could include surgery, chemotherapy, or radiotherapy, depending on the guidelines existing in practice (Tonetti et al., 2018). Among all the malignant bone tumors, osteosarcoma is the most frequent and affects mostly the adolescent and young adult age group. For its aggressiveness and metastatic potential, it is one of the tumors that arises from the osteoblasts and is often found in the long bones, particularly around the knee joint. Osteosarcoma typically presents with localized pain, swelling, and occasionally fracture. Its treatment typically involves a combination of surgery and neoadjuvant chemotherapy, the latter aimed at reducing tumor size before surgery and maximizing overall survival. Tumor response to chemotherapy is a significant prognostic factor, which guides further treatment and long-term survival (Tonetti et al., 2018). Due to the nature of osteosarcoma, both the medical as well as psychosocial issues of the affected patients are to be handled by a multidisciplinary team. Ewing's sarcoma is a second severe bone tumor that appears nearly exclusively in children and young adults with a unique histology and clinical course. Unlike osteosarcoma, Ewing's sarcoma arises from primitive neuroectodermal cells and has a predilection for flat bones or the pelvis. Characteristics typically include localized pain and swelling with concomitant systemic symptoms such as fever and weight loss. The treatment of Ewings sarcoma is usually a combination of chemotherapy, surgery, and radiotherapy to achieve complete resection and metastatic disease control. The prognosis of Ewing's sarcoma relies on several elements, including tumor size, location, and presence of metastasis at presentation (Casali et al., 2018). Consequently, ongoing developments in treatment and research are needed to optimize outcomes for patients with this devastating malignancy (Figure 11.2).

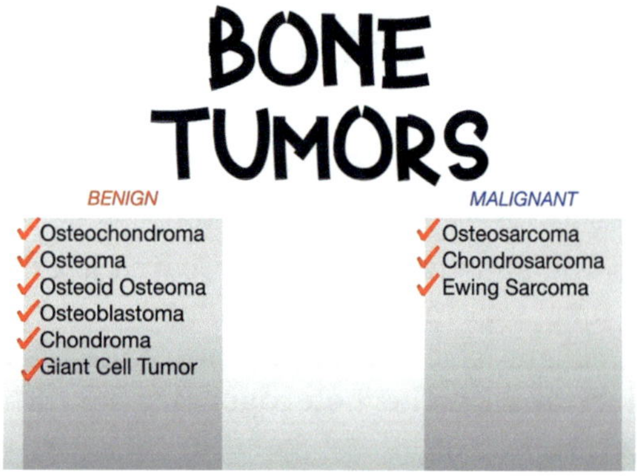

Figure 11.2. A diverse array of classifications exists, each presenting unique characteristics and clinical implications.

Source: https://i.ytimg.com/vi/YeW48XoXqKo/maxresdefault.jpg.

11.1.1. Primary Bone Tumors

The subclassification of the primary bone tumors has significance in appreciating their biology, treatment, and prognosis. The tumors are subclassified as benign and malignant with further subclassification by tissue of origin. The benign tumors such as osteochondromas and enchondromas are slower growing and non-metastasizing and thus possess a more favorable prognosis. In contrast, aggressive behavior and high metastatic rates are observed in malignant primary bone tumors like osteosarcoma and Ewing's sarcoma, which demand a more intensive treatment. It is critical for patients and doctors to recognize these distinctions because the nature of the tumor has a significant impact on the therapeutic regimen, such as surgery, chemotherapy, and radiation therapy. Primary bone tumor diagnosis is a multidisciplinary process of combining clinical evaluation, imaging examinations, and histopathological examination. Primary suspicion based on localized pain, swelling, or pathologic fractures occurs. Radiological examination using X-rays, MRI, and CT scans is essential in providing detailed information on the size, location, and character of the tumor. Following imaging, final diagnosis still relies on biopsy so that pathologists can properly classify the tumor and assess its aggressiveness. Improvements in imaging technology have increased diagnostic accuracy, enabling early detection and treatment, an element that is crucial in determining patient outcomes. Thus, convergence of clinical and pathological information is the basis for the best management of primary bone tumors. Treatment patterns of primary bone tumors are evolving, which is due to advancements in medical technology and research. Surgery remains the cornerstone of the management of malignant and benign tumors. In benign tumors, surgery is done with the intent of resecting the tumor without compromising the structures surrounding it, allowing for an acceptable outcome with minimal morbidity. In contrast, malignant tumors often require more aggressive intervention, including limb-salvage reconstruction or, most severely, amputation, followed by adjuvant therapy with chemotherapy or focused radiation. More advanced treatment modalities, including immunotherapy and gene-directed therapy, are being developed to enhance outcomes and minimize treatment-related morbidity. The ongoing research in attempts to find biomarkers will likely lead to more specific treatment protocols according to the tumor's biological profile, underlining the evolving nature of primary bone tumors management and the need for constant innovation in it (Tonetti et al., 2018) (Figure 11.3).

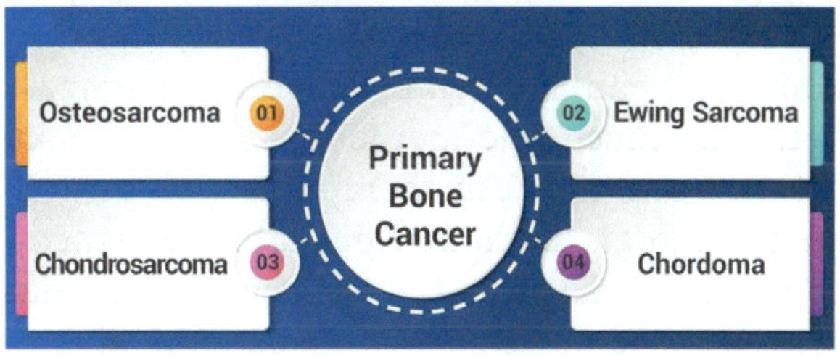

Figure 11.3. The classification of primary bone tumors.

Source: https://external-content.duckduckgo.com/iu/?u=https%3A%2F%2Factchealth.com%2Fimages%2Fbone-cancer-what-do-you-need-to-know23%2F02.webp&f=1&nofb=1&ipt=9de5e286afe501d25daa6b1d48f8321d2b3c14f0d54da0bf88b4eda507925060.

11.1.2. Secondary (Metastatic) Bone Tumors

Formation of secondary (metastatic) bone tumors is a severe problem in the broader context of bone and soft tissue tumors. Unlike primary bone tumors, metastatic bone tumors are formed from cancer cells that have spread from other organs, such as the breast, prostate, or lung. Metastatic bone tumors can have significant effects on the structural integrity of bones and may result in serious complications, such as fractures and debilitating pain. The metastatic bone disease diagnosis typically signifies advanced stages of cancer, which requires a treatment plan of several aspects dealing with the primary malignancy and symptom relief from pain in the bone. Complicated patients, for instance, need thorough evaluation and individualized pain management interventions to improve their quality of life in the face of unfavorable prognoses (Tang et al., 2025). Mutinous to the clinical environment, metastatic bone tumors can have various pain mechanisms and responses to treatment, at times requiring unique therapeutic approaches. It has been reported that 10% to 20% of cancer patients experience refractory cancer pain, which complicates their cases (Tang et al., 2025). Osteoporosis or a past history of skeletal injury is especially the case. Control of pain is often effective to encompass both pharmacologic methods, such as opioid titration and adjuvant therapy, as well as non-pharmacologic methods. Application of patient-controlled analgesia (PCA) technologies has proven to be efficacious with patients able to regulate pain control in real time while possibly preventing the incidence of extreme side effects. In addition, understanding the patient's personal pathology is important in optimizing outcomes, which calls for coordination of oncologists, pain specialists, and palliative care clinicians.

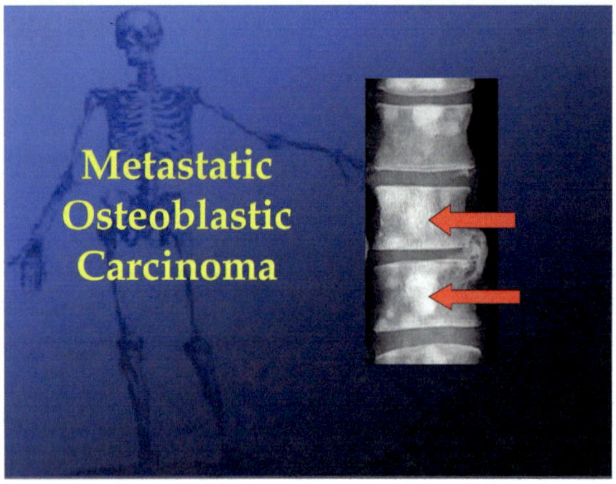

Figure 11.4. The emergence of secondary (metastatic) bone tumors.

Source: https://external-content.duckduckgo.com/iu/?u=https%3A%2F%2Fimage.slideserve.com%2F687179%2Fmetastatic-osteoblastic-carcinoma-l.jpg&f=1&nofb=1&ipt=c9b590baae5a49e942e1c82d0458e9a903655b5488c1de24089ce65ba6d035e1.

Despite medical advances, there exist significant disparities in the provision and use of palliative care treatment in metastatic bone cancer patients. Evidence has shown that socioeconomic and ethnic factors may have considerable effects on the likelihood of effective palliative interventions. Among pediatric populations, for instance, Black children and Hispanic children are less likely to be treated with palliative care compared to White children, thus exacerbating the challenges of pain management as well as total quality of life. The disparity not only marks the importance of future research to identify these barriers but also emphasizes the need for advocacy to attain equal access to healthcare. Mitigating such inequities is central to improving the palliative care environment for all patients so that pain relief and supportive therapies are accessible and tailored to various populations afflicted by secondary bone tumors (Figure 11.4).

11.1.3. Benign vs. Malignant Bone Tumors

This difference between bone tumors as benign and malignant is crucial for treatment and the prediction of patient outcomes. Benign bone tumors, such as osteochondromas and enchondromas, are typically characterized by slow growth, well-defined margins, and minimal aggression to adjacent tissues. They typically have no or minimal potential for metastasis and can remain asymptomatic for years, sometimes requiring intervention only after becoming a source of pain or functional impairment. Malignant bone neoplasms, including osteosarcoma and Ewing's sarcoma, can grow rapidly and invade locally with a high potential for metastasis to distant sites. Recognition of the contrast between these two tumors is essential to clinical management since, by early intervention, survival in malignant disease patients can be significantly improved. Diagnostic imaging plays a pivotal role in the differentiation between benign and malignant bone tumors using advanced technology to enhance precision. Magnetic Resonance Imaging

(MRI) has also become a trendy modality, with greater soft tissue contrast and the ability to investigate tumor characteristics non-invasively. Specific imaging biomarkers, such as kinetic rates Ktrans and Kep—revealing vascular permeability—have been effective in distinguishing malignant tumors from benign tumors (Sar et al., 2024). Apart from that, diffusion-weighted MRI can measure data related to tumors' cellularity in units of ADC values, which are typically lower in malignant tumors due to increased cellular density (Helal et al., 2024). By employing these imaging methods, physicians can properly classify the type of bone tumors and thereby formulate appropriate treatment plans and follow-up. The therapeutic importance of differentiation between malignant and benign bone tumors is significant, with implications for the management plan. Benign tumors are often amenable to observation, removal by surgery, or curettage if symptomatic, with the patient being able to maintain function with minimal morbidity. Malignant tumors, on the other hand, require multidisciplinary treatment, often involving a combination of surgery, chemotherapy, and radiotherapy, based on the aggressiveness and extent of the disease. Clinical management of malignant bone tumors needs a more intense approach because they are highly aggressive and have high metastatic potential and a poor prognosis if untreated. The consequence of misdiagnosis is serious, leading to improper treatment plans that negatively impact patient outcomes. Hence, accurate assessment and benign vs. malignant tumor differentiation are important in order to provide effective and timely intervention in the area of bone and soft tissue oncology.

11.2. Types of Soft Tissue Tumors

The histogenesis of soft tissue tumors is a critical part of their biology and clinical behavior. Broadly, soft tissue tumors are classified into benign and malignant tumors. Lipomas and hemangiomas are examples of benign soft tissue tumors and tend to have slow growth and sometimes may not present any symptoms, though in some cases they may need to be excised for cosmetic reasons or due to causing functional impairment. On the other hand, cancerous soft tissue tumors like sarcomas, like liposarcoma and synovial sarcoma are extremely difficult to treat due to their virulence and their potential to metastasize. The histopathological characteristics of the tumors play an important role in proper diagnosis and treatment, as the course of treatment usually relies on the nature of the tumor, the location of occurrence, and the grade of the tumor, which decides both clinical and overall survival rates. The site of soft tissue tumors within the anatomy also influences their presentation and prognosis. Tumors of the extremities, for instance, such as those of the ankle and foot, have been studied to present with some patterns within the demographics and tumor type. Such was the case in a study involving 72 patients, where 63 (87.5%) of the lesions presented as soft tissue tumors, and benign tumors predominated over malignant tumors by more than three to one. Interestingly, giant cell tumor was found to be the most frequent diagnosis, indicating the need for tumor type- and site-specific therapeutic interventions. Also, the median patient age and gender distribution observed, reflecting the prevalence of female patients with benign tumors, emphasize the role of demographic determinants in the clinical presentation as well as handling of soft tissue tumors (Azevedo et al., 2013). Psychological distress also plays a significant role in overall well-being among patients with soft tissue tumors. The prevalence of psychological distress was assessed in a population of patients with pre-operative bone and soft tissue tumors and determined that a high percentage of them had increased levels of anxiety and depression. This warrants more focus on overall care of the patient aside from the tumor treatment itself. Integration of risk factors such as age, gender, and tumor malignancy can assist healthcare workers in delivering personalized psychological care. Elderly patients and female patients with malignant tumors, for instance, were particularly vulnerable, which suggests integrating mental health evaluation into standard oncologic treatment (Ise et al., 2021). Treatment of these psychological aspects can be a significant factor to ensure enhanced patient outcomes and satisfaction during the entire treatment process (Figure 11.5).

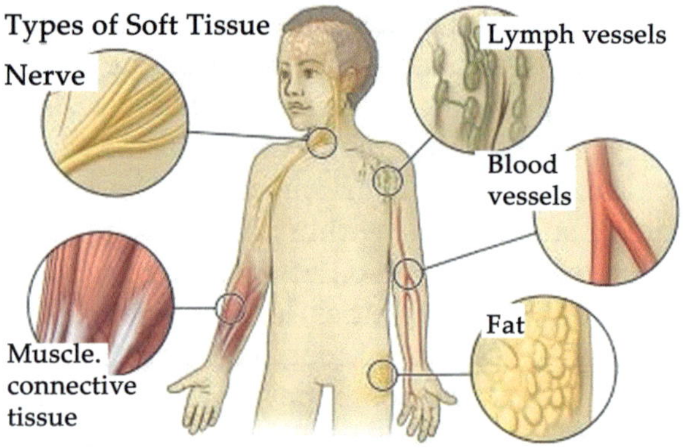

Figure 11.5. The classification of soft tissue tumors in body.

Source: https://external-content.duckduckgo.com/iu/?u=https%3A%2F%2Fwww.toplinemd.com%2Fadvanced-surgical-physicians%2Fwp-content%2Fuploads%2Fsites%2F14%2F2020%2F11%2F1.-What-Is-a-Soft-Tissue-Mass.jpg&f=1&nofb=1&ipt=8059297874fbae2ca30c1eb30706b411b581c0b69dbe991b8f876f8ec1614a2.c

11.2.1. Classification of Soft Tissue Tumors

Soft tissue tumor grouping is critical in facilitating accurate diagnosis and management. Tumors are typically grouped based on their histological characteristics, including the tissue of origin, cellular composition, and specific molecular alterations. The broad classification categorizes soft tissue tumors into benign and malignant. Benign soft tissue tumors such as lipomas and fibromas will also have well-defined margins with low growth potential, whereas malignant counterparts such as sarcomas have aggressive behavior and high metastatic risk. The advancing technology of molecules implies that the characterization of soft tissue tumors is no longer restricted to morphology but is now followed by genetic mutations and chromosomal aberrations that play a growing role in selecting treatment. Understanding of these classifications is vital to practitioners as it directly correlates with prognosis in patients and treatment plans, giving evidence of the significance of elaborative diagnostic techniques within soft tissue tumors (Baumhoer et al., 2024). Technological advancements have also cemented the establishment of the elucidation of soft tissue tumor classification through elaborate molecular characterization. Traditional diagnostic modalities, while necessary, are supplemented by molecular data that introduces specificity and accuracy to tumor classification. Fluorescence in situ hybridization and DNA sequencing give genetic alteration data helpful in the discrimination of tumor subtypes not apparent by histological examination alone. Immunohistochemical profiling has also been most useful in tumor type discrimination based on characteristic patterns of expression. These molecular results not only enable better diagnosis but also enable the development of specific therapies, marking the beginning of individualized medicine in oncology. In soft tissue tumors, however, such novel strategies are still most important since they can make possible more precise classification and treatment protocols on the basis of specific patient characteristics (Baumhoer et al., 2024). The clinical relevance of nomenclature in soft tissue tumors also extends to the treatment modalities. The heterogeneity of soft tissue tumors is best addressed by a particular form of therapy, often established by the tumor grade and type. Surgical resection is most often the initial treatment for confined tumors, but metastatic disease may necessitate the combination of surgery, radiation, and systemic therapies. Clinical practice guidelines now incorporate molecular profiling in the decision to treat, thus offering patients the most suitable regimens based on the classification of their tumor. Complication rates of various treatment modalities must also be considered, such as in trials of cryoablation procedures, wherein some tumors yielded varying rates of complications. These findings also highlight the importance of correct classification not only in treatment options but also in anticipating likely complications, the ultimate aim being to improve patient outcomes (Figure 11.6).

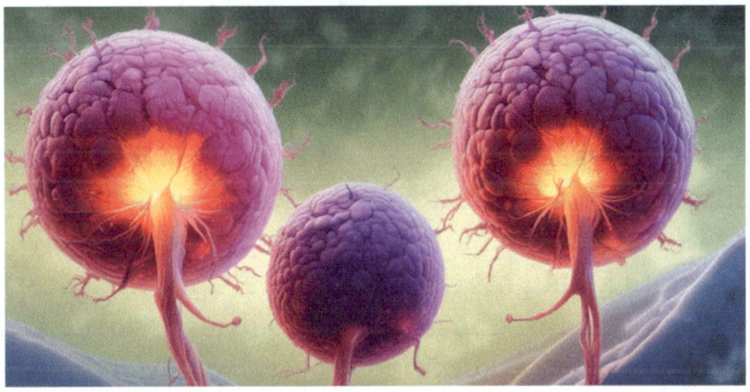

Figure 11.6. The classification of soft tissue tumors is paramount in facilitating appropriate diagnosis and treatment.

Source: https://external-content.duckduckgo.com/iu/?u=https%3A%2F%2Fassets.quizgecko.com%2Fcdn-cgi%2Fimage%2Fwidth%3D800%2Cquality%3D90%2Cformat%3Dwebp%2Fquiz%2F13980919f2e5772c52f04992aae33a2b.jpg&f=1&nofb=1&ipt=c565855f684212c5723dbd31b85b71739f16c63dbe6880a414aaba0db073f89e.

11.2.2. Common Types of Benign Soft Tissue Tumors

The group of benign soft tissue tumors includes many different histologic types, the most frequent being adipocytic tumors. These adipose tissue tumors are lipomas and liposarcomas, and the most frequent of the benign ones are the lipomas. They are typically well-circumscribed, movable nodules that can occur at any anatomic location but are more frequently found over the trunk and limbs. Histologically, lipomas are characterized by mature adipocytes, and thus their diagnosis is quite simple (Ratnaparkhi et al., 2025). The predominance of adipocytic tumors accounts for approximately 84% of benign neoplasms within soft tissues, according to intensive research. In addition, their prevalence is more prevalent among middle-aged people, with a high expression of a relationship between age and tumor incidence. In addition to adipocytic tumors, nerve sheath tumors also constitute a significant proportion of benign soft tissue tumors. These tumors include schwannomas and neurofibromas, with the latter occurring more often. Schwannomas typically arise from Schwann cells and typically present as asymptomatic masses that may lead to neurological symptoms depending on where they are located. Neurofibromas are frequently associated with neurofibromatosis and may appear as multifocal lesions (Scheele et al., 2024). Histological diagnosis is reliant on the utilization of immunohistochemical markers, primarily S-100 protein positivity, to assist in distinguishing them from other lesions. With nerve sheath tumors comprising about 10.5% of benign soft tissue tumors, their unique clinical and pathological features serve to underscore the importance of proper diagnosis to be able to distinguish them from their malignant counterparts. Vascular tumors, although less common, are also an important category of benign soft tissue tumors. Hemangiomas and lymphangiomas are the primary manifestations of this group. Hemangiomas, which represent an abnormal growth of blood vessels, occur most frequently in infancy and childhood and normally regress spontaneously. They may appear as red or purple cutaneous lesions, and although they are typically benign, enlargement may create complications that require treatment (Ratnaparkhi et al., 2025). Lymphangiomas are of lymphatic origin and are typically found in the axilla or neck. They are treatable with surgical excision, especially in symptomatic individuals. The variability in composition and clinical picture of vascular tumors highlights the significance of histopathological examination in arriving at a precise diagnosis and in guiding management against the backdrop of benign soft tissue tumors (Figure 11.7).

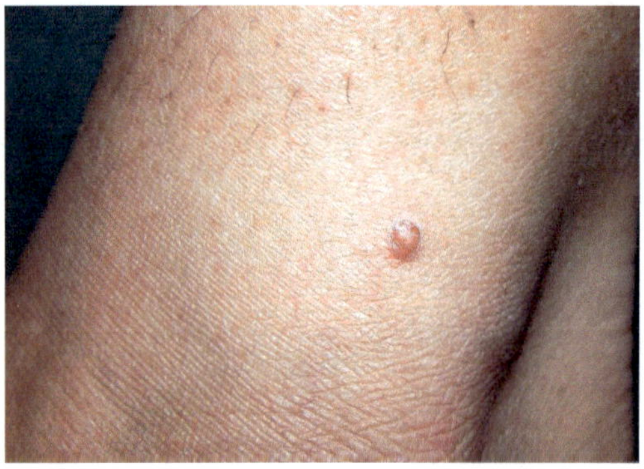

Figure 11.7. The spectrum of benign soft tissue tumors encompasses.

Source: https://external-content.duckduckgo.com/iu/?u=http%3A%2F%2Fwww.chicagoorthopath.net%2Fneurothecoma_gross.jpg&f=1&nofb=1&ipt=e383171ffbae80c1b48fbab5f7a4720670c8406c91cad0b3e47a8014e9f515c0.

11.2.3. Common Types of Malignant Soft Tissue Tumors

Soft tissue sarcomas, malignant neoplasms, form a heterogenous population of neoplasms originating from the mesenchymal tissues like fat, muscle, nerves, and blood vessels. Among these, one of the most common is sarcoma that occurs in significant histological diversity and biological virulence. For instance, liposarcoma, an adipose tissue malignancy, has different subtypes from well-differentiated to pleomorphic forms. Similarly, leiomyosarcoma arises from smooth muscle and can occur in various anatomical locations, including the uterus and retroperitoneum. The classification of these tumors significantly impacts treatment protocols and prognostic outcomes, with each subtype potentially responding differently to therapeutic interventions. In a general evaluation of these cancers, understanding the special characteristics that exist is required for each tumor type to enable effective clinical management and further research as well, involving pertinent active investigations into their molecular biology (Scheele et al., 2024). Another relevant category of malignant soft tissue tumors is rhabdomyosarcoma, the majority of which occur in children and young adults. This sarcoma develops from the skeletal muscle progenitor cell and is characterized by numerous histological variants, e.g., embryonal and alveolar types, which are associated with treatment and prognosis. Rhabdomyosarcoma can occur in a broad range of locations, from the head and neck to the urogenital tract, presenting individual diagnostic challenges. Recent studies indicate the effectiveness of multimodal therapeutic approaches, i.e., the combination of surgery, chemotherapy, and irradiation, particularly in localized tumor disease. With age-incidence and heterogeneous therapeutic response, the treatment of rhabdomyosarcoma underscores the necessity of interdisciplinary practice among oncology professionals in order to enhance the survival of patients and extend the understanding of tumor biology that may potentially direct future targeted treatments (Minervini et al., 2024). Synovial sarcoma is another important malignant soft tissue tumor with its characteristic genetic alteration in the form of the SYT-SSX fusion gene. This sarcoma occurs most frequently in young adults, often in the vicinity of the knee or at around joint spaces, thus making treatment difficult due to its local recurrence and virulence. The clinical presentation can mimic benign lesions, making early diagnosis a formidable obstacle that emphasizes the need for precise imaging and histopathological assessment. Surgical excision is the cornerstone of management, augmented by chemotherapy in the event of metastasis. Further research into the molecular pathways involved in synovial sarcoma is critical in the development of novel treatment protocols that would further increase patient survival (Scheele et al., 2024). As the science evolves, the integration of genomic data into practice could potentially lead to mechanisms of personalized medicine treatment strategies for this difficult malignancy and provide fuel for the discussion in the world of oncology.

11.3. Symptoms and Diagnosis

The diagnosis of bone and soft tissue tumors often begins with a general assessment of symptoms complained of by the patient. The common presentations are focal pain, swelling, and limited range of motion, which are usually characterized as chronic and progressively worsening. These symptoms can be secondary to the tumor compressing adjacent tissues and causing pain and impairment of function. In some cases, systemic symptoms such as fever, weight loss, and fatigue also appear along with the local symptoms, which suggest more systemic involvement of the disease process. Early diagnosis is critical because the time of diagnosis greatly affects the success of the treatment. With the symptomatic profile, clinicians can establish priorities for further diagnostic investigation to determine the pathology behind the musculoskeletal tumors. Diagnostic imaging plays a pivotal role in the evaluation of suspected bone and soft tissue tumors. Radiographic techniques such as X-rays, CT scans, and MRIs are employed to determine the size, location, and type of the tumor. Besides delineating the tumors morphology, these imaging modalities also aid in discriminating benign from malignant lesions. The presence of specific findings—such as periosteal reaction or soft tissue mass—may even raise suspicion of malignancy and need to be further investigated. Moreover, advanced imaging techniques can also evaluate related pathological changes, presenting an integrated image needed for an accurate diagnosis.

As seen from recent reports, an integrated process involving orthopedic oncologists and pathologists is needed for combined evaluation leading to the right diagnosis and decision. Once imaging tests suggest the possibility of a tumor, histological analysis is typically done to confirm the diagnosis, which in this instance is a tumor biopsy. This is necessary in determining if the tumor is malignant or benign and specifically what its subtype is, both of which determine treatment and clinical outcome. Biopsy techniques are not the same, needle biopsy or surgical excision being choices based on where the tumors are and the type of tumors. Following biopsy, pathologists analyze the tissue sample, often employing immunohistochemical staining and molecular studies to identify certain markers associated with different tumor types. The important diagnostic process identifies risk factors and guides the development of personalized treatment plans. As the landscape in cancer diagnosis keeps evolving, the integration of comprehensive clinical, radiological, and pathological evaluations remains crucial in advancing patient care in bone and soft tissue tumors (Siegel et al., 2019, 2021).

11.3.1. Common Symptoms Associated with Bone Tumors

Bone tumors, both benign and malignant, present with a variety of frequent signs and symptoms that have an important impact on the patient's quality of life. Localized pain is one of the key symptoms, which can emerge insidiously or suddenly and is usually worsened by movement or activity. For malignant tumors, this pain becomes persistent as a sign of advanced disease. Swelling and tenderness over the involved site can also be a sign of an underlying tumor. As the illness progresses, the physical presence of the tumor can lead to interference with the normal bone structure and cause fractures, even with minimal trauma. Such indications of structural issues and pain require sensitive clinical assessment to differentiate among various bone tumors and to determine the treatment regimen. The other frequent symptom associated with bone tumors is fatigue, which is a secondary result of the reaction of the body to the malignancy. The systemic impact could be compounded by the immunological response of the body in combating the tumor. Patients similarly report a feeling of overall malaise, which could be expressed as loss of weight and loss of appetite. With malignant tumors, systemic symptoms such as fever or night sweats can also occur, reflecting a more insidious disease progression. Systemic presentation emphasizes the importance of extensive evaluations since they are often associated with other illness conditions that can complicate treatment and plans for diagnosis. Recognition of these signs is of extreme importance, not only towards medical treatment but also towards the improved understanding of the patient's condition. Eventually, some patients will have neurological signs depending on where the tumor is located, particularly if it is near or compressing the spinal column or nerves. Symptoms can range from paresthesia or extremity tingling to more disabling presentations like weakness or loss of coordination. In other instances, if tumors are leading to compression on the surrounding structures, they can lead to compromises like spinal or radicular pain, severely limiting mobility and function. It is vital to identify such neurological symptoms since they could mean that urgent evaluation and/or treatment would be necessary. Due to the intricacy of bone tumor symptoms, diagnosis and treatment are best managed through a multidisciplinary team to determine accuracy as well as effectiveness, emphasizing the importance of early medical intervention in a bid to maximize patient outcomes (Siegel et al., 2019, 2021) (Figure 11.8).

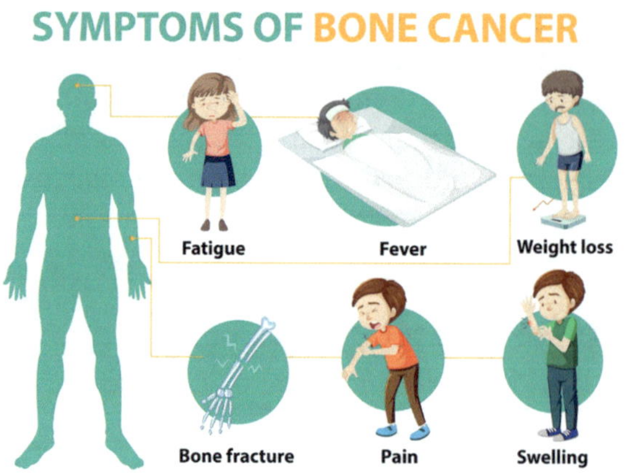

Figure 11.8. Common symptoms associated with bone tumors.

Source: https://external-content.duckduckgo.com/iu/?u=https%3A%2F%2Fimage.freepik.com%2Ffree-vector%2Fmedical-infographic-bone-cancer-symptoms_1308-47540.jpg&f=1&nofb=1&ipt=e6206e64a80d9c3dfddd0d5f98e232b5b112064569538ae94b590546a026daef.

11.3.2. Diagnostic Imaging Techniques

Use of appropriate diagnostic imaging modalities plays an essential role in the evaluation and characterization of bone and soft tissue tumors. Traditional radiography still remains the modality of choice due to its availability and the ability of the method to sufficiently portray bony details. Initial radiographs can show characteristic findings such as cortex involvement, periosteal reaction, and calcification that can indicate malignancy. However, when such results turn out to be indeterminate, magnetic resonance imaging (MRI) is increasingly being used for its higher soft tissue contrast and therefore for accurate visualization of the sizes of tumors and interfaces with adjacent structures. MRI is particularly helpful in defining the local spread of the tumors and involvement of marrow, which are critical factors in accurate diagnosis and therapy planning before any surgical intervention (Patra et al., 2018). Computed tomography (CT) is a useful imaging modality as an adjunct imaging tool, especially in the assessment of complex bony anatomy or suspected lung metastases in osteosarcoma and Ewing sarcoma. High-resolution imaging using CT is capable of precise delineation of fine details, such as cortical destruction and intramedullary calcifications, crucial in establishing a definitive diagnosis. Also, CT guidance permits biopsy procedures to be done, extracting exact samples from potential suspect lesions with reduced risks of contamination. Also, more recent imaging techniques like positron emission tomography (PET) and whole-body MRI are being used more frequently for staging and evaluation of response to treatment based on the detection of metastatic spread that conventional imaging may not detect, thereby affecting therapeutic decisions (Patra et al., 2018). Imaging test interpretation is an interactive process that brings radiologists and oncologists together to develop an integrated diagnosis plan. Each imaging modality offers specialized information regarding tumor biology and behavior, which in turn guides treatment. Three-dimensional imaging and molecular diagnostics are advanced technologies that are likely to further improve the accuracy of tumor characterization. With progressing diagnostic imaging, overcoming the tumor differentiation difficulties from benign lesions or conditions such as infection will be required with utmost care. Hence, multidisciplinary teams' collaborative synergy is essential to deliver patients with personalized therapeutic interventions that leverage the individual strengths of various imaging modalities (Casali et al., 2018).

11.3.3. Biopsy Procedures for Tumor Confirmation

Biopsy is also extremely critical in the diagnosis and characterization of tumors of the soft tissues and bones. By either an incisional or excisional method, these minimally invasive procedures allow clinicians to get tissue samples for histopathological study. Depending on the size, site, and imaging features before biopsy, the selection of the biopsy method will be determined. As in many clinical cases discussed, a correct evaluation of radiological results can significantly influence the choice of biopsy method. For example, an incisional biopsy was employed to diagnose an intraosseous ganglion cyst in a patient aged 60, who came with an osteolytic lesion of the proximal tibia, after imaging made several conditions likely (Giardini et al., 2020). Such mechanisms not only support definite diagnoses but also permit the development of effective treatment plans. Pathologists' interpretive skills in determining tumor type and behavior are of immense importance, placing a premium on accurate biopsy sampling. The pathologist's report on the biopsy sample allows critical assessment, revealing the underlying histological features informing treatment plans. In other cases, like xanthogranulomatous osteomyelitis, which later mimicked a neoplasm, a preoperative diagnosis was established only after analysis of the biopsy specimens (Lee et al., 2013). The distinction between benign and malignant tumors is crucial because it directly impacts management avenues, ranging from observation to more invasive surgical strategies. Thus, proper histopathological examination can ensure that patients receive the best appropriate and timely treatment, emphasizing the lasting significance of biopsy procedures as a necessary part of oncological diagnosis. The introduction of new biopsy techniques is continually enhancing diagnostic accuracy in the assessment of bone and soft tissue tumors.

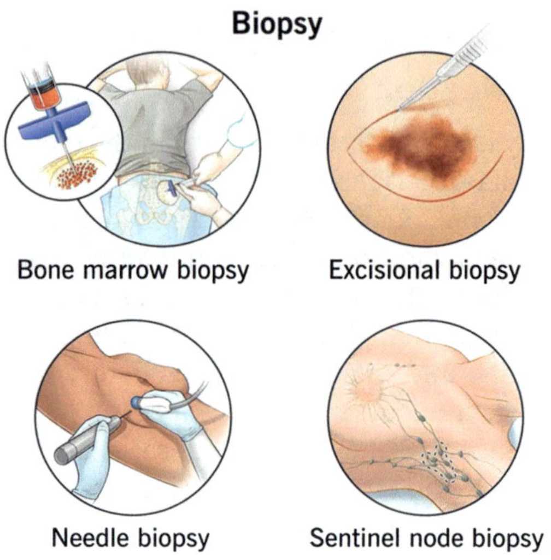

Figure 11.9. Biopsy procedures play a crucial role in the confirmation and characterization of tumors in bones and soft tissues.

Source: https://external-content.duckduckgo.com/iu/?u=https%3A%2F%2Fmy.clevelandclinic.org%2F-%2Fscassets%2FImages%2Forg%2Fhealth%2Farticles%2F15458-biopsy&f=1&nofb=1&ipt=f65bd91e53107360c0eb9bf3aa39f0f535966b845b9b8e9b6ed7038a292c8b75.

Technical improvements in imaging modalities such as MRI and CT scans have improved the visualization of lesions, allowing for more directed biopsies that reduce complications and increase yield. For instance, MRI results may indicate progressively more aggressive lesions; thus, a specific biopsy prevents misdiagnosis and the associated subsequent consequences of failing treatment (Giardini et al., 2020). Besides, biopsy procedures like ultrasound and fluoroscopy-guided biopsy have made clinicians increasingly able to sample hard-to-reach targets more precisely. Such ongoing refinement of biopsy procedures reaffirms the significance of biopsy procedures in tumor diagnosis to make sure that clinicians obtain data that enable them to develop sensible treatment plans and ultimately improve cancer patient outcomes (Figure 11.9).

11.4. Treatment Options for Bone Tumors

Treatment of bone tumors is generally found to necessitate the utilization of a multidisciplinary treatment approach involving more than one modality of treatment tailored specifically to the individual stage and type of tumor. Surgical therapy remains a cornerstone of treatment, particularly in primary malignancies of the bone such as osteosarcoma and Ewing's sarcoma. Surgery involves trying to resect the tumor completely while maintaining as much normal surrounding tissue as possible. For most cases, this is done with limb salvage surgery, which may preserve the function and mobility of the limb. Other than that, adjuvant therapy—such as chemotherapy or radiation therapy—is a crucial part of the treatment plan, particularly if the tumor is deemed aggressive or if it has metastasized. These adjunct therapies can be used to reduce preoperative tumor bulk or kill microscopic residual disease after surgery, potentially enhancing patient outcomes. Among benign bone neoplasms, procedures such as curettage and bone grafting have gained increased popularity since they are less invasive and effective. Therapy modalities for tumors such as the aneurysmal bone cyst (ABC) are mainly directed towards tumor removal with sparing of contiguous structures. Curettage is the shared procedure herein and can be supplemented with adjunctive measures such as phenol, liquid nitrogen, or even bone substitute to reduce recurrence rates. Current advancements also include minimally invasive techniques such as image-guided sclerotherapy, where sclerosing agents are utilized to promote lesion obliteration with minimal surgery. Emerging therapies, including monoclonal antibodies such as Denosumab, are being employed with a shift towards individualized medicine in the therapy front for bone tumors, catering to patients' needs and providing hope to them. Though the science of bone tumors is ongoing, the advancements in treatment are crucial for making a positive impact on patient outcomes. According to available statistics, the incidence of bone tumors has motivated increased study to rationalize existing treatment modalities and provide new approaches.

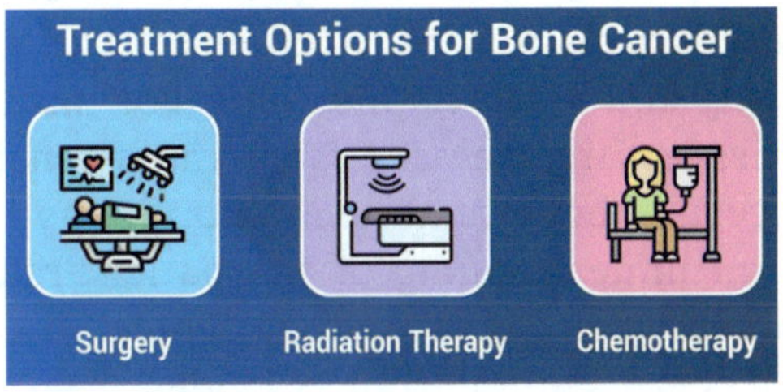

Figure 11.10. The management of bone tumors often necessitates a multidisciplinary approach.

Source: https://external-content.duckduckgo.com/iu/?u=https%3A%2F%2Factchealth.com%2Fimages%2Fbone-cancer-what-do-you-need-to-know23%2F04.webp&f=1&nofb=1&ipt=fe5cc536854f3a8e2f2c05d305324a0cbf2d5109d5597076779b114e3c65c455.

For example, the American Cancer Society is projecting an increase in the number of cancer cases overall, with tumor treatments involving the bones adapting according to these projections and disease pathology changes (Siegel et al., 2021). Besides surgical treatment, there is also greater emphasis on minimally invasive approaches, which can reduce recovery time and minimize complications. With ongoing research into bone tumor biology, the identification of new targets for therapy may make more effective treatment more likely. The future, thus, of bone tumor management, thus, is poised to transform and enhance the survival rate as well as health of patients with the condition (Restrepo et al., 2022) (Figure 11.10).

11.4.1. Surgical Interventions

Surgical interventions occupy an important role in the management of bone and soft tissue tumors, particularly in the management of locally advanced or aggressive neoplasms. The efficacy of surgical interventions is maximized by teamwork between multidisciplinary teams, which typically consist of surgeons, chemotherapists, and radiotherapists. This cooperative approach allows for the development of personalized treatment plans based on several factors, including tumor location, tumor type, and overall patient general health. Not only do these personalized treatments aim to accomplish complete resection of the tumor, but they also aim to preserve functional anatomy whenever that is possible. The use of advanced and innovative technologies in operations, such as the conservation of organs, greatly contributes to the guarantee of better results for the patient, reducing post-surgical complications and making recovery clearer. Additionally, anatomical reconstruction following tumor extirpations is an integral part of surgical procedures for bone and soft tissue tumors. Depending on recent evidence, the requirement for reconstructive plastic surgery is vast in accordance with the amount resected, as evidenced by dissimilar percentages for every operative field. For example, for segmental resections of long bones, the need for reconstruction is estimated at 28-32%, whereas the figures are significantly greater in the case of complex cases of soft tissue sarcomas and pelvic bone surgeries, where percentages reach up to 80% (Safin et al., 2024). These reconstructive procedures not only restore function and form but also contribute significantly to minimizing the chances of local recurrence, thereby enhancing overall treatment success and quality of life in postoperative patients. In addition to the physical challenges created by tumor resections, surgical methods must overcome factors responsible for higher postoperative complications. A study on musculoskeletal tumors revealed that preoperative assessments play a significant role in the outcome of surgery and in the definition of variables such as ASA status and bone tumors as determinantal causes of morbidity (Heesen et al., 2024). Therefore, it is essential to identify patient-specific risk factors and their impact on the success of surgery while personalizing surgical strategy. Through careful preoperative evaluation and utilization of benchmarking data, surgeons can minimize risks and enhance patient safety. Ultimately, though, the goal is not only to excise cancerous tumors but also to enhance the function and well-being of individuals afflicted by these challenging diseases (Figure 11.11).

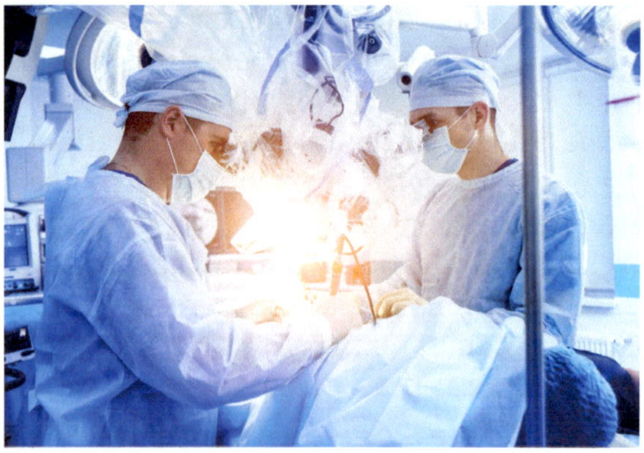

Figure 11.11. Surgical interventions.

Source: https://external-content.duckduckgo.com/iu/?u=https%3A%2F%2Fwww.curianmedical.co.uk%2Fwp-content%2Fuploads%2F2021%2F10%2Fsurgery-scaled.jpg&f=1&nofb=1&ipt=3e3604e58fe4224f7a858c48a46efe2c7447b9f7babadc87800d186826ac5477.

11.4.2. Radiation Therapy

The use of radiation therapy in the treatment of bone and soft tissue tumors provides a critical approach to the management of malignancies that have typically presented as complex clinical issues. Radiation therapy is typically used either as a pre- or post-operative adjunct to enhance local control and avoid recurrence. In the case of high-grade tumors, such as osteosarcoma or soft tissue sarcomas, radiation can be used in addition to surgery to ensure any residual microscopic disease is addressed following resection. According to research, the appropriate application of radiation therapy can lead to drastically improved survival rates alongside multimodal treatments, justifying its position within comprehensive oncological treatment (Casali et al., 2018). It is essential to understand the differential features of bone and soft tissue tumors while contemplating radiation therapy. Various types of tumors are differently radiosensitive, and this has treatment planning and result implications. For instance, soft tissue sarcomas are more radio-sensitive than certain bone tumors. A tailored approach with an understanding of the patient-related factors as well as the tumor biology, hence, assumes crucial importance. Evidence dictates that a team of multidisciplinary radiation oncologists, surgeons, and medical oncologists would all need to assess the potential benefits and harms of radiation therapy, particularly in larger, deeper, or comorbid conditions seen in patients with these malignancies (Casali et al., 2018). In addition, advancements in radiation treatment have enhanced its efficacy and minimized potential side effects, and therefore it has emerged as an increasingly sought-after therapy for bone and soft tissue malignancies. Technologies such as intensity-modulated radiation therapy (IMRT) and image-guided radiation therapy (IGRT) allow physicians to deliver the precise dose to the tumor with less destruction of surrounding healthy tissue. These technologies not only increase locoregional control rates but also lower radiation exposure-related complications, of which importance given the often young patients being treated for bone sarcomas. Their application in clinical practice requires ongoing research and evaluation to continue refining treatment recommendations, ultimately towards improved patient outcomes in the complex setting of bone and soft tissue tumors (Casali et al., 2018) (Figure 11.12).

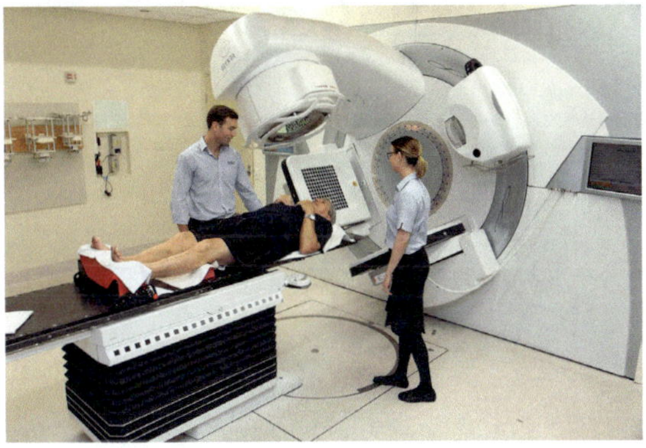

Figure 11.12. The integration of radiation therapy.

Source: https://external-content.duckduckgo.com/iu/?u=https%3A%2F%2Fhealthjade.com%2Fwp-content%2Fuploads%2F2018%2F06%2Fradiation-therapy.jpg&f=1&nofb=1&ipt=a493841dd45e0576ad80948a01705a638514a079dc0834ecd4b583698a72fa7a.

11.4.3. Chemotherapy and Targeted Therapies

The treatment scenario in cancer of soft tissues and bones has fundamentally altered, with chemotherapy and targeted therapy being the stars of tumor management. Chemotherapy remains the backbone in most pediatric sarcomas, which are notorious for their aggressiveness. The majority of these tumors, including osteosarcoma and rhabdomyosarcoma, generally respond very favorably at the outset to treatment with chemotherapeutic agents, leading to widespread necrosis of the tumor; however, this response does not always translate into permanent remission since some tumors have high recurrence rates. There is a need for more effective therapeutic protocols, particularly in patients who are resistant or unresponsive to standard chemotherapeutic protocols. Identification of predictive biomarkers that show a correlation with treatment response, as discussed in the study, can direct more personalized therapeutic choices that could potentially improve patient prognosis and improve survival rates in this at-risk population (Cheng et al., 2019). Targeted therapy has proven to be a significant innovation within the armory for the treatment of bone and soft tissue tumors, particularly through its potential to exploit specific molecular alterations present within cancer cells. Unlike conventional chemotherapy, which is given to all proliferating cells indiscriminately, targeted therapy was devised to inhibit the expression of certain signaling pathways that confer advantages for cancer growth and survival. In pediatric sarcomas, the detection of chromosomal abnormalities and copy number variants (CNVs) has revealed actionable genomic alterations that can be used in guiding treatment. For instance, by characterizing CNVs that correlate with sensitivity or resistance to chemotherapeutics, physicians can potentially tailor treatment regimens so that therapeutic effects can be optimized. The integration of genomic data into the clinic can enable oncologists to select drugs that specifically target each patient's unique genomic landscape in their tumor, thus giving a more personalized model of treatment (Cheng et al., 2019). Moreover, the advent of nanomedicine holds out a new horizon for chemotherapeutic and targeted drug delivery, using the potential of nanotechnology to optimize therapeutic results with minimal off-target effects. Through the use of nanoscale biomaterials, researchers are designing systems with capabilities to target drugs specifically to the site of tumors and optimize localized therapeutic impact while minimizing systemic toxicity. This innovative method has been shown to be effective in improving the pharmacokinetics and bioavailability of drugs targeted against bone and soft tissue cancers. Nanomedicine also provides the ability to co-deliver more than one therapeutic modality like immunotherapies and biologicals in order to improve the overall antitumor activity. As nanotechnology progresses with further breakthroughs, its use in drug delivery is certain to revolutionize treatment modalities with promise for better results in managing difficult cancers like osteosarcoma and Ewing's sarcoma (Figure 11.13).

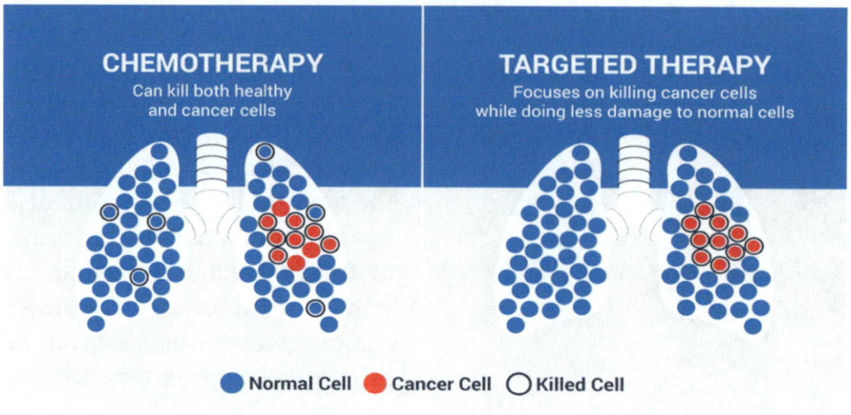

Figure 11.13. The treatment landscape for tumors of bones and soft tissues.

Source: https://external-content.duckduckgo.com/iu/?u=https%3A%2F%2Fwww.medicalcenterturkey.com%2Fwp-content%2Fuploads%2F2021%2F06%2Fchemotherapy-targeted-therapy-1160x609.png&f=1&nofb=1&ipt=4cb40e11f68b7e4c69f890af6e24aa7867890eb20d922f63e132ad1513839a4d.

11.5. Treatment Options for Soft Tissue Tumors

Treatment of soft tissue sarcoma is generally multidisciplinary in nature, and one must ideally use operation with chemotherapy and radiotherapy together. Operation remains the most important treatment, particularly for primary tumors. The aim is to achieve a complete resection with maximal preservation of normal surrounding tissue. The operation technique is based on tumor size, site, and grade, and there should be clear margins to reduce the risk of recurrence. For patients not receiving surgery, other modalities such as chemotherapy can be utilized, particularly for high-grade or metastasizing tumors. Chemotherapeutic regimens rely heavily on the tumor subtype, with doxorubicin and ifosfamide being the most frequently used drugs. Multimodal therapy is employed in attempts to customize treatment to specific patient needs, maximizing therapeutic response with a try to limit toxicity. Radiation treatment can also be extremely significant in the case of soft tissue tumors. Radiation can be employed preoperatively to decrease the size of tumors so that they might be excised surgically or postoperatively to destroy residual microscopic disease. In some cases, particularly in unresectable tumors, radiation may be delivered as a solitary treatment modality. Radiation therapy achieves its effects by inducing damage to the DNA of cancer cells and thereby stopping their growth and multiplication. It is interesting to note that innovative therapies have attracted significant attention in exploiting the inflammatory response to enhance therapeutic impacts. Inflammation-modulating approaches have demonstrated promising potential in developing new therapies. This includes agents modifying signaling cascades such as NF-kB and various cytokines that modify tumor microenvironments, which have important influences on treatment outcomes (Zhao et al., 2021). In addition, novel treatment modalities are being explored to complement traditional therapy for soft tissue tumors. The inhibition of the blood supply to the tumor that is required for tumor growth has become an area of interest with anti-angiogenic therapy. The treatments aim to disrupt tumor vascularization, thereby inhibiting their growth and metastatic potential. While they promise much, these treatments can be highly variable in their success, as evidenced by the heterogeneous nature of the responses found in various tumors (Lugano et al., 2019). Immunotherapy has been at the forefront of research in recent times as well, i.e., by using the body's immune system for the purpose of targeting and eliminating cancer cells. While early results show promise, much remains to be understood in terms of how best to select patients and schedule the treatments. Combined, these new forms of treatment herald the approach toward the personalized medicine required to improve outcomes in patients with soft tissue tumors.

11.5.1. Surgical Excision

Surgical excision is a primary mode of treatment for bone and soft tissue tumors, wherein the tumor is removed with maximal preservation of normal tissue. The procedure involves an accurate assessment of the characteristics of the tumor, including size, location, and invasion into surrounding structures, to decide on the surgical method. Most importantly, the establishment of negative surgical margins is crucial; this entails microscopically normal tissue encompassing the resected tumor, significantly improving the patient's outcome. Recent developments have highlighted the importance of having a multidisciplinary team where plastic and vascular surgical units collaborate, thereby expanding the indications for limb salvage procedures without compromising oncological principles. These coordinated efforts enhance the functional viability of reconstructions following tumor removal, aligning with the overall aim of surgery to provide tumor elimination without having an adverse impact on the quality of life of the patients (Gupta et al., 2025). Surgical excision is carried out through exhaustive preoperative planning, involving the attainment of accurate diagnostic data utilizing methods such as percutaneous core needle biopsies. Core needle biopsies offer major benefits compared to traditional open biopsies in the form of reduced invasiveness and decreased complication rates, hence facilitating early treatment and diagnosis. The precision of core needle biopsies, as depicted in existing studies, attains up to 96% in bone tumors and up to 92% in soft tissue tumors, which is highly in favor of surgical planning. These high accuracy rates are essential because they rule out unnecessary big resections, guiding surgeons to target only the diseased tissues. Furthermore, effective communication in a multidisciplinary environment enhances diagnostic success and enhances surgical excision outcomes (Cengiz et al., 2025).

Post-operative care following excision is essential in the overall cure process of tumors on bones and soft tissues. Patients can be subjected to additional therapies such as adjuvant chemotherapy or radiation to forestall recurrence, particularly if unfavorable margins were not achievable. Functional assessment tools, such as the Musculoskeletal Tumor Society Score, allow the comparison of surgical outcomes based on the improvement of mobility and function in the limb. It is established in research that patients who are provided with holistic care in the form of coordinated surgery and multidisciplinary treatment always demonstrate improved functional outcomes and quality of life. Finally, the strategic combining of surgical excision with additional adjuvant therapy assures not only tumor elimination but also the protection of the patients physical function and social relationships in the long term (Gupta et al., 2025) (Figure 11.14).

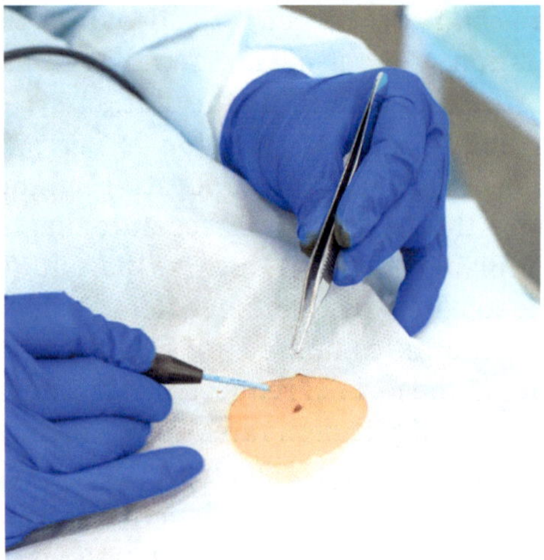

Figure 11.14. Surgical excision serves as a primary treatment modality for tumors of bones and soft tissues.

Source: https://external-content.duckduckgo.com/iu/?u=https%3A%2F%2Fbrightclinic.com.my%2Fcms%2Fwp-content%2Fuploads%2F2022%2F08%2Fsurgical-excision1.jpg&f=1&nofb=1&ipt=f8b403fea893aae0d1fe657a4b13dac9ad64e40a7fc876cc5a3a4321b7ac2f92.

11.5.2. Role of Radiation Therapy

Radiation therapy plays a multifaceted role in the treatment of bone and soft tissue tumors, particularly when surgery cannot be performed or the total resection cannot be achieved. This treatment utilizes high-energy particles or waves to kill cancer cells and diminish tumor size and spread of the disease. For bone cancers such as osteosarcoma, radiation therapy is employed as an adjunct to surgery or as a single modality in unresectable cases. Radiation therapy is further advocated by ongoing advances in techniques such as intensity-modulated radiation therapy (IMRT), which allows for increased accuracy in tumor cell targeting while sparing surrounding healthy tissues from unnecessary exposure. Thus, radiation therapy plays a vital role in enhancing the survival rate and preventing tumor growth in several clinical situations. Within the soft tissue sarcoma treatment profile, radiation therapy is a key ingredient, especially when tumors lie in anatomically problematic locations. Such tumors pose a series of special challenges because they tend to be in close relation to vital structures, such that a precisely planned radiotherapy course is needed to achieve maximal results. Preoperative radiation therapy is also commonly applied, allowing reduction of the tumor before surgery, which might also make resection more efficient and even keep healthy tissue from critical damage. Further, postoperative radiation has been shown to reduce recurrence rates, which would cure any residual cancer cells that might have been left behind during surgery. The addition of radiation therapy in a multimodal approach becomes essential in maximizing local control and overall prognosis in patients with soft tissue sarcomas, highlighting the relevance of individualized treatment protocols. Recent studies have also better explained the biological effect of radiation therapy, revealing its capability to maximize the effectiveness of immunotherapies in the treatment of bone as well as soft tissue malignancies. By its alteration of the tumor environment through processes such as increased antigen presentation and release of inflammatory cytokines, radiation therapy can synergistically enhance the body's immune response against cancer. It directs attention to the importance of multidisciplinary methods that combine radiation with immunotherapeutic agents to attain improved treatment outcomes. As evidenced by recent studies, the combination of these modalities is accompanied by the potential for personalized cancer treatment regimens that are maximally effective with minimal toxicity. Increasing applications of radiation therapy, especially its combination with novel immunotherapies, confirm its pivotal position in contemporary treatment of bone and soft tissue sarcomas, thus paving the way for more effective clinical applications in oncology (Figure 11.15).

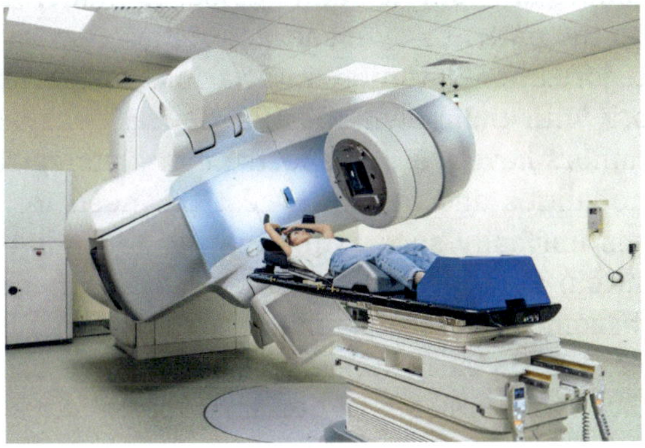

Figure 11.15. Radiation therapy plays a multifaceted role in the management of tumors of bones and soft tissues.

Source: https://external-content.duckduckgo.com/iu/?u=https%3A%2F%2Fstylebuzzer.com%2Fwp-content%2Fuploads%2F2024%2F01%2FRadiation-Therapy-in-Cancer-Treatment.webp&f=1&nofb=1&ipt=a7d2c0f8077f5cb60095871113ef041e003644e60740cd5a0b129e2bdcd07e38.

11.5.3. Emerging Therapies and Clinical Trials

The therapeutic profile of bone and soft tissue sarcomas is evolving based on a compelling necessity to improve outcomes in the field dominated by heterogeneity. Traditional treatment, such as surgery and radiation, often cannot address the malignant qualities of advanced sarcomas effectively, and there is a necessity to find new treatments. Ongoing clinical trials are investigating new modalities, including targeted therapy and immunotherapy, that leverage the potential of the immune system to recognize and combat sarcoma cells. The expectation of these emerging treatments is that they could redefine the treatment strategies of sarcomas and offer new hope for patients who have limited other options. In addition, large-scale genomic profiling studies are now beginning to inform tailored treatment strategies, underscoring the importance of personalized medicine in terms of elevating survival in such a unique cohort of patients (Gómez-Puerto et al., 2025). Also involved in new directions in therapy are advanced computational methods for maximizing the efficiency of clinical trials. One significant development in this area is the spatial quantitative systems pharmacology (spQSP) model, which is designed to simulate tumor growth and treatment interactions at both tissue and organ levels. This new approach allows for the investigation of the spatial heterogeneity of tumors and the way different regimens of therapy will create different responses in patients. By using real clinic trial spatial multi-omics data, researchers are able to validate model predictions and also maximize dosing regimens. These advancements will be critical to reveal potential biomarkers that have the potential to guide clinical decision-making in order to ultimately lead to better treatment outcomes for aggressive sarcoma patients (Zhang et al., 2023). As trials progress, the use of combination therapies is gradually emerging as a determining factor in the treatment of bone and soft tissue tumors. Current trials have set the scene for the fact that combinations of immunotherapies and targeted therapies can yield unprecedented clinical responses among well-characterized patient subsets. The analysis of these combinations, facilitated with computational models and large-scale biomarker analyses, will unlock the door to synergistic effects that enhance therapeutic benefit while minimizing side effects. Further refinement of these approaches in the clinic is the vision of scientists to not only extend survival rates but also to better the quality of life for these patients with such complex cancers. The future of therapy in this challenging area is based on state-of-the-art research and astute clinical advancement of studies that will efficiently transfer the results of the laboratory into effective therapeutic advances (Gómez-Puerto et al., 2025).

11.6. Prognosis and Outcomes

The prognosis and outcome of bone and soft tissue tumors are complex and subject to numerous factors, varying from the type and stage of the tumor to the patient's own characteristics. Accurate diagnosis is paramount, as it forms the basis for the categorization of tumors into various categories, varying from epithelial to bone and soft tissue tumors with their own specific clinical behavior and treatment responses. For instance, maxillofacial tumors have a broad spectrum of histological types, which can have an impact on management modalities and again suggest the need for a multidisciplinary management strategy. Management is normally successful when it depends on early diagnosis and initiation of appropriate intervention. Complications such as metastasis can significantly alter prognosis; thus, regular follow-up becomes necessary for improved results. By close monitoring, clinicians can identify any recurrence signs in early stages, and in the long term, enhance survival rates and patient quality of life for such cancers (Shawly et al., 2023).

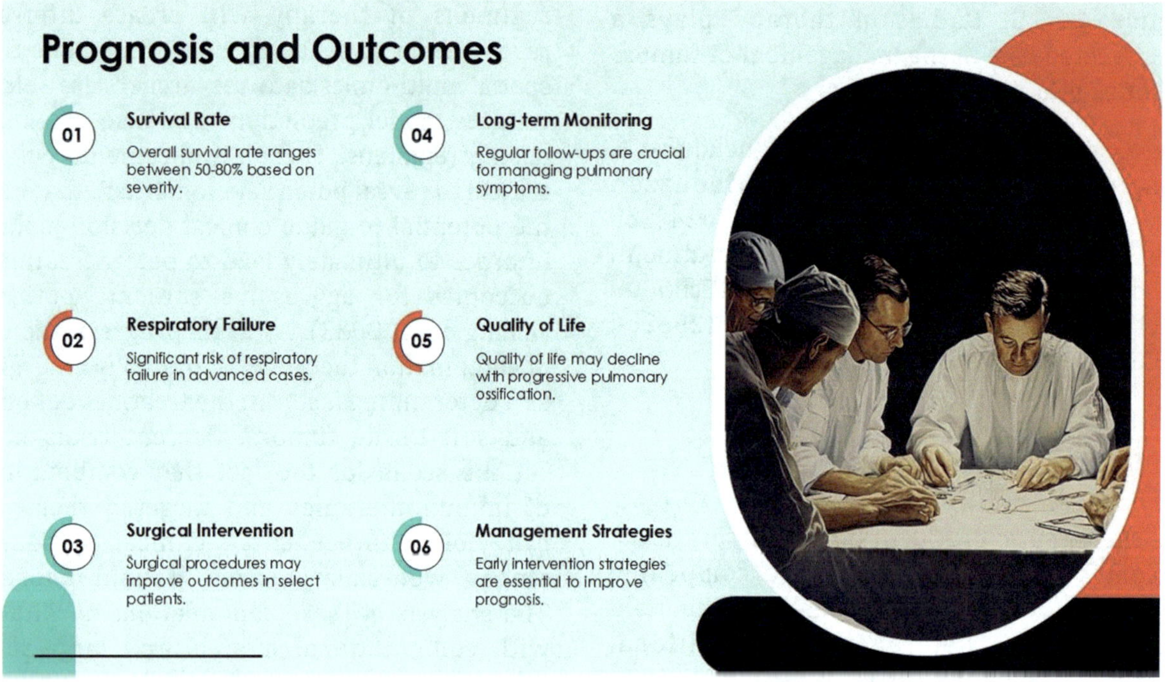

Figure 11.16. The prognosis and outcomes of tumors affecting bones and soft tissues.

Source: https://external-content.duckduckgo.com/iu/?u=https%3A%2F%2Fwww.slideteam.net%2Fmedia%2Fcatalog%2Fproduct%2Fcache%2F1280x720%2Fp%2Fr%2Fprognosis_and_outcomes_ossification_ppt_template_acp_slide01.jpg&f=1&nofb=1&ipt=3e25f1d6a5678af3afa74bb07b9210ad9a2d06b339466b07842d86d541c96eae.

In children, the prognosis for cancers like rhabdomyosarcoma (RMS) can be particularly daunting, considering that it is the most frequent of soft tissue tumors in children. With an incidence of 0.9 per 100,000 children, RMS is inclined to be diagnosed early at a mean age of five years and has the sinister tendency for far-advanced metastasis. The prognosis of leptomeningeal metastasis is particularly bleak, with reported evidence that approximately 25% of patients harbor such spread at the time of presentation. The combined treatment, comprising chemotherapy, radiation, and potential surgery, is promising, but the outcomes are not consistent. In a recent cohort study, nearly half of the patients were discovered to be alive post-treatment, with both prospects of improvement as well as the challenges revealed when complex treatment procedures are employed (Rodina et al., 2023). Maximum outcome in the management of bone and soft tissue tumors is possible only through an evolved understanding of prognostic variables. Patient tolerance to therapy can be infinitely different, based on reasons like the timing of the tumors at presentation and their inherent biological characteristics. Moreover, progress in therapeutic modalities, such as targeted therapy and refinement in surgical techniques, continues. These developments play a critical role in enhancing the survival rates and minimizing treatment-related complications for patients. Additionally, the integration of holistic care—such as rehabilitation and psychological support—is critical towards ensuring long-term success. As cancer research goes on, there will inevitably be greater understanding of fine-tuning interventions for each individual case, which will lead to improved prognoses and quality of life for tumor-bearing patients of bone and soft tissue (Rodina et al., 2023; Shawly et al., 2023) (Figure 11.16).

11.6.1. Factors Influencing Prognosis

Prognosis for bone and soft tissue tumors depends upon the intricate relationship among multiple factors, including histological type, grade, and location. Histological type is of primary concern since individual tumors exhibit various biological behaviors and also response to treatment. For instance, based on studies, chondrosarcoma and chordoma possess relatively good prognoses compared with osteosarcoma, which possesses a more aggressive clinical behavior and higher mortality. Understanding histological characteristics allows clinicians to develop more-targeted treatment approaches, hence the impact on survival outcomes. In addition, tumor grade is an important prognostic indicator: higher grades tend to have poorer prognoses since they are virulent and possess metastatic potential. Specifically, higher-level grading raises surgical resection and overall disease management risks, which directly affect patient prognosis and survival rates (Tsuchiya et al., 2025). Tumor size and locoregional extent also play a crucial role in establishing the prognosis for sarcoma patients. Larger or more extensive tumors are generally indicative of an advanced disease and pose a risk for complicating resection by surgery. Larger tumor size has been reported to be associated with increased local recurrence as well as poorer overall survival in both soft tissue sarcomas and bone tumors. Specifically, the more advanced stage of the tumor is a gloomy prognostic indicator, with worse outcomes customarily recorded for stage IV because of the development of metastasis. Furthermore, the spread into adjacent anatomical structures may complicate total surgical resection, deteriorating the prognosis. Resection margins, which are key to surgical success, have a great influence on recurrence risk; the surgical strategy must thus be planned meticulously to achieve the best benefit to the patient (Fromm et al., 2024). Moreover, the application of neoadjuvant treatment modalities, including chemotherapy and radiotherapy, has been shown to be a significant prognostic determinant. Application of combined neoadjuvant therapy is generally found to have increased tumor necrosis, which would theoretically enhance survival rates. However, while tumor necrosis after neoadjuvant chemotherapy has been predictive of therapeutic response, it is not uniformly linked with good outcomes in soft tissue sarcomas. In some instances, no correlation with overall survival in high grade tumors has been found, showing the multifactorial nature of predictors for good outcomes. Besides, the timing, type, and effectiveness of adjuvant therapy, the patient's age and general health status further complicate the prognostic scenario, necessitating an integrated and personalized approach to patient management (Fromm et al., 2024) (Figure 11.17).

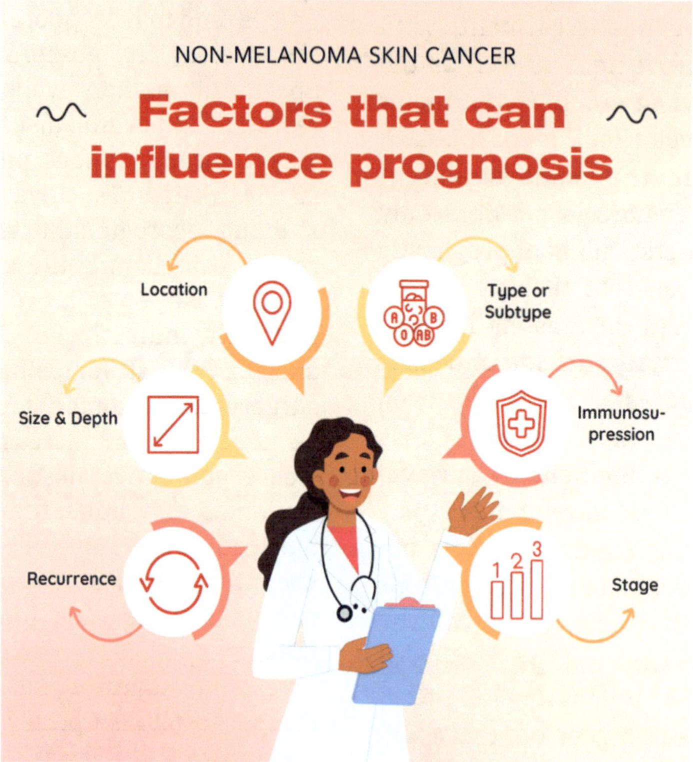

Figure 11.17. The prognosis of tumors of bones and soft tissues.

Source: https://static.wixstatic.com/media/e08cdc_7abd9f43b0014970a833267f7926fcc5~mv2.png/v1/fit/w_1096,h_1100,al_c/e08cdc_7abd9f43b0014970a833267f7926fcc5~mv2.png.

11.6.2. Survival Rates for Different Tumor Types

Survival rates for the different types of tumors vary significantly, which reflects the heterogeneity of cancers in the soft tissues and bones. Sarcomas, e.g., tumors of the connective tissues such as muscle, fat, and bone, usually have mixed survival outcomes. According to recent statistics, the overall five-year survival rate of patients with soft tissue sarcomas is approximately 65%, although this varies according to the size, location, and histological subtype of the tumor. Outcomes in patients are also determined by the amount of surgical resection achieved and the presence of metastasis at initial diagnosis; the prognostic environment for bone and soft tissue tumors is complicated and multi-dimensional. For tumors in the bone, the classification and staging of the tumor predict prognosis the most. In one of the more prevalent bone cancers, osteosarcoma, the five-year survival rate is about 70% if the tumor is localized, but it drops precipitously to about 30% if the tumor becomes metastatic. In contrast, less common tumors like chondrosarcoma do not have the same survival pattern, with low-grade variants having greater than 80% survival rates, and high-grade subtypes presenting a much poorer prognosis. These distinctions underscore the necessity of early diagnosis and tailored treatment options based on the characteristic features of the tumor and the need for overall management in optimizing patient outcomes for these challenging-to-treat cancers. Furthermore, maturation therapies have profoundly impacted rates of survival for different tumour forms.

The integration of targeted therapy and immunotherapy has transformed the paradigm for treating tumors, yielding new hope for difficult-to-treat soft tissue tumors and bone tumors. For example, the creation of novel combinations of drugs in soft tissue sarcomas has yielded a good prognosis for the patients, as optimization of surgery and adjuvant therapy in osteosarcoma improved survival chances. It can clearly be seen that there has been considerable improvement in lowering cancer mortality, e.g., a radical decline in tumor-specific fatalities, in line with the American Cancer Society, indicative of the ongoing developments in oncology (Siegel et al., 2024). With continued research effort and investment in precision medicine, the future looks good for an ongoing increase in survival rates among patients who are battling tumors of the soft tissues and bone (Siegel et al., 2021) (Figure 11.18).

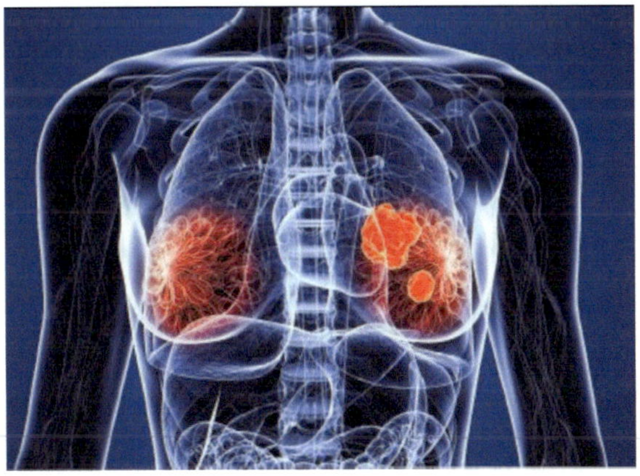

Figure 11.18. Survival rates for different tumor types vary significantly.

Source: https://www.wcrf.org/wp-content/uploads/2024/10/Breast-Survivors.jpg.

11.6.3. Long-Term Effects of Treatment

The late consequences of treatment for bone and soft tissue tumors are multifaceted, impacting the physical health as well as the quality of life of the survivors. Survivors tend to report a variety of chronic symptoms that persist well after the acute treatment, including pain, fatigue, and functional impairments. This prolonged symptomatology can be attributable to both the tumor as well as the aggressive treatment protocols that often include surgery, radiation therapy, and chemotherapy. In particular, treatments can lead to complications, such as nerve damage or scarring, that increase distress and limit mobility further. Thus, it is necessary to understand the general implications of post-treatment effects to address the needs of this patient population and to make certain that interventions are appropriately modified to address long-term health outcomes effectively. Moreover, some treatment methods entail unique hazards to long-term health that must be addressed with care. For instance, surgical operations may lead to structural damage or loss of function in engaged limbs, which pose long-term challenges to rehabilitation. The patients typically develop activity restrictions or limb weakness, which can restrict them from active engagement in life and enhance feelings of isolation. Additionally, chemotherapy may lead to delayed side effects, such as chemotherapy-induced peripheral neuropathy, which can significantly influence the patient's ability the performance of daily activities (Andrews et al., 2020). These physical and psychological issues demand a multidisciplinary approach to care that underscores the necessity for intensive rehabilitation services designed to maximize function and enhance quality of life in survivors facing the long-term sequelae of their treatment. Additionally, eliminating the differences in the outcomes of long-term treatment is essential in the management of bone and soft tissue tumors. Evidence indicates that there are certain demographic groups whose outcomes will be poor due to factors such as socioeconomic status and healthcare resource access. For instance, Black patients experience poorer mortality rates for certain cancers, and that can be complemented by system disparities in treatment quality and availability (Siegel et al., 2024). The application of tailored rehabilitation regimens can be crucial to reducing the long-term effects of treatment as well as improving outcomes for these disadvantaged populations. By ensuring equitable healthcare programming and optimizing access to supportive therapy, the medical community can more effectively work towards reducing the burden of long-term treatment effects, where each individual can have the opportunity to lead healthy, normal lives following treatment.

SUMMARY

In short, the progress in soft tissue and bone tumor diagnosis and treatment has transformed the traditional forms of treatment to a large extent. Amputation was the traditional approach to managing musculoskeletal tumors in the past, but the evolution of limb salvage surgery (LSS) has shifted the trend towards limb preservation with effective control of cancer. Evidence has shown that LSS yields comparable oncologic outcomes with amputation, combined with the benefit of enhanced quality of life among patients, particularly with successful rehabilitation. This adjustment represents the need for a multidisciplinary approach in tailoring treatment plans according to the unique needs of each patient, hence optimizing survivorship and also functional recovery (Muhammad et al., 2025). Further, correct histopathological examination remains necessary in the effective treatment of bone and soft tissue neoplasms. The ability to correctly identify the nature of such tumors, their histological details, as well as their potential genetic markers, forms a key consideration in the selection of the most efficacious treatment approach. Techniques such as trephine and core biopsies have been found to have high information content in providing adequate tissue samples for examination, influencing treatment plan and outcome directly. Developing biopsy techniques and imaging modalities has further enhanced the precision of the diagnosis so that patients are given personalized interventions that target their respective tumor types accurately (Saprykina et al., 2024). In the end, management of bone and soft tissue tumors involves ongoing research and development in therapeutic and surgical fields. As limb-salvage procedures have become the more routine choice for so many, though, complications and local recurrence remain an issue. Anything new in this vein will have to be driven by a commitment to enhancing surgical technique, imaging capabilities, and finding new adjuvant therapies that can optimize patients' potential for success. As our understanding of these complex tumors deepens, fostering collaboration between oncologists, radiologists, and pathologists will be vital in achieving comprehensive care that not only prioritizes survival but also prioritizes the quality of life for individuals affected by these conditions.

The study of tumors that develop in soft tissues and bones is a complex interaction of clinical and biological factors. At the heart of the understanding of these tumors is an appreciation for the activity of the extracellular matrix (ECM), which is an interacting group of macromolecules that not only plays a role in the structural integrity of tissues but also has dramatic effects on cellular function. Some of the key components of the ECM, such as collagens and glycoproteins, are involved in cell adhesion, migration, and differentiation, all of which are critical in tumorigenesis and tumor growth. Interestingly, any modification in the ECM composition can promote tumorigenesis and metastasis and thereby emphasize the need for the exploration of ECM-directed therapeutic strategies in bone and soft tissue tumors (Karamanos et al., 2021). Collaboratively, the uncovering of ECM relationships will enhance our understanding of the tumor microenvironment and present avenues for new therapies. Another crucial aspect of bone and soft tissue neoplasms is the potential for tumor dormancy and recurrence. Cancer cells typically disseminate from the original neoplasm, entering a period of dormancy for protracted periods, remaining undetectable until they re-engage an active state to form metastases. Recent research has outlined mechanisms by which cells re-enter a reactivation phase, with particular stress on the importance of inflammation and the production of neutrophil extracellular traps (NETs). Not only do NETs create a permissive environment for the re-awakening of the tumor, but they also structurally reorganize the ECM, facilitating growth transition from dormancy towards aggressiveness (Albrengues et al., 2018). This consciousness highlights treating not only the initial tumor but also processes of recurrence and dormancy in the treatment of bone and soft tissue tumors. Finally, the development of targeted therapies directed against the ECM and mechanisms of tumor reactivation is a promising frontier in oncology. New advances in molecular biology have revealed some ECM components and mechanisms in tumor growth and have unveiled potential therapeutic targets. For instance, disruption of NET assembly or interference with ECM remodeling may avoid the vicious reawakening of quiescent tumors, severely worsening patient outcome. This personalized treatment regimen is a paradigm change in oncology, where the microenvironment and its interaction with tumor cells are equally crucial as the identification of the type of tumor itself (Albrengues et al., 2018; Karamanos et al., 2021). Overall, the cellular and molecular intricacy involved in bone and soft tissue tumors has to be tackled in order to develop useful and innovative therapy plans.

CLOSER LOOK

RADIATION THERAPY

Radiation therapy is a medical treatment that uses high-energy radiation to destroy cancer cells, shrink tumors, and prevent the spread of disease. It works by damaging the DNA of rapidly dividing cancer cells, which inhibits their ability to grow and reproduce. Radiation therapy is commonly used in the treatment of various cancers, either alone or in combination with surgery and chemotherapy. There are two main types of radiation therapy: external beam radiation, where radiation is delivered from a machine outside the body, and internal radiation, or brachytherapy, where radioactive sources are placed inside or near the tumor. Treatment planning is highly precise, using advanced imaging techniques such as CT scans, MRI, and PET scans to target cancer cells accurately while minimizing damage to surrounding healthy tissues. Radiation therapy can be given before surgery to shrink tumors, after surgery to eliminate remaining cancer cells, or as a primary treatment when surgery is not feasible. It is also used for palliative care to relieve pain and improve quality of life in advanced cancer cases. Common side effects include fatigue, skin irritation, nausea, and localized tissue reactions, which vary depending on the treatment area. With modern technology and improved techniques, radiation therapy has become safer and more effective, offering better outcomes and improved survival rates for cancer patients.

REFERENCES

1. Ise, M., Nakata, E., Katayama, Y., Hamada, M., Kunisada, T., Fujiwara, T., Nakahara, R., Takihira, S., Sato, K., Akezaki, Y., Senda, M., & Ozaki, T. (2021). Prevalence of Psychological Distress and Its Risk Factors in Patients with Primary Bone and Soft Tissue Tumors. *Healthcare (Basel, Switzerland)*, *9*(5), 566. https://doi.org/10.3390/healthcare9050566 (accessed on 26th June 2025).
2. Albrengues, J., Shields, M. A., Ng, D., Park, C. G., Ambrico, A., Poindexter, M. E., Upadhyay, P., et al. (2018). Neutrophil extracellular traps produced during inflammation awaken dormant cancer cells in mice. *Science, 361*. https://doi.org/10.1126/science.aao4227 (accessed on 26th June 2025).
3. Andrews, C., Siegel, G., & Smith, S. R. (2020). Rehabilitation to improve the function and quality of life of soft tissue and bony sarcoma patients. *Patient Related Outcome Measures, 10*, 417–425. https://doi.org/10.2147/prom.s130183 (accessed on 26th June 2025).
4. Azevedo, C. P., Casanova, J. M., Guerra, M. G., Santos, A. L., Portela, M. I., & Tavares, P. F. (2013). Tumors of the foot and ankle: a single-institution experience. *The Journal of foot and ankle surgery : official publication of the American College of Foot and Ankle Surgeons, 52*(2), 147–152. https://doi.org/10.1053/j.jfas.2012.12.004(accessed on 26th June 2025).
5. Baumhoer, D., Hench, J., & Amary, F. (2024). Recent advances in molecular profiling of bone and soft tissue tumors. *Skeletal Radiology, 53*, 1925–1936. https://www.semanticscholar.org/paper/079fcdf4a1d16360238665d920c8742ff2776de4 (accessed on 26th June 2025).
6. Casali, P. G., Abecassis, N., Bauer, S., Biagini, R., Bielack, S., Bonvalot, S., Boukovinas, I., et al. (2018). Soft tissue and visceral sarcomas: ESMO–EURACAN Clinical Practice Guidelines for diagnosis, treatment and follow-up. *Annals of Oncology, 29*, iv51–iv67. https://doi.org/10.1093/annonc/mdy096 (accessed on 26th June 2025).
7. Casali, P. G., Bielack, S., Abecassis, N., Aro, H. T., Bauer, S., Biagini, R., Bonvalot, S., et al. (2018). Bone sarcomas: ESMO–PaedCan–EURACAN Clinical Practice Guidelines for diagnosis, treatment and follow-up. *Annals of Oncology, 29*, iv79–iv95. https://doi.org/10.1093/annonc/mdy310 (accessed on 26th June 2025).
8. Cengiz, T., Yurtbay, A., Muslu, O., Aydın Şimşek, Ş., Özbalci, A. B., Coşkun, H., Bariş, Y. S., et al. (2025). Evaluation of the diagnostic accuracy of percutaneous core needle biopsy in bone and soft tissue tumors. *Acta Chirurgiae Orthopaedicae et Traumatologiae Cechoslovaca, 91*(6), 376–384. https://www.semanticscholar.org/paper/dab7e3227c2c7f32da5b5ab3438c97308201cef0 (accessed on 26th June 2025).
9. Cheng, L., Pandya, P. H., Liu, E., Chandra, P., Wang, L., Murray, M. E., Carter, J., et al. (2019). Integration of genomic copy number variations and chemotherapy-response biomarkers in pediatric sarcoma. *BMC Medical Genomics, 12*. https://doi.org/10.1186/s12920-018-0456-5 (accessed on 26th June 2025).
10. Fromm, J., Klein, A., Kirilova, M., Lindner, L., Nachbichler, S., Holzapfel, B., Goller, S., et al. (2024). The effect of chemo- and radiotherapy on tumor necrosis in soft tissue sarcoma–Does it influence prognosis? *BMC Cancer, 24*. https://www.semanticscholar.org/paper/9e385f6a7c98466e36e805a739289de4cf26c32b (accessed on 26th June 2025).
11. Giardini, P., Menna, C., Barbareschi, M., & Molinari, M. (2020). Unusual osteolytic intraosseous

ganglion cyst of the medial tibial condyle in a patient affected by mild osteoarthritis of the knee. *Acta Bio Medica: Atenei Parmensis, 91*. https://www.semanticscholar.org/paper/abe0b875c1444efd44d28363db12c598c3ea00b8 (accessed on 26th June 2025).

12. Gómez-Puerto, D., Cicala, C., Valverde, C., & Serrano, C. (2025). Emerging treatments for sarcoma: From 2024 onward. *Expert Opinion on Emerging Drugs, 30*, 53–70. https://www.semanticscholar.org/paper/dc2300a99bdff25d6153e925c21301baad6f349f (accessed on 26th June 2025).

13. Gupta, P., Bansal, U., Thakuriya, A., & Rawat, S. (2025). Combined surgical team approach for limb salvage: To avoid amputations in skin, vessels, or nerve involvements in bone and soft tissue tumors. *Journal of Bone and Joint Diseases*. https://www.semanticscholar.org/paper/57e6cb6589590592c3e57d093fc5d8d559bf84ea (accessed on 26th June 2025).

14. Helal, A. A., Sakr, H., & Elsayed, S. S. M. (2024). Added value of diffusion-weighted magnetic resonance imaging in evaluation of musculoskeletal soft tissue masses. *QJM: An International Journal of Medicine*. https://www.semanticscholar.org/paper/b10529d2e7d7db8b5e9a05f379748a233f6e6fdd (accessed on 26th June 2025).

15. Johnson, D. E., Burtness, B., Leemans, C. R., Lui, V. W. Y., Bauman, J. E., & Grandis, J. R. (2020). Head and neck squamous cell carcinoma. *Nature Reviews Disease Primers, 6*. https://doi.org/10.1038/s41572-020-00224-3 (accessed on 26th June 2025).

16. Karamanos, N. K., Theocharis, A. D., Piperigkou, Z., Manou, D., Passi, A., Skandalis, S. S., Vynios, D. H., et al. (2021). A guide to the composition and functions of the extracellular matrix. *FEBS Journal, 288*, 6850–6912. https://doi.org/10.1111/febs.15776 (accessed on 26th June 2025).

17. Lee, S. H., Lee, Y. H., Park, H., Cho, Y., Song, H. T., Yang, W., & Suh, J. (2013). A case report of xanthogranulomatous osteomyelitis of the distal ulna mimicking a malignant neoplasm. *The American Journal of Case Reports, 14*, 304–307. https://www.semanticscholar.org/paper/bd9d216eac01958deab293fe7c6bddade4a919d4 (accessed on 26th June 2025).

18. Lugano, R., Ramachandran, M., & Dimberg, A. (2019). Tumor angiogenesis: Causes, consequences, challenges and opportunities. *Cellular and Molecular Life Sciences, 77*, 1745–1770. https://doi.org/10.1007/s00018-019-03351-7 (accessed on 26th June 2025).

19. Minervini, F., Sergi, C., Scarci, M., Kestenholz, P., Valentini, L., Boschetti, L., & Bertoglio, P. (2024). Benign tumors of the chest wall. *Journal of Thoracic Disease, 16*, 722–736. https://www.semanticscholar.org/paper/d5a6fcd4849c958aed095823a5011666f928178f (accessed on 26th June 2025).

20. Muhammad, R., Khan, S. A., Abdullah, S., Javaid, T., Umer, M., & Gull, H. (2025). Limb salvage surgery compared to amputation in bone and soft tissue tumors: A critical analysis of current evidence. *Journal of Medical & Health Sciences Review*. https://www.semanticscholar.org/paper/a915ac438cd8e238c9e0815d451082e14f83f230 (accessed on 26th June 2025).

21. Orsi, F., Hamiddin, A. S., Sattin, C., Pizzi, C., Varano, G., Della Vigna, P., Mauri, G., et al. (2024). Liquid nitrogen-based cryoablation: Complication rates for lung, bone, and soft tissue tumors cryoablation. *The British Journal of Radiology, 97*, 1863–1869. https://www.semanticscholar.org/paper/118f8161f755140493ddc45c2466dc17f4cb3671 (accessed on 26th June 2025).

22. Patra, J. K., Das, G., Fraceto, L. F., Campos, E. V. R., Rodriguez-Torres, M. del P., Acosta-Torres, L. S., Díaz-Torres, L. A., et al. (2018). Nano based drug delivery systems: Recent developments

and future prospects. *Journal of Nanobiotechnology, 16*. https://doi.org/10.1186/s12951-018-0392-8 (accessed on 26th June 2025).

23. Phan, P., Chidiac, C., Shalkow, J., & Rhee, D. S. (2025). Socioeconomic disparities in palliative care utilization among children with late-stage bone and soft tissue sarcomas: A National Cancer Database analysis. *Journal of Clinical Oncology*. https://www.semanticscholar.org/paper/e3c6911768b815cf74da5581bd021f40447b7f24 (accessed on 26th June 2025).

24. Ratnaparkhi, A. D., Anvikar, A., Deshmukh, B., Patil, P. S., Nene, P. K., & Gosavi, A. (2025). Clinicopathological profile of benign soft tissue tumors–A study of 256 cases. *Panacea Journal of Medical Sciences*. https://www.semanticscholar.org/paper/73c42d2f810a03bff554a6a0e0401ca836d96aa4 (accessed on 26th June 2025).

25. Restrepo, R., Zahrah, D., Pelaez, L., Temple, H. T., & Murakami, J. W. (2022). Update on aneurysmal bone cyst: Pathophysiology, histology, imaging and treatment. *Pediatric Radiology, 52*, 1601–1614. https://doi.org/10.1007/s00247-022-05396-6 (accessed on 26th June 2025).

26. Rodina, V., Polyakov, T., Gorbunova, S., Krylov, A. L., Kashanina, A., Merkulov, O. A., & Varfolomeeva, S. (2023). Risk of leptomeningeal metastasis in children with Para meningeal rhabdomyosarcoma with intracranial spread. *Russian Journal of Pediatric Hematology and Oncology*. https://www.semanticscholar.org/paper/c4d94a77e69785f90c1ede68b9ae6d8a2bc30e5e (accessed on 26th June 2025).

27. Safin, A., Rodionova, D. V., Rukavishnikov, R. S., Khasanov, A. M., Saifullin, R., Safin, R., & Khalikov, M. M. (2024). The reconstructive stage in the combined treatment of tumors of bones, soft tissues and skin. *Bone and Soft Tissue Sarcomas, Tumors of the Skin*. https://www.semanticscholar.org/paper/4f9156f913c1d687d9e337cbaae7c419ff51328c (accessed on 26th June 2025).

28. Saprykina, E. A., Teplyakov, V. V., Shaposhnikov, A., Lazukin, A. V., Ukhvarkin, A. P., & Dobrosotsky, S. V. (2024). Diagnostic efficacy of trephine biopsy and core biopsy of bone and soft tissue tumors. *Bone and Soft Tissue Sarcomas, Tumors of the Skin*. https://www.semanticscholar.org/paper/05f4bc6ec3127d1bfaf39ad1d3091d4df935dbb9 (accessed on 26th June 2025).

29. Sarı, S., Sarı, E. A., Balcı, A., Havıtçıoğlu, H., & Tuna, B. (2024). The role of perfusion magnetic resonance imaging in discrimination of benign vs malign character of musculoskeletal tumors. *Journal of Basic and Clinical Health Sciences*. https://www.semanticscholar.org/paper/9af0df60bb2f8397eaec0cdd39d124c613dace0a (accessed on 26th June 2025).

30. Scheele, N., Harrasser, S., Beischl, S., Dammerer, D., Lenze, F., Knebel, C., & Lenze, U. (2024). Distribution patterns of benign and malignant bone and soft tissue tumors and tumor-like lesions in the hindfoot and ankle: A 12.5-year analysis. *In Vivo, 38*, 2383–2389. https://www.semanticscholar.org/paper/dae99c15aafcd4b664590c246c8c9cb7b0209f0d (accessed on 26th June 2025).

31. Shawly, H., Softah, W. A., Sharrahi, H., Alenezi, A. H., Alshaibani, Z. M., Alruwili, R. A., Alotaibi, T. A., et al. (2023). Types, prevalence, management, and outcome of maxillofacial tumors. *International Journal of Community Medicine and Public Health*. https://www.semanticscholar.org/paper/9f45ecc84c426a204830f0faad06d969af2df401 (accessed on 26th June 2025).

32. Siegel, R. L., Miller, K. D., & Jemal, A. (2019). Cancer statistics, 2019. *CA: A Cancer Journal for Clinicians, 69*, 7–34. https://doi.org/10.3322/caac.21551 (accessed on 26th June 2025).

33. Siegel, R. L., Miller, K. D., Fuchs, H. E., & Jemal, A. (2021). Cancer statistics, 2021. *CA: A Cancer Journal for Clinicians, 71*, 7–33. https://doi.org/10.3322/caac.21654 (accessed on 26th June 2025).

34. Tang, J., Ding, F., Yu, M., & Cai, X. (2025). Analgesic treatment of refractory cancer pain caused by bone and soft tissue metastasis of lower esophageal and cardial adenocarcinoma: A case report. *Medicine, 104*. https://www.semanticscholar.org/paper/17e33556cd3e48784471cf99db8c805e977dbbca (accessed on 26th June 2025).

35. Tonetti, M. S., Greenwell, H., & Kornman, K. S. (2018). Staging and grading of periodontitis: Framework and proposal of a new classification and case definition. *Journal of Clinical Periodontology, 45*. https://doi.org/10.1111/jcpe.12945 (accessed on 26th June 2025).

36. Tsuchiya, R., Ogura, K., Ohtori, S., & Kawai, A. (2025). Statistics of primary malignant spine tumors in Japan: A retrospective study using the Bone and Soft Tissue Tumor Registry in Japan. *Spine*. https://www.semanticscholar.org/paper/c9369d5585a1ce32cdcb82434abdfb2a2b7a67b0 (accessed on 26th June 2025).

37. Turaga, K. K., & Girotra, S. (2020). Are we harming cancer patients by delaying their cancer surgery during the COVID-19 pandemic? *Annals of Surgery, 278*, e960–e965. https://doi.org/10.1097/sla.0000000000003967 (accessed on 26th June 2025).

38. Zhang, S., Deshpande, A., Verma, B., Wang, H., Mi, H., Yuan, L., Ho, W. J., et al. (2023). Informing virtual clinical trials of hepatocellular carcinoma with spatial multi-omics analysis of a human neoadjuvant immunotherapy clinical trial. *bioRxiv*. https://www.semanticscholar.org/paper/aefde4d576dcbe99a27ad905db67861bd9d6a4db (accessed on 26th June 2025).

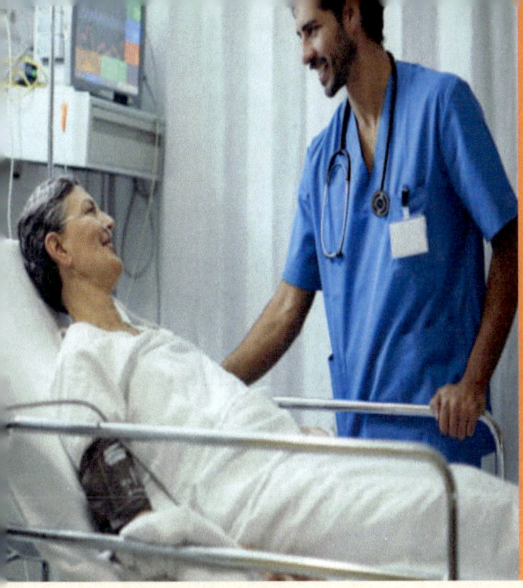

Chapter 12

POST-SURGICAL REHABILITATION

Contents

Introduction....369
12.1. Phases of Post-Surgical Rehabilitation....373
12.2. Assessment and Evaluation....376
12.3. Role of Healthcare Professionals....380
12.4. Rehabilitation Techniques and Modalities....383
12.5. Patient Education and Engagement....387
12.6. Psychological Aspects of Rehabilitation....390
12.7. Challenges in Post-Surgical Rehabilitation....393
12.8. Innovations in Rehabilitation Technology....397
Summary....401
References....404

Introduction

Postoperative rehabilitation is an important component of the continuum of healthcare, utilized to facilitate recovery following surgery. It is a systemic strategy to optimize healing, re-establish function, and enhance the patient's global quality of life. Rehabilitation is typically begun shortly following surgery, when the acute body response has not decreased, and continues through degrees of recovery. At this point, it is important to assess the individual requirements and special conditions of each patient to develop rehabilitation regimes to cater to them well. Rehabilitation may include educating patients regarding their body limitations and pain management strategies, keeping in view the need to adhere to prescribed rehabilitation exercises for maximum outcome. This multi-faceted approach not only fosters bodily healing but also allows patients to be empowered emotionally, where they can notably increase their self-efficacy and motivation towards rehabilitation. The intricacies of rehabilitation after surgery, however, largely rely on what surgery was performed and the role of multiple systems in the body. For instance, orthopedic surgeries tend to necessitate specialized intervention involving mobility, strength, and range of motion of affected limbs. On the other hand, regenerative rehabilitation following cancer treatment-related operations can be as complex as evaluation to address underlying complications, i.e., erectile dysfunction following a radical prostatectomy. There is evidence that interventions such as pelvic muscle training, among others, can be helpful in recovery, but results can be variable. Furthermore, evidence from (Asker et al., 2022) also indicates the challenge of restoring erectile function after nerve-sparing methods, which verifies the necessity of incorporating specialized rehabilitation techniques that target treating such very specific deficits during recovery. Thus, an individualized approach in rehabilitation not only optimizes physical outcomes but basically influences psychological status and quality of life as well.

The broader context of post-surgical rehabilitation extends beyond the individual recovery process to a collective understanding of patient care. While health professionals struggle with the realm of rehabilitation, adherence to given guidelines is paramount in the provision of impactful interventions. European Society of Cardiology (ESC) guidelines, as reported in Kirchhof et al. (2016), give high regard to the integration of current evidence-based practice in clinical interventions with a focus on patients. This means that physicians must engage in candid dialogue with patients to reach decision-making involving both clinical data and individual settings. With the balancing act between clinical acumen and more recent guidelines, healthcare professionals are able to develop overall rehabilitative environments geared towards meeting specific patient needs. Ultimately, with the facilitation of rehabilitation standards compliance, patients can maximize recovery trajectories and achieve enhanced health outcomes.

Definition and Importance

Postoperative rehabilitation is a multi-dimensional process to recover patients' pre-surgical functioning after surgery. It is a process that entails a range of therapeutic interventions with the goal of enhancing physical functioning, reducing pain, and enhancing general well-being. It typically includes physical therapy, strength conditioning, and patient education, each tailored to individualized recovery paths. The significance of having a programmatic rehabilitative program cannot be overstated, particularly when taking into account procedures such as autologous chondrocyte implantation (ACI). A study indicates that the patient's functional ability can be extremely significantly compromised in the early recovery phase, and thus there is a requirement for overall rehabilitative measures to address physical as well as psychological aspects of recovery (Howard et al., 2014). The importance of rehabilitation post-surgery extends beyond the simple reintroduction of body functions. It becomes the means to optimize recovery durations and enhance patients' quality of life. Throughout rehabilitation, patients are instructed on how to perform daily activities without worsening their condition and thus encouraging independence as well as self-confidence. Furthermore, rehabilitation is an effective stimulus that encourages patients to adhere to recovery programs and remain positive about improvement. The establishment that self-rated improvements in functioning sometimes precede physical alterations demonstrates the value of psychological aspects of formal programs of rehabilitation (Howard et al., 2014). Such an integrated view not only aids the recovery process but also addresses the greater aspects of health and well-being. Along with improvement in the physical state, effective postoperative rehabilitation is essential to minimize the risk of complications and ensure the long-term success of surgery. A well-planned schedule of rehabilitation can enable a gradual return to physical function, hence preventing issues such as muscle atrophy and stiffness of the joints. For example, ACI patients usually have challenges in achieving weight-bearing function during the first three months following surgery, which can be well managed by structured exercises and supervised therapy (Howard et al., 2014). The integrative nature of postoperative rehabilitation, where there is ongoing monitoring and modulations of interventions, is key to catering to the individualized needs of patients, finally resulting in a better recovery experience and enhanced long-term outcomes. Rehabilitation thus becomes a key aspect of the continuum of postoperative care, underlining its definition and role in holistic recovery (Figure 12.1).

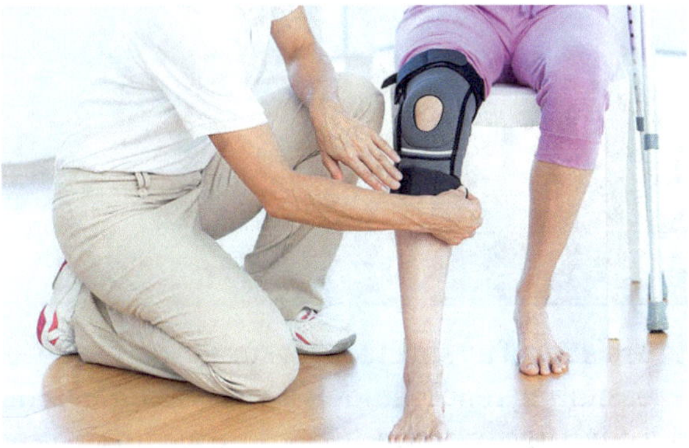

Figure 12.1. Post-surgical rehabilitation is defined as a multifaceted approach designed to restore patients' pre-operative functionality following surgical interventions.

Source: https://www.refitrehab.com/wp-content/uploads/2021/08/Pre-Post-Surgical-Rehabilitation.jpg.

Goals of Rehabilitation

In post-surgical rehabilitation, the overall objectives often encompass restoring function, alleviating pain, and enhancing patients' quality of life. For orthopedic surgery such as rotator cuff repairs, tailored rehabilitation programs can directly influence recovery outcomes. Some research indicates that patient-led, individualized rehabilitation may be more beneficial than conventional rehabilitation with rigid protocols. This shift of focus is intended to aid patients by allowing them to have an active part in their own healing process. By encouraging patients to move their arms as they are able and to guide their rehabilitation according to their own comfort levels, these individualized interventions may ultimately reduce shoulder pain and disability in a more favorable time frame, as can be observed especially at the 12-week mark after surgery (Bateman et al., 2024). Enhancing functional mobility is another crucial rehabilitative objective. Postoperative patients, particularly those who are recovering from major body surgery, often have problems extending beyond the immediate postoperative zone. For instance, patients with tetraplegia will require reconstructive upper extremity surgery, not only to try and restore physical function but also to promote psychosocial adjustment. As hinted at by the literature that reviewed treatment parameters, the process of decision-making for rehabilitative therapy is not simply determined by quantifiable improvement in health, i.e., range of motion, but also on the perception of rehabilitation intensity and satisfaction by the patient (Dahlgren et al., 2008). Through the incorporation of functional recovery with patient-centered goals, rehabilitation is an integrated process towards increased independence and health. Besides, the psychological components of rehabilitation are vital in nature and cannot be overlooked. Patients during post-surgical times often experience ups and downs in emotional response, ranging from frustration to demotivation due to physical debilitation and pain. Such psychological aspects need to be managed in order to achieve the objectives of rehabilitation. Incorporation of counseling and mental health support into the rehabilitation model can improve resilience and rehabilitation protocol compliance. Educating patients regarding probable recovery channels and creating support networks within communities can lead to a great extent in making the coping abilities of patients stronger. By coordinating the psychological and physical recovery goals, rehabilitation professionals can enable the patient to defeat setbacks and fully engage in their process of recovery and thereby deliver holistic care for post-surgical rehabilitation.

Types of Surgical Procedures Requiring Rehabilitation

The scope of surgical procedures that necessitate rehabilitation is wide and includes many orthopedic, gastrointestinal, and cardiovascular procedures. A very high-profile one that immediately comes to mind is Ulnar Collateral Ligament Reconstruction (UCLR), which is crucial for overhead sport athletes, for instance, baseball. Ultrasound collateral ligament damage usually occurs as a result of repetitive throwing sports stress. Following UCLR, patients can be expected to undergo a considerable recovery process with emphasis on both physical therapy and progressive return to sport-specific task performance. The invasiveness of the procedure is what makes the importance of the rehabilitation regimen clearly evident, wherein a well-planned regimen attempts to restore joint stability, mobility, and strength in the affected area, along with prevention of future damage. The intricacy of rehabilitation following such interventions emphasizes the necessity for personalized care programs that can be tailored to the unique requirements of the patient's lifestyle and sporting aspirations, thus allowing for maximum recovery outcomes and competitive return to play (Guy et al., 2019). Aside from orthopedic interventions, gastrointestinal surgeries also necessitate meticulous post-operative rehabilitation. An appropriate example is the management of Short Bowel Syndrome (SBS), which may follow extensive small bowel resections. Patients are likely to depend on parenteral nutrition to compensate for lost absorptive capacity. Operations that lengthen the bowel or reposition intestinal segments are of huge relief but must be supplemented with a long-term rehabilitation plan to allow nutritional absorption and gastrointestinal health. Rehabilitation in this instance does not just encompass physical recuperation; it goes as far as education, facilitating the patients' modification of their diet and optimization of their nutrition following surgery. Effective rehabilitation techniques are critical in avoiding complications and enhancing the overall quality of life of the patients via the upkeep of their symptom control as well as independence in their daily lives (Marino & Lauro, 2018).

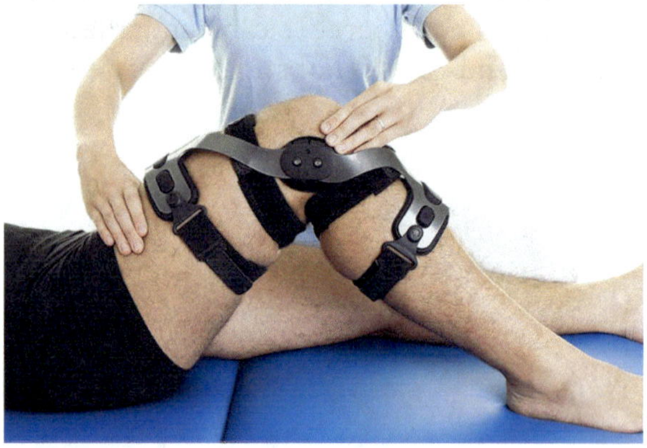

Figure 12.2. The spectrum of surgical procedures necessitating rehabilitation is vast, encompassing various orthopedic, gastrointestinal, and cardiovascular interventions.

Source: https://spinesportsmedicine.org/wp-content/uploads/2017/12/Post-surgical-rehabilitation2.jpg.

Cardiac surgeries, such as coronary artery bypass grafting (CABG), similarly point towards the necessity of structured post-operative rehabilitation. Both the physical and psychological strain on patients following such highly invasive procedures is significant, calling for a tailored rehabilitation program. Such programs typically incorporate cardiac rehabilitation, including monitored exercise regimens, lifestyle modification, and psychological counseling aimed at enhancing cardiovascular health as well as overall well-being. Exercise also enables the return of cardiac function, as well as checking the hazards of a postoperative sedentary lifestyle. With enhanced progressive exercise and cardio training, patients can establish confidence in their ability and effectively minimize long-term cardiovascular disease hazards. Thus, the role of rehabilitation in the process of recovery after CABG plays a crucial role in achieving full physical and emotional recovery, thereby improving health outcomes (Marino & Lauro, 2018) (Figure 12.2).

12.1. Phases of Post-Surgical Rehabilitation

Post-surgical rehabilitation stages are very important for the patients' transition from surgery to a maximum level of recovery. The initial stage, also referred to as the acute phase, normally begins in the postoperative period and may last for some days. The patient needs to remain stable, and complications such as infections, pain, and limitation of movements are prevented. During this phase, doctors typically utilize interventions that focus on mobilization and control of pain for the facilitation of recovery. Care is also necessary in attending to patients' nutritional needs in an effort to combat the body's physiological stresses brought by surgery. Effective management during this phase sets a sound base for the subsequent follow-up phases, where an active engagement of the patient becomes increasingly important. As patients progress beyond the acute phase, they reach the subacute or convalescent phase, typically of days to weeks post-surgery. During this period, there is a shift towards restoring function and enhancing the quality of life. Treatment during this phase typically involves physical rehabilitation therapy to restore strength and range of motion, aimed specifically at the procedure in question. Apart from this, patients may be provided with psychological and nutritional care as they surmount recovery challenges. Similar to this, for example, patients undergoing recovery from head and neck cancer can be supported by tailored nutrition methods, which indicates the relevance of multidimensional management (Wierzbicka et al., 2025). The integration of physical rehabilitation and psychosocial treatment comes into play as patients surmount functional and emotional changes brought on by surgery. Finally, the transition to the rehabilitation phase in the long term is an ongoing process that takes months or years after surgery. It involves repeated assessment and adaptation of rehabilitative goals as patients move toward independence and greater functionality. Multidisciplinary care remains necessary, with most healthcare teams having physical therapists, occupational therapists, dietitians, and mental health specialists working in consultation to address the complex needs of their patients (Sigfrid et al., 2021). As the patients acclimatize to their post-surgical conditions, individualized rehabilitation programs have the ability to make significant improvements to their overall quality of life. Thus, awareness regarding and proper application of the various phases of post-operative rehabilitation is essential for maximizing recovery results as well as for an all-encompassing patient care plan.

12.1.1. Immediate Post-Operative Phase

The post-operative phase, shortly after surgery, is of great importance where the primary recovery and rehabilitation of the patients commence. It is a time of intense observation and management of pain, vital signs, and potential complications arising post-operatively. Particularly with orthopedic procedures, such as meniscal repair surgeries, effective management of pain ensures early mobilization and initiation of rehabilitation activity. For instance, clinicians must consider specific biomechanical characteristics of the reconstructed structures, which dictate the post-operative rehabilitation plan. Adequate evaluation of patients' individual anatomical and functional characteristics allows healthcare specialists to create individualized rehabilitation protocols, which can significantly enhance the outcome of recovery. As such, it is imperative to make a well-planned recovery plan during this initial step for the most favorable rehabilitation processes and avoiding complications, the patients can regain functional independence in an efficient and effective way. Multidisciplinary collaboration among the healthcare team members, like surgeons, physical therapists, and nurses, is also needed in successful rehabilitation during the immediate post-operative period. This interdisciplinary approach allows for a comprehensive assessment of the patient's requirements, not only physical rehabilitation but also the mental aspects of recovery. An example would be emotional support being vital in life-changing surgeries such as transfemoral amputations, where adaptation to the loss of the limb has a very direct impact on mental health. Modern advances in postoperative care are putting greater emphasis on the integration of early prosthetic fitting into the rehabilitation plan, as immediate postoperative prostheses (IPOP) can facilitate mobilization and confidence during healing. Ultimately, good team communication ensures that patient condition changes are communicated instantly, and real-time rehabilitation protocols are adjusted based on evolving clinical knowledge to maximize the effectiveness of recovery. In conclusion, the initial post-surgical period is a critical point in successful post-surgical rehabilitation, this emphasizing the significance of personalized interventions and interdisciplinary teamwork. The precise application of protocols that take into consideration biomechanics, pain management, and psychological aspects can profoundly influence recovery trajectories. Under conditions such as posterior medial meniscus root tears, there can be a rehabilitative process that counteracts the risk of joint instability as indicated by the need for rehabilitation on a specialized basis using sound clinical principles (Monson & LaPrade, 2025). Similarly, with amputations, the novel strategies such as adaptive designs for the prosthetic socket prioritize reducing the dynamic fluctuations in a patient's status for a successful recovery (Pany et al., 2025). Regardless, the foundation here provides the foundation for restoration of functional capacity and also improving the general quality of life in surgical patients (Figure 12.3).

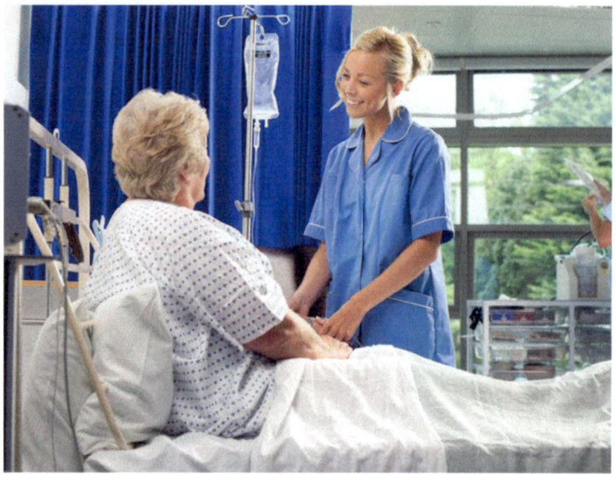

Figure 12.3. The immediate post-operative phase is a critical period wherein the initial recovery and rehabilitation of patients begin.

Source: https://media.post.rvohealth.io/wp-content/uploads/2020/08/postoperative-care_thumb.jpg.

12.1.2. Early Rehabilitation Phase

The early rehabilitation phase is a critical component of surgical recovery, which is the beginning of therapeutic interventions for enhancing post-surgical recovery. It typically begins days after surgery and is therefore determined largely by effective strategies that are customized to the underlying surgical condition. There are several reasons why early rehabilitation exists, such as prevention of disuse atrophy, reduction of pain, and enhancement of range of motion. Patients may be introduced to low-load blood flow restriction training (LLBFRT) at this stage, an intervention that has increasingly gained popularity owing to its musculoskeletal rehabilitation implications. This intervention is hypothesized to enhance muscle volume and endurance and thus provides a foundation upon which rehabilitation in the future will be done (Pany et al., 2025). Nonetheless, despite some studies showing positive effects of LLBFRT on muscle volume and strength, the overall efficacy of the technique is still operator- and response-dependent. Rehabilitation in the postoperative period after surgery also needs to include respiratory and functional abilities, especially in patients with extensive thoracic or spinal surgery. Scoliosis operations, for instance, can have a major impact on respiratory function deficits that can necessitate the use of specialized interventions such as inspiratory muscle training. This can enhance respiratory muscle strength and functional capacity in post-surgical patients through the use of structured exercises that facilitate pulmonary efficiency. Clinical evidence of improvements in six-minute walk distance and vital capacity in patients who are on inspiratory muscle training compared to those receiving conventional treatment has been indicated (Shabbir et al., 2025). Such findings underscore the importance of applying focused rehabilitation methods to counteract the multifaceted challenges presented during the early recovery phase. Multidisciplinary coordination is key to ascertaining optimal rehabilitation outcomes during the early stage of rehabilitation. By coordinating physical therapy treatment with breathing and function training, health providers are positioned to facilitate an integrated system of recovery that is conducive to long-term success. The proper evaluation and adjustment of rehabilitation plans must be done to address the varied progress and problems of patients. Physical therapists, occupational therapists, and other specialists working in a team form make the support system more distinct for overall care. Lastly, the first phase of rehabilitation is the foundation of subsequent rehabilitation programs, once more stressing the application of time- and target-oriented interventions that can have a strong impact on patterns of recovery and maximize the quality of life in postoperative patients (Figure 12.4).

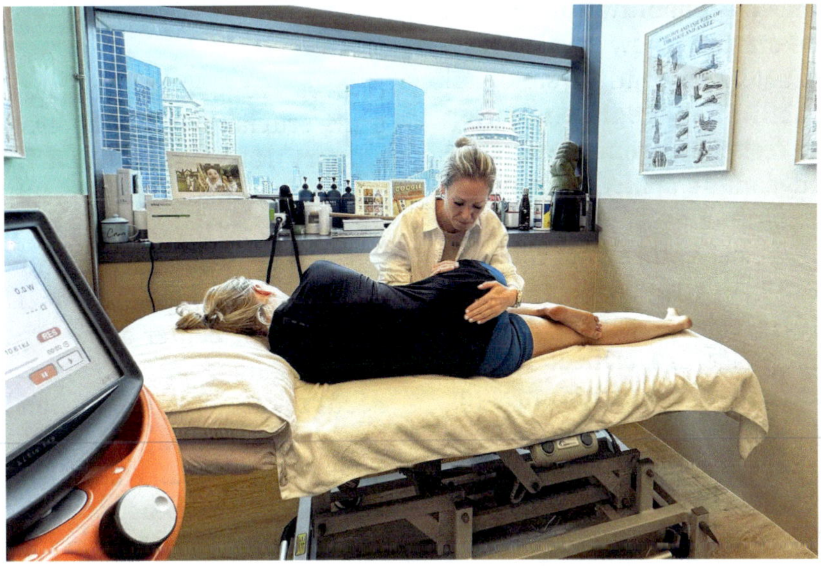

Figure 12.4. Early rehabilitation targets several objectives, including minimizing disuse atrophy, reducing pain, and enhancing range of motion.

Source: https://www.hellophysio.sg/wp-content/uploads/post-op-physiotherapy.jpg.webp.

12.1.3. Advanced Rehabilitation Phase

The Advanced Rehabilitation Phase is an important phase of the continuum of post-surgical rehab, particularly for sports participants who have had surgery such as Ulnar Collateral Ligament Reconstruction (UCLR). While earlier phases were focused on pain reduction and enhancing mobility, the Advanced Rehabilitation Phase heavily focuses on the rehabilitation of strength, flexibility, and functional ability. During this time, rehabilitation programs become more vigorous, utilizing sport-specific motions and neuromuscular training to enable advancement to a return to sports activity. Rehabilitation activities must be tailored specifically to the requirements of the sport being played to not only allow the athlete to effectively recover, but to return to the pre-injury level of performance. This phase is also marked by close monitoring to avoid re-injuries, and this speaks volumes about the necessity for an organized regimen to facilitate improved healing with minimal risk of re-injury. In UCLR, commitment to elbow stability and strengthening is paramount during the Advanced Rehabilitation Phase. This phase can be started a few weeks post-surgery to allow initial healing and physiological adaptation. Rehabilitation regimens often involve progressive resistance training exercises for enhancing the dynamic stability of the elbow joint, thereby conditioning athletes to cope with the stress of overhead throwing motions characteristic of sports like baseball. Since interventions at this level have been highlighted, treatments at this phase are critical for the restoration of confidence and function since the psychological aspect of rehabilitation remains equal in significance as physical recovery. Evidence-based practices ensure that the chosen therapeutic exercises are consistent with the best results documented in reconstructive surgery, thus facilitating an optimal and safe recovery for return to sport (Guy et al., 2019). Additionally, a thorough assessment is critical during the Advanced Rehabilitation Phase to gauge improvement and adjust rehabilitation plans accordingly. Biomechanical testing is often utilized by clinicians to assess the function of the reconstructed ligament and involved musculature to place athletes in a manner in which they are engaging in activity without compromising their surgical repair. This level of individualized attention not only facilitates monitoring of functional improvement but also plays a significant educational and motivational role for the athlete. Through being well-informed of their improvement and increasingly invested in their rehabilitation process, athletes are subsequently well-placed to adhere to prescribed programs. Despite the advancements in surgical technique outlined within research, diligent work undertaken during the Advanced Rehabilitation Phase remains paramount to addressing the shortfall between surgical treatment and successful reintegration into competitive sport (Lebert, 2017).

12.2. Assessment and Evaluation

Impressive evaluation and assessment are both crucial within the framework of post-surgery rehabilitation, particularly following procedures like joint replacements or tendon repairs. A stepwise process of evaluation not only directs the rehabilitation course but also adjusts interventions based on individual patient needs. At the center of the process is identifying certain clinical outcomes that the rehabilitation needs to tackle, e.g., reduction in pain, improved range of motion, and restored functional mobility. Clinicians usually use standardized instruments to measure such outcomes so that they can gather qualitative and quantitative data. Interdisciplinary techniques such as goniometry for assessing joint angles or standardized questionnaires to assess pain tolerance are imperative in providing a balanced description of a patient's rehabilitation process. Such evidence-based assessment forms the cornerstone for making informed clinical decisions and modifications in the rehabilitation protocol as appropriate. Finally, postoperative rehabilitation assessments ought to extend beyond simple physical recovery and incorporate psychosocial factors that can influence patient outcomes. Understanding the patient's psychological condition, social support structures, and adherence to rehabilitation regimens are needed for successful rehabilitation. Studies emphasize the significance of these factors in enhancing patient motivation and adherence throughout the rehabilitation process. According to the clinical guidelines, therefore, rehabilitation regimens must include regular reevaluations in consideration of these psychosocial factors in addition to standard physical evaluations. This combined system not only addresses the bodily aspect of rehabilitation but also provides a supportive setting that fosters patient involvement and compliance with their healing process. These integrative assessment practices assist in developing customized rehabilitation plans that can optimize recovery and minimize the chances of complications. Post-surgical rehabilitation regulation, particularly that of conditions such as Achilles tendon ruptures, prescribes the need for an organized method of assessment and evaluation. Although injuries such as these are prevalent in occurrence and the overall result with treatment is effective, disagreement regarding standardized practices for rehabilitation can be found, suggesting that this may perhaps be reflected through variations in clinical practice. Here, synergism between systematic reviews of the available literature and expert opinions can provide a framework for regulation of rehabilitation with the aim of improving the quality of care and utilization of resources for all patients (Oliva et al., 2018). Proper evaluation and assessment are thus inevitable in addressing this heterogeneity, where the rehabilitation process adheres to the best practices of the present time and evidence-based techniques. The continuous evaluation not only authenticates accountability in treatment interventions but also enables the patient by actively involving him/her in his/her journey of recovery, thereby leading to improved results (Thierry et al., 2013) (Figure 12.5).

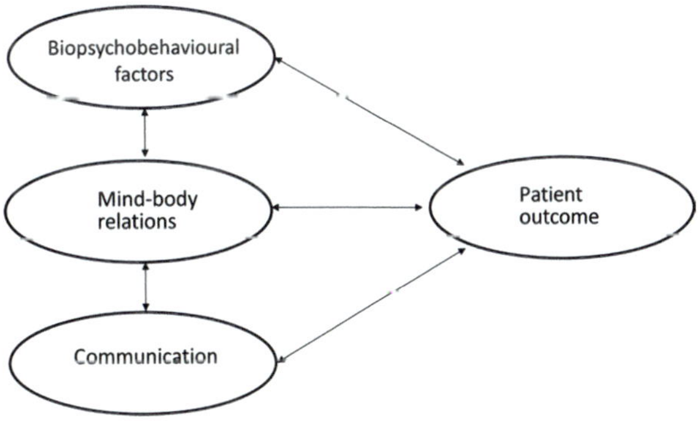

Figure 12.5. Understanding a patient's psychological state, social support systems, and adherence to rehabilitation protocols is crucial for successful recovery.

Source: https://media.springernature.com/full/springer-static/image/art%3A10.1057%2Fs41599-025-04359-0/MediaObjects/41599_2025_4359_Fig1_HTML.png.

12.2.1. Pre-Rehabilitation Assessment

The pre-rehabilitation assessment is a critical stage in post-surgical rehabilitation since it forms the basis for individualized intervention strategies. During this phase, professionals meticulously determine the patient's medical history, current physical state, functional capacity, and psychosocial factors that will influence healing. This comprehensive assessment equips healthcare professionals with the data necessary to determine specific rehabilitation needs and create personal goals that match the patient's needs and overall treatment. By addressing such factors early on, practitioners are able to optimize recovery times and optimize patient outcomes generally, as interventions are more intensely targeted and effective. Furthermore, a thorough understanding of the individual factors of each patient guides the selection of effective therapeutic modalities, so that rehabilitation is more tailored following surgery. A thorough pre-rehabilitation assessment is therefore an overall determinant in the success of the rehabilitation process. In addition, the pre-rehabilitation assessment plays a primary role in enabling open communication between healthcare staff and patients. It is not just about gaining clinical information but also developing a platform in which patients are encouraged to talk about their hopes and concerns relating to their rehabilitation. With collaboration, a feeling of ownership and accountability for the process of rehabilitation for the patients exists. By involving patients in conversations regarding their evaluation results and rehabilitation options, practitioners can enhance patient compliance with prescribed therapeutic interventions. Moreover, when patients are educated and actively participate in making decisions regarding their care, they are more likely to adhere to their rehabilitation plans, thereby improving rates of compliance and achieving maximum outcomes. Pre-rehabilitation evaluation is thus an active tool for enhancing communication and collaboration in the rehabilitation process. Clinical protocol and guideline consideration remain ongoing throughout the pre-rehabilitation assessment process so that interventions are evidence-driven and consistent with the latest research. The inclusion of established guidelines allows healthcare practitioners to make informed choices that are specific to a patient's condition and recovery process. As guided by relevant literature, a standardized pre-rehabilitation assessment procedure enables the identification of potential areas of healing resistance and determines the selection of guided therapies that address these concerns (Kuriakose & Xiao, 2020). Moreover, adherence to guidelines ensures consistency in service delivery and facilitates the use of standardized instruments for quantifying patient progress. This step-by-step process not only enhances the standard of rehabilitation but also supports the broader goal of enhancing clinical practice and outcomes (Habib et al., 2015). By putting evidence-based methods first during the pre-rehabilitation assessment, practitioners can facilitate better and more efficient streams of post-surgical recovery for patients.

12.2.2. Ongoing Evaluation Techniques

Routine evaluation techniques are the cornerstone of postoperative rehabilitation, allowing for tailored recovery for patients. These techniques encompass a variety of assessment instruments and techniques that enable healthcare practitioners to monitor the progress of patients with great care. Routine evaluations not only identify improvements in the physical dimension but also indicate potential setbacks, allowing intervention at the earliest moment. Functional assessments, for instance, such as range of motion and strength tests, provide quantifiable data to direct rehabilitation planning. Through these techniques, therapists can modify exercise regimens based on the patient's response, maintaining a care dynamic and adaptable. Responsiveness provides a healing climate that is conducive to optimal recovery, and it emphasizes the necessity of ongoing monitoring of patient status along the path of rehabilitation. In addition to physical examination, ongoing assessment strategies incorporate patient-reported measures that inform the subjective aspect of recovery. These tests, which may include pain level, emotional function, and quality-of-life questionnaires, give a better sense of the recovery process from the patient's perspective. Patient involvement with rehabilitation is key, as it enhances compliance and motivation in adherence to recommended interventions. Furthermore, research has determined that comprehensive assessment techniques can enhance the effectiveness of treatment overall, leading to enhanced long-term outcomes. Through the interaction of objective and subjective assessments, clinicians can have a fuller understanding of the condition of the patient's rehabilitation, encouraging collaborative decision-making essential to quality care. Moreover, ongoing evaluation procedures must be in line with standards established to ensure interventions are evidence-based and ethical.

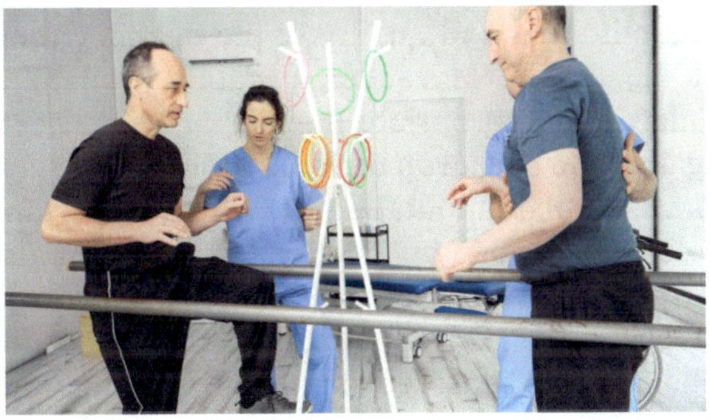

Figure 12.6. Ongoing evaluation techniques are fundamental in post-surgical rehabilitation, facilitating a tailored approach to patient recovery.

Source: https://motion-pt.com/wp-content/uploads/2024/04/Post-Surgical-Rehabilitation-3-1024x576.jpg.

For example, guidelines provided in modern clinical research highlight the integration of technology advancements in quantifying patient improvement. Through distance monitoring equipment and telehealth technology, therapists are now able to have constant interaction and assessment even in remote areas. These types of technologies allow for real-time modifications of care plans based on real-time feedback. In addition, healthcare professionals are also reminded to be cognizant of evolving guidelines and public health guidelines that can impact post-surgical rehabilitation regimes. This compliance with pre-established protocols not only facilitates the consistency of continuous evaluations but also consolidates the aggregate quality of care provided to patients throughout the process of their recovery (Kirchhof et al., 2016; Kuriakose & Xiao, 2020) (Figure 12.6).

12.2.3. Outcome Measurement Tools

The application of outcome measure tools is essential in surgical rehabilitation since they provide essential measures for evaluating recovery in patients. Through the measurement of various dimensions of functional performance and patient change, the tools enable clinicians to establish the effectiveness of rehabilitation interventions. Standardized scales and tools are typical measurements used to evaluate parameters like mobility, pain, and physical function in general.

Clinicians usually avail themselves of a wide array of options, thus reflecting considerable variation in the tools used in these measurements. The selection process is not necessarily systematic, however, resulting in variation of tools within different rehabilitation settings. Thus, the lack of common protocols can result in using non-standard measures that have no potential to actually assess patient outcomes, and it may be challenging to establish driving forces for optimizing rehabilitation strategies and recovery pathways for post-operative patients (Marek et al., 2023). Standard measurement tools of outcomes also find their significance in research settings, which helps develop evidence-based practice in rehabilitation. These tools facilitate systematic measurement of treatment effect, enabling researchers to aggregate and synthesize data from multiple studies. Results are synthesized at the center of establishing comprehensive rehabilitation protocols that can be applied in diverse clinical environments. Increased reliance on quantitative measures makes it possible to better understand the effectiveness of rehabilitation, facilitating better clinical decision-making and person-centered patient care practices. In addition, technological and methodological improvements also trigger the creation of new measurement tools that are further elevating the degree of objectivity as well as test validity. Together with innovations in artificial intelligence and customized measuring devices, rehabilitation professionals are better equipped to examine outcomes since they increasingly utilize measurements that have proven efficacious in orthopedic and neurological conditions (Marek et al., 2023). The successful incorporation of outcome measurement tools into postoperative rehabilitation regimes also mirrors more general standards and guidelines for healthcare. Healthcare professionals are continually urged to make use of such tools in order to enhance their clinical judgment and decision-making. Conformity with instituted guidelines not only aids in the objective evaluation of patient benefit but also ensures compliance with regimes optimized for maximal recovery results. Yet clinicians should bear in mind special patient needs and circumstances when employing these guidelines. Flexibility that is part of choosing proper measurement tools should be balanced with the need to follow evidence-based practice. The need for maintaining the rigor of outcomes assessment while providing individualized care necessitates that rehabilitation processes effectively functioning in patients post-surgery are stimulated.

12.3. Role of Healthcare Professionals

In the realm of post-operative rehabilitation, medical providers play a priceless part in recovery as well as in improving patient outcomes. Their care extends beyond routine follow-ups; they are active members of a multidisciplinary team that involves physical therapists, occupational therapists, and nurses, each possessing specialized skills contributing to the rehabilitation process. This synergy is critical, particularly in complex conditions such as recovery from a stroke, where studies indicate early and repeated rehabilitation interventions have an important role in shaping the motor and cognitive impairments of a patient. With the convergence of several therapeutic modalities, healthcare professionals can tailor the rehabilitation program to target unique patient needs, thereby optimizing physical rehabilitation and quality of life overall (Hong et al., 2024). Moreover, rehabilitation in a timely and appropriate manner is emphasized against the backdrop of some procedures, such as transtibial amputation (TTA). An important role is played by medical professionals, particularly prosthetists, in the initial stage of post-surgical treatment and rehabilitation. Their expertise is determinative regarding the decisions on prosthetic fit and patient care on an ongoing basis. For instance, differences in incision methods—i.e., the Sagittal Flap vs. the Posterior Flap—may influence prosthetic fitting time and hence the functional outcomes of the patient. Utilizing advanced postoperative treatment methods and state-of-the-art prosthetic technology, healthcare providers can maximize recovery periods and simplify the process from operation to rehabilitation (Johannesson & Rusaw, 2024). In addition to clinical practice, medical workers must also play a vital role in addressing the psychological and emotional aspects of post-operative recovery. The majority of patients experience anxiety, depression, or confusion throughout the rehabilitation process, which may severely impede their recovery. With emotional support and counseling, medical workers help patients overcome such adversities and establish a positive rehabilitation environment. Moreover, communication skills are of utmost importance; the healthcare professional must make things clear concerning the rehabilitation process, deal with realistic expectations, and encourage patient participation in their recovery process. This comprehensive approach, combined with physical and emotional care, ultimately creates resilience and allows patients to regain their independence and quality of life following surgical intervention (Johannesson & Rusaw, 2024).

12.3.1. Physical Therapists

Physical therapists occupy a key role in the image of post-surgical rehabilitation as initiators of the healing process following surgical interventions. With their education in human movement and body mechanics, physical therapists are qualified to individually tailor rehabilitation programs for postoperative individuals according to their individual conditions. By assessing the patient's condition, physical therapists can implement strategies that promote healing, enhance mobility, and prevent complications such as stiffness and muscle atrophy. Not only does this customized treatment assist with improving function, but it boosts the patient's confidence level in their body's ability post-surgery, leading to increased active participation in their rehabilitation process. Hence, the work of the physical therapists is not mere teaching; they are key support systems during the physical and emotional challenges of recovery. It has been established that early intervention by physical therapists significantly enhances clinical outcomes for post-operative patients. For instance, research indicates that the early initiation of rehabilitation interventions has been associated with reduced post-intensive care syndrome (PICS) physical impairment among patients who underwent critical surgery and were later admitted to intensive care. Outcomes of a multicenter prospective observational study indicate that early intervention by physical therapists is successful in the first week following surgery. Utilizing tools such as the ICU mobility scale, progress can be monitored and adjustments to the rehabilitation program made as needed. The significant association between early rehabilitation therapy and lower rates of PICS physical impairment puts a focus on integrating physical therapy as part of standard postoperative practice, with a resultant improved long-term patient outcome (Oku et al., 2025). Apart from facilitating physical rehabilitation, physical therapists facilitate multidisciplinary care in healthcare settings, particularly intensive care units (ICUs).

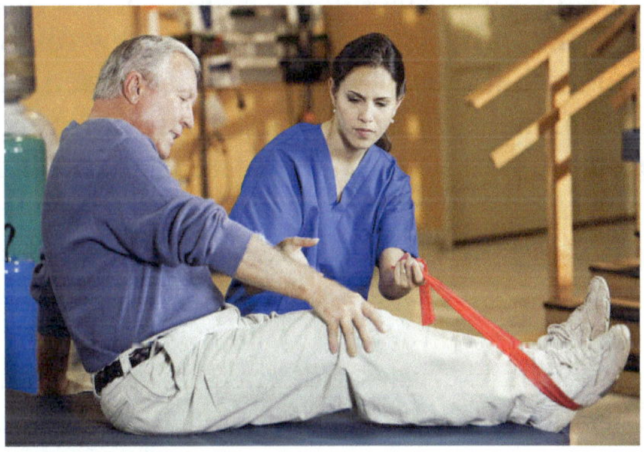

Figure 12.7. Physical therapists play a critical role in the landscape of post-surgical rehabilitation, acting as key facilitators in the recovery process following surgical interventions.

Source: https://www.nurseregistry.com/wp-content/uploads/2017/03/phyiscal-therapy-800.jpeg.

Their interventions ensure that patient care is collaborative and holistic in addressing the complicated needs of post-operative recovery patients. Research conducted in Saudi Arabian ICUs indicates the various roles of physical therapists that include respiratory care, mobilization at an early stage, and rehabilitation processes. With coordination with other healthcare professionals, physical therapists become key decision-making colleagues in patient outcome determination. Coordination not only improves the quality of care and patient satisfaction but also overall satisfaction. Ultimately, with healthcare systems in greater appreciation of the vital role physical therapists have to offer in post-surgical recovery, integration into practice becomes a necessity for optimal recovery and complication avoidance (Alokayli & Alkhaldi, 2024) (Figure 12.7).

12.3.2. Occupational Therapists

Occupational therapists are also crucial during post-operative rehabilitation since they provide patients with the necessary tools and skills to regain their functional capacities and self-sufficiency after surgery. The primary role of occupational therapy is to facilitate patients to perform meaningful daily activities, which may be compromised by pain, decreased mobility, or physical disabilities following surgery. By evaluating the unique needs and goals of each patient, occupational therapists establish individualized therapy programs involving therapeutic exercises, adaptive strategies, and environmental modifications. Such interventions not only benefit physical rehabilitation but also psychological well-being, encouraging patients to engage in activities critical to overall quality of life. In post-surgical rehabilitation, teamwork among healthcare practitioners cannot be stressed enough. Occupational therapists work closely with surgeons, physical therapists, and nursing staff to offer a comprehensive approach to patient care, rehabilitation of a physical as well as psychosocial nature. For instance, the installation of an effective program of rehabilitation, as suggested by expansive guidelines, involves the coordination of providers to offer the optimal level of education and support in recovery to patients. This interdisciplinary approach is important in managing possible complications and optimizing overall outcomes for patients, as reported in Ambrosetti et al. (2020). Effective communication and collaboration facilitate better management of expectations and improved patient compliance with the rehabilitation processes. To further optimize the effectiveness of post-surgical rehabilitation, occupational therapists apply evidence-based methods and continuously adapt their practices based on recent research findings. Such commitment to staying current with rehabilitation science advances is critical in the act of developing interventions for diverse patient populations, including those following orthopedic and cardiovascular surgery, and neurological conditions. The demand for properly planned rehabilitation programs can be highlighted on the basis of recommendations such as the European Stroke Action Plan, which emphasizes the requirement of organized care for various facets of recovery, as outlined in Norrving et al. (2018). These strategic methodologies not only improve recovery pathways but also help ensure that patients are empowered with the skills necessary to move within their spaces with ease, hence maintaining long-term success in their rehabilitative processes.

12.3.3. Physicians and Surgeons

The role of surgeons and doctors is the core of the healthcare situation, particularly as it relates to post-operative rehabilitation. These healthcare professionals are charged with diagnosing, treating, and ultimately managing patients pre- and post-surgical procedures. Their field of interest not only encompasses the surgeries themselves but also involves understanding the overall care that is required by patients during the recovery process. This general practice is of critical significance since the success of surgery often relies on successful techniques of rehabilitation that need to be either directly given or coordinated with other medical professionals by doctors and surgeons. What they lay is the foundation for how patients are going to deal with their recovery process, and therefore their role is critical not only to give back function but to improve the general quality of life after surgery (Bonica, 2017). In addition to their direct roles in surgery, physicians and surgeons play an equally important role in educating patients about the rehabilitation process. With proper communication and individualized guidance, they can set proper expectations of recovery duration and rehabilitation milestones. The educational component is instrumental in empowering patients and making them more involved in the rehabilitation process. It ensures compliance with advised rehabilitation protocols, which in turn can have a significant impact on recovery. Also, physicians and surgeons usually collaborate with physical therapists and rehabilitation physicians to organize lengthy postoperative rehabilitation in a multidisciplinary way, ensuring the patient's requirements are met with a multidisciplinary approach. Combined activity such as this acknowledges team effort as a means to achieve quality results after surgery (Thierry et al., 2013). Further, physicians and surgeons' consultations with their patients during rehabilitation extend beyond clinical governance. It encompasses emotional support and reinforcement, which are crucial in maintaining patient motivation and morale. After surgery, patients can suffer from physical impairment and psychological distress, and the availability of a sensitive healthcare provider can make a significant contribution towards the recovery process. Psychological resilience is particularly crucial in rehabilitation settings so that successful recovery may be ensured. Physicians and surgeons, therefore, must not only work on physical healing but also work on their patients' emotional well-being, ensuring a conducive environment for proper recovery. Therefore, their multifaceted role during post-surgical recovery is crucial in the building of full health and recovery (Bonica, 2017) (Figure 12.8).

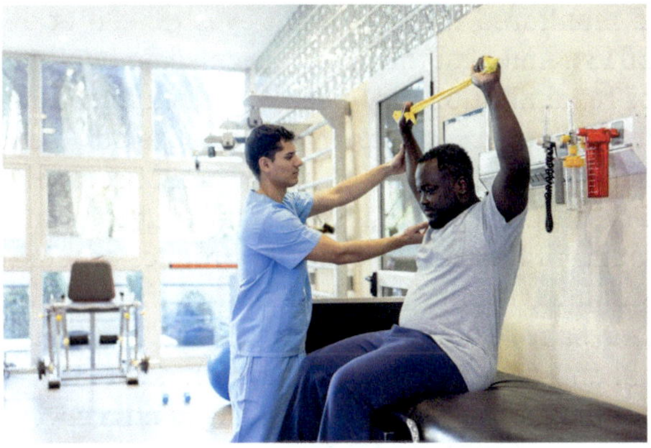

Figure 12.8. The role of physicians and surgeons is pivotal in the landscape of healthcare, particularly in relation to post-surgical rehabilitation.

Source: https://www.woosterhospital.org/wp-content/uploads/sites/229/2024/09/post-surgical_rehabilitation_blog-img.jpg.

12.4. Rehabilitation Techniques and Modalities

One of the essential elements of post-surgical rehabilitation is to use various techniques and modalities of rehabilitation to enable recovery. Of the techniques, the role of physical therapy is central, employing specific exercise regimes to optimize mobility and strength. Physical therapy is generally supported by the application of manual techniques, some of which may involve joint manipulation and soft tissue mobilization. These therapies focus on the correction of particular impairments following surgery and allow patients to regain functional movement patterns once again. With a multidisciplinary strategy, particularly in conditions like inguinal disruption, the foundation is established for better recuperation. Specialists recommend treatment onset with conservative therapy in the form of targeted physiotherapy such that symptoms are managed effectively and progress is monitored under vigilant eyes (Sheen et al., 2013). Amongst the most recognized modalities of rehabilitation, dry needling is employed for its high success rate in musculoskeletal pain management as well as promotion of recovery. Dry needling influences certain trigger points found in muscles in order to produce a neural stimulus, facilitating relaxation of the muscles and pain reduction. The advantage is not just enhancement of the range of motion but muscle oxygenation as well, thus enabling rapid recovery from surgery. Even as the use of dry needling has increased in popularity, incorporating dry needling into postoperative rehabilitation is a developing area of study, where findings indicate that the combination of dry needling with other therapies can provide even greater benefits. Such multi-modal treatment approaches increase the need for the individualization of rehabilitation protocols to the particular needs of the patient and synergy of treatment modalities (Kotze et al., 2019). Finally, technology incorporation into practice has revolutionized post-surgical recovery. Modalities like electrical stimulation, biofeedback, and ultrasound therapy have become increasingly fashionable as they have been shown to accelerate healing as well as enhance functional outcomes. These technologies not only assist in reducing pain but also permit muscle activation under a controlled environment, thereby accelerating recovery. Evidence does indicate that the incorporation of such innovative modalities with the more traditional rehabilitation regimes can improve patient outcomes. As technology evolves, the integration of new rehabilitation modalities becomes increasingly significant in the development of effective, evidence-based rehabilitation interventions. Thus, the establishment of an integrated and individualized rehabilitation protocol becomes essential in providing patients' recovery processes while optimizing their physical function (Sheen et al., 2013).

12.4.1. Manual Therapy

Manual therapy has emerged as a key ingredient of post-surgical rehabilitation due to its plethora of advantages. Manual therapy involves hands-on treatment modalities such as mobilization, manipulation, and soft tissue techniques for pain relief and function improvement. It proves to be of special value in the treatment of soft tissue damage and musculoskeletal pain that are secondary to surgery. By decreasing muscle tension and joint stiffness, manual therapy can potentially enable a greater range of motion and aid the body in natural healing processes. Furthermore, there is evidence to suggest that manual therapy could complement physical therapy and be an effective adjunctive treatment (Joglar et al., 2023). This systemic approach is not merely interested in the body's physical rehabilitation but also in the psychological healing since decreased anxiety and good mood have been observed in patients following sessions of therapy. Besides its physical application, manual therapy is also important in preventing post-surgery complications. Adhesions and scarring inside the body may result from surgery, and if handled improperly, they can lead to a decline in movement and cause chronic pain. Manual therapy treatments, administered during the rehabilitation process, can effectively eliminate these complications by promoting tissue mobility and facilitating the circulation of blood. This not only enhances pain reduction but also contributes significantly to enhancing overall recovery rates (Burton et al., 2021). The touch-based concept of manual therapy can significantly empower patients as it allows them to have an active role in their own rehabilitation process. This empowerment can help instill a sense of agency, which is paramount to mental health and adherence to rehabilitation regimens. Additionally, the integration of manual therapy into postoperative rehabilitation regimens is concordant with a patient-centered philosophy. Individualized care plans that consider each patient's unique needs have the potential to enhance satisfaction and adherence to treatment. This individualization is vital in addressing specific concerns such as degrees of pain, movement limitations, and previous medical conditions. Manual skills therapists can test and adapt their techniques based on direct patient feedback, thereby optimizing rehabilitation experiences. Evidence also continues to show the effectiveness of such personalized treatment, calling its potential to improve functional outcomes and reduce rehabilitation time (Joglar et al., 2023). Finally, as medicine becomes more advanced, the focus on incorporating manual therapy in postoperative rehabilitation is an expansion of the concept of total care to include a better physical and emotional recovery path (Figure 12.9).

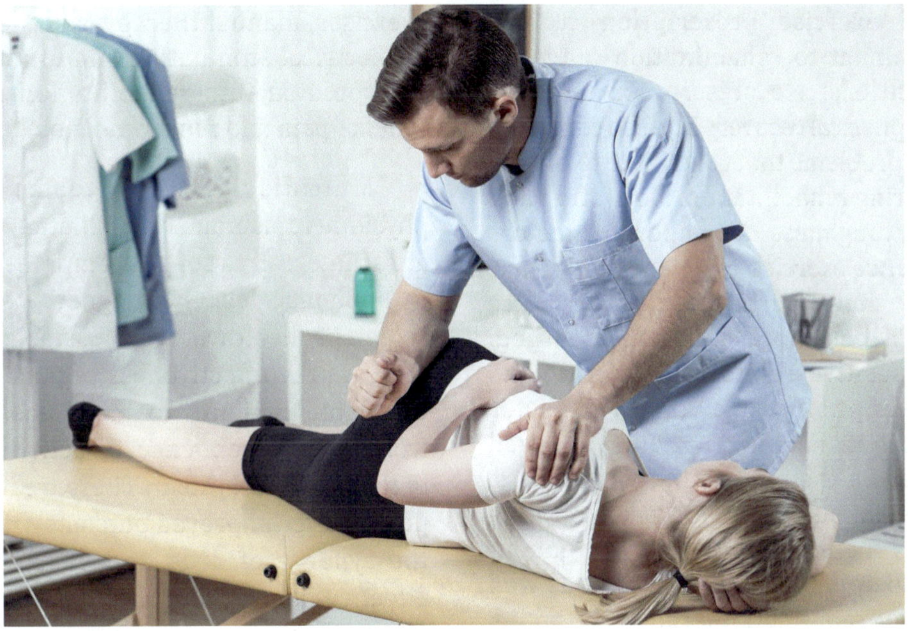

Figure 12.9. Manual therapy encompasses hands-on techniques such as mobilization, manipulation, and soft tissue techniques aimed at alleviating pain and restoring function.

Source: https://physiozonebd.com/wp-content/uploads/2024/08/manual-therapy.jpg.

12.4.2. Exercise Prescription

An effective exercise prescription is an integral component of rehabilitation after surgery, designed to facilitate recovery and restore functional independence. An effort that involves an individualized method taking into account the patient's specific clinical conditions, surgical history, and personal goals, for instance, patients of cardiovascular surgery recover significantly better with exercise regimens geared towards enhancing cardiovascular fitness, strength, and flexibility. Research allows clinicians to develop precise exercise regimens that improve physiology with low risks of complications. Against this backdrop, the work of experts like Yasunori Suematsu demonstrates the ever-increasing yearning to develop exercise prescriptions further by incorporating non-invasive estimates of exercise intensity and thereby enabling effective patient rehabilitation (Suematsu, 2025). Moreover, the strategic utilization of mild aerobic exercise is greatly essential in rehabilitation, particularly in patients with lower limb injuries. Lower limb injuries may result in extreme disability in mobility and quality of life when left untacked. Mild aerobic exercises such as walking and cycling are effective in the enhancement of blood flow and muscle strength and therefore in hastening the process of healing. It has been discovered that aquatic exercise can be particularly beneficial through the hydrodynamic characteristics, which minimize strain but maximize muscle function (Akhoondian, 2025). Aquatic exercise enables patients to increase range of motion and strength without exacerbating injury, demonstrating how optimal exercise prescription can be highly determinant to rehabilitation outcome. A personalized exercise prescription not only addresses the physical recovery but also considers psychological problems that contribute to overall well-being during rehabilitation. Motivation and psychological toughness are important factors that can influence exercise regimen compliance. Clinicians are therefore inclined to introduce strategies of a behavioral kind, such as goal setting and positive reinforcement, into the exercise prescription framework. This.factor is also critical in keeping patients engaged and stimulated in their rehabilitation process. Future studies should then focus on refining such protocols of exercise to suit varying patient populations, to optimize physical effects as well as psychosocial remission, thereby reinforcing the broader rationale for individualized exercise prescription for postoperative rehabilitation.

12.4.3. Modalities for Pain Management

Effective pain management is a crucial part of post-surgical rehabilitation, with both healing phases and patient satisfaction implications. Options for managing post-surgical pain range from pharmacologic interventions to physical therapies and adjuvant techniques. The pharmacologic options are typically non-steroidal anti-inflammatory agents (NSAIDs), narcotics, and adjuvant medications for nerve pain relief. Application of a multimodal analgesia strategy—with drugs of multiple mechanisms—has the potential to enhance pain relief and possibly minimize the side effects of individual agents. The strategy recognizes that postoperative pain can be mediated through more than one mechanism, thus necessitating an individualized strategy to optimize benefits to patients and promote early mobilization, which is highly desirable in rehabilitation. In addition to pharmacological measures, physical therapies are also important in bringing relief from pain during post-surgery recovery. Therapeutic exercises, manual therapy, and modalities such as electrical stimulation and ultrasound can be incorporated into rehabilitation protocols for relief of pain and functional mobility restoration.

Multidisciplinary teams, including physiotherapists and rehabilitation professionals, are an integral part of this comprehensive process. By applying specially designed physical therapy regimens, healthcare professionals are able to increase the effectiveness of pain management to enable patients to more easily transition from drug dependence to active management of their own treatment. These treatments have a potential for improved outcomes, demonstrating the synergy of drug and physical therapy in effective control of post-operative pain. Other treatments may also warrant consideration as adjuncts to standard pain management. Mechanisms such as acupuncture, massage therapy, and cognitive behavior therapy are more widely recognized for their ability to enhance standard measures in reducing pain perception and facilitating emotional adjustment during recuperation. Consensus has focused on the merit of a holistic treatment incorporating these modalities, particularly in the case of chronic pain sufferers. The multidisciplinary strategy—combining medical and therapeutic interventions—is an appreciation that pain is a complex phenomenon requiring multifaceted management regimes. Lastly, as the science of pain management evolves further, ongoing research and consensus among practitioners, such as in studies such as those documented in Sheen et al. (2013), will increasingly inform techniques and determine the optimal approaches to the treatment of patients through post-surgical recovery (Figure 12.10).

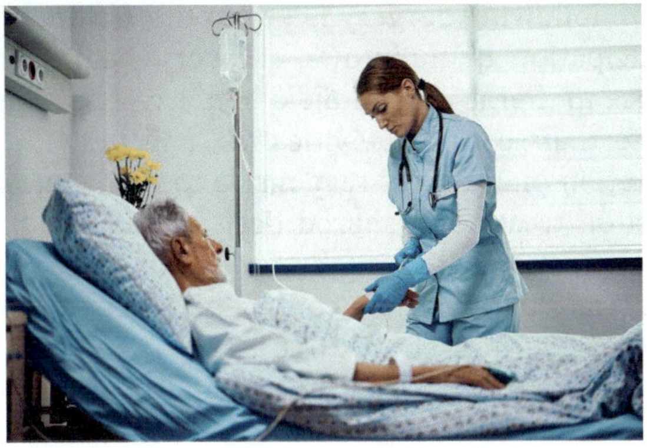

Figure 12.10. Effective pain management is a crucial component of post-surgical rehabilitation, influencing recovery times and overall patient satisfaction.

Source: https://sukinohealthcare.com/wp-content/uploads/2023/06/Post-operative-cares.jpg.

12.5. Patient Education and Engagement

Effective patient education and communication are critical components of postoperative rehabilitation, closing the intervention from clinical instruction to patient understanding. Involvement of the patient in the rehabilitation process enhances compliance with rehabilitation programs, as well as autonomy, which is key to optimal outcomes. Comprehensive education involves a clear explanation of the procedure, the course of recovery, and the specific rehabilitation program to be followed. According to current guidelines, emphasizing the role of engaging the patient in treatment decisions based on social determinants of health is crucial in optimizing recovery. This joint decision-making can truly empower the patient to become better satisfied and compliant with ordered regimens. Without this educational foundation, patients can struggle to understand their role in recovery, compromising the effectiveness of their rehabilitation protocol and longer recovery periods. Moreover, the benefits of patient education are evidenced in the literature and show better physical and psychological outcomes throughout the recovery process. Informing patients with pertinent information regarding their condition and prognosis of recovery reduces tension and enhances rehabilitation exercise compliance. The use of detailed guidelines, such as those reported in the recent systematic reviews, lends support to adding structured educational interventions to rehabilitation programs. These treatments can include not only the medical rehabilitative elements, i.e., pain management and mobilization, but also emotional support channels. The 2023 AHA/ACC/ACCP/ASPC/NLA/PCNA Guideline emphasizes the importance of developing personalized education plans that resonate with patients' interests and daily habits, hence optimizing their engagement in rehabilitation activities (Virani et al., 2023).

In addition to promoting patient autonomy and emotional well-being, effective educational strategies can avoid repetitive post-surgery complications, such as elderly falls. Current evidence highlights that falls and their outcomes adversely impact functional independence and quality of life, particularly among high-risk populations. Heterogeneous recommendations have impeded knowledge of risk for falls, which may detract from total rehabilitation strategies (Montero-Odasso et al., 2022). By incorporating targeted patient education on fall prevention and putting it into practice in the recovery process, healthcare teams are in a better position to equip patients with the information and tools they require to move around safely. Consequently, incorporating these educational aspects not only enhances safety but also fosters a healthier recovery process. An integrated approach to patient education and engagement is thus key in achieving maximum post-surgical rehabilitation outcomes.

12.5.1. Importance of Patient Involvement

The integration of patient involvement in rehabilitation following surgery is key to the facilitation of optimal outcomes of recovery. With patient participation in their own recovery, healthcare professionals can enhance the level of patient adherence to therapy and build a better relationship. Patient-centered practice allows patients to articulate their own issues, desires, and individual preferences, hence formulating a customized rehabilitation plan that is responsive to their unique needs. As seen through the study of erectile dysfunction treatment, shared decision-making has been noted to be vital in enhancing treatment satisfaction and facilitating better health outcomes. Involved patients are likely to comply with post-surgical routines that contribute to successful rehabilitation and overall satisfaction with care received (Burnett et al., 2018).

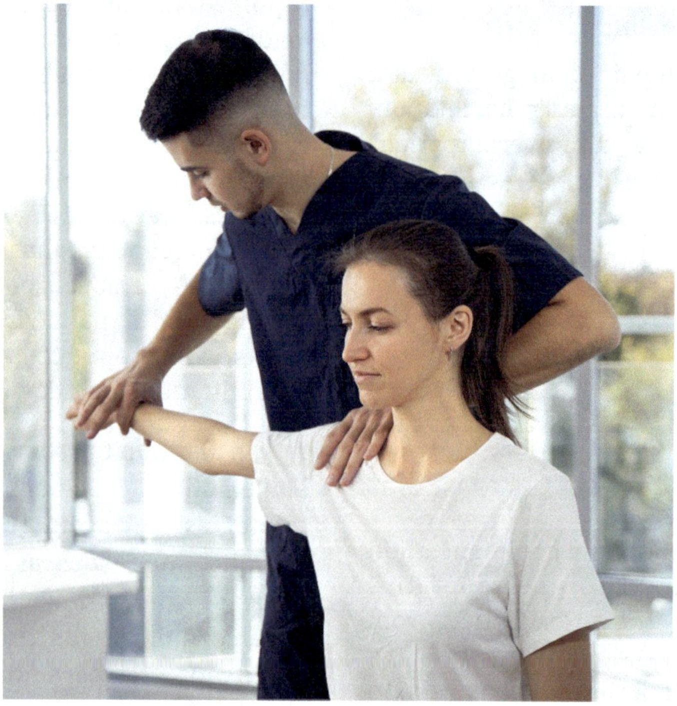

Figure 12.11. By actively engaging patients in their rehabilitation journey, healthcare professionals can enhance patient adherence to prescribed therapies and establish more meaningful relationships.

Source: https://www.southgatephysio.co.uk/wp-content/uploads/2023/10/medium-shot-woman-getting-help-scaled.jpg.

12.5.2. Strategies for Effective Communication

Successful communication becomes essential during the rehabilitation phase after surgery since it enhances patient understanding of the recovery process. Such an understanding is vital to encouraging patient involvement and following rehabilitation protocols. Proper communication starts with doctors who must deliver complex medical data in a way that is concise and comprehensible. By using simple language, images, and exhibits, health workers can facilitate easier comprehension, which raises the likelihood of patients adhering to ordered rehabilitation plans. Evidence shows that where patients have been educated on their rehabilitation timetables, they become more inclined to take ownership of their rehabilitation processes, hence, yielding better outcomes and reduced complications in their post-operative lives (Liang et al., 2020). In addition, a participating component of effective communication is the act of listening. Healthcare providers are to engage patients through setting them at ease to express their worries, questions, and sentiments regarding rehabilitation. This bidirectional dialogue not only establishes trust but also allows providers to tailor rehabilitation plans to address unique patient needs. If patients are listened to and heard, they are likely to have fewer worries and higher motivation throughout the healing process. Moreover, engaging patients actively in planning their treatment leads them to articulate their own expectations and goals. This collaboration ultimately maximizes the success of the rehabilitation process, leading to improved satisfaction and results for healthcare professionals and patients alike (Cardoso et al., 2018). Last but not least, follow-up communication is essential in post-surgical rehabilitation. Regular follow-ups through scheduled visits, calls, or digital means are used to remind patients of details discussed during initial consultations and monitor their progress. Follow-up provides an opportunity to discuss challenges patients face in adhering to their rehabilitation timetables, allowing providers to make necessary adjustments accordingly. This open communication does not merely promote accountability but also guarantees that patients are assured of receiving their care actively. The use of technology, such as patient portals and telehealth visits, can enhance accessibility and responsiveness between visits, making for a stronger support system during the recovery phase. This efficient means of communication ensures a smoother recovery process from surgery to rehabilitation and ultimately contributes to improved patient outcomes as well as general satisfaction with the recovery process (Liang et al., 2020).

12.5.3. Resources for Patient Education

Successful patient education is an essential element of post-surgical rehabilitation, enabling patients to understand their recovery processes and actively engage in their care. Education materials for patients typically include a range of materials, including leaflets, educational films, and computer systems that provide rehabilitation advice. Tailored education can help to ensure optimal compliance in a patient's adherence to prescribed exercises for rehabilitation and health practice. This empowerment translates to improved treatment outcomes and a strengthened therapeutic relationship between patients and healthcare professionals. With healthcare systems in the world focusing more on patient-centered interventions, the incorporation of individualized education materials is not merely beneficial but imperative to improve the rehabilitation process after surgery. These materials serve as scaffolding for patients to build their knowledge and confidence in the post-surgical period. Apart from standard learning materials, internet-based resources are playing an increasingly important role in post-surgical rehabilitation. Virtual networks and mobile applications offer easy access for patients to receive ongoing education and support, particularly where onsite attendance may be limited. This is boosted by a growing literature that distinguishes the efficacy of digital interventions in health settings. For instance, physiotherapists have reported effective application of virtual training programs for people who are being rehabilitated after surgery, as seen from the e-survey that indicates global practice in terms of pediatric ataxia rehabilitation following posterior fossa tumor surgery (Hartley et al., 2019). Such content can include interactive tutorials, exercise diaries, and discussion forums for patient interaction, all combining to form an overall support network during recovery. In addition, it is also the responsibility of healthcare practitioners to apply these learning materials efficiently. By evaluating the patient's individual learning needs and styles, clinical professionals can adapt learning materials for better understanding and retention. This not only responds to the diversity in learning styles among patient populations but also takes into consideration the psychosocial and emotional issues encountered by patients after surgery. Education must also entail the education of the participants regarding the possible hindrances to rehabilitation, such as reduced access to physiotherapy upon discharge, as perceived through concerns raised in existing research (Hartley et al., 2019). Through deliberate focus on the delivery of appropriate resources in collaboration with the participants, healthcare workers can promote comprehension and adherence to rehabilitation regimens, leading to improved health outcomes during the post-operative period (Figure 12.12).

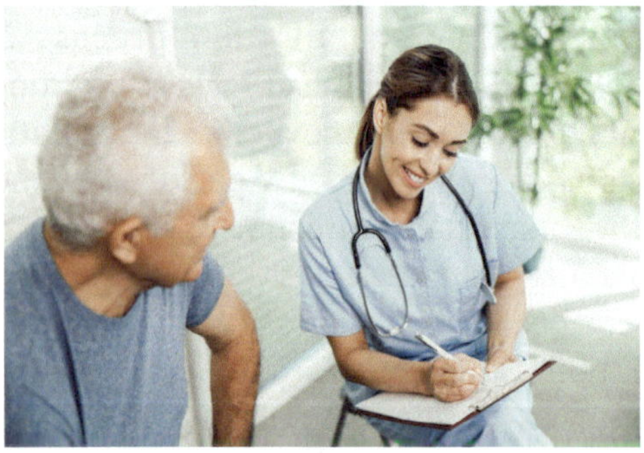

Figure 12.12. Effective patient education is pivotal in post-surgical rehabilitation, supporting patients understanding of their recovery processes and enabling active participation in their care.

Source: https://aihcp.net/main/wp-content/uploads/2024/02/Depositphotos_499564196_S.jpg.

12.6. Psychological Aspects of Rehabilitation

Psychological rehabilitation factors also play a pivotal role in the overall process of recovery following surgery. The patient can undergo profound psychological transformation as he or she adapts to the outcomes of surgery, from a span of discontent to permanent alterations of bodily functions. The emotional after-storm that follows could also manifest itself as anxiety, depression, or even post-traumatic stress disorder, hindering the individual from an active engagement in the rehabilitation program. These psychological challenges must be addressed, as mental health is a key factor in the outcomes of physical rehabilitation. By establishing a positive mental status, healthcare professionals can improve motivation and compliance with rehabilitation treatments and protocols, thereby supporting a more totalistic recovery process. Additionally, the incorporation of psychological care into rehabilitation treatment has been observed to result in better outcomes. Counseling, psychotherapy, and group therapy sessions may provide patients with useful coping strategies to endure the emotional consequences of surgery. Research indicates that psychological support results in higher attendance in their rehab program and less pain experience and more rapid functional restoration (Kuriakose & Xiao, 2020). Moreover, fostering a patient's social support group—family, friends, and caregivers—can cultivate a stronger foundation for psychological resilience. This holistic model not only addresses short-term psychological needs but also the basis of long-term mental health, with implications for the success of interventions during post-surgical recovery. Finally, understanding the interplay between psychological and physical mechanisms of recovery is essential for practitioners providing post-surgical rehabilitation. It becomes apparent that each patient's psychological experience is unique and is shaped by many factors, such as personal history, coping, and the character of the surgical process itself. Stroke patients, for instance, might have distinct psychological issues requiring tailored interventions (Pelliccia et al., 2020). Following this, a balanced approach that unites psychological testing and body rehabilitation methods can optimize recovery outcomes. In the end, placing greater emphasis on psychological factors in postoperative rehabilitation not only encourages the overall health of the patient but also reaffirms the fundamental relationship between mind and body during recuperation.

12.6.1. Coping with Post-Surgical Pain

Post-operative pain management is a multifaceted issue that has a direct impact on the rehabilitation process of patients. The nature of the operation, patient tolerance to pain, and psychological problems all contribute to pain experience after surgery. Worth noting is the reality that psychological aspects of anxiety and depression have a critical bearing on the perception and management of patient pain. Evidence indicates that those patients who arrive at surgery with high levels of pre-operative anxiety are more likely to have high levels of post-operative pain and anxiety, showing a direct relationship between psychological status and pain control. Therefore, knowledge of these psychological factors is the most critical consideration for health professionals to develop effective pain management care that targets physical as well as emotional support throughout recovery. In addition to this, post-operative pain can hinder not only a patient's physical recovery but also their psyche. With acute pain, the majority of patients suffer from increased levels of depression and anxiety, which further exacerbate their pain. This creates a vicious circle wherein unchecked pain fosters mental distress, which makes recovery all the more difficult. Of note, resolution of these psychosocial elements is necessary for effective post-surgical treatment. An integrative approach that incorporates both pain management modalities and psychosocial management can help facilitate an integrated recovery process. Evidence exists to support such care includes improving rehabilitative outcomes, enabling patients to regain normal functionality sooner (Mafo Degge et al., 2017). Finally, issues faced by the individuals managing postoperative pain must be mitigated through comprehensive care measures. Healthcare systems have to prioritize the development of standardized packages of treatment that include both pain management and psychological support. It is essential to do this in an effort to address the complex impact of pain on patients' lives, which may extend beyond the body (Mafo Degge et al., 2017). Besides, ongoing education of healthcare providers on the complex interaction between emotional and bodily aspects of pain is key. As continued research sheds light on the correlation between these dimensions, improved care processes are likely to be developed, resulting in improved patient outcomes and an enhanced rehabilitative experience following surgery (Figure 12.13).

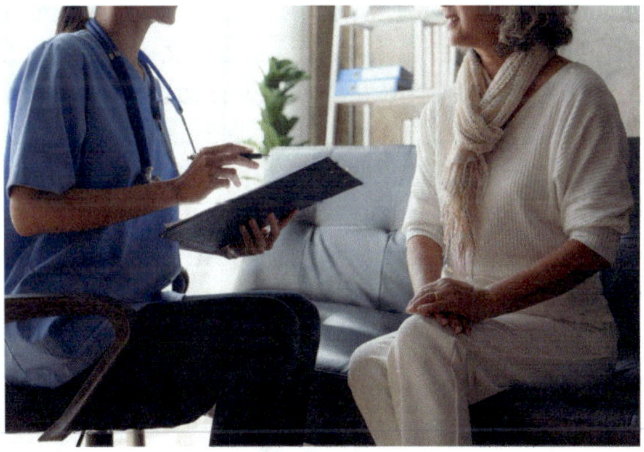

Figure 12.13. Coping with post-surgical pain is a multifaceted challenge that significantly impacts the rehabilitation process for patients.

Source: https://aihcp.net/main/wp-content/uploads/2024/02/Depositphotos_622838168_S-1-1.jpg.

12.6.2. Addressing Anxiety and Depression

Anxiety and depression are prevalent among post-surgical rehabilitation patients, influencing recovery trajectories and patient outcomes in major ways. Psychological and emotional consequences of surgery can heighten underlying issues or precipitate new ones, hence the importance of extensive psychological evaluation during rehabilitation. Following surgery, particularly when it involves trauma such as severe burns, the intricacy of emotional recovery must be managed with utmost delicacy. According to recent literature, the psychological impact of such injuries can lead to a higher risk of anxiety and depression, which require immediate and ongoing psychological care across the rehabilitation continuum. Healing from such concerns of mental well-being not only adds to overall well-being but also augments patient engagement and compliance with rehabilitation protocols, thereby making the environment more supportive for physical healing. The role of health workers towards the detection and treatment of depression and anxiety in this case cannot be overstated. Effective rehabilitation requires clinicians not only to cater to patients' physical recuperation but also to ascertain their psychological status. For instance, studies have established that patients who view their disease as threatening and resort to passive coping strategies report increased rates of anxiety and depression, an indication of the need for targeted psychological therapies. By incorporating screening protocols, such as the Hospital Anxiety and Depression Scale (HADS), clinicians can identify vulnerable patients early in their rehabilitation program so that psychological support can be tailored to suit their individual needs. The preventative measures alleviate the emotional stresses felt by patients and improve rehabilitation outcomes, offering a holistic approach that treats body and mind equally. Also, collaborative models of care that bring in mental health specialists are essential in the management of the multifaceted problems surrounding post-surgical anxiety and depression. By incorporating a multidisciplinary model, healthcare groups can assess and manage the psychological dimensions of recovering from surgery more efficiently. Cognitive-behavioral therapy, psychoeducation, and coping skills training interventions have proven to be successful in reversing maladaptive coping skills and boosting resilience in rehabilitation patients. Additionally, repeated assessments of illness perception and its association with mental health—particularly among severely injured individuals—emphasize the importance of constant monitoring and treatment during the process of recovery from surgery. Such interventions are not only advantageous psychologically but also facilitate a smoother rehabilitation process transition, ultimately leading to better patient outcomes and quality of life as established in the literature (Kuiper et al., 2023; Merchant et al., 2025).

12.6.3. Building Motivation and Resilience

The rehabilitation process after surgery normally relies on the ability of the patients to create motivation and resilience. Rehabilitation requires more than the healing of the body; it requires a psychological acceptance of healing. Patients tend to struggle with emotional factors, for example, fear of pain or anxiety about their physical ability. These emotions can discourage them and require creating an environment that supports personal investment in the rehabilitation process. Adjusting rehabilitation protocols, not only to individual physical needs but also to psychological wellness, is an important motivational factor. Incorporating psychological support elements such as counseling or motivational interviewing can assist professionals in developing an attitude for recovery and resilience. It promotes not only compliance with rehabilitation procedures but also the formation of an active attitude by patients in striving to regain their health. Constructing resilience during post-surgical rehabilitation involves intentional interventions that prepare the patient to cope with setbacks. Resilience is the ability to recover from distress and to positively adapt to adversity. When individuals begin rehabilitation, setbacks such as reversals in progress or unexpected physical limitations have the potential to discourage them. Effective rehabilitation courses emphasize goal setting and incremental milestones en route, milestones that are being achieved and celebrated along the way. Each small success reaffirms a patient's faith in their ability to succeed and stimulates further motivation. Furthermore, self-awareness and mindfulness patients are more likely to recognize their emotional responses to set situations and hence have more control of their recovery process. By instilling an environment where resilience can be fostered, clinicians build more resilient patients to address the complexity of rehabilitation. Emerging technologies also play an important part in building motivation and resilience for post-surgery rehabilitation. The application of digital health tools, such as mobile health apps and telemedicine, is an emerging wave in the pattern of personalized medicine. These devices, as well as allowing remote tracking of rehabilitation progress, also allow for real-time feedback and patient education to further ensure compliance with recovery protocols. Moreover, the integration of human digital twins (HDT) in rehabilitation practices can offer a tailored representation of an individual's health status, real-time interfacing with their physiological and emotional conditions (Chen et al., 2023). Such advancements can help patients visualize their progress and sense the impact of their efforts, reinforcing intrinsic motivation. The integration of technology with treatment regimens strengthens an effective coping approach, leaving patients feeling more engaged in their rehabilitation process. Through the leverage of these technologies, post-operative rehabilitation then becomes an even more active and empowering experience for patients (Figure 12.14).

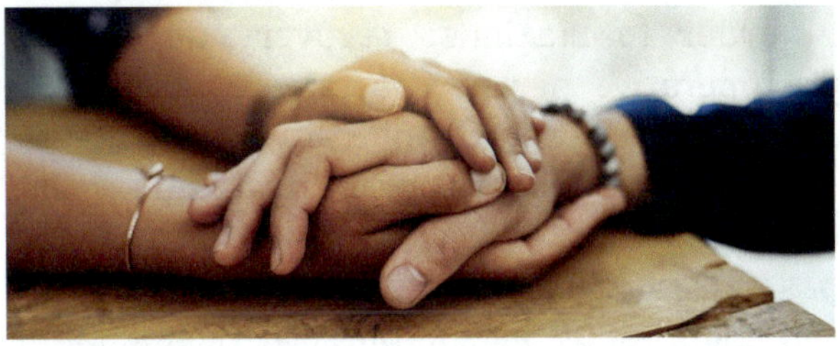

Figure 12.14. Patients frequently confront emotional challenges, such as fear of pain or anxiety about their physical capabilities.

Source: https://www.hopkinsmedicine.org/-/media/images/health/_-images-to-be-filed/anxiety_header_4/anxiety_header 4/how_to_help_someone_with_anxiety_hero/how_to_help_with_anxiety_hero_image.jpg?h=500&iar=0&mh=500&mw=1300&w=1290&hash=B588C6F6EF843A18868C1929391EE41B.

12.7. Challenges in Post-Surgical Rehabilitation

The rehabilitation process after surgery is riddled with numerous complications that involve the healing process and overall recovery results. One major impediment is the physiological reaction of patients to surgery, including different complications such as inflammation and metabolic dysregulation. For instance, patients undergoing severe trauma under surgery can undergo augmented inflammatory and hypermetabolic states, similar to post-burn patients. This physiological response could take a long time, and thus the rehabilitation process becomes complicated. Additionally, these patients can be required to have individually customized nutritional care in order to balance high energy requirements with metabolic complications, such as hyperglycemia. Individual differences in the response demand an individually tailored rehabilitation approach depending on the need to constantly evaluate and adjust the approach in order to maximize recovery during the postoperative period (Osborne et al., 2023). Another significant post-operative rehabilitation challenge is the psychological impact surgery has on patients. Emotions and psychiatric disturbances post-surgery, including anxiety and depression, can significantly impair physical rehabilitation results. Patients are disturbed by uncertainty about how their recovery will progress, leading to issues with motivation and rehabilitation participation. It is crucial to pay heed to the psychological problems because they can cause poor compliance with rehabilitation protocols and can hinder the progress. Incorporating psychological support in the shape of counseling or group therapy with physical rehabilitation can empower patients, enable resilience, and improve overall outcomes (Kuriakose & Xiao, 2020).

In addition, logistical limitations such as the availability of facilities for rehabilitation and also socioeconomic factors are likely to influence recovery following surgery. The majority of the patients are mostly discharged from the general acute care hospitals and sent back home, where there is possible limited access to specialized rehabilitation facilities. The geographic disparity has a likelihood of causing inequalities during recovery, particularly in the case of rural patients or economically marginalized patients. Besides that, the economic cost of ongoing therapy, coupled with potential poor health insurance coverage, leads to many patients refusing required rehabilitation. These system problems need to be solved in order to improve access to quality post-surgical rehabilitation services. By supporting policies that promote fair access and resources, healthcare systems can offer improved recovery results for all patients irrespective of their socioeconomic status or location (Osborne et al., 2023).

12.7.1. Common Barriers to Recovery

Recovery following surgical procedures can be significantly hindered by a number of impediments to care experienced by patients during the rehabilitation period. Of first concern is the lack of treatment protocols, which will lead to variability in the management of post-surgical conditions. For example, in Achilles tendon rupture (ATR), the lack of standard protocols leads to uncertainty among the caregivers regarding the best way to manage patients. This inadequacy not only affects the recovery process but also raises the cost to society due to prolonged rehabilitation and unsuccessful attempts at recovery. Enhancing the precision and concordance of treatment modalities is imperative to achieve the optimum level of patient recovery and rehabilitation process (Kuriakose & Xiao, 2020). Psychological factors also find a significant place in the process of recovery. Patients are likely to have difficulty with anxiety, depression, and fear of re-injury, which could decrease motivation and adherence to rehabilitation protocols. For instance, survivors of stroke primarily encounter psychological problems that prevent them from rehabilitation, thereby affecting their overall recovery. It is for this reason that mental health support should be included together with physical rehabilitation to provide an environment that is conducive to healing and recovery. Tackling these psychological barriers with proper counseling and care systems can ensure that patients overcome mental barriers, thereby encouraging them to undergo the recovery process (Kuriakose & Xiao, 2020). Lastly, the socioeconomic status of patients must also be taken into consideration as a pertinent barrier in the recovery process. Individuals from lower socioeconomic status typically face limitations in accessing healthcare facilities, consequently developing hesitations in rehabilitation processes. Regular constraints, such as lack of transportation, financial issues, and insufficient time after work obligations, can exclude timely rehabilitation and follow-up treatment. This limitation can lead to disproportionate recovery results, particularly for those undergoing rehabilitation after major surgery. Integration of the support networks and resources of the community is essential in breaking these barriers, providing all patients with equal access to the rehabilitation interventions needed for successful recuperation (Dams et al., 2019) (Figure 12.15).

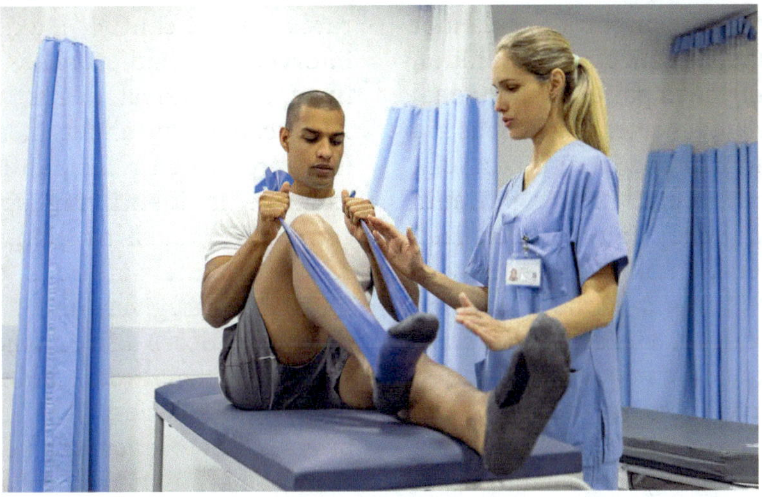

Figure 12.15. Recovery following surgical procedures can be significantly hindered by various barriers that patients face during the rehabilitation process.

Source: https://wp02-media.cdn.ihealthspot.com/wp-content/uploads/sites/393/2024/03/ACL-Surgery-Rehabilitation.jpg.webp.

12.7.2. Managing Complications

Rehabilitation after surgery is a critical phase in the healing process, which not only enhances the functional abilities of patients but also reverses complications due to surgery. Management of complications needs a coordinated effort through the implementation of physiotherapy, education, and individualized care plans. Complications like pain, limited mobility, and psychological distress commonly encountered by patients tend to complicate their rehabilitation goals. A strategic management system has the capacity to identify potential post-surgical complications at an early stage, precluding prolonged hospital stays and readmission. For instance, rehabilitation teams are able to assess and adjust treatment plans based on the shifting needs of patients at a dynamic level, establishing the environment which ensures recovery is the ultimate priority and general quality of life during the post-surgical period is even higher. Management of specific complications such as postoperative peritonitis (PP) is particularly vital in abdominal surgery environments. Literature indicates that PP remains among the most challenging complications, with mortality ranging from 22.3% to 90% in affected patients (Droniak, 2019). Surgical interventions, including laparoscopic lavages and ultrasound-guided drainage, are usually required to manage such complications effectively. The occurrence of acute complications, including respiratory failure and cardiovascular insufficiency, nevertheless renders recovery hard and requires concentrated rehabilitation methods. Understanding the pathophysiology and clinical presentation of such complications enables effective deployment of intensive rehabilitation protocols by healthcare teams, not only addressing the physical rehabilitation but also the psychological and emotional rehabilitation, thereby maximizing outcomes for such patients with such apparently insurmountable issues. The correlation between successful rehabilitation and the management of complications cannot be overestimated. Individualized rehabilitation protocols considering each patient's individual situation and underlying medical conditions are required to control risks and ensure recovery. For example, spinal cord injury patients following the earthquake require specialized physiotherapy intervention that deals with their specific impairments without causing secondary complications. Moreover, constant assessment and adjustment of rehabilitation measures must be conducted to attain optimal recovery patterns and to improve long-term outcomes. Thus, post-surgical rehabilitation success is ultimately based on an integrated approach in which complication prevention is made a priority and patients are provided with holistic treatment to allow them to return to their maximum health and function.

12.7.3. Addressing Patient Compliance

Patient compliance with rehabilitation after surgery is necessary to maximize the benefits of recovery. Noncompliance can result in longer healing times, potential adverse reactions, and overall less satisfaction with surgical interventions. Patients' knowledge of rehabilitation activities and viewing such activities as significant are often compliance determinants. Educational initiatives preparing patients for the post-operative setting have the potential to be at the core of enhancing compliance. By explaining the rationale for the rehabilitation interventions and projected time frames in a clear way, health professionals allow patients to take an active role in their own rehabilitation. This collaborative approach can foster feelings of responsibility, perhaps surmounting frustration and helplessness related to the rehabilitation process. Patient-focused care plans that consider the idiosyncratic requirements and limitations of individual patients may also reduce compliance rates significantly. Making rehabilitation interventions and exercises cater to a patient's lifestyle, physical needs, and psychological state can bring about increased compliance with prescribed rehabilitation activity. A good example is identifying specific barriers to compliance, such as pain, so that clinicians can formulate solutions that are relevant. Engaging caregivers and family members in the care process also enhances support so that patients stay motivated and encouraged to finish their rehabilitation. This multimodal method proves to be particularly beneficial in complex cases, where patient involvement is crucial to achieving the best outcome in rehabilitation. Numerous motivational methods can also be used to create compliance and cooperative behaviors in surgery follow-up rehabilitation. Literature indicates that positive reinforcement, goal setting, and follow-up appointments can be significant predictors of patient motivation. Commemorating little achievements not only boosts morale but also reinforces the patient's resolve to adhere to their rehabilitation regimen. Furthermore, realistic, attainable goals instill a sense of accomplishment, and this can be particularly beneficial for those patients recovering from complicated operations. From multi-disciplinary case reports, for instance, from nasal rehabilitation following basal cell carcinoma or orthopedic surgery in children with cerebral palsy, evidence is provided to attest to the necessity of a holistic approach in tackling the problem of compliance. Ultimately, continued research into personalized and innovative methods of rehabilitation will prove crucial in escalating patient compliance and optimizing post-operative outcomes (Shami, 2024; Barakati et al., 2025) (Figure 12.16).

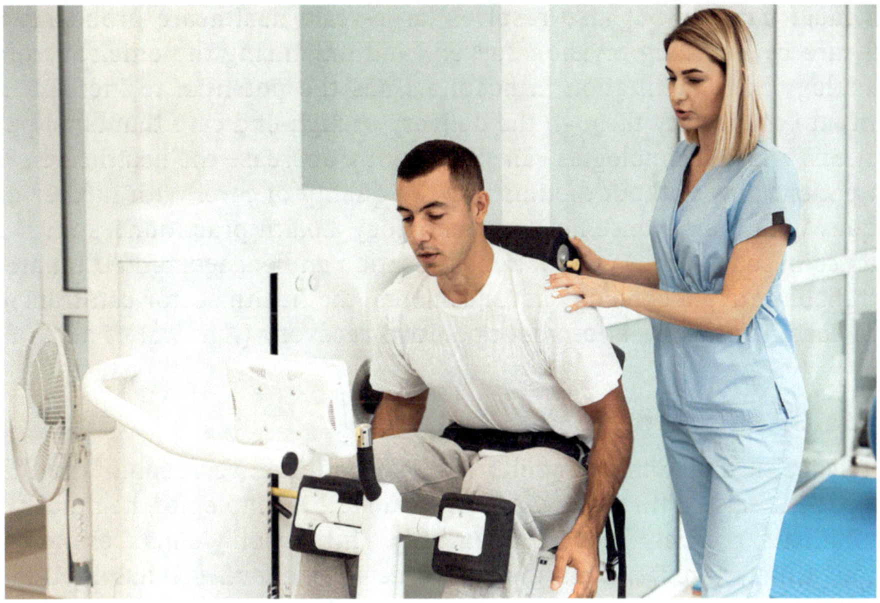

Figure 12.16. Educational initiatives aimed at informing patients about the post-operative process can play a pivotal role in enhancing adherence.

Source: https://rerouteandreboot.com/wp-content/uploads/2024/05/pre-post-surginer.png.

12.8. Innovations in Rehabilitation Technology

Integration of rehabilitation technology advances is an essential part of enhancing patients' outcomes after surgery. The development and application of wearable technologies, such as smart braces and motion sensors, inform clinicians more than ever about the physiological responses of patients as they recover. The devices allow for movement patterns to be monitored in real time, allowing therapists to develop personalized rehabilitation protocols for personalized requirements and track recovery successfully. Through the revolution of traditional rehabilitation to a more responsive, information-driven process, these innovations assist patients in recovering function and mobility with better effectiveness. As healthcare technology keeps advancing, technology's interaction with tailored care will transform the antiquated paradigms of rehabilitation, building a participatory setting in which patient engagement and monitoring are focal points, ultimately leading to enhanced long-term recovery outcomes (Agrawal et al., 2025). Besides wearable technology, artificial intelligence and robotics are revolutionizing postoperative rehabilitation. Robotic-enhanced technologies, particularly in orthopedic procedures such as total knee arthroplasty, enhance surgical precision and have a direct impact on rehabilitation protocols. Such advanced systems provide real-time feedback regarding patient movement and recovery parameters, allowing therapists to make evidence-based decisions during recovery phases. With better alignment and fewer postoperative complications, faster healing rates and less postoperative pain are advantageous for the patients. Moreover, the advent of robotic systems has led to the shift towards more individualized rehabilitation approaches, specifically designed to treat heterogeneous patient groups. With advancing technology, their capability to normalize the rehabilitation process while ensuring optimal functional outcomes cannot be overstated (Aneja et al., 2024). Integrating innovations in rehabilitation technology not only helps individual patients but also resolves large-scale healthcare problems. It reduces the cost of medical care by lowering revision surgery and enhancing the efficiency of rehabilitation programs. Technology in rehabilitation in hospitals has the potential to increase the number of patients brought into the facility through the delivery of high-end care that is on par with current healthcare practices. These technologies can significantly decrease the healthcare system's burden by speeding up patient flow without diminishing the quality of care. With further development of therapy techniques with the advancement of technology, health practitioners must be adaptive in embracing evidence-based practice with patient education and engagement. Ultimately, through the exploitation of rehabilitative technology advancements, the health sector can transition towards a better and more sustainable system of post-operative recovery (Agrawal et al., 2025).

12.8.1. Telehealth and Remote Monitoring

Integration of telehealth and remote monitoring in postoperative rehabilitation is a significant development in patient care. With the application of digital technologies, healthcare providers can closely observe patients' recovery processes remotely. This not only enhances patient involvement but also facilitates timely interventions that are crucial to effective rehabilitation. For instance, remote monitoring devices can allow clinicians to be able to monitor patients' vital signs, pain scores, and overall progress without frequent visits to the clinic. Such frequent interaction can lead to improved compliance with rehabilitation programs and, in turn, improved patient outcomes in postoperative care (Kale, 2023).

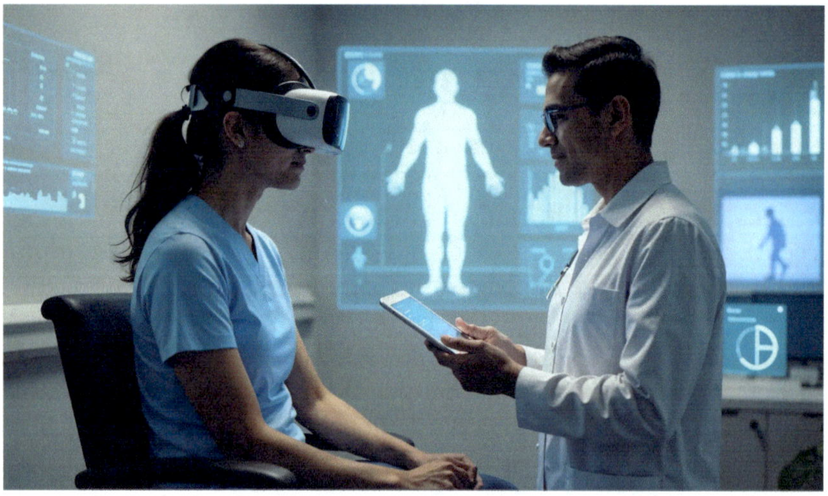

Figure 12.17. The integration of telehealth and remote monitoring into post-surgical rehabilitation represents a significant advancement in patient care.

Source: https://sparshmindinnovations.com/wp-content/uploads/2025/01/How-VR-is-Revolutionizing-Physiotherapy.webp.

Telehealth is generally a valuable intervention for individuals who may struggle to receive traditional care due to a variety of obstacles. Geographical limitations, specifically in rural or underserved populations, can significantly hinder patients from receiving needed follow-up care after surgery. Telehealth serves as a connection by providing online consultations, wherein patients can connect with their healthcare providers without having to travel long distances. This not only saves time and resources for patients and healthcare systems but also upholds health equity as it provides assurance that patients, regardless of their region, gain timely access to necessary medical care (Bywood, 2013). Telehealth use during post-surgical rehabilitation also refers to the role of personalized care plans developed based on the specific needs of each patient. With remote monitoring, practitioners can gather data on patient progress and adapt care strategies accordingly. Ongoing evaluation facilitates early identification of potential complications or setbacks prior to their occurrence as significant issues. In addition, utilization of telehealth promotes a patient-centered approach with active engagement of individuals in the recovery process. With the progress in healthcare, growing reliance on telehealth and remote monitoring heralds a revolutionary transformation towards more accessible and patient-centered post-surgical rehabilitation practices that would prove to raise the level of care provided to patients (Kale, 2023) (Figure 12.17).

12.8.2. Wearable Technology

The advent of wearable technology has begun to revolutionize the post-surgical rehabilitation world, creating avenues for enhanced patient tracking and customized treatment. The smartwatches, fitness trackers, and specialized biometric sensors monitor real-time data on physiological measures such as heart rate, activity levels, and indicators of recovery. By applying this data, healthcare professionals can tailor back-end recovery procedures to manage the specific needs of individual patients in such a way that rehabilitation is not merely effective but also patient-tailored. In addition, wearables enable remote monitoring such that clinicians can act at the earliest indicator of deviation from anticipated recovery curves, hence preventing complications and readmissions. One of the fields that has emerged in wearable technology is integrating sensors in rehabilitation devices, and this has been promising in the improvement of patients' outcomes. An example is the manufacturing of opto-electronic sensors, which has led to the manufacturing of pressure-sensitive insoles that can measure human-robot interaction in rehabilitation exoskeletons, and therapy becomes more efficient. This technology facilitates a more detailed prognosis of patient progress and points of focus, with observations perhaps too subtle for conventional systems. Due to advancements in wearables, their application in postoperative rehabilitation will increase steadily, and an active and dynamic rehabilitation process directed toward personalized patients' needs will become a reality (Koopman et al., 2013). Besides, the potential of wearable technology to bridge care gaps and promote multidisciplinary rehabilitation can be viewed in the case of UPPERCARE. The technology utilizes ICT to amplify self-care and facilitate rehabilitation plan compliance through interactive interfaces as well as group support. By integrating various actors, e.g., healthcare professionals, as well as kin, UPPERCARE optimizes patients' responsibility and motivation during recovery. This holistic approach is particularly important in the context of an aging population, in which rehabilitation methods are key to maintaining mobility and autonomy. With the increasing sophistication of wearable technology, its role in facilitating holistic care will be pivotal in addressing both the technical and social obstacles that face post-operative patients (Paredes et al., 2017).

12.8.3. Virtual Reality in Rehabilitation

Virtual reality (VR) in post-surgical rehabilitation is a groundbreaking technique that enhances patient outcomes and ensures maximum therapy adherence. Traditional forms of rehabilitation, even though beneficial, cause disengagement among patients since the exercises are monotonous and repetitive. VR technology innovatively addresses this drawback by recreating real-life scenarios in engaging and interactive settings to engage patients in them. For instance, they have noted higher levels of compliance and motivation among patients being treated with VR-based therapy, increasing the chances of recovery as well as satisfaction with the rehabilitation process. Such high levels of engagement are because VR contains the gamification factors that can transform rehabilitation tasks into less of a chore and more of a pleasure, hence an improved healing and recuperation environment. In addition, VR use in rehabilitation has been confirmed by early research with its application even in specialized areas of pediatric rehabilitation. A recent e-survey of physiotherapists who have special training in rehabilitating children after surgery to correct ataxia showed that traditional treatments like balance training and gait re-education are the norm (Hartley et al., 2019). However, with the inclusion of VR, these simple techniques may be improved upon through visual and spatial stimulation that is not possible with traditional methods. As it becomes learned by clinicians, there lies the possibility to individualize the rehabilitation program to meet unique demands, optimizing efficiency and facilitating a more specifically tailored rehabilitation process. This adaptability can become crucial in addressing the array of issues pediatric patients face post-surgery, allowing for a simpler rehabilitation process. Moreover, as technology continues to progress, the future of rehabilitation can be anticipated to further enhance with the inclusion of AR to VR to create a much more immersive therapy experience. While more research is still being developed, implications for both learning and application in rehabilitation are considerable (Obagi et al., 2020). The combination of these technologies enables the simulation of various environments in a safe and controlled environment, accelerating functional recovery in an efficient as well as stimulating manner. With the clinicians adopting these emerging tools, the potential for improved clinical outcomes becomes more pronounced. Adopting VR and AR can not only overcome the current shortcomings of conventional rehabilitation but also potentially lead to a new paradigm of patient-focused care that prioritizes engagement, flexibility, and technology-driven innovation in post-surgical recovery (Figure 12.18).

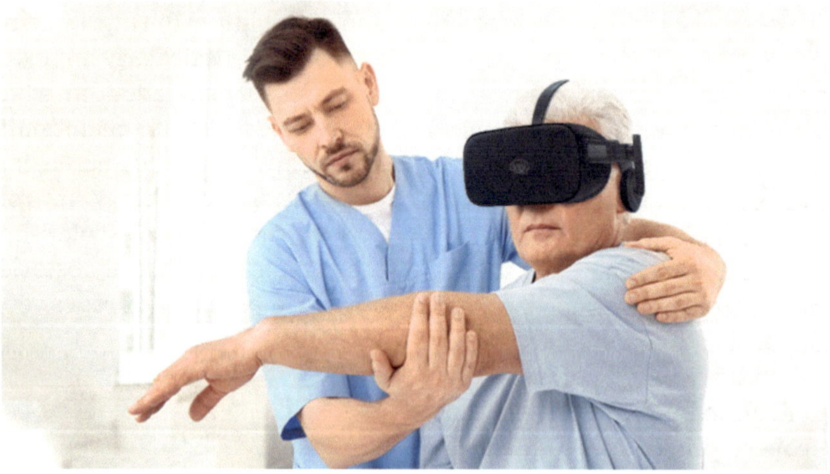

Figure 12.18. The integration of virtual reality (VR) into post-surgical rehabilitation represents a transformative approach aimed at enhancing patient outcomes and optimizing therapy engagement.

Source: https://rewinhealth.com/wp-content/uploads/2024/08/role-of-virtual-reality-for-stroke-rehabilitation.jpg.

SUMMARY

The introduction to Post-Surgical Rehabilitation in overview emphasizes the essential role played by rehabilitation in the recovery process after surgery. According to numerous studies, it has been concluded that therapy designed specifically for individual patients can be significantly effective in enhancing a patient's pattern of recovery, finally leading to improved bodily function and improved overall wellness. For instance, in the analyzed patients with lung cancer, precursory or subsequent pulmonary rehabilitation has been shown to appreciably increase walking distance and lung capacity measures, thus affirming the time and tailored strategy principle as an active ingredient of effective rehabilitation methods (Mosquera et al., 2024). It is a precious item of information for clinicians who develop post-operative care plans to optimize patient results. Moreover, awareness of the nuances of rehabilitation based on the type of surgery performed is essential to maximize healing. While in the case of elbow fractures, the research did not find that post-operative rehabilitation was always beneficial to improve outcomes in terms of range of motion, it also indicated that early post-operative rehabilitation might be a consideration to avoid complications such as stiffness of the joint. This refers to the intrinsic intricacy of rehabilitation treatments and refers to the need for individualized care based on the patient's specific surgical situation and status. Because of this, medical professionals need to put much focus on comprehensive assessments and adaptive rehabilitation programs such that patients are able to receive the most effective interventions after surgery (Donati et al., 2024). Finally, the overall message conveyed in the conclusion is the importance of ongoing research and evidence-based practice in post-surgical rehabilitation. As medical technology and surgery continue to evolve, so too will the approaches to rehabilitation have to adapt to meet the changing needs of patients as well. Regular evaluation of rehabilitation efficacy through systematic reviews and meta-analyses will provide clinicians with important knowledge for optimizing post-surgical care. By encouraging a culture of inquiry and compromise, the medical community can enhance recovery protocols and ultimately improve patient outcomes across many surgery situations, thus reinforcing the central role of rehabilitation in modern medicine.

In postoperative rehabilitation, understanding the nuances of the condition being treated is essential. One such case is in the case of inguinal disruption (ID), more commonly used in contemporary medical literature, where focus is placed on the consequences of abnormal tension in the groin area and not on the traditional concept of hernia. This shift in attitude, solidified by agreement involving physiotherapy, radiology, and surgical professionals, reinforces the importance of multidisciplinary treatment. As ID has been characterized by particular tissue pathology and potential tears, individualized physiotherapy emerges as an important initial treatment that may maximize the benefits of recovery for surgical patients with this condition (Sheen et al., 2013). A complex comprehension of the medical history thus has a direct relevance to the process of rehabilitation and serves to emphasize the role of interprofessional collaboration. The role of physiotherapy extends beyond mere rehabilitation; it is an approach to post-operative healing that involves physical as well as psychological mechanisms of healing. After surgery, physiotherapy aims towards recovery of strength, enhanced movement, and restriction of the likelihood of reinjury, alongside encouraging patient-oriented care that is sensitive to variable recovery patterns. This process acknowledges the complexity of human physiology and varied response patterns towards surgical intervention and imposes the necessity of individually designed rehabilitation programs

(Morris, 2002). In addition to surgical techniques such as mesh repair or suture reinforcement, physiotherapy is an early route for patients to regain functionality and confidence following surgery, in effect ushering them back into their day-to-day lives and sports activities. Furthermore, the use of standardized rehabilitation regimens not only enhances patient outcomes but also augments the quality of care within healthcare systems. Instituting national registries, as would be recommended by specialists, could make complete data compilation on surgery and rehabilitation results later possible. This way, better surveillance of recovery patterns would become possible in addition to finding out the best practices that correlate with predetermined standards of quality (Morris, 2002). By such a commitment to improvement and through the leverage of knowledge acquired through empirical evidence, healthcare professionals are able to enhance the efficiency and credibility of post-operative rehabilitation and thereby, ultimately, increase patient satisfaction levels and make the healthcare system stronger.

A CLOSER LOOK

REHABILITATION

Rehabilitation is a structured process aimed at restoring physical, psychological, and social functioning after injury, illness, surgery, or disability. Its primary goal is to help individuals regain independence, improve quality of life, and return to daily activities as safely and effectively as possible. Rehabilitation involves a multidisciplinary approach, often including doctors, physiotherapists, occupational therapists, speech therapists, psychologists, and social workers. Physical rehabilitation focuses on improving strength, flexibility, balance, coordination, and mobility through therapeutic exercises, manual therapy, and assistive devices. Occupational therapy helps individuals relearn daily living skills such as dressing, eating, and working, while speech and cognitive therapy support communication and mental functioning in patients with neurological conditions. Rehabilitation programs are personalized based on the patient's condition, age, functional level, and recovery goals. Early initiation of rehabilitation is crucial, as it prevents complications such as muscle wasting, joint stiffness, and reduced mobility. Emotional support, motivation, and patient education are also essential components that encourage active participation in the recovery process. In chronic conditions and long-term disabilities, rehabilitation promotes adaptation, independence, and social integration. Preventive rehabilitation strategies, including ergonomic training, fitness programs, and lifestyle modifications, help reduce the risk of future injuries. Overall, rehabilitation plays a vital role in comprehensive healthcare by supporting holistic recovery and long-term well-being.

REFERENCES

1. Abiodun, A., Andrews, T., Aylard, P., Barczak, A., Barriball, L., Beck, M., Bergen, S., et al. (2005). Patient experiences of anxiety, depression and acute pain after surgery: A longitudinal perspective. https://core.ac.uk/download/76097.pdf (accessed on 26th June 2025).
2. Agrawal, A., & Chandrakar, K. (2025). Biomechanical impacts of wearable and implantable technologies in post-surgical rehabilitation. *Journal of Neonatal Surgery*. https://www.semanticscholar.org/paper/fa6f62090b5710b9dc90ac5ac422504376c3e953 (accessed on 26th June 2025).
3. Akhoondian, M. (2025). Effect of mild aerobic exercise on the rehabilitation of lower limb injuries: A narrative review. *Journal of Sports and Rehabilitation Sciences*. https://www.semanticscholar.org/paper/a51ae30a55dd247198b4b37441880a87abace6c1 (accessed on 26th June 2025).
4. Al Shami, A. (2024). A comprehensive review of rehabilitation strategies post-orthopedic intervention in pediatric cerebral palsy. *Journal of Musculoskeletal Surgery and Research*. https://www.semanticscholar.org/paper/46c3b06a22b7e5ce42afcacef390f71deaf14eda (accessed on 26th June 2025).
5. Alokayli, W. T., & Alkhaldi, S. M. (2024). An investigation into the role of physical therapists in Saudi intensive care units. *International Journal of Physical Education & Sports Sciences*. https://www.semanticscholar.org/paper/d4221ebcfaf430c514c789b6074d70635a7bb4ae (accessed on 26th June 2025).
6. Ambrosetti, M., Abreu, A., Corrà, U., Davos, C. H., Hansen, D., Frederix, I., Iliou, M. C., et al. (2020). Secondary prevention through comprehensive cardiovascular rehabilitation: From knowledge to implementation. *European Journal of Preventive Cardiology, 28*, 460–495. https://doi.org/10.1177/2047487320913379 (accessed on 26th June 2025).
7. Aneja, K., Rudraraju, R. T., & Shyam, A. (2024). Robotic-assisted total knee arthroplasty: Innovations, precision, and the future of joint reconstruction. *Journal of Orthopedic Case Reports, 14*, 4–7. https://www.semanticscholar.org/paper/7accda304b125db7b2771ac0d74c553d640befef (accessed on 26th June 2025).
8. Asker, H., Yilmaz-Oral, D., Öztekin, Ç. V., & Gür, S. (2022). An update on the current status and future prospects of erectile dysfunction following radical prostatectomy. *The Prostate, 82*, 1135–1161. https://doi.org/10.1002/pros.24366 (accessed on 26th June 2025).
9. Bailey, J. F., Berven, S. H., Burch, S., Chu, J., et al. (2019). ISSLS Prize in Bioengineering Science 2019: Biomechanical changes in dynamic sagittal balance and lower limb compensatory strategies following realignment surgery in adult spinal deformity patients. https://core.ac.uk/download/323062549.pdf (accessed on 26th June 2025).
10. Barakati, T., Ehsan, H., Humkar, O., Shadab, H., & Ibrahimkhil, M. A. (2025). Nasal rehabilitation in a patient after basal cell carcinoma and radiotherapy: A case report. *Clinical Case Reports, 13*. https://www.semanticscholar.org/paper/cb052bd9d9a5cbc071b500356cc1c0ca1a166afc (accessed on 26th June 2025).
11. H. Paredes et al., "UPPERCARE: A community aware environment for post-surgical musculoskeletal recovery of elderly patients," 2017 IEEE 21st International Conference on Computer Supported Cooperative Work in Design (CSCWD), Wellington, New Zealand, 2017, pp. 251-256, doi: 10.1109/CSCWD.2017.8066703. (accessed on 26th June 2025).

12. Bateman, M., Connan, Z., Drew, S., Fakis, A., et al. (2024). Clinical and cost-effectiveness of individualised (early) patient-directed rehabilitation versus standard rehabilitation after surgical repair of the rotator cuff of the shoulder: Protocol for a multi-center, randomized controlled trial with integrated Quintet Recruitment Intervention (RaCeR 2). https://core.ac.uk/download/603245781.docx (accessed on 26th June 2025).

13. Berney, C. (2020). Enforced smoking cessation programmed prior to elective surgery. *ANZ Journal of Surgery, 90*. https://www.semanticscholar.org/paper/049bf25df0e70fe9020758be2cd8b21d5d1319a0 (accessed on 26th June 2025).

14. Bonica, M., Students of Health Management 721.01, University of New Hampshire. (2017). *Healthcare Management Primer*. https://core.ac.uk/download/215509297.pdf (accessed on 26th June 2025).

15. Morris C. (2002). A review of the efficacy of lower-limb orthoses used for cerebral palsy. *Developmental medicine and child neurology, 44*(3), 205–211. https://doi.org/10.1017/s0012162201001943(accessed on 26th June 2025).

16. Bowers, R., NHS Quality Improvement Scotland (Funder), & Ross, K. (2009). Best practice statement: Use of ankle-foot orthoses following stroke. https://core.ac.uk/download/9025419.pdf (accessed on 26th June 2025).

17. Retnaningsih, R., Budiyono, A., Ismail, R., Tugasworo, D., Danuaji, R., Syahrul, S., & Gunawan, J. (2023). Robotics Applications in Neurology: A Review of Recent Advancements and Future Directions. Journal of Instrumentation, Automation and Systems, 10(1), 25–33. https://doi.org/10.5281/zenodo.8062306 (accessed on 26th June 2025).

18. Hartley, H., Carter, B., Bunn, L., Pizer, B., Lane, S., Kumar, R., & Cassidy, E. (2019). E-Survey of Current International Physiotherapy Practice for Children with Ataxia Following Surgical Resection of Posterior Fossa Tumour. *Journal of rehabilitation medicine. Clinical communications, 2*, 1000020. https://doi.org/10.2340/20030711-1000020(accessed on 26th June 2025).

19. Burnett, A. L., Nehra, A., Breau, R. H., Culkin, D. J., Faraday, M. M., Hakim, L., Heidelbaugh, J. J., et al. (2018). Erectile dysfunction: AUA guideline. *The Journal of Urology, 200*, 633–641. https://doi.org/10.1016/j.juro.2018.05.004 (accessed on 26th June 2025).

20. Burton, M. J., Ramke, J., Marques, A. P., Bourne, R., Congdon, N., Jones, I., Ah Tong, B. A. M., et al. (2021). The Lancet Global Health Commission on global eye health: Vision beyond 2020. *The Lancet Global Health, 9*, e489–e551. https://doi.org/10.1016/s2214-109x(20)30488-5 (accessed on 26th June 2025).

21. Bywood, P. T. M. (2013). Allied health video consultation services. https://core.ac.uk/download/43335675.pdf (accessed on 26th June 2025).

22. Cardoso, F., Senkus, E., Costa, A., Papadopoulos, E., Aapro, M., André, F., Harbeck, N., et al. (2018). 4th ESO–ESMO International Consensus Guidelines for Advanced Breast Cancer (ABC 4). *Annals of Oncology, 29*, 1634–1657. https://doi.org/10.1093/annonc/mdy192 (accessed on 26th June 2025).

23. Chen, J., Yi, C., Okegbile, S. D., Cai, J., & Shen, X. (2023). Networking architecture and key supporting technologies for human digital twin in personalized healthcare: A comprehensive survey. *IEEE Communications Surveys & Tutorials, 26*, 706–746. https://doi.org/10.1109/comst.2023.3308717 (accessed on 26th June 2025).

24. Cruz Mosquera, F. E., Rios Murillo, S., Naranjo Rojas, A., Perlaza, C., Castro Osorio, D., & Liscano, Y. (2024). Effect of exercise and pulmonary rehabilitation in pre- and post-surgical patients with lung cancer: Systematic review and meta-analysis. *Medicina, 60*. https://www.semanticscholar.org/paper/1632ff019afca23e16209315266bd90dcb976f8b (accessed on 26th June 2025).

25. Dahlgren, A., Donelly, C., Murphy, C., McDowell, C. L., Rushton, D. N., Maynard, F. M., Snoek, G. J., et al. (2008). Decision for reconstructive interventions of the upper limb in individuals with tetraplegia: The effect of treatment characteristics. https://core.ac.uk/download/pdf/11479809.pdf (accessed on 26th June 2025).

26. Dams, O. C., van den Akker-Scheek, I., Diercks, R. L., Wendt, K. W., Bosma, E., van Raaij, T. M., Munzebrock, A. V. E., et al. (2019). The recovery after Achilles tendon rupture: A protocol for a multicenter prospective cohort study. *BMC Musculoskeletal Disorders, 20*. https://doi.org/10.1186/s12891-019-2437-z (accessed on 26th June 2025).

27. Sheen, A. J., Stephenson, B. M., Lloyd, D. M., Robinson, P., Fevre, D., Paajanen, H., de Beaux, A., Kingsnorth, A., Gilmore, O. J., Bennett, D., Maclennan, I., O'Dwyer, P., Sanders, D., & Kurzer, M. (2014). 'Treatment of the sportsman's groin': British Hernia Society's 2014 position statement based on the Manchester Consensus Conference. *British journal of sports medicine, 48*(14), 1079–1087. https://doi.org/10.1136/bjsports-2013-092872(accessed on 26th June 2025).

28. Obagi, Z. A., Rundle, C. W., & Dellavalle, R. P. (2020). Widening the scope of virtual reality and augmented reality in dermatology. *Dermatology online journal, 26*(1), 13030/qt6mz1s20x. (accessed on 26th June 2025).

29. do Valle Varela, J. P., Paes de Moura, J., Andrade, R. F., Monfradini da Silva, J., Monteiro, S. T., Duccini, F. Z., Samorini, T. D., et al. (2025). Breast reconstruction after mastectomy. *Health and Society*. https://www.semanticscholar.org/paper/561053037bb5487ab07923a13d4e02d369938503 (accessed on 26th June 2025).

30. Donati, D., Aroni, S., Tedeschi, R., Sartini, S., Farì, G., Ricci, V., Vita, F., et al. (2024). Exploring the impact of rehabilitation on post-surgical recovery in elbow fracture patients: A cohort study. *Musculoskeletal Surgery, 109*, 33–39. https://www.semanticscholar.org/paper/58354406759dae8abd6dd89c2e76775d81af80bb (accessed on 26th June 2025).

31. Droniak, M. (2019). Management of postoperative peritonitis in low-resources services. https://core.ac.uk/download/301580706.pdf (accessed on 26th June 2025).

32. Dunnigan, M. G., & Pollock, A. M. (2003). Downsizing of acute inpatient beds associated with private finance initiative: Scotland's case study. *BMJ (Clinical research ed.), 326*(7395), 905. https://doi.org/10.1136/bmj.326.7395.905(accessed on 26th June 2025).

33. Howard, J. S., Mattacola, C. G., Mullineaux, D. R., English, R. A., & Lattermann, C. (2014). Patient-oriented and performance-based outcomes after knee autologous chondrocyte implantation: a timeline for the first year of recovery. *Journal of sport rehabilitation, 23*(3), 223–234. https://doi.org/10.1123/jsr.2013-0094(accessed on 26th June 2025).

34. Guy, K. D., McDermott, B. P., Gallagher, K., & Washington, T. (2019). Ulnar Collateral Ligament Reconstruction with Traditional Docking Compared to Novel Surgical Techniques. Health, Human Performance and Recreation Undergraduate Honors Theses Retrieved from https://scholarworks.uark.edu/hhpruht/70(accessed on 26th June 2025).

35. F Oliva, A., Forte, A. M., De Carli, A., Anna, C., et al. (2018). I.S.Mu.L.T. Achilles tendon ruptures guidelines. https://core.ac.uk/download/168405702.pdf (accessed on 26th June 2025).

36. Habib, G., Lancellotti, P., Antunes, M. J., Bongiorni, M. G., Casalta, J. P., Del Zotti, F., Dulgheru, R., et al. (2015). 2015 ESC Guidelines for the management of infective endocarditis. *European Heart Journal, 36*, 3075–3128. https://doi.org/10.1093/eurheartj/ehv319 (accessed on 26th June 2025).

37. Mafo Degge, H., Hayter, M., & Laurenson, M. (2017). An integrative review on women living with obstetric fistula and after treatment experiences. *Journal of clinical nursing, 26*(11-12), 1445–1457. https://doi.org/10.1111/jocn.13590c(accessed on 26th June 2025).

38. Hong, R., Li, B., Bao, Y., Liu, L., & Jin, L. (2024). Therapeutic robots for post-stroke rehabilitation. *Medical Review, 4*, 55–67. https://www.semanticscholar.org/paper/1f7c5b57aa8da20e3976a65073f7f8179ac29502 (accessed on 26th June 2025).

39. Joglar, J. A., Chung, M. K., Armbruster, A. L., Benjamin, E. J., Chyou, J. Y., Cronin, E. M., Deswal, A., et al. (2023). 2023 ACC/AHA/ACCP/HRS guideline for the diagnosis and management of atrial fibrillation. *Circulation, 149*. https://doi.org/10.1161/cir.0000000000001193 (accessed on 26th June 2025).

40. Johannesson, A. G., & Rusaw, D. F. (2024). Prosthetists' perspective on surgical intervention, postoperative treatment, and prosthetic assessment following transtibial amputation. *Journal of Surgery*. https://www.semanticscholar.org/paper/e8232a4c6adb2df1966a1789980fbd033456fece (accessed on 26th June 2025).

41. Kale, M., et al. (2023). Telemedicine revolution: Bridging gaps in access to healthcare. https://core.ac.uk/download/596247489.pdf (accessed on 26th June 2025).

42. Kirchhof, P., Benussi, S., Kotecha, D., Ahlsson, A., Atar, D., Casadei, B., Castellá, M., et al. (2016). 2016 ESC Guidelines for the management of atrial fibrillation developed in collaboration with EACTS. *European Heart Journal, 37*, 2893–2962. https://doi.org/10.1093/eurheartj/ehw210 (accessed on 26th June 2025).

43. Thierry C. Gillebert, Nicholas Brooks, Ricardo Fontes-Carvalho, Zlatko Fras, Pascal Gueret, Jose Lopez-Sendon, Maria Jesus Salvador, Renee B. A. van den Brink, Otto A. Smiseth, Reinhard Griebenow, Peter Kearney, Alec Vahanian, J. Bauersachs, J. Bax, H. Burri, A.L.P. Caforio, F. Calvo, P. Charron, G. Ertl, F. Flachskampf, P. Giannuzzi, S. Gibbs, L. Gonçalves, J.R. González-Juanatey, J. Hall, D. Herpin, G. Iaccarino, B. Iung, A. Kitsiou, P. Lancellotti, T. McDonough, J.J. Monsuez, I.J. Nuñez, S. Plein, A. Porta-Sánchez, S. Priori, S. Price, V. Regitz-Zagrosek, Z. Reiner, L.M. Ruilope, J.P. Schmid, P. A. Sirnes, M. Sousa-Ouva, J. Stępińska, C. Szymanski, D. Taggart, M. Tendera, L. Tokgözoğlu, P. Trindade, K. Zeppenfeld, L. Joubert, C. Carrera, European Society of Cardiology, Observer on behalf of the UEMS (Cardiology Section):, Review Coordinators:, Contributors and reviewers:, ESC staff:, ESC Core Curriculum for the General Cardiologist (2013), European Heart Journal, Volume 34, Issue 30, 7 August 2013, Pages 2381–2411, https://doi.org/10.1093/eurheartj/eht234c(accessed on 26th June 2025).

44. Koopman, B., Giovacchini, F., Podobnik, J., Donati, M., Carrozza, M. C., De Rossi, M., Munih, M., et al. (2013). A flexible sensor technology for the distributed measurement of interaction pressure. https://core.ac.uk/download/pdf/11486644.pdf (accessed on 26th June 2025).

45. Kotze, K. (2019). The pairing of trigger points dry needling with rehabilitation techniques. https://core.ac.uk/download/213463742.pdf (accessed on 26th June 2025).

46. Kuiper, H., Leeuwen, C. V., Stolwijk-Swüste, J., & Post, M. W. M. (2023). Does the disposition of passive coping mediate the association between illness perception and symptoms of anxiety and depression in patients with spinal cord injury during first inpatient rehabilitation? *Disability and Rehabilitation, 46*, 4368–4376. https://www.semanticscholar.org/paper/a530432a2237560e308fde235e6c24d2109830d8 (accessed on 26th June 2025).

47. Kuriakose, D., & Xiao, Z. C. (2020). Pathophysiology and treatment of stroke: Present status and future perspectives. *International Journal of Molecular Sciences, 21*, 7609–7609. https://doi.org/10.3390/ijms21207609 (accessed on 26th June 2025).

48. Marino, I. R. & Lauro, A (2018). Surgeon's perspective on short bowel syndrome: Where are we? *World J Transplant*. 2018;8(6):198-202. doi:10.5500/wjt.v8.i6.198. https://core.ac.uk/download/288122098.pdf (accessed on 26th June 2025).

49. Lebert, A. (2017). SLAP lesion in overhead athletes. https://core.ac.uk/download/154745976.pdf (accessed on 26th June 2025).

50. Liang, Z., Chong, M., Sim, M. A., Lim, J. L., Castañeda, P., Green, D. W., Fisher, D., et al. (2020). Surgical considerations in patients with COVID-19. *Journal of Bone and Joint Surgery, 102*, e50. https://doi.org/10.2106/jbjs.20.00513 (accessed on 26th June 2025).

51. Marek, K., Redlicka, J., Miller, E., & Zubrycki, I. (2023). Objectivizing measures of post-stroke hand rehabilitation through multi-disciplinary scales. *Journal of Clinical Medicine, 12*, 7497. https://doi.org/10.3390/jcm12237497 (accessed on 26th June 2025).

52. Merchant, M., Hu, S. B., Miller, C., Ahmadi, T., Garcia, E., & Smith, M. I. (2025). Comprehensive management of severe burn injuries: A multidisciplinary approach from resuscitation to rehabilitation. *Emergency Care and Medicine*. https://www.semanticscholar.org/paper/d3dc30e79094bfa550ca88cb6570fb63174073da (accessed on 26th June 2025).

53. Monson, J., & LaPrade, R. F. (2025). Posterior medial meniscus root tears: Clinical implications, surgical management, and post-operative rehabilitation considerations. *International Journal of Sports Physical Therapy, 20*, 127–136. https://www.semanticscholar.org/paper/f171daa05cf529805355b89d288fcfcd61dbbbcb (accessed on 26th June 2025).

54. Montero-Odasso, M., van der Velde, N., Martin, F. C., Petrović, M., Tan, M. P., Ryg, J., Aguilar-Navarro, S. G., et al. (2022). World guidelines for falls prevention and management for older adults: A global initiative. *Age and Ageing, 51*. https://doi.org/10.1093/ageing/afac205 (accessed on 26th June 2025).

55. Norrving, B., Barrick, J., Dávalos, A., Dichgans, M., Cordonnier, C., Guekht, A., Kutluk, K., et al. (2018). Action plan for stroke in Europe 2018–2030. *European Stroke Journal, 3*, 309–336. https://doi.org/10.1177/2396987318808719 (accessed on 26th June 2025).

56. Oku, S., Hatakeyama, J., Liu, K., Tojo, K., Idei, M., Inoue, S., Yamakawa, K., et al. (2025). Early rehabilitation interventions by physical therapists for severe COVID-19 patients were associated with decreased incidence of post-ICU physical impairment. *Annals of Rehabilitation Medicine, 49*, 49–59. https://www.semanticscholar.org/paper/72cb23e36df5e24fd5342448e8fb36719c2cef6d (accessed on 26th June 2025).

57. Osborne, T., Wall, B. A., Edgar, D. W., Fairchild, T. J., & Wood, F. (2023). Current understanding of the chronic stress response to burn injury from human studies. *Burns & Trauma, 11*. https://doi.org/10.1093/burnst/tkad007 (accessed on 26th June 2025).

58. Pany, T. K., Sahoo, P., Parween, N., Swargiary, N., & Narayan, L. (2025). Affordable multi-axial adjustable socket for immediate post-operative prosthesis: Enhancing early rehabilitation in developing countries. *International Journal of Science and Healthcare Research*. https://www.semanticscholar.org/paper/4b2ae6d4ef038fe2c994ec08994c25ac5263ec96 (accessed on 26th June 2025).

59. Pelliccia, A., Sharma, S., Gati, S., Bäck, M., Börjesson, M., Caselli, S., Collet, J. P., et al. (2020). 2020 ESC Guidelines on sports cardiology and exercise in patients with cardiovascular disease. *European Heart Journal, 42*, 17–96. https://doi.org/10.1093/eurheartj/ehaa605 (accessed on 26th June 2025).

60. Ricco, J. B., Bartelink, M. L., Björck, M., Brodmann, M., Cohnert, T., Czerny, M., De Carlo, M., et al. (2017). 2017 ESC Guidelines on the diagnosis and treatment of peripheral arterial diseases, in collaboration with the European Society for Vascular Surgery (ESVS). *European Heart Journal, 39*, 763–816. https://doi.org/10.1093/eurheartj/ehx095 (accessed on 26th June 2025).

61. Santos-Pérez, D., Ochiana, N., Carrasco-Páez, L., & Martínez-Díaz, I. C. (2025). Effects of low load blood flow restriction training on post-surgical musculoskeletal patients: A systematic review and meta-analysis of randomized controlled trials. *Applied Sciences*. https://www.semanticscholar.org/paper/721081361df7205db1bf21ffa666d7cd7c4f64a3 (accessed on 26th June 2025).

62. Shabbir, H., Shafi, M. T., & Mushtaq, M. H. (2025). Effects of inspiratory muscle training on respiratory strength and functional capacity in post-operative patients with scoliosis during maximum protection phase. *The Healer Journal of Physiotherapy and Rehabilitation Sciences*. https://www.semanticscholar.org/paper/325b42e23f24ea1b0015e01218dbca895978b38c (accessed on 26th June 2025).

63. Sigfrid, L., Cevik, M., Jesudason, E., Lim, W., Rello, J., Amuasi, J., Bozza, F., et al. (2021). What is the recovery rate and risk of long-term consequences following a diagnosis of COVID-19? A harmonized, global longitudinal observational study protocol. *BMJ Open, 11*. https://www.semanticscholar.org/paper/93c41a5c8fe6a2900bfc6060ffc0d2065e995dcb (accessed on 26th June 2025).

64. Slawomirski, L., & Klazinga, N. (2022). The economics of patient safety. *OECD Health Working Papers*. https://doi.org/10.1787/761f2da8-en (accessed on 26th June 2025).

65. Soares, C. L. A., Magalhães, J., Faria-Fortini, I., Batista, L. R., Lima, L. A. O., & Faria, C. (2024). Barriers and facilitators to access post-stroke rehabilitation services in the first six months of recovery in Brazil. *Disability and Rehabilitation, 46*, 5601–5607. https://www.semanticscholar.org/paper/98c1d9c27ab568b414119548c5d3d9c9d27cd5eb (accessed on 26th June 2025).

66. Suematsu, Y. (2025). Development of myocardial oxygen consumption index using non-invasive continuous blood pressure monitor and practical application of optimal exercise prescription algorithm. *Impact*. https://www.semanticscholar.org/paper/c8cff8fa731ad688f345e7ebee5082e7f3bc54b2 (accessed on 26th June 2025).

67. Virani, S. S., Newby, L. K., Arnold, S. V., Bittner, V., Brewer, L. C., Demeter, S. H., Dixon, D. L., et al. (2023). 2023 AHA/ACC/ACCP/ASPC/NLA/PCNA guideline for the management of patients with chronic coronary disease. *Circulation, 148*. https://doi.org/10.1161/cir.0000000000001168 (accessed on 26th June 2025).

68. Wierzbicka, M., Kiszka, M., Barnaś, S., Jeziorny, M., Zając, B., Dwornikowska-Dąbrowska, M., & Jędruchniewicz, N. (2025). The Ready for Safe Cancer Treatment (RESET) tool: Enhancing quality and optimizing timely and safe discharge with transitional care adjustments for head and neck cancer patients. *Otolaryngologic Polska: The Polish Otolaryngology, 79*(3), 1–7. https://www.semanticscholar.org/paper/da515e7cb371148b489c30d2c809737079fcaec4 (accessed on 26th June 2025).

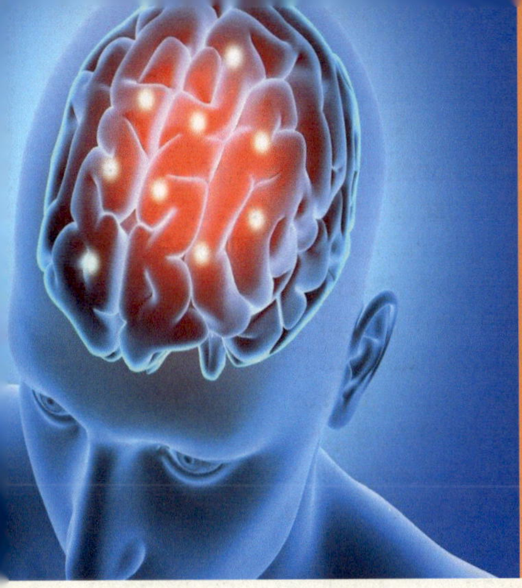

Chapter 13

NEUROLOGICAL DISORDERS WITH ORTHOPEDIC IMPLICATIONS

Contents

Introduction....411

13.1. Functional Neuroanatomy Relevant to Physiotherapy....415

13.2. Common Neurological Conditions....420

13.3. Other Neurological Disorders....424

13.4. Signs and Symptoms of Neurological Disorders....428

13.5. Principles of Neuroplasticity....432

13.6. Assessment and Diagnosis of Neurological Disorders....436

Summary....441

References....444

Introduction

The intersection of neurological illness and orthopedic outcomes represents a complex and intricate area of research in medical science as well as clinical practice. It is important to understand how neurological diseases such as cerebral palsy, multiple sclerosis, and spinal cord injury lead to musculoskeletal disease in the treatment plan design. As these conditions have a tendency to impede motor control and coordination, patients develop secondary orthopedic impairments in the form of joint deformities, spasticity in muscles, and osteoporosis. For instance, cerebral palsy patients will require certain orthopedic interventions, such as orthopedic surgery or bracing, to address mobility issues and provide a better quality of life. Research has put more emphasis on the need for an overall approach that, besides treating the primary neurological issue, also considers the orthopedic complications arising from it that patients may experience. Also, diverse presentation and course patterns of the majority of neurological disorders necessitate a multidisciplinary approach for optimal management.

This is particularly so in diseases such as Mucopolysaccharidosis VI, where the combined expertise of geneticists, orthopedic surgeons, physical therapists, and other healthcare providers is essential to optimal management. Management of such disorders involves routine observation, assessment of functional ability, and relief interventions for both neurological as well as concomitant orthopedic issues. In fact, in the process, mounting evidence exists to suggest that using targeted therapies can result in a significant change in ambulation and enhance the quality of life for orthopedic outcomes of neurological disorders. Maximal interaction amongst healthcaregivers is thus essential in the treatment of such interlocking conditions. Moreover, advancements in research in the field of neurological disorders with orthopedic implications have facilitated the formation of evidence-based guidelines that help bridge the discovery-to-implementation gap. Guidelines play a significant role in informing the care practices and ensuring that the patient receives comprehensive management per his or her personalized needs. By combining expert opinion and clinical evidence, health professionals are in a position to establish best practices for treatments as diverse as physical therapy to surgery. The relevance of the guidelines is underscored by consensus-building processes, which permit the integration of patient experience with clinical expertise to ensure that the treatment landscape remains dynamic and relevant. The development of such frameworks is essential in the improvement of both patient satisfaction and clinical outcomes in the scenario of neurological disorders bearing orthopedic relevance.

Structure of the Central Nervous System

Interactions between the central and peripheral nervous systems form the foundation of an entire view of neurological function and disease. The central nervous system (CNS), or the spinal cord and brain, is the central control for stimulus processing and response. On the contrary, the peripheral nervous system (PNS) includes all the neural tracts outside the CNS, including cranial and spinal nerves that are engaged in the communication of information from/to the CNS and the rest of the body. This intricate interaction provides a means for information exchange essential to body functions, including motor control and sensory perception. A disruption in this organization can have profound consequences, occurring in such neurological conditions as stroke, which causes focal brain damage, or multiple sclerosis, in which the immune system attacks myelin sheaths. Information regarding this organization is most important for clinicians who diagnose and treat neurological diseases (Welch et al., 2020). Functional neuroanatomy provides valuable information on how specific areas of the nervous system contribute to movement and sensation, information which is especially relevant to physiotherapy clinics. An example is the motor cortex located in the frontal lobe, which coordinates voluntary movement by providing commands through the spinal cord to muscles. Similarly, the somatosensory cortex located in the parietal lobe processes touch information, which enables us to understand our environment. Assessment of UMN and LMN damage can help physiotherapists prepare goal-oriented rehabilitation interventions. Weakness and spasticity are signs of UMN lesions that can be found in stroke patients, and flaccid paralysis in peripheral nerve injury patients can be a sign of LMN lesions. Therefore, the understanding of neuroanatomical structures is important to create efficient intervention strategies in the area of physiotherapy (Barrow & Bendok, 2019). The principles of neuroplasticity stress the plasticity of the CNS in response to injury or learning, leaving windows of hope for effective rehabilitation from neurological diseases. Neuroplasticity is the capacity of the brain to reorganize itself by forming new connections between brain cells throughout an individual's lifetime, allowing recovery from damage even after a severe injury. The process can be observed in conditions such as Parkinson's disease, in which treatment often aims to harness neuroplasticity to improve motor function and slow decline. For this purpose, brain reorganization eliciting exercises can achieve enhanced mobility and strength in the subject with SCI and other disorders. Use of neuroplastic principles in physiotherapy is not only capable of enhancing symptom management but also of empowering the patient by enhancing independence and quality of life. Finally, the understanding of the intricate structure of the CNS and its mechanisms forms the foundation of successful treatments in numerous neurological disorders (Welch et al., 2020) (Figure 13.1).

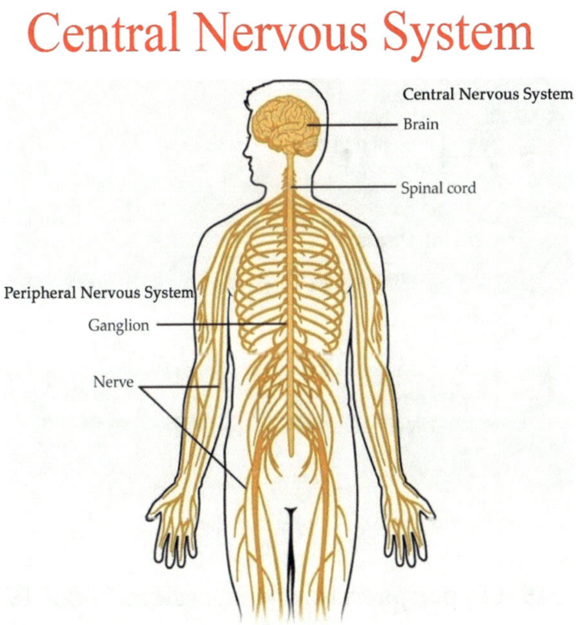

Figure 13.1. Central nervous system.

Source: http://www.karunayoga.in/wp-content/uploads/2017/09/cns.jpg.

Structure of the Peripheral Nervous System

The complex interaction between all the components of the nervous system is what maintains body functions and responding to stimuli outside the body. The peripheral nervous system (PNS) is a critical extension of the central nervous system (CNS), regulating motor and sensory input through the entire body. The PNS, consisting of cranial and spinal nerves, is separated into the somatic and autonomic nervous systems. The somatic nervous system regulates voluntary movements, providing the neural pathways over which sensory data can be transmitted to the CNS and motor instructions can be executed. The autonomic nervous system regulates involuntary processes like heart rate and digestion through its sympathetic and parasympathetic branches. The awareness of the organization of the PNS enhances our knowledge concerning how injury, like in common neurological disease, disrupts routes of communication so that symptoms and signs supervene and impact patient management and rehabilitative treatments. Functional neuroanatomy of the PNS is even more relevant when applied to neurological disorders. For instance, injuries of the spinal cord (SCIs) might lead to interruption in nerve conduction to and from the limbs, resulting in widespread motor and sensory loss. Multiple sclerosis (MS) and Parkinson's disease include demyelination or degeneration of both central and peripheral tracts and thus make diagnosis and treatment more difficult. Clinical manifestations of signs and symptoms observed with upper motor neuron (UMN) and lower motor neuron (LMN) lesions allow one to know the site and extent of neural damage. UMN lesions may manifest with spasticity and hyperreflexia, whereas LMN lesions may be presented by weakness of the muscles and atrophy. Hence, an in-depth knowledge of PNS anatomy assists clinicians in differentiating these neurologic conditions and formulating particular rehabilitation protocols. Besides, the principles of neuroplasticity emphasize the nervous system's flexibility, particularly in the PNS. Neuroplasticity allows for reorganization and restitution of function following injury, applicable to conditions like stroke and traumatic injury. Rehabilitation therapy that is based on neuroplastic mechanisms can facilitate regeneration of neuronal pathways as well as optimize restoration of function. For example, following peripheral nerve injury, the re-routing of injured axons to the target tissue is crucial for functional recovery. Familiarity with PNS anatomy is useful in guiding physiotherapists in how to plan interventions through repetitive task practice and sensory feedback to enhance the healing process. By integrating awareness of the PNS and mechanisms of neuroplasticity, practitioners are better positioned to manage the difficulties imposed by diverse neurological disorders, enhancing patient outcome and quality of life for individuals affected (Figure 13.2).

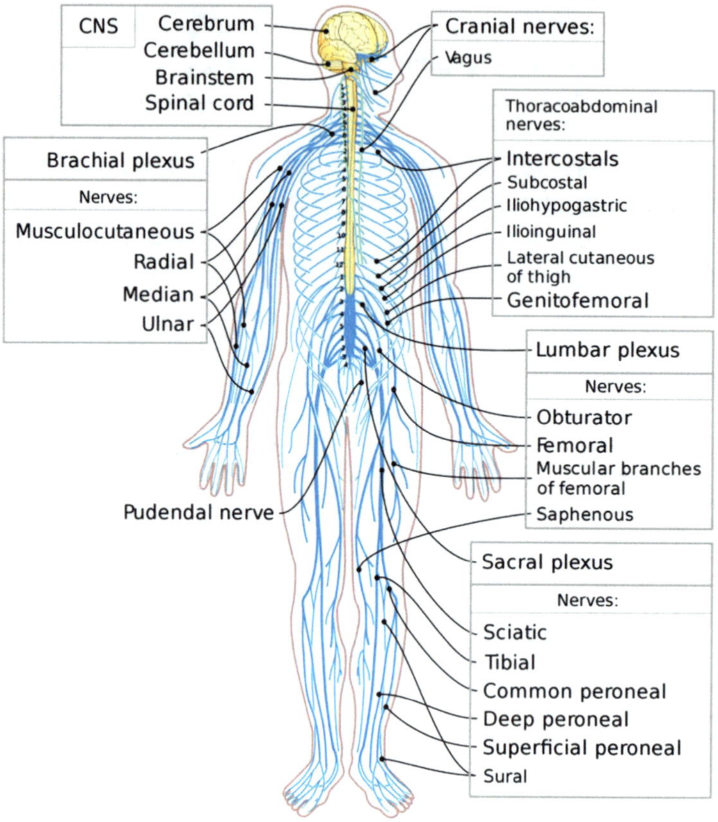

Figure 13.2. Peripheral-nervous-system.

Source: https://healthjade.net/wp-content/uploads/2019/05/peripheral-nervous-system-768x849.jpg.

Functions of the Nervous System

It is the intricate interaction of the peripheral and central nervous systems that sustains the innumerable functions governing the body and behavior of humans. The central nervous system (CNS), comprised of the brain and spinal cord, plays a critical role in processing sensory information and organizing responses. It serves as the central command center to integrate incoming information from the peripheral nervous system (PNS), comprising nerves that extend throughout the body. This higher-level network of communication facilitates essential activities such as motor function control, reflexes, and homeostatic regulation. The functional significance of the neuroanatomy is particularly vital in fields like physiotherapy, where the goal is restoring function and avoiding secondary effects of neurological disease on motor function and coordination, to close the gap between anatomy and rehabilitative practice (Barrow & Bendok, 2019). The role of neuroplasticity is a key characteristic of the nervous system's operation, showing the capacity to respond to injury or neurological disease. Neuroplasticity refers to the brain's ability to reorganize itself through the formation of new neural connections throughout a person's life in reaction to learning, experience, or injury. This plasticity can assist recovery in conditions such as stroke, spinal cord injury (SCI), and multiple sclerosis (MS), where neural circuits can be interrupted. Furthermore, treatment methods often capitalize on this effect to generate improved recovery by initiating compensatory mechanisms for lost function. For instance, rehabilitation techniques can involve multiple repetitions of motor capabilities that trigger neuroplastic changes so that patients can regain independence in activities of daily living. Thus, knowledge about the mechanisms of neuroplasticity is essential to develop effective interventions to optimize functional recovery in individuals with neurological disorders (Azzalini et al., 2019). Knowledge about the UMN and LMN lesion signs and symptoms is necessary for diagnosing and treating a variety of neurological disorders. UMN lesions commonly lead to heightened muscle tone, hyperreflexia, and the presence of pathological reflexes, reflecting disturbances in the CNS pathways. However, LMN lesions are characterized by muscle weakness, decreased reflexes, and muscle atrophy, reflecting localized disturbances in lower motor neurons. Parkinson's disease and cerebral palsy are examples of the varied presentations of such lesions, impacting motor function and overall well-being. When physiotherapists and medical professionals analyze such symptoms, they can plan treatments based on related deficits in particular, which enhances overall management of patients with neurological disorders. Thus, measuring the functional implications of both UMN and LMN categories is crucial in effective diagnosis and targeted therapeutic interventions in neurorehabilitation (Barrow & Bendok, 2019).

13.1. Functional Neuroanatomy Relevant to Physiotherapy

In the understanding of the complex relationship between the nervous system and movement, functional neuroanatomy is an important physiotherapy key. The central nervous system (CNS), comprising the brain and spinal cord, plays a fundamental role in the processing of sensory information and the management of motor responses. In contrast, the peripheral nervous system (PNS) connects the CNS with limbs and organs for communication throughout the body. This intricate web not only governs voluntary movement but also reflex movement, an area of great relevance to rehabilitation. By mapping these systems in detail, physiotherapists can tailor interventions that optimize recovery through the optimization of nervous system function. This is crucial in the management of neurological conditions such as muscular dystrophies, in which weakening of muscles needs special rehabilitation to improve the quality of life and mobility, as in the case of early ambulatory stage Duchenne Muscular Dystrophy (Chitlange et al., 2024). Physiotherapy also addresses a population of diffuse neurological disorders, each with unique challenges and symptoms. For instance, diseases such as stroke, spinal cord injury (SCI), and Parkinson's disease exhibit a variety of manifestations that express both upper motor neuron (UMN) or lower motor neuron (LMN) injury. UMN injury characteristically manifests as spasticity of the muscles, weakness, and hyperreflexia, whereas LMN injury characteristically manifests as muscle wasting, flaccid paralysis, and reduced reflexes. An appreciation of such differences allows physiotherapists to devise intervention strategies aimed at re-establishing mobility and function. Additionally, symptoms like ataxia in most neurological conditions bring to the fore the importance of highly coordinated muscle control, most particularly concerning the cerebellum. This region of the brain has an important role to play in coordinating sensory input with smooth locomotion, which brings into perspective the need for intensive therapeutic exercises in this regard to address gait abnormalities (Sivhugwana, 2021). Neuroplasticity, when applied in the context of rehabilitation, is a characteristic principle that illustrates the brain's capacity to reorganize and react to disease or injury. Treatment with physiotherapy utilizes this feature to initiate recovery through stimulating neural pathways and exercising functional motor patterns. Task-oriented training, repetitive practice, and neuromuscular facilitation are all key methods that facilitate the promotion of neuroplastic adjustments in the brain as well as spinal cord. Interestingly, these approaches are especially efficient when integrated with individually tailored treatment plans, considering the patient's specific neurological status and functional objectives. As researchers learn more about how neuroplasticity works, physiotherapy will increasingly integrate these findings into practice, optimizing the chances for effective rehabilitation in a spectrum of neurological disorders (Figure 13.3).

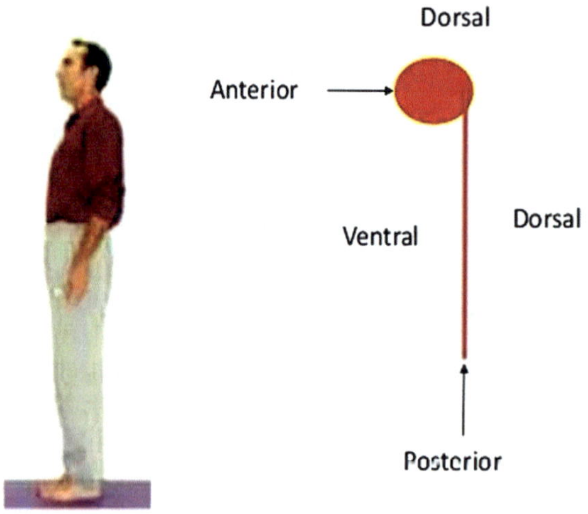

Figure 13.3. Basics-of-functional-neuroanatomy.

Source: https://image.slidesharecdn.com/functionalneuroanatomy-150409090214-conversion-gate01/95/basics-of-functional-neuroanatomy-7-638.jpg?cb=1550198069.

13.1.1. Key Brain Regions and Their Functions

The intricate brain architecture has countless specialized regions, all working together to form an enormous network of functions needed for human action. The limbic system, as well as specific regions like the hippocampus and amygdala, play a significant role in emotion control, memory, and emotional response processing. Evidence suggests that structural abnormalities in these areas could produce varied psychological disorders, and an understanding of their functions within the context of neurological disorders is highly suggested. Awareness of the way in which alterations in the limbic system manifest themselves as symptoms of mood disorder or memory loss informs both diagnostic procedures and treatment processes, illustrating the intimate connection between anatomy and clinical practice for physiotherapy and rehabilitation (Azzalini et al., 2019). Also, the cerebellum, formerly in the primary role of motor function, has been reclassified as a central part of the cognitive process. New discovery reveals it to be active in emotional regulation and higher-order thought, which has implications of unprecedented importance for the explication of conditions like the cerebellar cognitive affective syndrome. Such shifting in perspective sets its focus on the interdependence between motor and cognitive capabilities and, as such, maximizes the area of treatment for coordination disorders or mental loss. Treatment procedures could be augmented through the knowledge of how cerebellar function contributes to more universal aspects of conduct, i.e., interventions in these aspects may have favorable impacts not only in movement but even in cognitive rehabilitation techniques (Schmahmann et al., 2019). Lastly, the cerebral cortex, consisting of the frontal, parietal, temporal, and occipital lobes, plays an important role in processing sensory information, sustaining executive function, and allowing linguistic function. These regions collaborate to enable higher-level behavior in the form of problem-solving, decision-making, and social interaction. Damage to any one region can result in particular neurological disorders, making precise diagnostic workups imperative in clinical practice. As an example, left temporal lobe lesions can result in language production or reception deficits with symptoms requiring specific therapeutic treatments. Understanding the diverse functions of such essential brain structures simplifies adopting a more complex approach to rehabilitation interventions in physiotherapy, actually promoting better patient outcomes as part of the bigger picture of neurological rehabilitation (Schmahmann et al., 2019) (Figure 13.4).

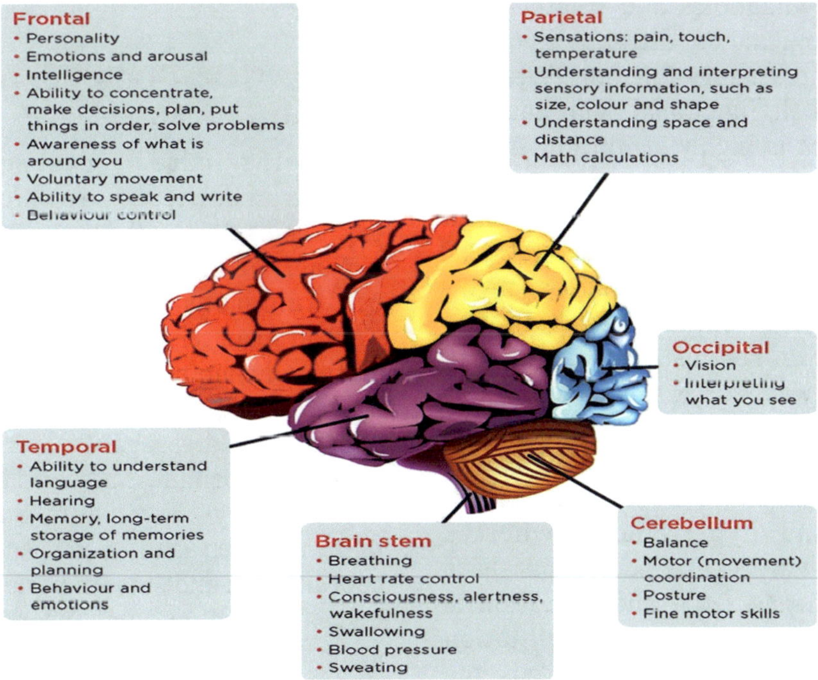

Figure 13.4. Regions of the brain and their function.

Source: https://biofeedback-neurofeedback-therapy.com/wp-content/uploads/Brain-regions-and-function.jpg.

13.1.2. Spinal Cord Anatomy and Function

The anatomical complexity of structures within the spinal cord plays a pivotal function in facilitating nervous system function as well as body homeostasis. The spinal cord, a critical component of the central nervous system (CNS), is composed of segments parallel to the vertebral column and each segment arises to become spinal nerves serving distinct parts of the body. This mechanism allows sensory input to shift from peripheral nerves into the spinal cord, where it is processed prior to being transmitted to the brain. Additionally, the spinal cord consists of both upper motor neurons (UMNs) and lower motor neurons (LMNs) necessary for voluntary movement. Damage to these pathways may result in extreme motor disability, manifesting in weakness or paralysis, depending on damage location and extent. Thus, learning the spinal cord anatomy is crucial in the diagnosis and treatment of various neurological conditions involving motor control and sensory function (Welch et al., 2020). Above all, functional neuroanatomy of the spinal cord is highly significant from a clinical perspective, especially in physiotherapy. Rehabilitation and management of neurological conditions such as spinal cord injury (SCI) or multiple sclerosis (MS) are based on an in-depth knowledge of spinal cord pathways and their functions. For instance, variation in presentation between UMN and LMN lesions should be familiar to physiotherapists, as this will determine therapeutic interventions and influence prognoses. UMN lesions can contribute to spasticity and hyperreflexia, whereas LMN lesions usually cause flaccid paralysis and reduced reflexes. Such differentiation is imperative when developing rehabilitation plans intended to promote neuroplasticity, the brains ability to modify itself in reaction to disease or injury. This malleability underlies numerous therapy practices employed in the management of diseases of the spinal cord and related motor tracts (McCoyd et al., 2019). A thorough understanding of spinal cord anatomy not only aids in neurological disease diagnosis, but it also allows healthcare professionals to construct effective rehabilitation strategies that utilize neuroplasticity. Conditions like Parkinson's disease and cerebral palsy possess specific complexities that are dependent on the underlying spinal cord anatomy and their relationship with the motor cortex and peripheral nervous system. Rehabilitative interventions must be crafted to account for these anatomical connections in order to facilitate optimal recovery. By applying principles of neuroplasticity, patients are often able to regain lost function or learn to compensate for loss, illustrating the ability of the nervous system to adapt. Such information also highlights the importance of interdisciplinary care between neurologists, physiotherapists, and occupational therapists to optimize patient outcomes through evidence-based practice (Welch et al., 2020).

13.1.3. Neurotransmitters and Their Role in Movement

The intricate interaction among neurotransmitters and movement is an expression of underlying neuroanatomical principles and is central to the understanding of numerous neurological disorders. Neurotransmitters like dopamine, acetylcholine, and gamma-aminobutyric acid (GABA) are crucial in mediating motor control so that neurons can convey messages to target tissues. For instance, dopamine is involved in the modulation of voluntary movements and functions in pathways such as the basal ganglia that regulate coordination and smooth performance of motor tasks. Dopamine signaling perturbations can generate clinical features of neurological disease, such as Parkinson's disease, where dopamine deficiency causes motor features such as tremor, rigidity, and bradykinesia. Thus, comprehending the mechanism of neurotransmitters is at the heart of exploring therapies for restoring movement in patients afflicted by such a disruption. Moreover, neurotransmitter disorders are driven by a myriad of causes, like genetic mutations affecting the synthesis or movement of these critical molecules. DTDS is a clear demonstration of how a mutation in the SLC6A3 gene leads to reduced reuptake of dopamine and ultimately to drastic motor and psychiatric dysfunction. It is a prototype for the complex interplay between neurotransmitter dysfunction and motor dysfunction, so that therapeutic targeting is a requirement. In addition, certain neurotransmitters are not observers; they have an active role in synaptic plasticity, which modifies synaptic strength, a learning prerequisite for motor habits. A comprehension of such mechanisms is fundamental to designing effective rehabilitation methods that implement neuroplasticity to enhance movement recovery in neurological-disordered patients, thereby highlighting the importance of customized physiotherapy approaches.

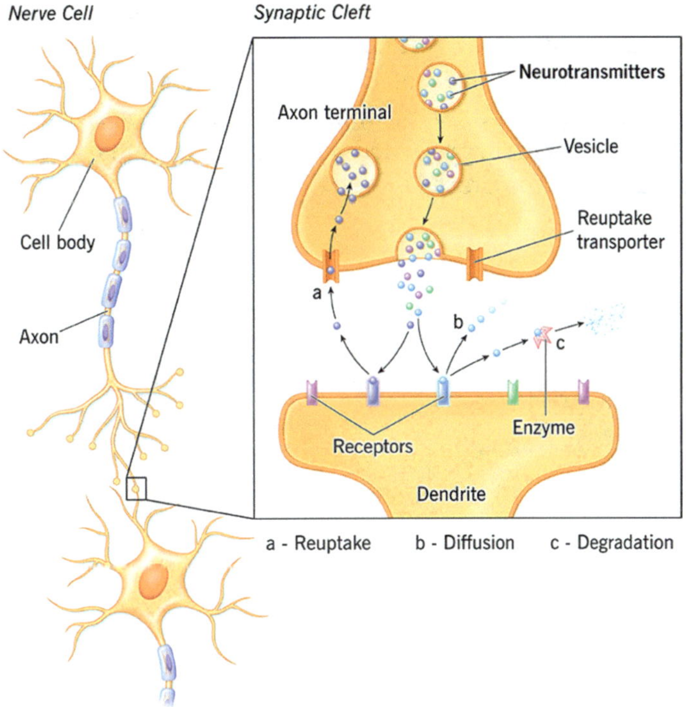

Figure 13.5. Neurotransmitters and their functions.

Source: https://my.clevelandclinic.org/-/scassets/images/org/health/articles/22513-neurotransmitters.

The role of neurotransmitters in movement is more than simple communication between neurons; it is complex biological mechanisms that have to be entered by many proteins and factors. The N-ethylmaleimide-sensitive factor (NSF) plays a key role in synaptic function, a function that aids synaptic vesicle cycling required for the release of neurotransmitters. NSF's interaction with SNARE proteins suggests its pivotal role in exocytosis and endocytosis, processes that are fundamental in neurotransmitter dynamics in synapses. Defining these interactions is of significance since NSF aberrations have been associated with diseases such as Alzheimer's disease and Parkinson's disease, where movement and cognition are seriously impaired. In this case, investigating the mechanistic activities of NSF may open up new therapeutic avenues for addressing the underlying cause of neurotransmitter-associated disorders. By recognizing these mechanisms, more effective measures can be devised to reverse the functional consequences of impaired neurotransmission and enhance rehabilitation success for those affected (Figure 13.5).

13.2. Common Neurological Conditions

The effects of common neurological disorders vary from a broad range, affecting individuals' functional ability and overall quality of life. Stroke represents one of the leading causes of long-term impairment globally. It occurs when the flow of blood to a portion of the brain is interrupted, leading to neuronal damage and ultimate functional impairment. The patients may present with varied symptoms depending on the area of the brain involved, including impairment of motor function, speech, and cognitive dysfunction. Clinical presentation is classified into upper motor neuron (UMN) and lower motor neuron (LMN) lesions, which aids in determining the type and extent of rehabilitation to be administered.

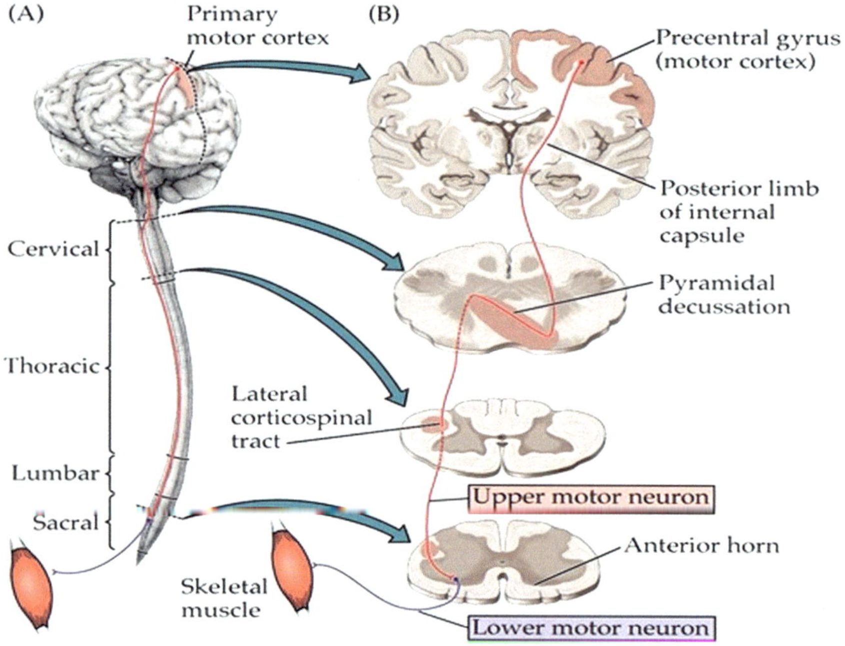

Figure 13.6. Upper-lower-motor-neuron-lesions.

Source: https://www.howtorelief.com/wp-content/uploads/2017/07/upper-lower-motor-neuron-lesions.jpg.

Understanding the neuroanatomy underpinning such conditions is crucial for physiotherapists, who play a critical role within the rehabilitation process, employing targeted strategies that facilitate neuroplasticity and recovery. Multiple sclerosis (MS) is another prevalent neurological disorder linked with autoimmune-mediated demyelination of the central nervous system. MS symptoms can be extremely heterogeneous, ranging from sensory impairment to motor deficit and cognitive impairment, consistent with its unpredictable nature. Patients typically experience exacerbation and remission phases, making them problematic to treat. Neuroanatomically, the damage is primarily in white matter pathways and impairs communication between various regions of the brain. Understanding MS pathophysiology is necessary for therapeutic intervention development, particularly with increasing interest in the role of the microbiota-gut-brain axis in shaping the immune response and inflammation. This also encompasses understanding the manner in which microbial metabolites can affect neuroinflammation and potentially influence disease course, an area which continues to be extremely significant in current research (Cryan et al., 2019). Within the framework of neurodegenerative disease, Parkinson's disease is an excellent example of the important role that progressive degeneration of specific neuronal subpopulations plays in affecting motor function and daily living. The hallmark of Parkinson's is the degeneration of dopaminergic cells in the substantia nigra, causing characteristic clinical features of tremor, rigidity, and bradykinesia. There are also cognitive impairments that arise in advanced disease but are underreported in early detection. The symptomatology has been categorized into UMN and LMN lesions, and this allows for more personalized treatment of specific impairments. Research into the pathophysiological mechanisms of Parkinson's has expanded to include potential biomarkers of disease progression, the role of neuroanatomical and clinical measurements in the guidance of treatment (Marshall et al., 2018). An extensive understanding of these common neurological diseases, rooted in neuroanatomy, is thus essential to effective clinical practice (Figure 13.6).

13.2.1. Stroke: Types and Impact

An awareness of the intricacy of neurological diseases means it is critical to learn closely how different types of strokes develop and affect patients subsequently. Strokes can be categorized into ischemic and hemorrhagic types, each having special challenges and aftereffects. Ischemic strokes due to occlusion of vessels typically result in immediate death of brain cells due to a lack of oxygen and nutrients. Conversely, bleeding strokes occur as a consequence of a ruptured blood vessel leading to bleeding within or around the brain. The brain's reaction to such sudden events is largely a function of the areas and severity of the insult. Thus, the severity of functional impairment, ranging from locomotion to mental impairments, is a function of stroke type and area of brain damage. The interplay of these factors is complex and suggests the need for considering each of the different stroke types in the context of general neurological wellness. Stroke impacts extend far beyond acute health issues, substantially affecting the patient's life as well as that of his or her caretaker. Patients who are affected by a stroke may have an avalanche of physical and emotional sequelae that ensue, such as paralysis and speech difficulty, as well as emotional sequelae such as depression and anxiety. These are usually the result of disrupted neural networks that are irreversibly altered in the course of the stroke event, initiating big neuroplastic changes within the brain. Rehabilitation is not an easy process since it's not only a physiological process of recovery but also psychological support to address the multi-dimensional effects of a stroke. Knowledge of these effects, particularly in a medical setting, is of great significance to medical practitioners, such as physiotherapists, who play a crucial role in the rehabilitation and enhancement of quality of life among stroke survivors. The integration of advanced neuroanatomical information into the treatment of stroke patients emphasizes the need for an understanding of the biological processes at stake. This is illustrated, for instance, by the duplicated representation of motor abilities within the cerebellum, which involves complex neural gradients so that stroke victims may require varying levels of rehabilitation based on areas of their brain affected (Guell et al., 2018). Apart from that, the interaction between the nervous system and immune functions shows that stroke may not only damage neuronal function but also influence systemic immune processes, and this could further worsen effects on recovery (Pavlov et al., 2018). This novel information highlights the importance of developing goal-directed interventions in individualized patient profiles and guides new therapeutic approaches, emphasizing that a nuanced appreciation of neuroanatomy and its cross-talk with stroke recovery can drive more effective rehabilitation strategies in the context of neurological disease.

13.2.2. Spinal Cord Injury (SCI): Causes and Consequences

The multi-dimensional nature of spinal cord injury (SCI) encompasses a vast range of etiologies and vast impacts that affect individual lives as well as healthcare systems. Traumatic causes such as motor vehicle accidents, falls, and sports injuries are among the leading causes of SCI. Non-traumatic causes, including diseases like multiple sclerosis or tumors, are also relevant. Interestingly, the effects of SCI reach further than the direct physical trauma caused by the event. The resulting compromise of the central nervous system can have a ripple effect, creating a cascade of secondary complications, including chronic pain, spasticity, and autonomic dysfunction, making patient rehabilitation even more challenging. Understanding of the processes by which these injuries are established and subsequently affect body function positions clinicians for improved therapeutic management and underscores the demands for ongoing research in these central areas. Study of SCI consequences illustrates far-reaching influence upon physical and psychosocial health. The sensory and motor impairments that result from spinal cord injury can result in great limitation in mobility and activities of daily living, typically rendering them more dependent on caregivers and healthcare services. Moreover, the patient will find it difficult to handle emotional and psychological challenges like depression and anxiety as they live with a severe disability. These psychosocial variables need to be addressed through a multidisciplinary treatment, and not only are the physiological symptoms addressed, but also the emotional and social effects of SCI. Rehabilitation therapists need to integrate concepts of neuroplasticity into treatment environments, employing adaptive procedures to capitalize on the brain's ability to reorganize and compensate for lost function in order to maximize overall quality of life for individuals with SCI.

The neuroanatomical contribution to the understanding of spinal cord injury highlights central and peripheral nervous system interaction during rehabilitation. Functional neuroanatomy adds clarity to the clinician's grasp of how injury at different levels of the spinal cord can lead to either upper motor neuron (UMN) or lower motor neuron (LMN) lesions, both with different signs and symptoms, guiding diagnosis and treatment. Clinicians would be able to use the understanding of these differences to tailor rehabilitation programs aimed at neuroplasticity and functional gains. For instance, the application of targeted treatments can effectively manage spasticity from UMN lesions or muscle atrophy from LMN lesions (Pöyhönen et al., 2019). These findings into patient presentation subsequently mean more personalized and effective therapy interventions in the area of neurological rehabilitation (Schmahmann et al., 2019) (Figure 13.7).

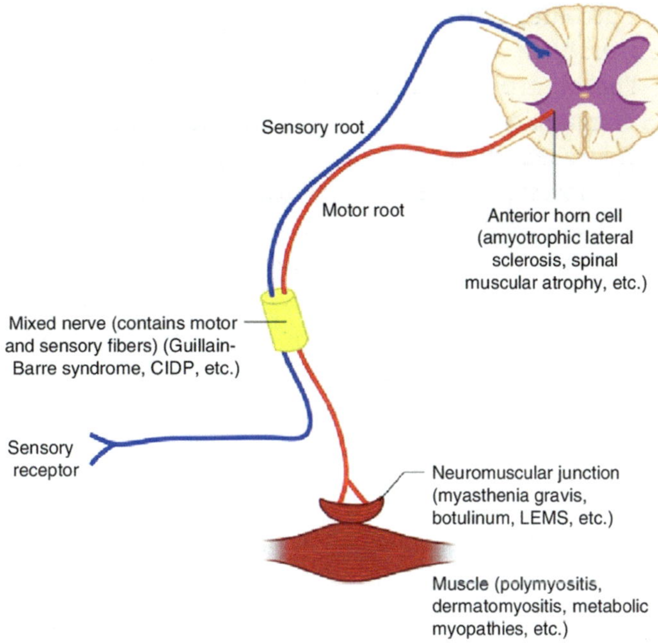

Figure 13.7. Lower motor neuron injury.

Source: https://www.researchgate.net/profile/Hani-Almoallim/publication/348257338/figure/fig1/AS:977973867982848@1610178548057/The-four-anatomic-stations-underlying-lower-motor-neuron-weakness.png.

13.2.3. Multiple Sclerosis (MS): Symptoms and Management

Multiple Sclerosis (MS) is a multifaceted presentation with a variety of symptoms in the range, which vary significantly from person to person, hence making it challenging to diagnose and manage. Neurological symptoms are primarily due to demyelination of central and peripheral nervous system neurons, thereby resulting in a multitude of challenges in the form of visual disturbances to motor disability, sensory impairment, etc. Fatigue, cognitive impairment, depression, and pain are particularly prevalent, with the co-occurrence of these symptoms suggesting shared underlying biological substrates. These entail modifications of the brain and related structures at a neuroanatomical level, and hence healthcare practitioners must be well versed in functional neuroanatomy relevant to MS so that they may design appropriate physiotherapy and management protocols suitable for their patients, including both physical and psychological features of this disease (Chitnis et al., 2022). MS must be treated with multi-modal intervention involving pharmacological as well as non-pharmacological interventions. Disease-modifying treatments seek to reduce the frequency and severity of relapses by acting on the immune system and reducing inflammation, thereby preventing further damage to neurons. In addition to medication, rehabilitative efforts are also a key part, including physiotherapy for enhancing movement and functional daily abilities. Cognitive behavioral therapy (CBT) is also useful in reducing associated symptoms such as depression and anxiety, thereby improving overall quality of life. Aside from this, additional evidence favors lifestyle change as a means of alleviating fatigue and enhancing neurological function through exercise and nutrition. Understanding the complementary approach to treating MS is necessary for contributing to better outcomes in patients with this disabling neurological condition (Chitnis et al., 2022). The neurobiological interaction underlying MS complexity resonates with the need for holistic research in this endeavor. As observed, pathological processes underlying fatigue, cognitive impairment, and mood disorders are often found to originate from shared biological mechanisms such as neuroanatomical change and pro-inflammatory cytokine release. These findings not only shed light on MS pathophysiology but also emphasize the necessity for a multifactorial treatment strategy. Investigations of these correlated symptoms can lead to new treatment strategies that address MS in an integrative way, hopefully discovering common pathways to therapy. Advancement toward elucidating MS through these neuroanatomy and neurobiology insights may ultimately translate into treatment strategies, setting the stage for improved management of both the physiological and psychological features of the disease that patients encounter (Chitnis et al., 2022).

13.3. Other Neurological Disorders

The multifaceted nature of neurological illness encompasses a wide variety of illnesses beyond the well-known sickness. Among them, illnesses such as autism spectrum disorder, schizophrenia, and Alzheimer's disease illustrate the complexity of neurodevelopmental and neurodegenerative diseases. Research continues to disclose the interplay of genetic risk factors and environmental forces in regards to these diseases. For instance, the gut-brain axis has emerged as a field of study, connecting the gut microbiota to brain function and behavior. With recent studies revealing that disturbances of the axis may play a role in the causation of various neurological disorders, the significance of an exhaustive understanding of neuroanatomy and physiology as it pertains to such complex associations has become apparent (Cryan et al., 2019). By considering both neuroanatomical and psychosocial factors, clinicians are better able to address the individualized states of patients with these diverse disorders. Understanding of complexity of other neurological disorders relies on consideration of epigenetic factors and their effects on intergenerational transmission of trauma. According to the described research, prenatal maternal stress can cause extreme alterations in the offspring's neurology due to epigenetic programming (Yehuda et al., 2018). The effects can be manifested in the form of behavioral disorders as well as cognitive impairments, which can lead to more severe neurologic disorders during adulthood. Significantly, such epigenetic changes can be carried forward through generations, evidence of the profound influence of early environmental experiences on brain physiology. The interplay between genetics and environmental pressures offers a window of opportunity for forthcoming studies directed towards therapeutic intervention and prevention procedures, thereby highlighting both the significance of neuroanatomy and the possibility of neuroplastic adjustment in the instance of such disorders. The implications of the other neurological disorders extend to rehabilitation, particularly for physiotherapy treatment. Neuroplasticity is central to understanding how the central and peripheral nervous systems can reorganize following injury or neurological impairment. For example, certain rehabilitation treatments may improve recovery through the strengthening of new neural pathways and compensation. With traumatic brain injuries and spinal cord injuries, neuroplasticity concepts allow physiotherapists to access the brain's natural ability to reorganize and adapt. In addition, working with disorders like multiple sclerosis and Parkinson's disease requires an individualized approach to physiotherapy with close attention to the unique symptoms and functional impairment resulting from the engagement of the upper motor neurons

(UMNs) and lower motor neurons (LMNs). With the integrated combination of knowledge of neuroanatomy, history of the patient, and ongoing research in other neurological illnesses, physiotherapy can help the healing process of the sufferer to a great extent (Figure 13.8).

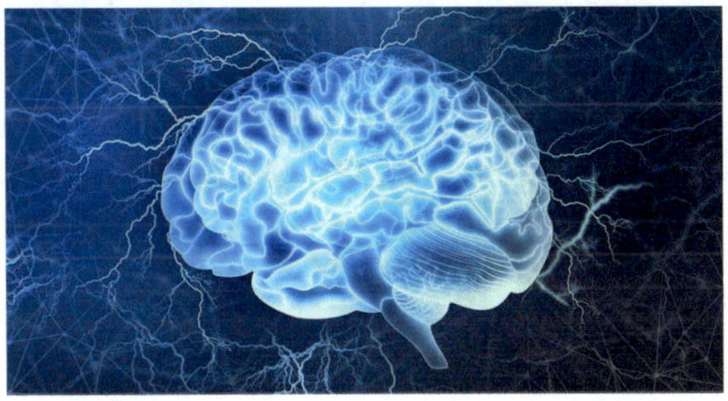

Figure 13.8. The intricate nature of neurological disorders.

Source: https://external-content.duckduckgo.com/iu/?u=https%3A%2F%2Fregionalneurological.com%2Fwp-content%2Fuploads%2F2019%2F11%2FAdobeStock_172813720.jpeg&f=1&nofb=1&ipt=2e53207fa54aad11117a49bcb742f87d960372ba55d38755cb0de2202bbff164.

13.3.1. Cerebral Palsy (CP): Overview and Treatment

The very intricate spinal cord and brain architecture is at the root of both causes and management of neurological disorders, such as Cerebral Palsy (CP). CP, a group of disorders that impact posture and movement, results from abnormal brain or central nervous system damage during fetal development or early infancy. The functional neuroanatomy of CP is of considerable importance for effective treatment planning. Practitioners ought to be able to grasp the fact that impairments of balance, coordination, and motor control are generally manifestations of occult neurological breaks, which can result in lesions of the upper motor neuron (UMN). These features of CP necessitate combined clinical assessment and customized rehabilitation protocols based on each patient's unique requirements and degree of condition, eventually highlighting the importance of having a complete grasp of neuroanatomy for the development of the best treatment regimens. Management of the issues of CP is carried out through a multidisciplinary approach, which includes therapeutic interventions and assistive equipment. Physiotherapy is one of the essential elements used in the treatment of patients with CP and is founded on the principles of neuroplasticity, which are dependent on the capacity of the brain to reorganize itself following injury and experience. Treatments are directed towards enhancing motor capacity, strength, and coordination and diminishing spasticity and symptomatic manifestations. Through various techniques such as targeted exercises, gait training, and hydrotherapy, the physiotherapists try to achieve enhanced functional mobility and overall well-being for the patients. Also, the addition of newer forms of treatments like robotic-assisted therapy and neuromuscular electrical stimulation reflects the dynamicity of CP rehabilitation practice with a constantly shifting theme of treatment options blending traditional and modern approaches. Emerging technology, for example, silent speech interfaces (SSIs), is promising advances in the enhancement of speech for people with severe speech disorders, often linked with CP. SSIs use non-acoustic biosignals to detect silenced speech intentions, providing a valuable additional mode of communication for individuals with barriers posed by their condition. The potential of these innovations calls for cooperation among clinicians, researchers, and technologists in designing feasible solutions that meet the unique requirements of individuals with CP. Ultimately, the increasingly accepted dynamic interplay between neuroanatomy and therapeutic modalities is a paradigm shift in how healthcare professionals will approach rehabilitation, focusing on individualized, evidence-based interventions that harness the latest technology and neuroplasticity research (Figure 13.9).

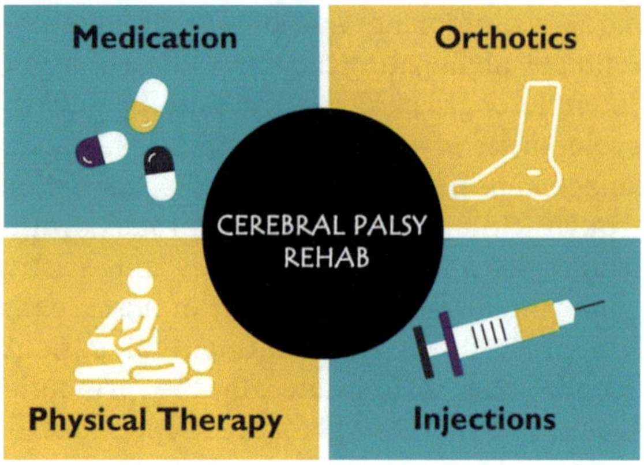

Figure 13.9. Cerebral palsy.

Source: https://external-content.duckduckgo.com/iu/?u=https%3A%2F%2Ftse2.mm.bing.net%2Fth%3Fid%3DOIP.oyLW28hjAKFlUP-WdDLc3gHaFG%26r%3D0%26pid%3DApi&f=1&ipt=660eeb22aedf65b1a37f0a14e9034beadb5a6aa7a5f0098ac8a85aec83c96c5c.

13.3.2. Parkinson's Disease: Pathophysiology and Symptoms

The intricate relationship between the central and peripheral nervous systems is critical in the diagnosis of such ailments as Parkinsons Disease (PD). As a neurodegenerative condition, PD primarily affects the substantia nigra, which is a region within the brain that has the function of synthesizing dopamine. This specific degeneration corresponds to a tremendous reduction in the balance of neurotransmitters that reaches its peak in quintessential symptoms such as bradykinesia, rigidity, and tremors. The pathophysiology of PD is characterized by Lewy bodies, which are the abnormal protein aggregates that disrupt the normal functioning of neurons. The progressive nature of this disease underscores the necessity of careful evaluation for the victims, most particularly in diagnosing and treating initial signs and symptoms. It is crucial to understand the neuroanatomical consequences not only for clinical evaluation but also for the establishment of useful therapeutic interventions that are patient-specific. As Parkinson's Disease progresses, it manifests a varied array of symptoms in addition to the motor impairments commonly seen in the disorder. Cognitive deficit, mood disorder, and disturbances of sleep are frequently underrated features of PD, particularly because they can greatly affect patients' quality of life. There has been new evidence of high rates of neuropsychiatric symptoms and sleep-wake disturbances in PD patients, which result in excessive daytime sleepiness and nocturnal sleep fragmentation. The effects result from pathophysiologic alterations of neurotransmitter systems other than dopaminergic ones, for example, serotonin and noradrenaline.

Understanding these multifaceted symptoms requires a multidimensional approach that respects both the neurologic and the psychosocial dimensions, leading towards a comprehensive management plan and research towards mechanistic-targeted therapies that can enhance such non-motor symptoms. Also, the exploration of sex differences in the expression and progression of Parkinson's disease brings one more new aspect into the understanding of this disease. Research has revealed that there are certain neuroanatomical and neurochemical differences on the basis of hormone-dependent factors, which can have dissimilar effects on disease course and expression in men and women. These sex differences should be recognized because they can also influence the efficacy of treatments as well as the development of treatment-specific interventions. For instance, the sex difference in symptomatology necessitates dissimilar clinical approaches in monitoring PD and treating it. The recognition of sex as an intrinsic variable for use in research and in clinical practice can promote more targeted treatments that are attuned to biological and psychosocial impacts, ultimately providing a greater understanding of Parkinson's disease and improved clinical outcomes (Zagni et al., 2016).

13.3.3. Epilepsy: Types and Treatment Options

Central and peripheral nervous system complexities are of primary concern in the understanding of neurological diseases such as epilepsy. This is a disease brought about by abnormal neuronal activity, leading to recurrent seizures that have immense life-quality implications for an individual. Triggered in various forms, epileptic seizures are mostly graded as focal and generalized. Focal seizures start in one region of the brain, with generalized seizures occurring in both hemispheres. Detection of these differences is essential for adequate planning of therapy. More sophisticated neuroimaging techniques, such as the application of 7 T MRI, enable doctors to visualize abnormalities in brain structure and function, which enables accurate classification and diagnosis of epilepsy, ultimately causing enhanced patient outcomes (de Vries et al., 2025).

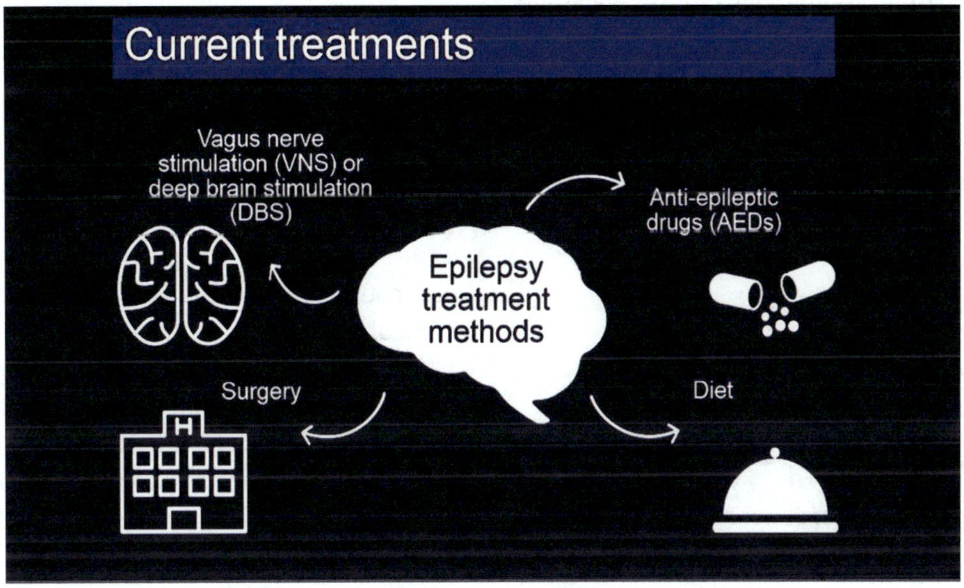

Figure 13.10. Epilepsy – seizure types, symptoms and treatment.

Source: https://i.ytimg.com/vi/UFlw89Sudec/maxresdefault.jpg.

An in-depth understanding of functional neuroanatomy is critical to delineate the networks involved in seizure generation and propagation. Management of epilepsy is complex and must be personalized for the type of seizure and etiology. Currently, more than 30 antiepileptic drugs have been approved by the U.S. FDA, with a wide range of pharmacologic therapeutic options. However, approximately one-quarter of individuals with epilepsy remain refractory to these medications, providing a significant challenge to treatment (Waris et al., 2024). This resistance then precludes other forms of treatment, including diet, neuromodulation techniques, and even surgery in refractory cases. Furthermore, there has been an emerging body of research investigating the use of herbal medicine as a therapeutic agent, wherein multiple plant extracts show potent anticonvulsant activity. These choices underscore the necessity of an inclusive system for controlling epilepsy, particularly in low and middle-income countries where access to standard treatments is generally still restricted. Research further illuminates the multifactorial pathogenesis of epilepsy, emphasizing that management approaches must address not merely the phenomena of the seizures but also the underlying disease biology. The potential of neuroplasticity—the capacity of the brain to reorganize itself functionally and structurally—opens a promising path for new treatment modalities. It is important to explore how various therapies can tap into the brains natural ability to change, which could lead to enhanced functional restoration and seizure reduction. Enlarging the horizons of epilepsy treatment, the combination of traditional treatments with systemic plant therapies could be targeted at several pathways of convulsive activity (Waris et al., 2024). While more is learned, the interaction between traditional and emerging interventions could propel towards more effective and complete management of epilepsy in neurological disease (Figure 13.10).

13.4. Signs and Symptoms of Neurological Disorders

The clinical presentation of neurological disorders is diverse and representative of extensive clinical presentations, with the utmost significance being to establish the neuroanatomical impairment underlying these. The patient may present with loss of motor, sensory, or cognitive functions that signify the manifestation of a malfunction of the central nervous system (CNS) or peripheral nervous system (PNS). Motor signs tend to indicate upper motor neuron (UMN) lesions with spasticity, hyperreflexia, and weakness most often, while lower motor neuron (LMN) lesions would more likely cause flaccid paralysis, atrophy, and decreased reflexes. Further, sensory disturbances such as paresthesia, loss of proprioception, or acute pain might indicate pathological processes affecting peripheral nerves, such as multiple sclerosis or diabetic neuropathy. Proper knowledge of these symptoms and signs is mandatory for accurate diagnosis and successful intervention practices in therapeutic settings. An early detection of neurological symptoms plays a substantial role in managing diseases such as stroke or Parkinson's disease. For instance, a stroke may suddenly appear in association with unilateral weakness, speech disorder, or change of vision. Recognition of these signs in time can go a long way in the outcomes, as early medical treatment can minimize brain damage and increase chances of recovery. On the other hand, long-term conditions like Parkinson's take their toll over time, beginning with tiny alterations in walking, tremors, or muscle stiffness.

Then patients experience loss of fine movements and cognitive functions, for which compensatory skills to carry out daily tasks become necessary. These symptoms are directly associated with specific neuroanatomical changes, illustrating the utility of the incorporation of functional neuroanatomy in clinical assessment and rehabilitation methods utilized to manage neurological patients. Proof has indicated that patterns of growth in the brain may be useful in describing signs and symptoms of neurological illness. To illustrate, neuroanatomical abnormality in patterns of brain growth has been detected in autistic children, as confirmed by longitudinal MRI research. Results indicate that gray and white matter growth continues at a heightened rate in affected toddlers, particularly in key brain regions such as the frontal and temporal cortices. In addition to being a window of understanding into the neural underpinnings of autism, this abnormal course also points to the clinician's utility in monitoring neurodevelopmental milestones. This data is important for clinicians interested in applying neuroplasticity principles, as detection of the signs and symptoms early on can permit intervention based on the brain's potential to adapt and heal, leading to better patient outcomes in neurological rehabilitation (Schumann et al., 2010) (Figure 13.11).

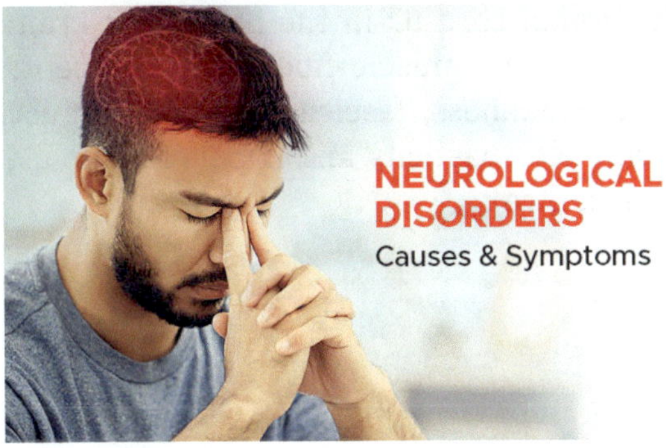

Figure 13.11. Common neurological disorders: causes & symptoms.

Source: https://external-content.duckduckgo.com/iu/?u=https%3A%2F%2Fpsrihospital.com%2Fwp-content%2Fuploads%2F2023%2F10%2FPSRI-Blog-banner-2.jpg&f=1&nofb=1&ipt=77e5b243be6a83c1c3e04afd51dbf7ac06669272b13f528fc238e3f68c6cf80c.

13.4.1. Upper Motor Neuron (UMN) Lesions: Characteristics

In the complex interplay between the central and the peripheral nervous systems, UMN lesions are of particular interest in the investigation of numerous neurological disorders. Described as damage to the corticospinal tracts within the central nervous system, UMN lesions tend to have definite clinical features that differentiate them from LMN lesions. The characteristic presentation of UMN lesions involves increased muscle tone, hyperreflexia, and the development of pathological reflexes such as the Babinski sign. These signs appear due to the disruption of descending motor tracts that play a role in modulating voluntary movement. The knowledge of these features is important to clinicians as it is the basis for treatment and rehabilitation, particularly in conditions like stroke and multiple sclerosis, in which UMN lesions are the common finding. UMN lesions have implications beyond their simple clinical presentation; they play an important role in affecting the motor function and quality of life of the patient. There can be spasticity, which is a pathological increase in muscle tone leading to rigidity and automatic contractions. Rehabilitation is made difficult by the spasticity, and functional activities of daily living are challenging. Hyperreflexia, or exaggerated reflex responses, can be a symptom and also a barrier to functional recovery since one cannot coordinate movements. The awareness of the aforementioned characteristics and their contribution to motor control is key to the design of effective physiotherapeutic interventions and emphasizes the necessity of specially targeted therapy exercises for both strength and flexibility to overcome the functional impairments of UMN lesions. Additionally, neuroplasticity explains recovery from UMN lesions, which highlights the central nervous system's ability to reorganize and adapt following injury. Even though upper motor neuron damage initially lowers motor function, the process of neuroplasticity offers hope for rehabilitation. With repetitive task-specific training, new circuits for motor function and partial restoration of lost functions can be attained. The integration of the principles of neuroplasticity into rehabilitation therapy is essential in order to optimize the outcome of patients. Interventions that encourage neuroplastic changes have the potential to result in improved motor control and increased independence of patients with UMN lesions. Similarly, familiarity with the characteristics of these lesions not only helps in proper diagnosis but also directs the techniques employed in treatment procedures aimed at modulating neuroplasticity and aiding recovery of function in neurological patients.

13.4.2. Lower Motor Neuron (LMN) Lesions: Characteristics

It is important to know Lower Motor Neuron (LMN) lesions in the differential diagnosis of various neurological disorders, especially in the context of their significance in clinical practice and rehabilitation. LMN lesions are due to damage to motor neurons in the anterior horn of the spinal cord or in the brainstem cranial nerve nuclei. This lesion impairs the communication between the muscle fibers and the central nervous system, yielding characteristic symptoms such as weakness, fasciculations, and muscle atrophy. Unlike Upper Motor Neuron (UMN) lesions, which yield spasticity and hyperreflexia, LMN lesions result in flaccid paralysis due to the loss of motor control.

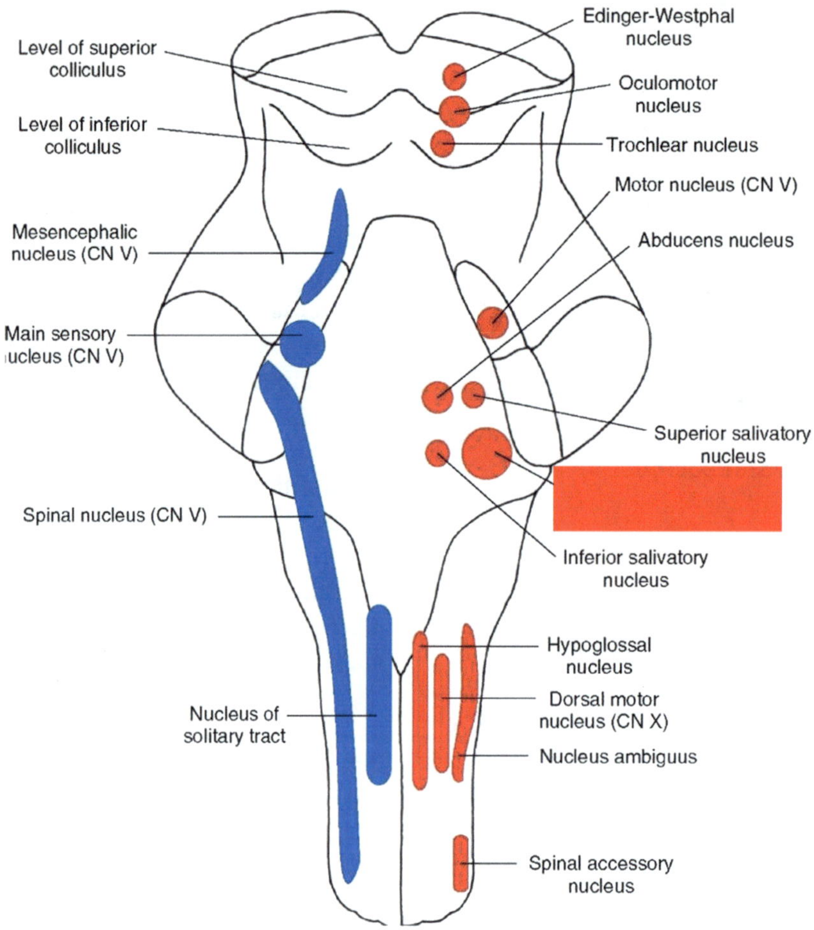

Figure 13.12. Cranial nerves, brainstem, dorsal

Source: http://humanphysiology.academy/Neurosciences%202015/Images/3/cranial%20nerve%20 nuclei.jpg.

These distinctive signs profoundly redefine management planning in diseases such as amyotrophic lateral sclerosis (ALS) and polio, where LMN signs predominance necessitates specially tailored physiotherapy interventions to optimize patient outcomes. Physicians must rely heavily on a thorough neurological examination that incorporates history-taking and physical examination in diagnosing LMN lesions. The neurological localization process is significant as it allows clinicians to accurately diagnose affected areas and predict functional impairment potentially secondary to LMN damage. The strength testing of muscles and reflex examination are valuable components that make up this evaluation. The variance in LMN and UMN lesions determines treatment strategies because LMN lesions are likely to call for careful observance of the accumulation and adaptation mechanisms to reverse the ensuing functional impairment in patients. In addition, determination of the muscles affected and the neural pathways is critical. It directs decisions where rehabilitation programs are concerned and emphasizes utilization of neuroplasticity principles for enhancing motor recovery in affected patients (Roy, 2022). Moreover, understanding the underlying biological mechanisms that initiate and propagate LMN lesions can give clues to potential therapeutic lines of intervention. For instance, the promise of neuroinflammation's role in LMN diseases to suggest therapeutic approaches that may involve anti-inflammatory medications or nutritional chemicals, such as flavonoids, that have been shown to impact neuroprotection and degeneration prevention. Evidence confirms that these compounds have an impact on the pathways involved in oxidative stress and mitochondrial pathology, which is prevalent in conditions like ALS (Mhalhel et al., 2023). This kind of interaction of lesions in LMN with biochemical factors enables better insight into neuroanatomy and its application to therapeutic techniques in physiotherapy. Heightened sensitivity to these factors will not only direct clinical decisions but also optimize patient care in the expanding field of neurological rehabilitation (Figure 13.12).

13.4.3. Diagnostic Approaches for Neurological Symptoms

Within neurologic assessment, diagnostic procedures play a crucial role in efficiently detecting underlying conditions. The assessment of the central and peripheral nervous systems requires a comprehensive approach involving clinical assessments and advanced imaging modalities. Clinical assessments tend to rely on patients' medical history, neurological examination, and standardized rating scales for determining the occurrence of symptoms specific to conditions such as stroke, multiple sclerosis (MS), and Parkinson's disease. Neurologists may also utilize advanced neuroimaging methods such as magnetic resonance imaging (MRI) and computed tomography (CT) scans in an attempt to see brain anatomy and establish any pathological alterations. Imaging methods are crucial, particularly in the ability to differentiate between upper motor neuron (UMN) and lower motor neuron (LMN) lesions, as they will be better positioned to guide treatment and rehabilitative protocols. Other diagnostic innovations include both imaging and functional assessment, particularly for patients with dysphagia, increasingly recognized as a major challenge in older individuals. Application of clinical swallow tests and instrumental tools like video fluoroscopy and fiberoptic endoscopic evaluation of swallowing is reflective of the modern multi-phased approach to diagnosis. Despite being effective, conditions like oropharyngeal dysphagia often go undiagnosed, especially in the elderly, due to strained resources and awareness in health facilities. Awareness of the connection between neurological disease and dysphagia is necessary because untreated cases can lead to severe complications like aspiration pneumonia and malnutrition, exponentially escalating morbidity and mortality risk among vulnerable populations (Baijens et al., 2016). Thus, an effective diagnostic model that can handle these complexities is essential. The addition of new methods of diagnosis continues to transform the picture of neurological symptom assessment. Sex and gender differences, as a case in point, speak of differences in the presentation and progression of symptoms across populations, ending in the suggestion of personalized therapeutic and diagnostic approaches (Meng-Lai et al., 2014). Further, principles of neuroplasticity that develop are in favor of early and correct diagnosis, which can facilitate improved rehabilitation techniques following neurological trauma. With clinical professionals seeking to keep up with innovations, attention is necessary for rigorous screening protocols. Having such procedures in place ensures neurological signs are detected early on, and the optimal opportunity for recovery and quality of life for the patient is increased.

13.5. Principles of Neuroplasticity

The ability of the brain to reorganize itself due to injury, learning, or environmental changes is a staggering aspect of neurobiology known as neuroplasticity. It is particularly significant in the case of neurological diseases, where the central nervous system tries to compensate for lost functions. A good example of such a process is in patients with diffuse low-grade gliomas (DLGG), where even with the tumor present, the brain shows compensatory processes that reorganize the functional architecture over time. In a study of 101 patients with DLGG, direct electrostimulation mapping allowed researchers to document and study dynamic cortical reorganizations over the course of multiple surgeries, with areas like the dorsolateral prefrontal cortex and supplementary motor area showing particular promise for neuroplastic adaptation. This adaptability emphasizes the importance of understanding neuroplastic concepts in designing rehabilitation plans for patients with various neurological disorders, thereby enhancing the recovery chances (Ng et al., 2023). Besides this response to tangible damage, neuroplasticity is also crucial in the role that emotional and cognitive experiences can play in restructuring neural pathways. Positive affect has been shown to have a powerful influence on the processing of artistic concepts in the brain and, in turn, impacts significant areas of learning such as attention, memory, and motivation. From this observation, one would predict that artistic activity may cause neuroplastic changes conducive to cognitive processes in rehabilitation and recovery in neurological disorders. By embracing the principles of neurasthenics, professionals can incorporate therapeutic arts interventions into rehabilitation therapy, wherein clients can harness their affective experience to activate cognitive enhancement. This way, understanding the intricate interdependence between cognition and emotions enhances the treatment options for clients with neurological deficits, providing an integrated treatment approach (Halkiopoulos et al., 2023). Lastly, the principles of neuroplasticity reveal the brain's great power of adaptation as the basis for new therapeutic approaches in physiotherapy. In diseases such as stroke, spinal cord injury (SCI), and multiple sclerosis (MS), rehabilitation can be tailored to exploit neuroplastic mechanisms. With adequate stimulation and therapeutic engagement, potentiation of the pathways of neural networks can be employed for recovery and functional gain of motor functions and cognitive tasks. As highlighted by the DLGG study, the identification of high-potential neuroplastic regions in the brain offers an opportunity to apply rehabilitation interventions with targeted precision.

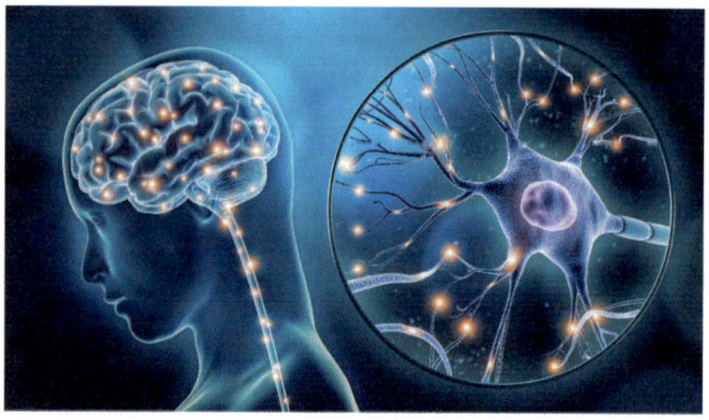

Figure 13.13. Principles of neuroplasticity.

Source: https://external-content.duckduckgo.com/iu/?u=https%3A%2F%2Fwww.lethealthbeyourguide.com%2Fwp-content%2Fuploads%2F2022%2F12%2FNeuroplasticity-Part-1.png&f=1&nofb=1&ipt=30abc85b3b3fdc3e9b928d3e31d9059c66fc7286814b6a0aa3597977bf01bc1a.

The research into neuroplasticity's underpinnings that continues to unfold is critical to advancing the treatment strategies of neurological disorders, not just to recover lost functions, but to enhance the quality of life in affected individuals as well (Figure 13.13).

13.5.1. Definition and Importance of Neuroplasticity

With respect to neuroanatomy and neurological disease, the process of neuroplasticity is arguably the most potent mechanism underlying the plasticity of the nervous system. This adaptability is not merely a theoretical construct but has very tangible implications for recovery and rehabilitation from neurological damage. Through the process of neuroplasticity, the brain can reorganize itself through the formation of new neural connections in response to experience, learning, and change in the environment. Such structural and functional changes are important in various stages of development and have future therapeutic potential in diseases such as stroke and spinal cord injury. With continuous studies on such adaptive plasticity, it is progressively becoming evident that neuroplasticity is very important in enhancing neurodevelopment and recovery, indicating its promise in therapeutic applications where restoration of function is the primary objective.

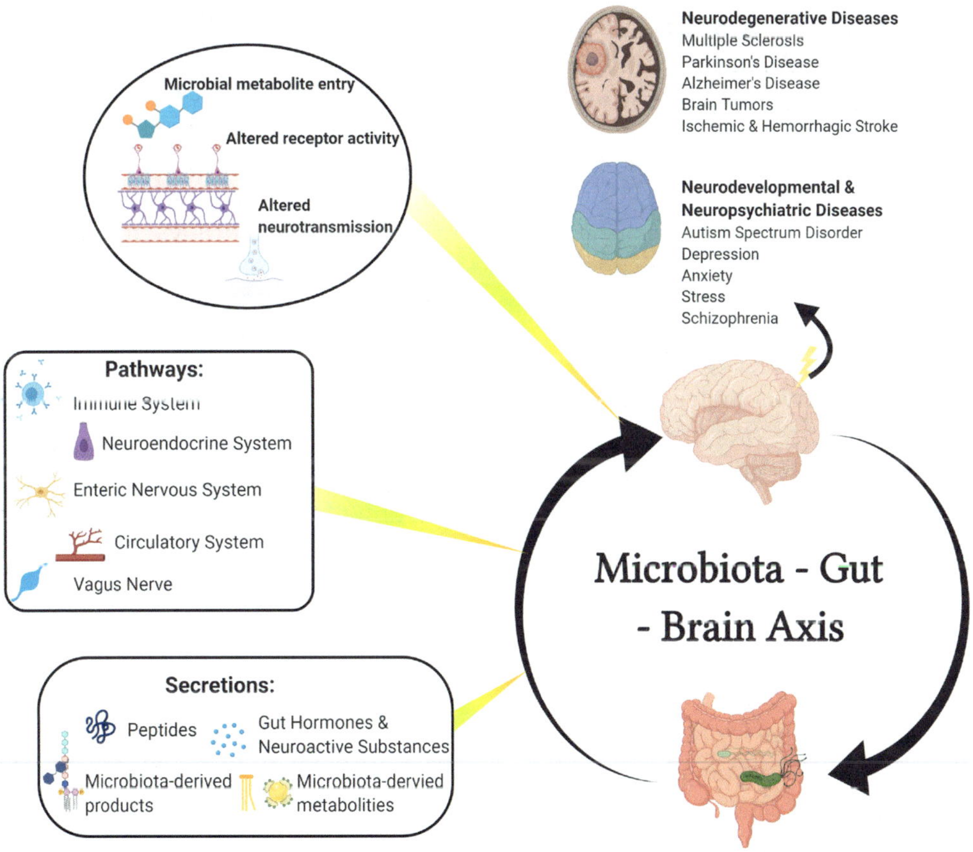

Figure 13.14. Microbiota and the gut-brain axis.

Source: https://www.thelancet.com/cms/attachment/ce443f82-cefe-4a35-a8ea-18a11bf34a5a/gr1_lrg.jpg.

The role of neuroplasticity is particularly evident when it comes to environmental determinants of brain function and development. Research indicates that enriched environments with provocative interaction and movement of the body can cause neuroplastic changes that not only facilitate normal neural development but also recovery from central nervous system damage. These findings demonstrate the dynamic interaction of extrinsic forces and intrinsic neuron readaptations, and a multifaceted relationship governing function throughout life. Additionally, different levels of development differ in their reaction to such external inputs, highlighting the role of timing in capitalizing on environmental gain for recovery. The ability of enriched environments to enhance learning and memory function ultimately contributes to a better appreciation of preventive and rehabilitative strategies in neuroanatomy, a topic deserving comprehensive study within the domain of neurological disorders (Han et al., 2022). In addition, neuroplasticity is increasingly defined in relation to the microbiota-gut-brain axis, and it provides a fresh frame of reference for understanding the association between physiological well-being and neural functioning. This new research direction recognizes how gut microbiota can influence brain physiology and behavior, and suggests that dietary interventions have the potential to influence brain health through neuroplastic mechanisms. Understanding these intricate relationships has significant future implications for the development of novel therapeutic strategies for the modulation of gut microbiota and neurological function. By doing so, it indicates the importance of a multidisciplinary approach with nutrition, environment, and neurological rehabilitation in optimizing brain recovery and development. As fields advance, future studies on neuroplasticity will enlighten us on pathways not only for the management of existing neurological disorders but also for enhancing overall cognitive wellness (Murciano-Brea et al., 2021) (Figure 13.14).

13.5.2. Mechanisms of Neuroplasticity in Recovery

The intricate arrangement of the nervous system, with its central and peripheral components, makes it remarkably flexible through neuroplasticity, particularly during recovery from disease or trauma. Neuroplasticity is the brain and nervous system's capacity to reorganize and generate new neural circuits as a result of experience, environment, or damage. This phenomenon can prove to be useful in rehabilitation following neurological disorders such as stroke and spinal cord injury (SCI), where damaged neural paths can often be supplemented or re-established. It can manifest as functional restoration of cortical maps or altered synaptic efficacies within the recovering nervous system, both of which enable the potential recovery of lost functions, thereby enhancing therapeutic advantages. These mechanisms highlight the significance of functional neuroanatomy in physiotherapy to allow the clinician to modify interventions that make use of these adaptive capabilities in an optimal way. The principles of neuroplasticity optimize the brain's incredible ability to reorganize itself structurally and functionally within a time frame. Factors that influence neuroplasticity are the nature of the injury, the age of the patient, and the dose and timing of rehabilitation therapy. For instance, in cerebral palsy (CP) or multiple sclerosis (MS), there are some neuroplastic issues that can be present. These could be demyelination or disruption in neural pathways, which makes recovery much more complex. Interventions like constraint-induced movement therapy and task-specific training are necessary to really employ neuroplastic mechanisms. These procedures provide not only extensive practice but also promote the participation of intact brain regions, activating neural circuit functions and even repairing defects, thereby consolidating the target process of functional recovery required for outcomes in patients. Current research into neural mechanisms has illuminated the participation of cranial nerve tracts and peripheral nervous system activation to improve neuroplasticity. New treatments such as cranial nerve stimulation offer new possibilities for improvement in cognitive and motor function by targeted neuromodulation. For instance, Adair et al. (2020) stress that these treatments drive axon pathway-specific brain networks involved in cognitive processing, which makes them relevant for recovery from neurological disorders. Also, procedures that have been obtained from traditional modalities, such as acupuncture, illustrate the body's intrinsic ability to trigger self-cures and restore homeostasis through regulated immune activities. Wang et al. (2023) believe that activation of acupoints could also cross-interact with neuroanatomical flows and hence augment neuroplastic responses. By the implementation of such diverse strategies, practitioners can leverage such mechanisms in a bid to create recovery and enhance rehabilitation outcomes for multiple neurological disorders, tending toward an overall and holistic recovery process (Figure 13.15).

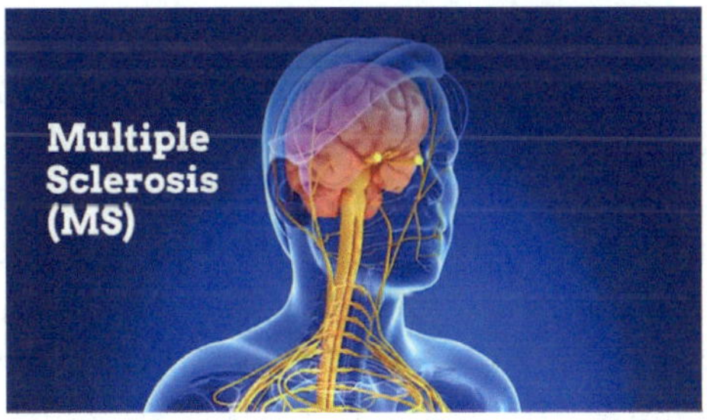

Figure 13.15. Multiple sclerosis.

Source: https://external-content.duckduckgo.com/iu/?u=https%3A%2F%2Fvinmec-prod.s3.amazonaws.com%2Fimages%2F20191203_041035_139621_maxresdefault.max-1800x1800.jpg&f=1&nofb=1&ipt=99863f31abb40fa0966a5df2f83b356709a01d980d482bc3907f8a077719f438.

13.5.3. Implications for Rehabilitation and Therapy

It is challenging to grasp the details of neurological illnesses, particularly to develop good rehabilitation strategies. The basis of recovery lies in the idea of neuroplasticity, in which the nervous system can reorganize and make up for itself following damage or disease. Rehabilitation procedures based on this capacity can result in remarkable recovery in patients' abilities. For instance, the stimulation of cognitive and physical therapies tailored to an individual's specific deficits has been shown to optimize gains in recovery. The use of neuroanatomical principles in therapy planning ensures that the interventions are adequately targeted, addressing discrete areas that could benefit from more precise rehabilitation. This individualized approach, supported by ongoing research and developments in neuroanatomical understanding, underscores the benefit of interdisciplinary collaboration in optimizing the therapeutic management of neurological patients. The cerebellum's evolving role in regulating not only motor performance but also cognitive and affective processes opens new avenues for rehabilitation management. Recent findings show that the cerebellum plays an important role in cognitive affect regulation and is therefore a therapeutic target for dysmetria of thought and emotion, the concern of the cerebellar cognitive affective/Schmahmann syndrome. This view of the cerebellum as an integration center in distributed neural circuits underlies therapies that enlist both motor and cognitive rehabilitation. Through the development of integrative treatment programs for these interconnected functions, practitioners can optimize patient outcomes in an integrated way. The future potential of personalized treatments aimed at the interconnection of cognitive, emotional, and motor rehabilitation will increasingly become essential in clinical practice, driving the advancement of effective therapeutic protocols in neurology. Moreover, disorders like primary progressive aphasia (PPA) show the importance of targeted interventions in neurological rehabilitation. PPA encompasses heterogeneous syndromes that require precise clinical strategies for assessment and treatment. For instance, proper knowledge of characteristic features of the prototypical variants of PPA allows therapists to develop specific strategies that are appropriate to the language impairments of each syndrome. Through the employment of a diagnostic pathway composed of potential pitfalls, clinicians can optimize treatment interventions derived from precise neuroanatomical data and functional assessments of the patient's capabilities. Emphasis on generic information processing impairment in identifying new pathophysiological biomarkers can provide groundbreaking treatments for enhancing communication and cognitive functions, ultimately influencing the paradigm for rehabilitation in patients with progressive aphasias and other similar neurological disorders.

13.6. Assessment and Diagnosis of Neurological Disorders

The intricate interaction between the peripheral and central nervous systems is the foundation of understanding the evaluation and diagnosis of neurological disorders. Neurological disorders, ranging from stroke to cerebral palsy (CP), each require nuance in diagnostic approach toward managing a series of clinical presentations. In early identification, especially of CP, the clinician is encouraged to identify clinical signs much earlier than the traditional time frame because increasing evidence indicates that outcomes are significantly enhanced by early intervention. For instance, the use of neuroimaging and standardized assessment, like that through the use as the Hammersmith Infant Neurological Examination, allows for the identification of risk factors for CP earlier than six months of age. Such prophylactic intervention not only guarantees prompt intervention but also stimulates neuroplasticity, therefore optimizing motor and cognitive growth, which is of paramount significance for the concerned patient (Novak et al., 2017). Familiarity with functional neuroanatomy is a core part of neuropsychological evaluations, guiding clinicians towards a diagnosis. Clinical neuropsychologists are supposed to apply various assessment strategies to make effective assessments of cognitive disorders via fixed or flexible battery methods based on the symptoms evident. Clinical neuropsychology requires immense knowledge in neuroanatomy but also behavioral neurology as well and cognitive neuroscience. With knowledge in these areas, neuropsychologists can conduct differential diagnoses effectively in discriminating between many neurological disorders. For example, discrimination between upper motor neuron (UMN) lesions and lower motor neuron (LMN) lesions is critical in the diagnosis of multiple sclerosis or Parkinson's disease because treatment as well as management varies greatly (Hill & Westervelt, 2015). The assessment techniques employed in the determination of neurological disorders vary with time, reflecting developments in neuroplasticity and assessment technologies. Technologies such as advanced neuroimaging devices enhance the accuracy of diagnosis through deeper brain structure and function visualizations. More recently, the inclusion of standardized assessment tools has been shown to increase predictive validity in high-risk infant populations for neurological conditions. These tools allow practitioners to assess developmental milestones and neurological function effectively, thereby establishing an effective treatment plan. In addition, the role of the caregiver and his or her understanding of these tests are increasingly regarded as essential, highlighting the importance of simultaneous methods that consider both patient and caregiver. Subsequently, integrative treatment methods may lead to enhanced results for individuals dealing with neurological disorders (Figure 13.16).

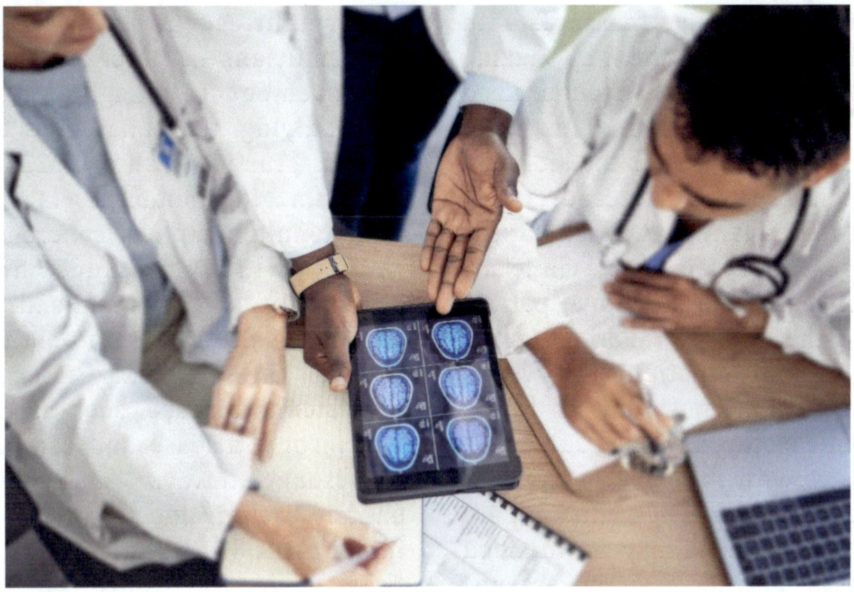

Figure 13.16. Assessment and diagnosis of neurological disorders.

Source: https://synopticmedical.com/wp-content/uploads/2023/03/the-diagnosis-and-treatment-of-neurological-diseases.jpeg.

13.6.1. Clinical Evaluation Techniques

An effective clinical evaluation technique is crucial in diagnosing and understanding neurological illnesses, particularly with the nervous system's intricate nature. An understanding of the central nervous system and peripheral nervous system allows clinicians to apply effective assessment techniques for a disorder. Techniques such as thorough patient history and physical examination are the cornerstones of the evaluation process, providing input into upper motor neuron (UMN) and lower motor neuron (LMN) lesions. Proper evaluation also involves interpretation of signs and symptoms related to various pathologies, from stroke to multiple sclerosis. As neurology becomes more and more in touch with machine learning technology, the clinical evaluation process is evolving. Uses of algorithms that have been created for processes such as medical imaging analysis enhance diagnostic accuracy and help clinicians distinguish between simulating symptomatology in various neuroanatomical contexts (Valliani et al., 2019). Additionally, neuroimaging developments provide essential information that complements clinical evaluations. Equipment such as Magnetic Resonance Imaging (MRI) and Computed Tomography (CT) scans has a pivotal role to play in imaging brain structures so that conditions like ischemic stroke can be differentiated from hemorrhage. Neuroimaging is not only essential in making the primary diagnosis but is also critical in the evaluation of disease changes and treatment response. The importance of combining these imaging modalities with clinical presentation cannot be overstated since it provides a more comprehensive picture of a patient's neurological condition. Medical imaging advancements are matched with theories on neuroplasticity, where practitioners can understand how the nervous system can recover or compensate following injury. This understanding informs rehabilitation following injury like traumatic brain injury or stroke (Sacco et al., 2013). Combining quantitative measures with clinical evaluations enhances them by making them stronger and more reliable. Standardized testing devices, such as the National Institutes of Health Stroke Scale (NIHSS) or the Modified Ashworth Scale for spasticity measurement, enable the objective quantification of patient status and change. These tools enable clinicians to set treatment goals from individual patient baselines, setting the stage for tailored therapy regimens. Coupled with patient interviews and qualitative evaluations, what is hence offered is a holistic picture in which subjective experience merges with measurable data. As more complex clinical means of evaluation are developed, they will increasingly be founded upon sophisticated technological convergence and rigorous empirical validation in an effort to ensure effective diagnosis and treatment of neurological disorders. Multi-mode analysis has potential for improved patient outcomes in neurology's intricate arena.

13.6.2. Imaging Techniques in Neuroanatomy

The role of contemporary imaging techniques cannot be overlooked in the research of neurological disorders. They are important both in the diagnosis and therapy of central and peripheral nervous system diseases alike. Functional magnetic resonance imaging (fMRI) is a case in point, as it allows an individual to study brain activity in terms of monitoring changes in blood flow, providing feedback on which areas of the brain become active during specific activities. This is particularly beneficial in disorders like stroke and multiple sclerosis (MS), whereby visualization of affected areas is enabled and individualized rehabilitative strategies can be facilitated. Furthermore, imaging evidence correlated with the clinical presentations of upper motor neuron (UMN) and lower motor neuron (LMN) lesions enhances a better understanding of neuromuscular abnormalities, directing physiotherapists and clinicians in practice. The technological advancement in imaging is significant in demystifying neuroanatomy's complexities in clinical practice (Polito, 2022). Underpinning these imaging modalities is the evolution of high-definition optical coherence tomography (OCT), which provides high-resolution assessments of the retina and optic nerve. As a subspecialty of neuro-ophthalmology, OCT provides an opportunity to explore the effect of systemic disease, such as that present in Parkinson's disease and cerebral palsy (CP), on visual pathways. The imaging technology enhances clinicians' abilities to relate visual impairment with related neurological status, thus promoting more holistic treatment regimens. Furthermore, continued advances in imaging technology facilitate greater understanding of neuroplasticity principles to guide rehabilitation planning. With precise evaluation of the neuroanatomical changes, clinicians are capable of optimizing treatment approaches to leverage the brain's adaptation capacity, thereby enhancing recovery from such injuries as spinal cord injury (SCI) and stroke. Advanced imaging thus plays a significant role in management as well as diagnosis in neuroanatomy (Kawasaki, 2010). Though there are plenty of advantages, the application of imaging techniques in neuroanatomy carries its limitations and considerations. Imaging findings need to be interpreted using specialist knowledge of neuroanatomy to prevent misinterpretation and inappropriate management and diagnosis. Excessive reliance on imaging can also diminish the role of clinical evaluation in ascertaining the overall picture of a patient's neurological status. Clinicians must reconcile the application of these imaging modalities with comprehensive expertise in clinical abilities to assess and manage neurological disorders optimally. Ethical considerations also apply to access to very advanced imaging technologies, as there can be health disparities that affect the quality of care received by those with neurological disorders. Though imaging technology will keep advancing, ongoing education and interprofessional practice will be fundamental to leveraging its full potential in optimizing outcomes in the practice of neuroanatomy (Polito, 2022) (Figure 13.17).

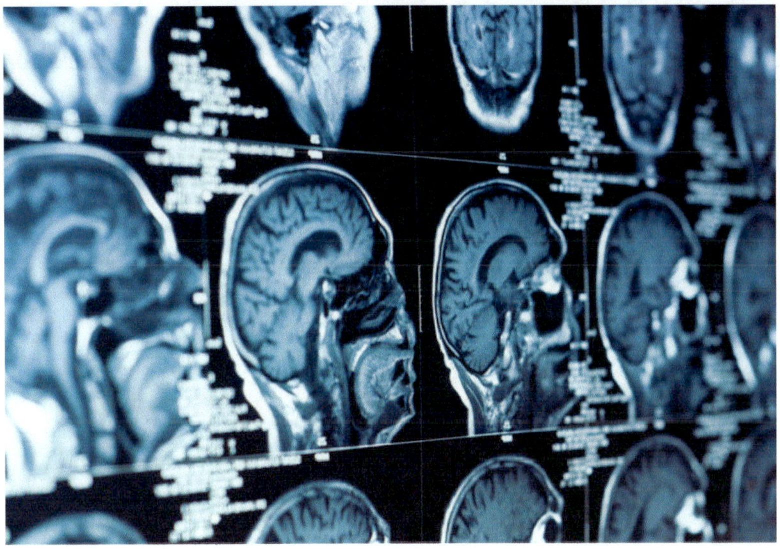

Figure 13.17. Imaging techniques in neuroanatomy.

Source: https://atlantaneurology.net/images/header/brain_scan_mobile.jpg.

13.6.3. Neuropsychological Assessments

It is crucial to appreciate the intricacies of neuropsychological testing as they are critical for evaluating and treating neurological diseases, as testing provides a very good understanding of cognitive processes and behavior. They quantify several cognitive functions, from attention and memory to executive function and language, which prove helpful for the diagnosis of disorders such as stroke, multiple sclerosis (MS), and Parkinson's disease. Through standardized testing and clinical interviews, clinicians are able to measure individual deficits patients may be experiencing so that therapeutic interventions can be tailored to optimize neuroplasticity. Flexibility in the nervous system is perhaps most crucial in physiotherapy, when rehabilitation programs tailored to the individual patient can optimize functional outcome. Neuropsychological tests are not only valuable as diagnostic instruments but also as a baseline measure for tracking improvement with treatment. The neural correlate of cognitive function assessed by neuropsychological measures is complex and inextricably intertwined with the structural and functional neurosciences of the central and peripheral nervous systems. Executive functions, for instance, are founded on a network of frontal-subcortical circuits to enable goal-directed behavior and cognitive flexibility, as highlighted in the literature (Cullum, 2013). These circuits can be disrupted by a range of neurological disorders, an indication of the necessity for rigorous testing in acknowledging the sophistication of cognitive impairment. In addition, neuroimaging techniques may utilize conventional testing procedures to image patterns of brain activity and identify maladaptive changes observed with neurological disease. Through this multi-dimensional approach, clinicians can better make sense of test outcomes and project the probable outcome of specific interventions, optimizing patient care in neuropsychology. Neuropsychological tests are not only for diagnostic purposes, as they establish a baseline for cognitive functioning, they also inform clinicians what treatment interventions work. For instance, cognitive rehabilitation and training methods aimed at enhancing flexibility can be guided by the results of neuropsychological testing, as these identify which cognitive function should receive targeted intervention (Uddin, 2021). The major priority remains individualization, particularly in cerebral palsy (CP) or spinal cord injury (SCI) patients, where cognitive dysfunction is compounded by physical disability. By continued observation of cognitive change with follow-up testing, clinicians have the ability to make evidence-based adjustments to treatment plans and therefore improve overall patient outcomes and recovery. Neuropsychological tests are thus indispensable tools within neurological practice, making the way for improved management and rehabilitation of a vast array of neurological disorders.

SUMMARY

While establishing the complex interconnection between neurological diseases and their orthopedic implications, the need is to embrace a multiple-faceted strategy in the effective management of the patient. The effect of neurological diseases on musculoskeletal health is huge and is likely to induce complications that necessitate a multimodal treatment regimen. For instance, conditions such as cerebral palsy pose mobility challenges not only to impede daily functioning but also contribute to patients' susceptibility to musculoskeletal deformity and pain. As emphasized in regard to relevant literature, successful interventions require an understanding of neurological as well as orthopedic principles, pointing towards the imperative of interdisciplinary interaction among healthcare professionals. This co-management not only aims to treat physical symptoms but also enhances the general quality of life, hence integrating functional restoration with emotional and psychological fulfillment. Furthermore, the enhancement in treatment methods for neurological disorders, particularly those that have underlying orthopedic considerations, has opened the door for greater patient outcomes. Evidence-based guidelines, as seen in the creation of those for Mucopolysaccharidosis IVA, which include elaborate management plans, are intended to facilitate evidence-informed cascades of decision-making that can be adopted by practitioners. The consensus development highlights the importance of having tailor-made treatment plans that address patient-specific needs in various areas, from physical therapy to surgeries, as well as ongoing follow-up. These interventions try to reverse the cumulative complexities of both neurological and orthopedic challenges, thereby placing value on a multidisciplinary approach to treatment. Ultimately, ongoing research and innovation in management plans are necessary to overcome the intricacies presented by neurological issues with orthopedic consequences. This ever-developing specialty requires constant updates to treatment protocols based on new data and clinical experience. As emphasized by current literature, there continues to be a need for innovations in clinical practice to meet evolving patient care needs. Future studies need to target areas that have existing deficits in knowledge, with an emphasis on ensuring that innovations in therapies and interventions are translated into meaningful clinical benefit. Finally, improving the quality of life in patients through integrated care is the ultimate aim of all stakeholders dealing with the treatment of neurological disorders with orthopedic issues.

A comprehensive understanding of the interactions between neurological conditions and orthopedic outcomes is crucial in the formulation of effective treatment regimens. One crucial finding reveals the effectiveness of myofascial release (MFR) for patients with upper extremity and cervical spine orthopedic and peripheral nerve conditions. Research has demonstrated that MFR significantly decreases pain and disability and enhances passive range of motion, strength, and overall function in the affected. The results are supported by evidence obtained from a systematic review of 23 articles as well as other trials. Surprisingly, the clinicians who wrote about their study reported attaining a high degree of knowledge regarding the efficacy of MFR, indicating the necessity for continuous education and further research towards optimizing treatment procedures using occupational therapy to a greater extent. This understanding of MFR highlights the significance of incorporating manual interventions into treatment regimens for neurological disorders that impact orthopedic health. Additionally, the role of a physiotherapist in the therapy of patients suffering from neurological disorders such as Parkinson's disease (PD) is significant. Physiotherapy aims to enhance quality of life and functional mobility through customized rehabilitation activities targeting motor as well as non-motor symptoms. Findings from randomized controlled trials indicate that interventions in physiotherapy provide significant improvements in gait parameters, functional mobility, and clinician-rated disability in comparison to no intervention. Specifically, findings show significant improvement in walking speed and balance parameters, thus enhancing the overall independence of PD patients. Despite some heterogeneity in quality among the trials reviewed, there is a unanimous opinion: physiotherapy treatments form an integral part of the total management of neurological disorders because they significantly decrease disability and increase independence. Myofascial release combined with physiotherapy forms part of a larger movement toward multidisciplinary models of treatment for patients with neurological disorders and their orthopedic presentation. Therapists are encouraged to utilize these evidence-based techniques, modifying them to fit the specific patient's needs. Additionally, there is an emerging requirement for more high-quality studies to determine the long-term effectiveness of various physiotherapeutic interventions and myofascial release in various regions of the body. This quest for greater therapeutic effectiveness is in keeping with the urgent need to more effectively address the complex character of neurological impairments through the use of a comprehensive approach that combines both rehabilitative and support interventions. These efforts not only attempt to enhance clinical success but also strive to enhance the overall quality of life for patients afflicted by these complex diseases.

CLOSER LOOK

NEUROPSYCHOLOGICAL CARE

Neuropsychological care focuses on understanding and treating the relationship between brain function and behavior. It involves the assessment, diagnosis, and rehabilitation of individuals with cognitive, emotional, and behavioral difficulties resulting from brain injury, neurological disorders, developmental conditions, or mental health issues. Neuropsychologists use standardized tests, clinical interviews, and behavioral observations to evaluate areas such as memory, attention, language, executive functions, perception, and emotional regulation. This specialized field plays a crucial role in conditions such as traumatic brain injury, stroke, epilepsy, dementia, learning disabilities, attention deficit hyperactivity disorder (ADHD), and neurodegenerative diseases. Based on detailed assessments, personalized intervention plans are developed to support cognitive rehabilitation, emotional adjustment, and functional independence. Interventions may include cognitive training exercises, behavioral therapy, coping strategies, and family counseling. Neuropsychological care also assists in treatment planning, educational support, and vocational rehabilitation by identifying strengths and limitations. Emotional support and psychotherapy help patients and families manage stress, anxiety, and changes in personality or functioning. Early assessment and intervention significantly improve recovery outcomes and quality of life. Overall, neuropsychological care provides a holistic, patient-centered approach that integrates brain science and clinical practice to enhance cognitive functioning, emotional well-being, and everyday performance across the lifespan.

REFERENCES

1. Adair, D., Truong, D. Q., Esmaeilpour, Z., Gebodh, N., Borges, H., Ho, L., Bremner, J. D., et al. (2020). Electrical stimulation of cranial nerves in cognition and disease. *Brain Stimulation, 13*, 717–750. https://doi.org/10.1016/j.brs.2020.02.019 (accessed on 26th June 2025).

2. Al Sari, R. R., Thalib, H. I., Imad, S. S., Khan, S., Haidar, S., Al Zoabi, B. M. K., Fadda, S. H., et al. (2025). A comparative exploration of monoamine neurotransmitter transport disorders: Mechanisms, clinical manifestations, and therapeutic approaches. Journal of Medicine and Life, 18, 188–195. https://www.semanticscholar.org/paper/d7539ab6d9fafa78509bf8baad03f27dad91c269 (accessed on 26th June 2025).

3. Azzalini, D., Rebollo, I., & Tallon-Baudry, C. (2019). Visceral signals shape brain dynamics and cognition. *Trends in Cognitive Sciences, 23*, 488–509. https://doi.org/10.1016/j.tics.2019.03.007 (accessed on 26th June 2025).

4. Baijens, L. W. J., Clavé, P., Cras, P., Ekberg, O., Forster, A., Kolb, G., Leners, J. C., et al. (2016). European Society for Swallowing Disorders – European Union Geriatric Medicine Society white paper: Oropharyngeal dysphagia as a geriatric syndrome. Clinical Interventions in Aging, 11, 1403–1428. https://doi.org/10.2147/cia.s107750 (accessed on 26th June 2025).

5. Barrow, D. L., & Bendok, B. R. (2019). Introduction: What is neurosurgery? *Operative Neurosurgery, 17*, S1–S2. https://doi.org/10.1093/ons/opz071 (accessed on 26th June 2025).

6. Bölte, S., Girdler, S., & Marschik, P. B. (2018). The contribution of environmental exposure to the etiology of autism spectrum disorder. Cellular and Molecular Life Sciences, 76, 1275–1297. https://doi.org/10.1007/s00018-018-2988-4 (accessed on 26th June 2025).

7. Cano-de-la-Cuerda, R., Blázquez-Fernández, A., Marcos-Antón, S., Sánchez-Herrera-Baeza, P., Fernández-González, P., Collado-Vázquez, S., Jiménez-Antona, C., et al. (2024). Economic cost of rehabilitation with robotic and virtual reality systems in people with neurological disorders: A systematic review. Journal of Clinical Medicine, 13. https://www.semanticscholar.org/paper/66bb34bad6934d0ad51ccf80d8b502ba48cd3561 (accessed on 26th June 2025).

8. Chitlange, N. M., Hullumani, S., Sasun, A. R., & Raghuveer, R. (2024). Effect of dynamic neuromuscular stabilization and rehabilitation strategies in six-year child with Duchenne muscular dystrophy: A case study. https://doi.org/10.20944/preprints202404.0620.v1 (accessed on 26th June 2025).

9. Chitnis, T., Vandercappellen, J., King, M. L., & Brichetto, G. (2022). Symptom interconnectivity in multiple sclerosis: A narrative review of potential underlying biological disease processes. Neurology and Therapy, 11, 1043–1070. https://doi.org/10.1007/s40120-022-00368-2 (accessed on 26th June 2025).

10. Cook, J. L., Green, C. R., Lilley, C. M., Anderson, S. M., Baldwin, M. E., Chudley, A. E., Conry, J., et al. (2015). Fetal alcohol spectrum disorder: A guideline for diagnosis across the lifespan. Canadian Medical Association Journal, 188, 191–197. https://doi.org/10.1503/cmaj.141593 (accessed on 26th June 2025).

11. Cryan, J. F., O'Riordan, K. J., Cowan, C. S. M., Sandhu, K. V., Bastiaanssen, T. F. S., Boehme, M., Codagnone, M. G., et al. (2019). The microbiota-gut-brain axis. Physiological Reviews, 99, 1877–2013. https://doi.org/10.1152/physrev.00018.2018 (accessed on 26th June 2025).

12. Cullum, C. M. (2013). Neuropsychological assessment. In *Cambridge University Press eBooks*. https://doi.org/10.1017/cbo9781139016919.026 (accessed on 26th June 2025).

13. de Vries, E., Hagbohm, C., Ouellette, R., & Granberg, T. (2025). Clinical 7 Tesla magnetic resonance imaging: Impact and patient value in neurological disorders. *Journal of Internal Medicine, 297*, 244–261. https://www.semanticscholar.org/paper/476e852ab6f06be55c48618c4a0fe232de906c12 (accessed on 26th June 2025).

14. Egger, J., Gsaxner, C., Pepe, A., Pomykala, K. L., Jonske, F., Kurz, M., Li, J., et al. (2022). Medical deep learning—A systematic meta-review. Computer Methods and Programs in Biomedicine, 221, 106874–106874. https://doi.org/10.1016/j.cmpb.2022.106874 (accessed on 26th June 2025).

15. Friston, K. (2022). Computational psychiatry: From synapses to sentience. Molecular Psychiatry, 28, 256–268. https://doi.org/10.1038/s41380-022-01743-z (accessed on 26th June 2025).

16. Geocadin, R. G., Callaway, C. W., Fink, E. L., Golan, E., Greer, D. M., Ko, N., Lang, E., et al. (2019). Standards for studies of neurological prognostication in comatose survivors of cardiac arrest: A scientific statement from the American Heart Association. Circulation, 140. https://doi.org/10.1161/cir.0000000000000702 (accessed on 26th June 2025).

17. Godoy, L. D., Rossignoli, M. T., Delfino-Pereira, P., Garcia-Cairasco, N., & de Lima Umeoka, E. H. (2018). A comprehensive overview on stress neurobiology: Basic concepts and clinical implications. Frontiers in Behavioral Neuroscience, 12. https://doi.org/10.3389/fnbeh.2018.00127 (accessed on 26th June 2025).

18. González, J. A., Gomez-Alanis, A., Martín-Doñas, J. M., Pérez-Córdoba, J. L., & Gómez, Á. M. (2020). Silent speech interfaces for speech restoration: A review. IEEE Access, 8, 177995–178021. https://doi.org/10.1109/access.2020.3026579 (accessed on 26th June 2025).

19. Guell, X., Schmahmann, J. D., Gabrieli, J. D. E., & Ghosh, S. (2018). Functional gradients of the cerebellum. eLife, 7. https://doi.org/10.7554/elife.36652 (accessed on 26th June 2025).

20. Halkiopoulos, C., Gkintoni, E., & Antonopoulou, H. (2023). Neuroeducation and artistic expression: An overview from the biopsychology viewpoint. *Technique Education and Humanities, 3*, 38–49. https://doi.org/10.47577/teh.v3i1.8235 (accessed on 26th June 2025).

21. Han, Y., Yuan, M., Guo, Y. S., Shen, X. Y., Gao, Z. K., & Bi, X. (2022). The role of enriched environment in neural development and repair. Frontiers in Cellular Neuroscience, 16. https://doi.org/10.3389/fncel.2022.890666 (accessed on 26th June 2025).

22. Hill, B. D., & Westervelt, H. J. (2015). Clinical neuropsychology. In *The Encyclopedia of Clinical Psychology*. https://doi.org/10.1002/9781118625392.wbecp412 (accessed on 26th June 2025).

23. Jiang, C. C., Lin, L., Long, S., Ke, X., Fukunaga, K., Lu, Y. M., & Han, F. (2022). Signaling pathways in autism spectrum disorder: Mechanisms and therapeutic implications. *Signal Transduction and Targeted Therapy, 7*. https://doi.org/10.1038/s41392-022-01081-0 (accessed on 26th June 2025).

24. Kannan, S., Dutta, A., & Das, A. (2024). Sleep disorders in functional neurological disorder–A systematic review and meta-analysis. Neurological Sciences, 46, 1573–1580. https://www.semanticscholar.org/paper/4aa9770572c0d45c879aea2b2d3da7f38b185254 (accessed on 26th June 2025).

25. Kawasaki, A. (2010). Neuro-ophthalmology: Through a wide-angle lens. *Frontiers in Neurology, 1*. https://www.semanticscholar.org/paper/0b4c38674117b7eb088b937b140bfc5f2718c4f3 (accessed on 26th June 2025).

26. Lai, M. C., Lombardo, M., Auyeung, B., Chakrabarti, B., & Baron-Cohen, S. (2014). Sex/gender differences and autism: Setting the scene for future research. Journal of the American Academy of Child & Adolescent Psychiatry, 54, 11–24. https://doi.org/10.1016/j.jaac.2014.10.003 (accessed on 26th June 2025).

27. Marshall, C. R., Hardy, C. J. D., Volkmer, A., Russell, L. L., Bond, R. L., Fletcher, P. D., Clark, C. N., et al. (2018). Primary progressive aphasia: A clinical approach. *Journal of Neurology, 265*, 1474–1490. https://doi.org/10.1007/s00415-018-8762-6 (accessed on 26th June 2025).

28. McCoyd, M., Salardini, A., & Biller, J. (2019). The neurological examination. Operative Neurosurgery, 17, S3–S16. https://doi.org/10.1093/ons/opz066 (accessed on 26th June 2025).

29. McEwen, B. S., & Gianaros, P. J. (2010). Central role of the brain in stress and adaptation: Links to socioeconomic status, health, and disease. *Annals of the New York Academy of Sciences, 1186*, 190–222. https://doi.org/10.1111/j.1749-6632.2009.05331.x (accessed on 26th June 2025).

30. Mhalhel, K., Sicari, M., Pansera, L., Chen, J., Levanti, M., Diotel, N., Rastegar, S., et al. (2023). Zebrafish: A model deciphering the impact of flavonoids on neurodegenerative disorders. Cells, 12, 252–252. https://doi.org/10.3390/cells12020252 (accessed on 26th June 2025).

31. Murciano-Brea, J., Garcia-Montes, M., Geuna, S., & Herrera-Rincón, C. (2021). Gut microbiota and neuroplasticity. Cells, 10, 2084–2084. https://doi.org/10.3390/cells10082084 (accessed on 26th June 2025).

32. Ng, S., Valdés, P. A., Moritz-Gasser, S., Lemaitre, A. L., Duffau, H., & Herbet, G. (2023). Intraoperative functional remapping unveils evolving patterns of cortical plasticity. Brain, 146, 3088–3100. https://doi.org/10.1093/brain/awad116 (accessed on 26th June 2025).

33. Novak, I., Morgan, C., Adde, L., Blackman, J. A., Boyd, R. N., Brunstrom-Hernandez, J., Cioni, G., et al. (2017). Early, accurate diagnosis and early intervention in cerebral palsy. *JAMA Pediatrics, 171*, 897. https://doi.org/10.1001/jamapediatrics.2017.1689 (accessed on 26th June 2025).

34. Pavlov, V. A., Chavan, S. S., & Tracey, K. J. (2018). Molecular and functional neuroscience in immunity. Annual Review of Immunology, 36, 783–812. https://doi.org/10.1146/annurev-immunol-042617-053158 (accessed on 26th June 2025).

35. Polito, J. M. (2022). Review of "Oxford Textbook of Neurocritical Care," edited by Martin M. Smith, Giuseppe G. Citerio, and W. Andrew I. Kofke. *The Neurodiagnostic Journal, 62*, 181–182. https://www.semanticscholar.org/paper/1ada2c64339d866efbe20962af2db1293e0e2087 (accessed on 26th June 2025).

36. Pöyhönen, S., Er, Ş., Domanskyi, A., & Airavaara, M. (2019). Effects of neurotrophic factors in glial cells in the central nervous system: Expression and properties in neurodegeneration and injury. Frontiers in Physiology, 10. https://doi.org/10.3389/fphys.2019.00486 (accessed on 26th June 2025).

37. Roy, G. B. (2022). Neurological localization in clinical practice. *Journal of Family Medicine and Disease Prevention, 8*. https://doi.org/10.23937/2469-5793/1510144 (accessed on 26th June 2025).

38. Sacco, R. L., Kasner, S. E., Broderick, J. P., Caplan, L. R., Connors, J. J., Culebras, A., Elkind, M. S. V., et al. (2013). An updated definition of stroke for the 21st century. Stroke, 44, 2064–2089. https://doi.org/10.1161/str.0b013e318296aeca (accessed on 26th June 2025).

39. Sandsmark, D. K., Elliott, J. E., & Lim, M. M. (2017). Sleep-wake disturbances after traumatic brain injury: Synthesis of human and animal studies. *SLEEP*. https://doi.org/10.1093/sleep/zsx044 (accessed on 26th June 2025).

40. Schmahmann, J. D., Guell, X., Stoodley, C. J., & Halko, M. A. (2019). The theory and neuroscience of cerebellar cognition. Annual Review of Neuroscience, 42, 337–364. https://doi.org/10.1146/annurev-neuro-070918-050258 (accessed on 26th June 2025).

41. Schumann, C. M., Bloss, C. S., Barnes, C. C., Wideman, G., Carper, R. A., Akshoomoff, N., Pierce, K., et al. (2010). Longitudinal magnetic resonance imaging study of cortical development through early childhood in autism. *Journal of Neuroscience, 30*, 4419–4427. https://doi.org/10.1523/jneurosci.5714-09.2010 (accessed on 26th June 2025).

42. Sivhugwana, Innocentia (2022). Factors related with the functional outcome of patients who sustained tibial plateau fractures. Dissertation (MSc (Physiotherapy))--University of Pretoria, 2022. https://core.ac.uk/download/565849089.pdf

43. Stassart, R. M., Möbius, W., Nave, K.-A., & Edgar, J. M. (2018). The axon-myelin unit in development and degenerative disease. Frontiers in Neuroscience, 12. https://doi.org/10.3389/fnins.2018.00467 (accessed on 26th June 2025).

44. Sunkin, S. M., Ng, L., Lau, C., Dolbeare, T., Gilbert, T. L., Thompson, C. L., Hawrylycz, M., et al. (2012). Allen Brain Atlas: An integrated spatio-temporal portal for exploring the central nervous system. Nucleic Acids Research, 41, D996–D1008. https://doi.org/10.1093/nar/gks1042 (accessed on 26th June 2025).

45. Uddin, L. Q. (2021). Cognitive and behavioural flexibility: Neural mechanisms and clinical considerations. Nature Reviews Neuroscience, 22, 167–179. https://doi.org/10.1038/s41583-021-00428-w (accessed on 26th June 2025).

46. Valliani, A., Ranti, D., & Oermann, E. K. (2019). Deep learning and neurology: A systematic review. *Neurology and Therapy, 8*, 351–365. https://doi.org/10.1007/s40120-019-00153-8 (accessed on 26th June 2025).

47. Wang, M., Liu, W., Ge, J., & Liu, S. (2023). The immunomodulatory mechanisms for acupuncture practice. Frontiers in Immunology, 14. https://doi.org/10.3389/fimmu.2023.1147718 (accessed on 26th June 2025).

48. Waris, A., Ullah, A., Asim, M., Ullah, R., Rajdoula, M. R., Bello, S. T., & Alhumaydhi, F. (2024). Phyto therapeutic options for the treatment of epilepsy: Pharmacology, targets, and mechanism of action. *Frontiers in Pharmacology, 15*. https://www.semanticscholar.org/paper/67239cc6cd6e110e055f5f1883dd6ee07aafe39f (accessed on 26th June 2025).

49. Welch, M. C., Yu, J., Larkin, M. B., Graves, E. K. M., & Mears, D. (2020). A multimedia educational module for teaching early medical neuroanatomy. MedEdPORTAL. https://doi.org/10.15766/mep_2374-8265.10885 (accessed on 26th June 2025).

50. Yang, J., Kong, L., Zou, L., & Liu, Y. (2024). The role of synaptic protein NSF in the development and progression of neurological diseases. Frontiers in Neuroscience, 18. https://www.semanticscholar.org/paper/ff139e444e53efc5cdc5efbab61fbcadcaa0ccc1 (accessed on 26th June 2025).

51. Yehuda, R., & Lehrner, A. (2018). Intergenerational transmission of trauma effects: Putative role of epigenetic mechanisms. World Psychiatry, 17, 243–257. https://doi.org/10.1002/wps.20568 (accessed on 26th June 2025).

52. Zagni, E., Simoni, L., & Colombo, D. (2016). Sex and gender differences in central nervous system-related disorders. *Neuroscience Journal, 2016*, 1–13. https://doi.org/10.1155/2016/2827090 (accessed on 26th June 2025).

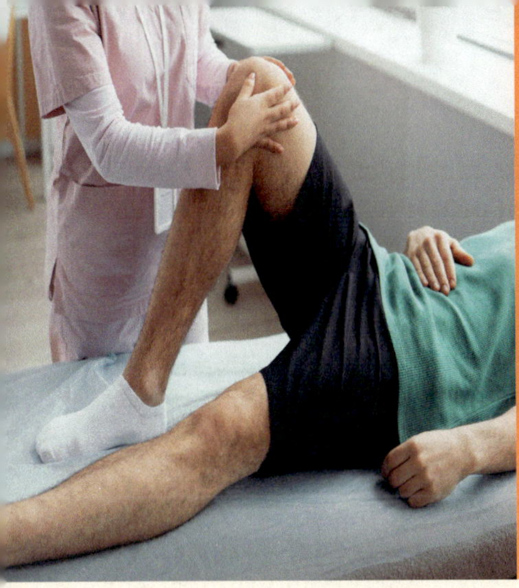

Chapter 14

PAIN MANAGEMENT IN ORTHOPEDIC PHYSIOTHERAPY

Contents

Introduction....449
14.1. Understanding Pain....451
14.2. Assessment of Pain....455
14.3. Treatment Modalities....460
14.4. Role of Exercise in Pain Management....463
14.5. Patient Education and Self-Management....467
14.6. Challenges in Pain Management....470
Summary....474
References....477

Introduction

The management of pain is also a vital component of orthopedic physiotherapy, encompassing various strategies to alleviate pain and facilitate functional rehabilitation for musculoskeletal disorder patients. Orthopedic physiotherapists play a critical role in assessing and managing pain through individualized treatment regimens. These may involve the integration of manual therapy, therapeutic exercises, and modalities like heat or cold application. Moreover, practitioners must understand the biopsychosocial model of pain because it describes the psychological and emotional factors that can influence a patient's perception of pain. Taking an holistic approach, physiotherapists can develop a pain management plan that not only facilitates physical rehabilitation but also emotional well-being, which is included in recovery. The evolution of pain management protocols has been increasingly guided by research enhancements and clinical guideline advice. Evidence-based models, including those contained within Enhanced Recovery After Surgery (ERAS) protocols, provide a coherent approach to perioperative care that can be of particular utility in orthopedic settings. This model centers on multimodal analgesia, which employs a variety of pharmacological and non-pharmacological mechanisms to decrease pain with reduced reliance on opioids. For example, ERAS guidelines encourage opioid-sparing medication and early mobilization to enhance recovery outcomes, proving the shift towards less invasive procedures and more support in pain management techniques. The application of these techniques not only makes patient comfort achievable but also facilitates quicker functional restoration, which leads to better long-term outcomes and reduced healthcare expenses. In conclusion, optimal pain management in orthopedic physiotherapy is a multi-dimensional task that demands consideration of both up-to-date research and patient-specific requirements. By utilizing novel pain management strategies and conforming to evidence-based guidelines, physiotherapists are well-positioned to maximize the recovery process for their patients. As the discipline further develops, keeping abreast of current knowledge through continued education and familiarization with novel approaches will be critical to maximizing treatment results. The inclusion of integrated approaches and advanced measures, as emphasized by the ERAS guidelines, promises to usher in a bright future for pain management in orthopedic physiotherapy. Through the delivery of an environment conducive to nurturing and thorough treatment methods, orthopedic physiotherapists stand to best address the complex issue of pain in their client base.

Importance of Pain Management in Orthopedic Care

Effective pain management in orthopedic care is essential to produce optimal outcomes for the patient and enhance the quality of life as a whole. Pain management strategies in orthopedics are essential not only to reduce pain during the process of rehabilitation, but also to promote adherence to exercise therapy protocols. When pain is left unrelieved, patients become less engaged in their own rehabilitation, which can subsequently lead to longer recuperation time and the risk for secondary complications. Effective pain management can similarly permit earlier mobilization and function return, ultimately saving healthcare costs in the form of longer hospital stays and repeated interventions. Accordingly, effective pain control is an integral part of the success of orthopedic physiotherapy and the patient's recovery process. The pain in the orthopedic patient is often multifaceted in nature and could be managed by a multidisciplinary approach. Orthopedic disorders such as fractures, arthritis, and soft tissue injuries can manifest as either acute or chronic pain and thus need to be managed by particular management strategies. A multidisciplinary approach can include pharmacological interventions, physiotherapy, and self-management skill education to facilitate the empowerment of patients during recovery procedures. Additionally, the integration of novel technologies, such as the use of surface electromyography (sEMG) for muscle and biofeedback assessment, has also been found to enhance the effectiveness of pain management programs (Campanini et al., 2020). By providing immediate feedback, the devices may empower patients to be more sensitive to their pain origins, leading to improved pain control and increased effectiveness in movement. Inter-professional working among healthcare professionals thus facilitates far better pain management in orthopedic care. Understanding the specific characteristics associated with various orthopedic conditions is central to creating successful pain management methods. Diseases such as X-linked hypophosphatemia (XLH) have intricacies that require keen evaluations and individualized therapies to reduce pain and its resultant complications. The multidisciplinary management proposed for such diseases is such that pain is addressed from a multipronged perspective, with regard to input from metabolic bone disease experts and physiotherapists who work hand in hand to maximize patients' outcomes (Haffner et al., 2019). In addition, patient education is integral since well-educated patients have a better chance to engage in their treatment, recognize patterns of pain, and adhere to treatment protocols. Such a comprehensive understanding of pain mechanics and orthopedic care is the ideal foundation of a holistic model of treatment in orthopedic physiotherapy that further enhances the efficacy of customized pain management interventions towards facilitating patient healing and wellness (Figure 14.1).

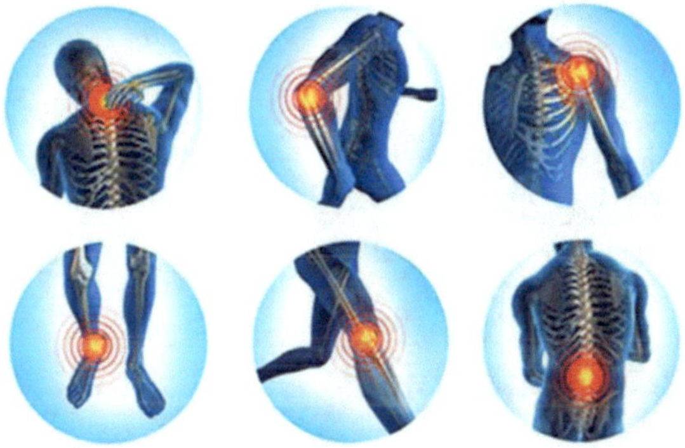

Figure 14.1. Illustration of orthopedic pain points.

Source: https://www.theorthopedicandpainpractice.com/wp-content/uploads/2023/05/12-1.jpg.

14.1. Understanding Pain

The pain sensation is multifactorial, caused by a multifaceted interplay between physiological, psychological, and social aspects. In orthopedic physiotherapy, it is important to understand this multifactorial nature of pain in order to design efficient treatment and management strategies. Pain typically serves as an evolutionary signal that alerts the body to impending damage; yet chronic pain might occur even without any visible injury. This chronic pain can persist due to maladaptive neural adaptations, and this can create a chronic cycle of pain and disability. Pain management is not merely the relief of pain symptoms but also considers the biopsychosocial model that recognizes the role of emotional and social factors in pain experience and adaptation. Without this interdisciplinary knowledge, treatments will be less effective at minimizing patient suffering and maximizing overall quality of life. The role of the physiotherapist in managing pain extends beyond addressing the physical aspects of injury. His or her expertise in creating customized rehab programs is essential to establishing patient resilience and improving functional outcomes. Interventions such as therapeutic exercises, mobilization of soft tissues, and manual therapy are classically employed to alleviate symptoms and restore motion. Importantly, the integration of cognitive-behavioral methods can be equally crucial in facilitating patients to reinterpret and adapt their pain experience. For instance, pain neuroscience education educates patients on pain mechanisms, thereby enabling them to become active participants in the process of recovery. The adoption of these strategies is underscored by a recognition that chronic pain, like that of conditions like frozen shoulder, may need a multidisciplinary intervention to best improve patient function in the long term (Chul-Cho et al., 2019). Further, the development of evidence-based guidelines contributes significantly to informing clinical practices among orthopedic physiotherapy. For instance, the 2016 SOSORT guidelines define principal conservative treatment modalities for conditions such as idiopathic scoliosis, prioritizing individualized exercise regimens and bracing. These recommendations are formulated after profound reviews of the literature that ensure new approaches reflect present scientific evidence in pain management and the best outcomes of treatment. Such guidelines provide physiotherapists with firm foundations for optimizing outcomes in their patients with pain disorders. Nevertheless, despite the wealth of new evidence, it remains challenging to standardize treatment protocols to ensure greater consistency and generalizability across patient populations. Ongoing application of high-quality research into practice will ultimately maximize the interventions delivered in orthopedic physiotherapy, which will enhance the overall management and understanding of pain (Négrini et al., 2018).

14.1.1. Types of Pain: Acute vs. Chronic

It is crucial to learn the distinction between acute and chronic pain so that one can properly handle pain in orthopedic physiotherapy. Acute pain is best defined as being directly caused by injury or surgery and serves a protective function, alerting the individual to potential harm. It tends to be of limited duration, between a few seconds and several weeks, and typically resolves once the initial cause is addressed. Acute pain in orthopedic environments is commonly caused by fractures, sprains, or post-surgery convalescence.

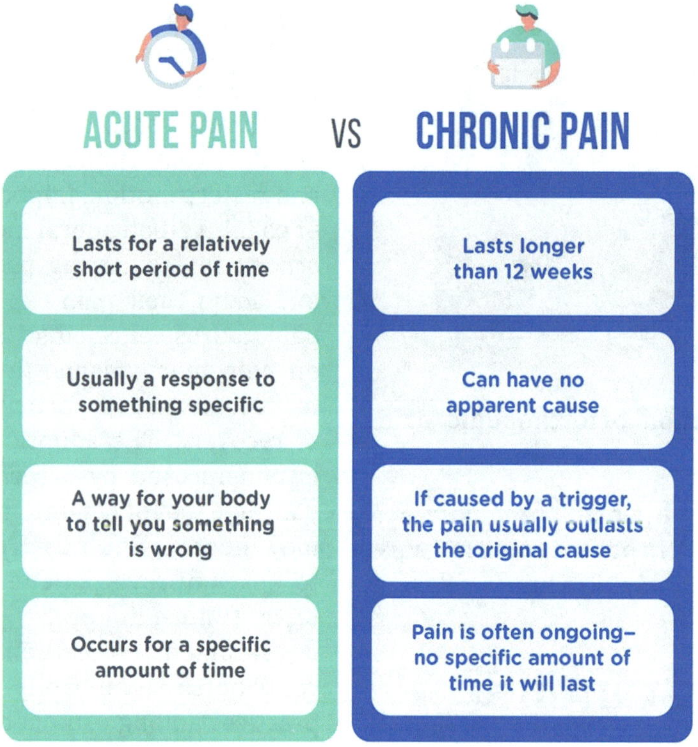

Figure 14.2. Acute vs. chronic pain.

Source: https://www.facebook.com/photo.php?fbid=1374582469668586&id=345182969275213&set=a.1009305922862911.

The treatment at this phase normally involves the alleviation of pain, improving mobility, and achieving functional autonomy through interventions such as manual therapy and patient education, thus enhancing the recovery process and lifestyle. Chronic pain, however, takes longer than anticipated to heal, persisting for months or even years. It may occur without a clear-cut initial trauma or continue well after recovery from injury, complicating treatment. Chronic pain might be associated with conditions such as osteoarthritis or chronic low back pain and typically tends to establish a pain-disability cycle that severely impacts daily living. Physiotherapists play a critical role in the management of chronic pain through the application of multidisciplinary approaches, integrating therapeutic exercise, psychological therapy, and lifestyle modification. Careful heed also needs to be paid to the psychosocial factors that affect pain perception, as chronic pain patients may become anxious or depressed, making their journey towards recovery more difficult. The following have far-reaching implications, touching the whole method of orthopedic physiotherapy. Acute pain management can center on short- and immediate physical interventions and outcomes, such as functional mobility and activity tolerance, whereas chronic pain management generally centers on long-term outcomes, balancing physical and psychological aspects simultaneously. Additionally, using objective measuring tools, as identified in surface electromyography (sEMG) literature, will assist practitioners in determining the degree of pain and the state of rehabilitation, bridging the gap between clinical practice and evidence-based research. By building a culture that encourages evidence-based practice, orthopedic physiotherapists can then contribute directly to improved patient outcomes in both chronic and acute pain conditions, hence making the field more effective overall (Campanini et al., 2020; Sivhugwana, 2021) (Figure 14.2).

14.1.2. Physiological Mechanisms of Pain

Physiological mechanisms of pain may be traced through a series of complex relationships between various biological elements, starting with mechanisms for the transmission of pain stimuli. Nociceptors, specialized sensory receptors, detect potentially harmful stimuli and convert them into electrical impulses. These impulses are conveyed through peripheral nerves to the spinal cord, which may either continue up to the brain for processing or be modulated at this stage. These simple mechanisms are central to the understanding of pain mechanisms, particularly in orthopedic physiotherapy, wherein therapists aim to alleviate pain and restore function. A beneficial approach to the treatment of pain relies on an understanding of the peripheral and the central mechanisms of perception of pain, which could direct therapeutic interventions for specific physiological pathways. At the center of pain detection is the brain's activity, that is, in areas responsible for sensory processing, emotion regulation, and coping strategy development. Following the delivery of nociceptive inputs, the brain processes and places such information, ultimately producing the perceptual phenomenon of pain. Interpretation is strongly modulated by history, psychological state, and social context. This realization leads to the significance of the biopsychosocial model within orthopedic physiotherapy, where professionals consider not just the physical injury but also the psychological and emotional roots of pain. Proper management of pain thus exists in the form of multifaceted interventions that consider both the physiological mechanisms and the biopsychosocial mechanisms of a patient's experience, enabling holistic treatment. Recent progress in our understanding of intervertebral disc disease also continues to describe the physiological mechanisms of pain caused by musculoskeletal disorders. Intervertebral disc disease generally manifests as lumbar back pain that is the consequence of complex interactions between spinal elements and related soft tissues. Progress in diagnostic tools, including noninvasive imaging and biomarkers, has revealed the pathophysiological basis, so that individualized treatment approaches are more favorable in orthopedic physiotherapy.

By separating pain treatment methods into conservative and invasive modalities, clinicians can better treat the multifaceted character of pain from intervertebral disc pathology. Knowledge of this information is critical, as targeted interventions must be used to optimize patient outcomes and foster recovery, demonstrating the pivotal role of knowledge of physiological mechanisms in effective pain management (Wu et al., 2020) (Figure 14.3).

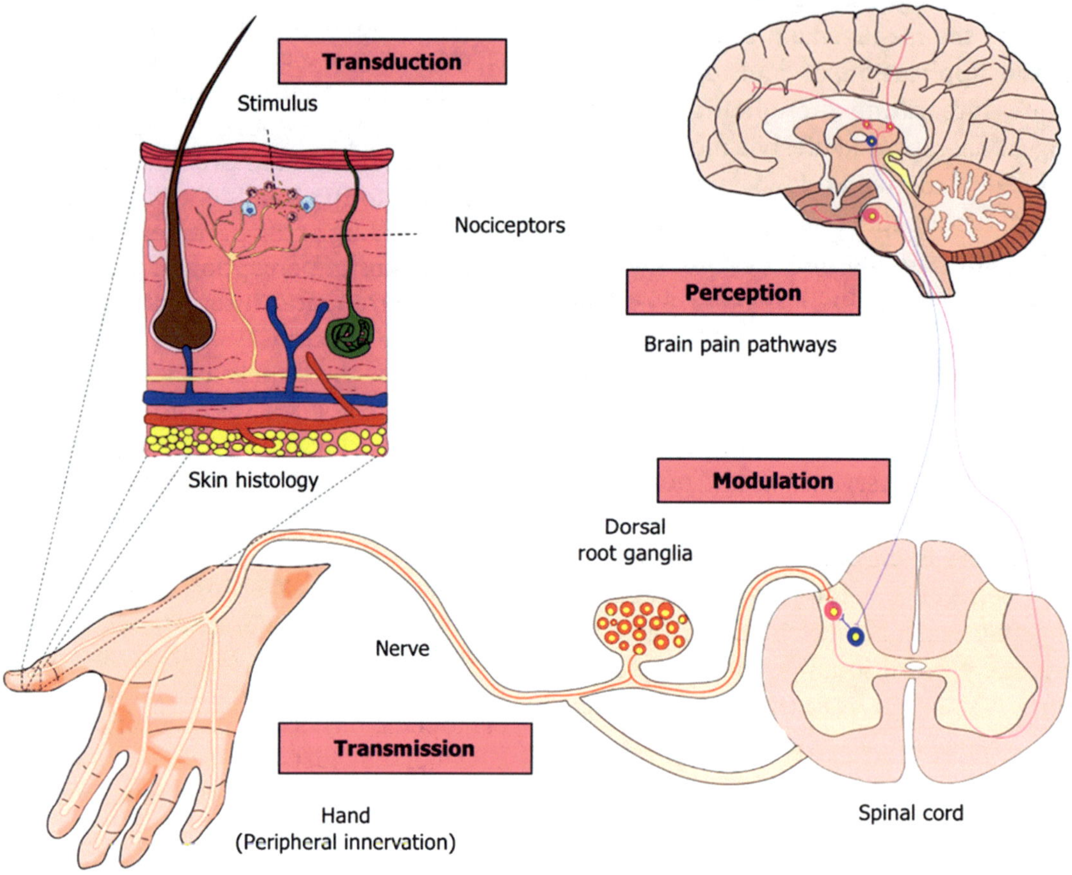

Figure 14.3. Pain mechanism.

Source: https://www.researchgate.net/profile/Geovana-Martelossi-Cebinelli/publication/376810683/figure/fig1/AS:11431281214418281@1703561126521/Pain-mechanism-Representative-diagram-of-anatomical-levels-involved-in-the-steps-of-pain.ppm.

14.1.3. Psychological Factors Influencing Pain Perception

Pain perception is a multifaceted phenomenon that is determined by a number of psychological factors with direct consequences to patients who are receiving orthopedic physiotherapy. Cognitive appraisal, or the process by which individuals evaluate and interpret their pain experiences, is crucial to pain perception. Patients who interpret pain as threatening build heightened anxiety, leading to heightened sensitivity to pain and debilitating effects. Moreover, the surrounding environment in which one is feeling pain may make it stronger or weaker. For example, patients who feel they are undergoing a process of healing will report less pain compared to those who are helpless. Such cognitive reframing is capable of empowering patients, making them more willing to conduct therapeutic exercises, which supports recovery. Thus, awareness of these psychological factors is important to physiotherapists as they develop tailored pain management programs that suit the unique requirements of patients. Emotional status also plays a significant role in the perception of pain, making it challenging to treat in orthopedic physiotherapy. Depression and anxiety have been seen to boost the perception of pain, leading to a vicious cycle of worsening disability and poor emotional well-being. For example, patients who are depressed will tend to experience pain more negatively, potentially undermining their commitment to therapy and labor objectives. Science documents that negative affect is likely to activate stress response mechanisms, further raising sensitivity to pain and making rehabilitation more difficult. Physiotherapists must then ensure that they consider a holistic approach that is sensitive to these affective responses in developing treatment interventions. By working on emotional health simultaneously with physical rehabilitation, practitioners can improve pain control and promote psychological resilience, ultimately improving patient outcomes. Social support and environmental influence also greatly influence pain experiences. Patients who possess good support systems report lower levels of pain because both emotional and informational support can lower stress and enhance coping ability. Research has shown that individuals who feel they are being listened to and understood will respond favorably to their rehabilitation. Conversely, being away from their loved ones makes them feel alone, resulting in higher reports of pain. It is the social process that makes it essential to incorporate family and friends into the rehabilitation process. As orthopedic physiotherapy often requires changes in lifestyle and the ongoing motivation to recover, the development of supportive environments can significantly affect a patient's course. Physiotherapists should thus be actively engaged in building strong social relationships in their treatment plans to foster physical as well as emotional rehabilitation.

14.2. Assessment of Pain

The assessment of pain is a critical aspect in orthopedic disorder treatment as it influences the therapeutic strategy used by physiotherapists directly. Subjective and objective measurements are carried out in an effort to experience the patient's pain phenomenon in totality. Subjectively, healthcare practitioners make use of self-assessed pain scales, which enable patients to measure their distress. Objective evaluation can include physical exam and imaging tests to measure underlying musculoskeletal pathology. Both strategies foster the concurrent comprehension of pain as a manifestation of disease and as constructed by psychosocial influences, allowing for customized treatment to address patient-specific requirements. Besides, the fact that pain is also characterized by emotional and psychological factors means efficient evaluation is a matter of evaluating co-morbidities such as depression or anxiety, thereby enhancing the treatment process overall (Khachane et al., 2019). The complexity of evaluation for pain is also brought out by the problem of chronic pain, which is usually refractory to conventional methods of treatment. Chronic pain, particularly orthopedic pain, may not be linked with any detectable physiological damage, and practitioners need to use a multidimensional approach to manage it effectively. This involves identifying the pain's characteristics—i.e., severity, length of time, and impact on function—and the psychosocial determinants of pain. Comprehensive patient history is typically conducted by physiotherapists through an integration of medical, psychological, and activity history to grasp the complex nature of chronic pain syndromes. Such extensive assessment methods allow for the identification of the relieving and aggravating pain factors, ultimately deciding the selection of the correct interventions. By thoroughly taking into account the physiological and psychological dimensions of pain, physiotherapists can provide more effective and humane care (Maher et al., 2019). One of the most important aspects of pain examination in orthopedic physiotherapy is the implementation of evidence-based methods to obtain the optimal outcome. Recent literature emphasizes the importance of standardized pain assessment measures, which improve consistency and reliability in the evaluation of pain across different patient populations. Standardized measures such as the Visual Analog Scale (VAS) or Numeric Rating Scale (NRS) can facilitate effective, concise communication between practitioners and patients, thus enhancing the efficacy of treatment. Moreover, recent studies highlight the need for interdisciplinary working in pain care, encouraging an interprofessional approach that includes physiotherapists, physicians, psychologists, and other professionals. The interprofessional collaboration provides an effective team approach to assess pain better, eventually resulting in customized treatment plans that are able to manage both acute and chronic pain states effectively. By embracing a holistic process of evaluation that encompasses subjective, objective, and evidence-based methodologies, physiotherapists can improve outcomes in pain management in their practice of orthopedics (Khachane et al., 2019) (Figure 14.4).

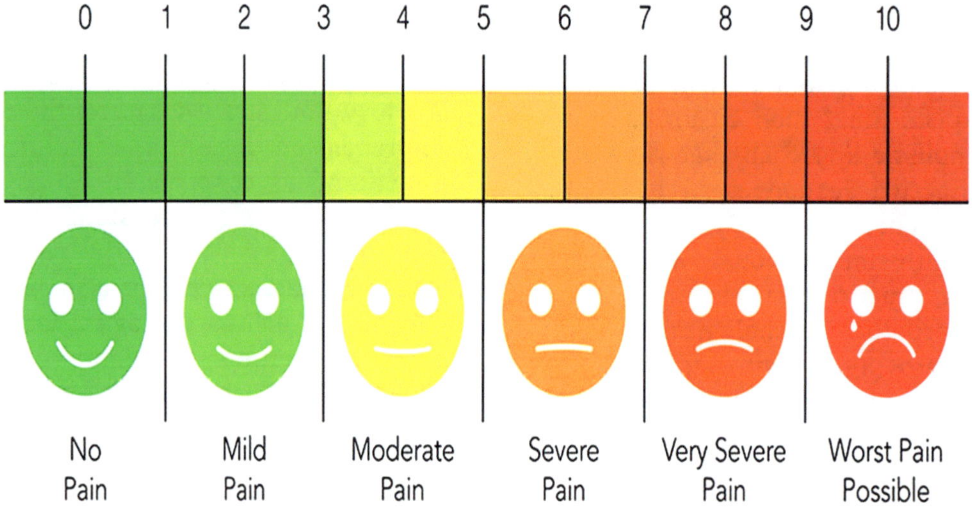

Figure 14.4. Pain scale.

Source: https://d1zxene68j3keg.cloudfront.net/sites/default/files/Resouces/images/Manage%20 Pain.jpg.

14.2.1. Tools and Techniques for Pain Assessment

Pain measurement during orthopedic physiotherapy is important to guide effective management. Various devices and methods can be employed to measure and quantify pain such that clinicians can tailor interventions to unique patient requirements. Patient-reported measures such as the Visual Analog Scale (VAS) and Numeric Rating Scale (NRS) render the patient an active partner in their communication of pain intensity, and thus enable subjective perception of pain to be measured. These measuring tools are widely used due to their simplicity and ease of administration. Additionally, observational tools, particularly in populations that cannot communicate their discomfort, rely on behavioral signs to assess the presence and intensity of pain. Consequently, the use of multiple pain measuring tools is mandatory in the provision of a full understanding of the patient's condition that subsequently enhances more effective pain management interventions within orthopedic physiotherapy (Figure 14.5).

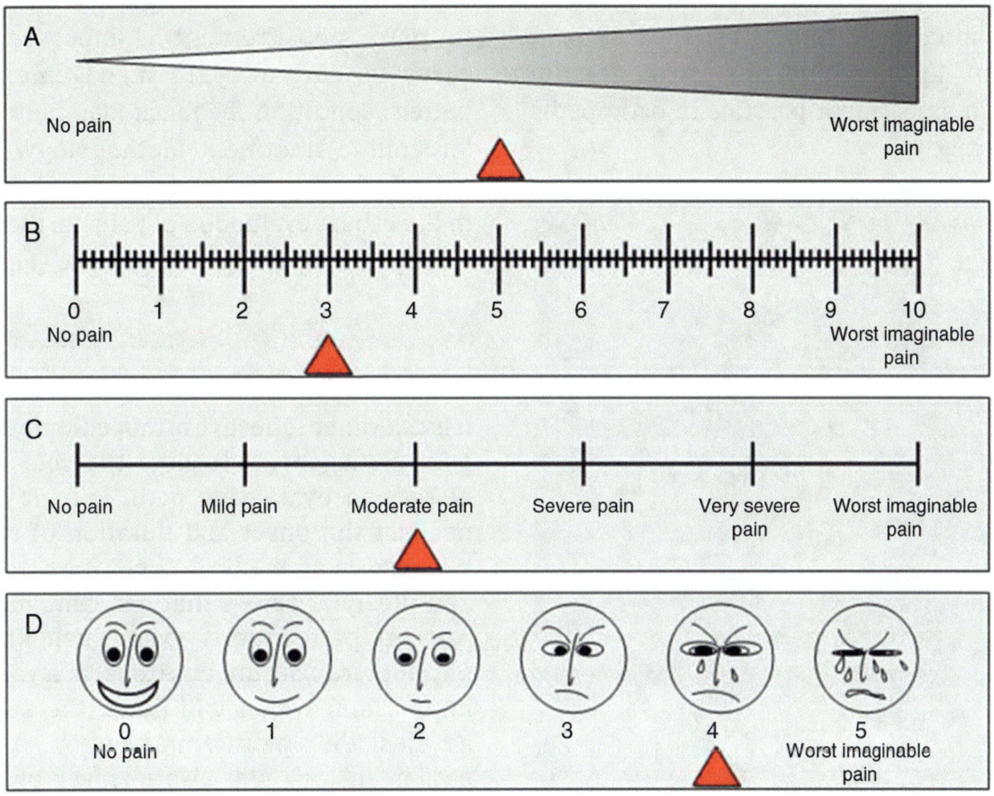

Figure 14.5. One-dimensional pain scales depicting examples of pain ratings. Pain is assigned to a range between 0 and 100 mm (VAS), a selection of possible answers (VRS), a numerical value between 0 and 10 (NRS), or a facial expression (SAS). (A) Visual analogue scale (VAS). (B) Numerical rating scale (NRS). (C) Verbal rating scale (VRS). (D) The 'Smiley' analogue scale (SAS).

Source: https://www.researchgate.net/profile/Bjoern-Bruecher/publication/259847648/figure/fig1/AS:267587510599735@1440809242912/One-dimensional-pain-scales-depicting-examples-of-pain-ratings-Pain-is-assigned-to-a.png.

Aside from self-report and observational measures, clinician-rated pain rating scales have emerged as a valid means of measuring pain in orthopedic patients. The McGill Pain Questionnaire and the Brief Pain Inventory are some of these scales that encompass sensory, affective, and evaluative dimensions of pain and offer a multidimensional approach to the understanding of the patient's experience. These scales not only fine-tune clinicians' ability to pick up the qualitative characteristics of pain but also inform treatment planning by helping to clarify the impact of the pain on daily living. As highlighted in earlier work, the choice of assessment instrument must be informed by individual patient factors and the specific context in which the assessment is taking place so as to optimize the accurate portrayal of pain. Finally, the integration of different assessment tools makes the evaluation more powerful, enabling the development of a tailored strategy for effective pain management. Moreover, modern technologies, such as pain assessment applications, can dramatically change pain assessment practice in orthopedic physiotherapy.

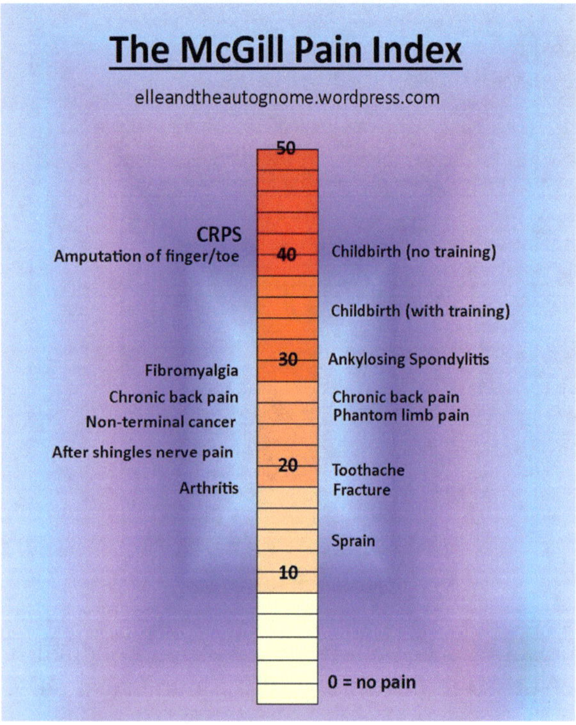

Figure 14.6. McGill Pain Scale.

Source: https://www.reddit.com/media?url=https%3A%2F%2Fi.redd.it%2Fr1yjgt9o2qf91.jpg.

Online platforms are likely to incorporate artificial intelligence and machine learning elements, enabling the creation of huge amounts of patient data over time and improving the efficiency and accuracy of the assessments. For instance, such software is capable of tracking pain pattern changes and response to treatment, providing valuable information to the clinicians. Having real-time information at hand, physiotherapists are able to make informed decisions regarding therapeutic interventions and corresponding adjustments. According to recent studies, technological implementation in pain measurement is most relevant to cases of chronic pain management, where patient condition feedback may help clinicians streamline treatment methodology. Thus, the advent of computerized tools is a significant leap in the robust evaluation of pain, further enabling orthopedic physiotherapy practice (Figure 14.6).

14.2.2. Role of Patient History in Pain Evaluation

It is relevant to effective orthopedic physiotherapy pain management to note the role of patient history in evaluating pain. Patient history is not just the onset and duration of symptoms, but also past medical conditions, treatments, and lifestyle factors that can contribute to the present pain status. From such knowledge, physiotherapists are able to form a valid clinical impression, which will guide the selection of an ideal therapeutic intervention. A thorough patient history will also uncover psychosocial variables that influence pain assessment and response to treatment. Once these connected variables are understood, clinicians are able to develop a more individualized and effective pain management plan that acknowledges the complexity of musculoskeletal pain. Systematically taking patient history is a cornerstone for differentiating between types of pain, i.e., nociceptive versus neuropathic pain. Different pain mechanisms require unique assessment strategies and treatment protocols. For instance, chronic pain syndromes like Complex Regional Pain Syndrome (CRPS) may present differently from one another because of their complex etiology and variable presentation. In these situations, it is important to assess patient history for information about previous diagnostic encounters and treatments received, which may affect current responses to pain. With the intricacies that are at play, physiotherapists will need to accept the confines of research that has been conducted up until now, draw understanding from a variety of sources in order to clarify practice effectively, as noted in previous work on this subject (Harden et al., 2022). Furthermore, the integration of the understanding that has been gained from an in-depth patient history can serve to constructively support communication and rapport between patient and physiotherapist. This therapeutic connection is paramount in orthopedic physiotherapy, in which active participation by patients is essential to the success of treatment. The greater the sense of being heard and understood regarding their pain experiences, the greater their adherence to recommendations for treatment. By utilizing modern approaches, such as virtual reality and augmented reality, as outlined in up-to-date literature, one can not only contribute to the healing process by allowing physical therapy to occur but also provide didactic support for patients in comprehending their condition and treatment options (Mishra et al., 2022). Thus, the role of patient history transcends information gathering; it is an integral, active part of an interdisciplinary approach to pain treatment that fosters understanding and collaboration (Figure 14.7).

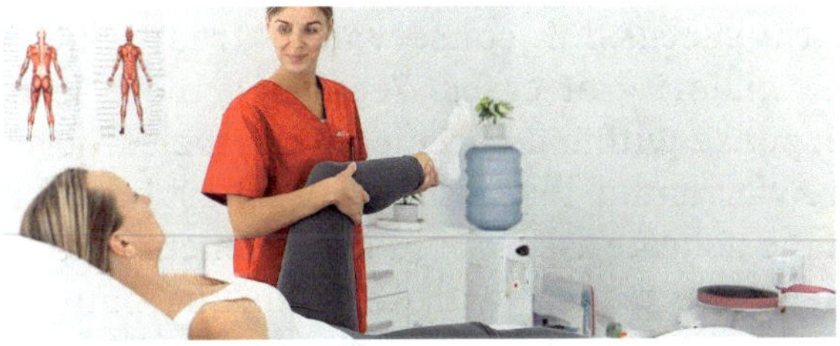

Figure 14.7. Pain management.

Source: https://firstresponsehealthcare.com/blog/wp-content/uploads/2022/03/pain_management_8420d87dbd.webp.

14.2.3. Importance of Objective Measures in Assessment

In orthopedic physiotherapy, and more so pain management, the use of objective measures in the evaluation process is imperative. Object measures provide clinicians with precise information that quantitatively assesses a patient's functional ability and degree of pain, thereby facilitating improved treatment planning. Unlike subjective scales, where their responses can vary based on mood and personal interpretation, objective measurement gives consistent information that can be replicated time and time again and compared over time. For instance, the use of standard scales and technological advancements in quantifying pain allow clinicians to accurately plot improvement, adjust therapeutic maneuvers, and eventually enhance outcomes in their patients. With this consideration, objective measurements not only serve to decrease biases but also increase the transparency of treatment efficacy within pain management regimens. Additionally, the application of objective measures is even more crucial in maintaining patient compliance with exercise regimens prescribed to them. Home exercise regimes adherence is typically problematic, with nonadherence standing as high as more than 50% (Argent et al., 2018). This phenomenon has the potential to lead to suboptimal clinical outcomes, since regular exercise is crucial to pain relief and rehabilitation. Therefore, utilizing connected health technologies, including mobile apps and wearable technology, can assist in enhancing compliance by creating real-time feedback as well as tracking compliance. By using such objective measures, clinicians can learn about patient behavior and tailor interventions to overcome major determinants of non-adherence, e.g., motivational problems or knowledge of the benefits of exercise. By so doing, the use of data functions empowers the clinicians and the patients alike and hence optimizes the effectiveness of pain management initiatives. Finally, objective measures in assessment are also recognized in clinical guidelines, for example, from the International Scientific Society on Scoliosis Orthopedic and Rehabilitation Treatment (SOSORT) (Négrini et al., 2018). The society emphasizes evidence-based protocols for assessment in conservative treatment methodologies, as well as stressing the application of standardized methods for assessment of the effectiveness of treatment. Through the synthesis of various literature reviews and consensus-driven suggestions, these guidelines stress the role of objective measures in both the assessment of treatment outcomes and the making of clinical decisions. This strict approach not only guarantees that patients are receiving the most effective and individualized care but also assists in bridging the gap between clinical practice and research. Lastly, emphasizing objective standards within the framework of assessment is important for the advancement of pain management in orthopedic physiotherapy, which leads to improved patient outcomes and satisfaction.

14.3. Treatment Modalities

In orthopedic physiotherapy, modalities play an important role in managing pain effectively. Physiotherapists apply several interventions based on the requirements of the patients with the intention of enhancing mobility and reducing pain. Modalities such as manual therapy, therapeutic exercise, and heat or cold modalities have proven to be of serious significance in preventing pain and facilitating recovery. Among these, therapeutic exercises are typically emphasized as they not only cure pain but also provide functional independence. Incorporation of these exercises in a complete treatment plan can help restore strength, flexibility, and overall joint function, which are important in the management of osteoarthritis and post-surgical rehabilitation. This multifaceted strategy emphasizes the importance of individualized therapy in providing maximal outcomes in patients with orthopedic disorders. Another increasingly known treatment approach includes the application of sophisticated technologies like surface electromyography (sEMG). Though it has the potential to maximize the outcomes of rehabilitation, sEMG is less used in clinics for a variety of reasons, ranging from cultural to educational and technical, to overcome. The evidence suggests that including objective measurements in physiotherapy will encourage evidence-based practice, maximizing the efficiency of treatment plans. Nevertheless, the divide between research breakthroughs and their applicability remains. More sophisticated education programs for enhancing the preparation of physiotherapy practitioners in the proper utilization of such technologies are urgently required. Closing this gap would lead to significant advances in treating orthopedic pain disorders and, consequently, enhance the quality of care provided to patients across different clinical environments (Campanini et al., 2020). Individual cases such as frozen shoulder (FS) illustrate the complexity of treatment modalities in orthopedic physiotherapy. FS is assessed with pain and restricted range of motion, necessitating extended treatment, which can be by conservative methods like physiotherapy or invasive procedures like arthroscopic capsular release. Heterogeneity in the success of treatment is reported in existing literature, with successful conservative treatment in the majority of cases. Yet, when there is no response within a specified time, the surgeries are warranted. Physiotherapists must be aware of the delicate aspect of FS management because they have to deal with the thin line between non-surgical and surgical treatments. This is a testament to the call for ongoing studies and revision of treatment methods to ensure they are aligned with the latest research and most effective practice in orthopedic physiotherapy (Chul-Cho et al., 2019).

14.3.1. Physical Therapy Techniques for Pain Relief

Physical therapy techniques play a key role in pain control, and especially in orthopedic physiotherapy, where pain reduction is typically the primary goal. Among the various techniques, manual therapy can prove particularly beneficial, with hands-on techniques to mobilize joints and tissues. In addition to reducing pain, it also enhances mobility and function. For instance, mobilization techniques can decrease stiffness developed due to conditions such as adhesive shoulder capsulitis, involving excessive scarring of tissue around the glenohumeral joint. Evidence also suggests that utilization of such techniques can result in greater range of movement and control of pain, with consequent benefit to overall functional status among patients (Khachane et al., 2019). Furthermore, the therapeutic advantages of manual therapy may even enhance a sense of teamwork between the patient and therapist, ensuring active involvement in the recovery process. Therapeutic exercises are also a very important part of physical therapy for pain relief. These exercises are carefully devised for strengthening the concerned muscles, stabilizing the joints, and enhancing the body's overall functional ability. By incorporating specific movements into treatment, physical therapists allow for controlled loading of tissues, which is critical to accomplish in the healing process. To illustrate, strength training can be used for patients undergoing post-surgical shoulder rehabilitation to encourage proper muscle activation and recovery. Evidence shows that patients receiving certain programs of exercise exhibit lower pain levels along with better functional capacity, hence reinforcing the effectiveness of exercise therapy for pain management (Khachane et al., 2019). Furthermore, the psychological benefits obtained through partaking in a systematic program of exercise could also promote adherence to therapy, a crucial aspect in long-term recovery. Modalities such as heat, cold, ultrasound, and electrical stimulation also find their place in physical therapy for the facilitation of relief from pain in orthopedic disorders. Heat therapy, for instance, can relax muscles and circulate blood, relieving pain in muscle strains. Cold therapy lessens swelling and numbs sharp pain, providing immediate relief from injury. In addition, ultrasound therapy can aid in tissue healing by strong thermal effects, while electrical stimulation can aid in the management of pain by interfering with pain signals sent to the brain. The combination of these modalities makes it possible for therapists to tailor treatment according to the specific needs of the patient and the conditions being addressed. By successful utilization of these approaches, physical therapists become significant contributors to overall pain management strategies in orthopedic physiotherapy, enhancing overall patient care (Le et al., 2016) (Figure 14.8).

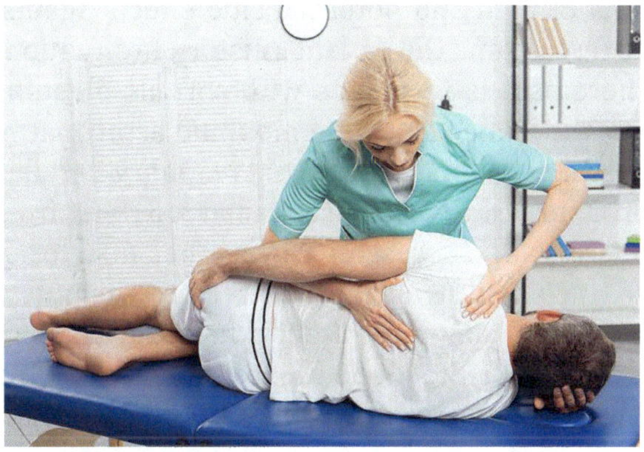

Figure 14.8. Expert physiotherapist for pain treatment.

https://www.google.com/url?sa=i&url=https%3A%2F%2Fpanoramahillsphysio.stck.me%2Fpost%2F269665%2FExpert-Physiotherapist-For-Pain-Treatment-Finding-Relief-at-Panorama-Hills-Physio&psig=AOvVaw3DAw4m3Pq7Ws4Yk_ntE-Nq&ust=1749380699331000&source=images&cd=vfe&opi=89978449&ved=0CBcQjhxqFwoTCOjAmY-V340DFQAAAAAdAAAAABAL.

14.3.2. Pharmacological Interventions in Pain Management

Pharmacology of pain management for orthopedic physiotherapy is made complex by the variety of patient requirements for varied pain syndromes. Non-steroidal anti-inflammatory drugs (NSAIDs) are most commonly utilized due to their potency as anti-inflammatory and analgesic compounds. In acute situations, recovery from surgery or acute traumatic musculoskeletal injury, these medications can significantly enhance patient comfort and recovery rate. Though chronic NSAID use is fraught with risks like gastrointestinal hemorrhage and cardiovascular events, it demands careful monitoring of the patient. So too is acetaminophen, widely recommended based on safety, utilized as a first-line for mild to moderate pain, particularly in those patients predisposed to the adverse effects of NSAIDs. These drugs are employed guardedly, balancing relief of pain and potential side effects against the disease and the patient's history. In situations where pain is severe, as with chronic bleeding into the same joint in hemophilic arthropathy, more intense pharmacologic weaponry is called for. Opioids are often prescribed for relief from severe pain, successful when other analgesics have failed. Although opioids can provide potent pain relief, long-term use is a cause for concern due to possible dependence, tolerance, and abuse. Therefore, orthopedic physiotherapists must exercise caution in prescribing these drugs as part of an overall, multidisciplinary pain management program. Opioids can be employed synergistically with adjunct treatments, like corticosteroids—intra-articular injections for inflammation pain in a local area—to enhance therapeutic effect with less risk of opioid side effects. This demands appropriate coordination between health professionals to develop overall treatment plans that deliver maximum pain relief outcomes. New pharmacologic therapies are also possible in the evolving situation of pain management. For instance, non-factor treatments for hemophilic arthropathy, which are capable of addressing such associated pain without the anticoagulant effect of traditional management, represent a new trend. Moreover, the application of cyclooxygenase-2 (COX-2) inhibitors is a therapeutic method that eliminates pain with the potential to reduce the adverse effects of the conventional NSAIDs. Lastly, effective pain treatment in orthopedic physiotherapy requires individualization of the drug therapy to a person's unique variables and the nature of pain under management. Effective pain practice management should integrate pharmacologic and non-pharmacologic interventions, including physiotherapy and patient education, to optimize mobility and quality of life for patients while treating them within the individual needs of the therapeutic environment (Gualtierotti et al., 2022; Geroin et al., 2023) (Figure 14.9).

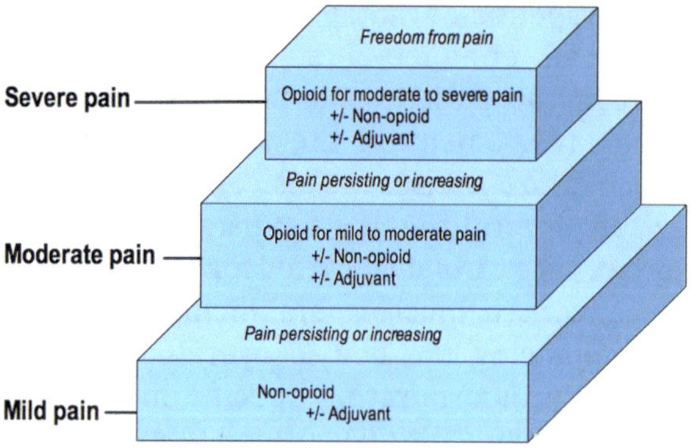

Figure 14.9. Pharmacological management of pain.

Source: https://www.researchgate.net/profile/Sadeq-Quraishi/publication/312576362/figure/fig2/AS:452639491137538@1484929072897/Pharmacological-management-of-pain-Adapted-from-the-World-Health-Organization-Pain.png.

14.3.3. Complementary Therapies and Their Effectiveness

With the advanced evolution of orthopedic physiotherapy, complementary treatments have been given much attention due to the assumed effectiveness of pain alleviation. These consist of treatments like acupuncture, massage, and mindfulness. They perform their functions by alleviating pain and improving the well-being of patients with musculoskeletal issues. For instance, acupuncture has come forth with possible effectiveness in reducing pain and improving mobility, particularly in patients suffering from lower back pain and arthritis. By fostering insight into other therapeutic modalities, the physiotherapist can offer a fuller variety of treatment that includes the psychological and emotional dimensions of pain and thereby constructs enhanced healing results within the patient population. The use of complementary therapies in orthopedic physiotherapy can also be influenced by more recent developments in clinical techniques, particularly in patient education and participation. Research has indicated that the impact of such treatments is increased when the patient is an active participant in creating their own pain management plans, as this provides a sense of agency and collaboration within the treatment process. Treatments such as sEMG can be utilized to provide objective measures of muscle function and dysfunction as adjunct treatments. This holistic approach is also part of a greater shift towards Evidence-Based Medicine, where the combination of various therapeutic approaches can lead to optimal patient benefit. Thus, equipping practitioners with knowledge regarding these complementary approaches not only strengthens orthodox practice but also the overall body of orthopedic physiotherapy in general. Furthermore, the effectiveness of complementary interventions may be heavily influenced by individual patient factors, including age, comorbidities, and even diagnoses like intervertebral disc diseases. Lower back pain is also common among older people, and intervertebral disc diseases are a common source of pain and disability. Understanding the pathophysiology of these disorders and the outcome measures of these complementary therapies permits individualized intervention strategies to meet specific patient needs. Technological advancements in noninvasive diagnostic tools are permitting more informed treatment decision-making. Lastly, the encouragement of the integrated partnership of complementary therapies and conventional orthopedic physiotherapy has the potential to create an integrated management system that supports the quality of care for chronic pain patients (Campanini et al., 2020; Wu et al., 2020) (Figure 14.10).

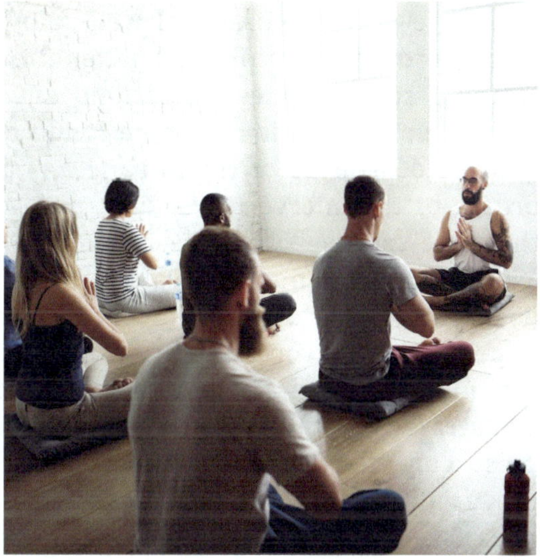

Figure 14.10. Complementary therapy.

Source: https://files.nccih.nih.gov/files/yoga-class-meditation-ThinkstockPhotos-637955386-square.jpg.

14.4. Role of Exercise in Pain Management

Exercise as part of pain management programs in orthopedic physiotherapy is critical, given its established effectiveness in alleviating pain caused by most orthopedic conditions. Regular physical activity has been established to stimulate the immune system to release endorphins, which are naturally produced body chemicals with pain-relieving properties. The biochemical effect has been established to be crucial in reducing the perception of pain and in enhancing general mood. While the patient exercises specifically designed for his or her requirements, they not only address the physical issues related to pain but also assist with improved functioning and mobility. Interestingly, exercise is capable of reversing the detrimental effects of immobilization due to lack of movement, which is common in people with chronic pain. By promoting movement, exercise makes it possible for the maintenance of musculoskeletal well-being as well as improvement to prevent patients from developing secondary complications due to disuse and immobilization. In some conditions, such as osteoarthritis of the knee (KOA) and disorders of the intervertebral disc, engaging in the right exercise programs becomes even crucial. KOA, the most prevalent form of osteoarthritis, impacts a high percentage of the older population and contributes to an enormous rate of morbidity and disability. Research has demonstrated that consistent low-impact exercise can effectively alleviate symptoms, improve joint function, and slow disease progression in KOA patients and thus enhance quality of life (Geng et al., 2023). Similarly, patients with diseases of the intervertebral discs are commonly faced with crushing lower back pain, the relief of which can be obtained by adopting systematic exercise programs. These programs can assist in lumbar and core strengthening, stabilizing the spine, along with relief to intervertebral discs (Wu et al., 2020). Therefore, individualized exercise intervention in the framework of orthopedic physiotherapy emerges as the cornerstone of integrated pain management. Additionally, the multifaceted benefits of exercise go beyond pain alone, such as improvement in psychological well-being as well as patient adherence to rehabilitation protocols. Active exercise patients have higher chances of self-reporting enhanced mood and decreased anxiety levels, which can change the basic pain experience. This is particularly useful in cases where chronic pain has led to mental distress, creating a cycle of added physical limitations. Effective exercise programs not only reduce pain but also self-efficacy patients by inducing feelings of control and motivation toward healing. By adding education concerning the role of exercise in controlling pain and its overall health value, medical providers are able to best enable patients to make well-educated choices regarding their treatment regimens. Thus, the role of exercise within orthopedic physiotherapy extends beyond mere symptom control to serve as a crucial part of comprehensive pain management protocols.

14.4.1. Benefits of Exercise in Orthopedic Rehabilitation

Exercise takes a pivotal role in orthopedic rehabilitation because it caters to both the physical and psychological areas of recovery. Exercise programs targeting the damaged sections enhance joint movement, strength, and promote tissue repair. A case in point is with conditions such as frozen shoulder, where a gradual rehabilitation program in the form of exercises to restore range of motion can successfully minimize pain and prevent further loss of function. Conservative treatment methods like physiotherapy typically yield better results without the interference of surgical intervention when done in a systematic way. The method puts high importance on exercise in the recovery of musculoskeletal normalcy, showing the effectiveness as an isolated form of pain management, especially in the context of orthopedic physiotherapy, where recovery of function is held above all else (Chul-Cho et al., 2019). Moreover, the practice of exercise during rehabilitation heals not only the physical manifestations of orthopedic injuries but also their psychological impact. Physical activity regularly will help to reverse the depression and anxiety so frequently found in association with long-standing illness or pain. Relief of pain by the release of endorphins associated with exercise, plus an overall sense of well-being, is a bonus. Specific exercise therapy, such as physiotherapeutic scoliosis-specific exercises (PSSE), has proven to be effective in improving spinal function and quality of life for patients with idiopathic scoliosis. The findings are highlighted against the need for rehabilitation protocols to be prioritized in favor of evidence-guided principles for organized exercise programs, as sanctioned by the latest guidelines from institutions committed to conservative treatment modalities (Négrini et al., 2018). Further, long-term benefits of exercise involve injury prevention and general musculoskeletal well-being. Exercise is a factor in learning stronger muscles and enhanced coordination, essential in the prevention of falls and subsequent injury, particularly for the elderly.

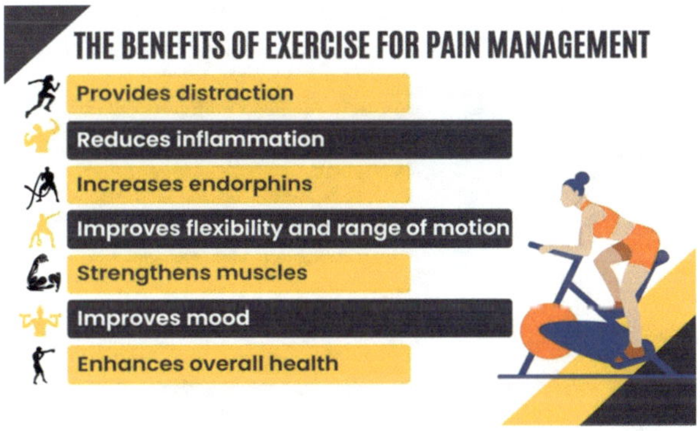

Figure 14.11. benefits of exercise for pain management.

Source: https://skalefitness.com/wp-content/uploads/2023/03/exercise-for-pain-1024x655.webp.

Exercises in orthopedic rehabilitation often revolve around balance, strength, and flexibility, making rehabilitation a holistic process. This forward-looking strategy not only addresses pain relief in the short term but also maintains long-term gain in terms of mobility and independence. The placement of exercise within orthopedic rehabilitation thus becomes a cornerstone not only for enhancing short-term recovery but also for maximizing lifetime health and function, thus significantly expanding the discipline of orthopedic physiotherapy (Figure 14.11).

14.4.2. Types of Exercises for Different Orthopedic Conditions

Effective exercise prescription is a key component in the management of several orthopedic disorders since it has the ability to reduce pain and also improve function dramatically. Patients with disorders such as osteoarthritis need to be prescribed low-impact exercises such as cycling and swimming, which reduce joint stress but improve mobility via them. Strengthening is also required because it improves the muscles encircling a joint so that it will be better protected during activity. Individualized rehabilitation exercises can employ a progressive treatment technique, targeting specific muscle groups to enhance stability and strength, allowing for slow rehabilitation and avoiding injury. Additionally, incorporating flexibility training is essential to assist in joint range of motion, which will decrease stiffness involved in orthopedic cases. Taken as a whole, the synergy between aerobic, strength, and flexibility training can be an effective foundation for orthopedic physiotherapy pain management and rehabilitation. In cervical or lumbar disc diseases, exercise training should emphasize core stabilization and extension of the spine to minimize pain and accelerate healing. One study highlighted that patients suffering from intervertebral disc diseases gain significant advantages from an organized exercise regimen, which may include pelvic tilts and abdominal bracing exercises to enhance spinal support strength and reduce the pressure on discs (Wu et al., 2020). Besides, professionally guided stretching exercises are designed to enhance the flexibility of the back muscles, reducing pain and increasing range of motion. Physical therapists tend to use modalities such as manual therapy along with specific exercises to obtain the best possible outcomes. This range-of-treatment process not only addresses pain management but also allows patients to be empowered through active participation in their rehabilitation, creating a general atmosphere that will lead to continued wellness. In pediatric populations, particularly those with cerebral palsy, exercise interventions must be specifically tailored to meet the unique developmental needs and capabilities. Therapeutic exercises can range from gross motor skill development to more complex functional motions, helping in muscle tone and coordination regulation. Proper physical exercise has been shown to significantly increase the quality of life and functional outcomes in cerebral palsy (Paul et al., 2022). Physiotherapy protocols usually involve enjoyable and game-like techniques in a drive to encourage young patients, enhancing compliance with exercise' guidelines and recommendations. Additionally highlighted are strengthening and stretching exercises aimed at improving balance and flexibility that are vital to preventing contractures and facilitating mobility. By enabling an environment where children can experience enjoyable aspects of exercise, physical therapists themselves take a front-line position in pain management and enhancement of functional capability among pediatric orthopedic disorder patients (Figure 14.12).

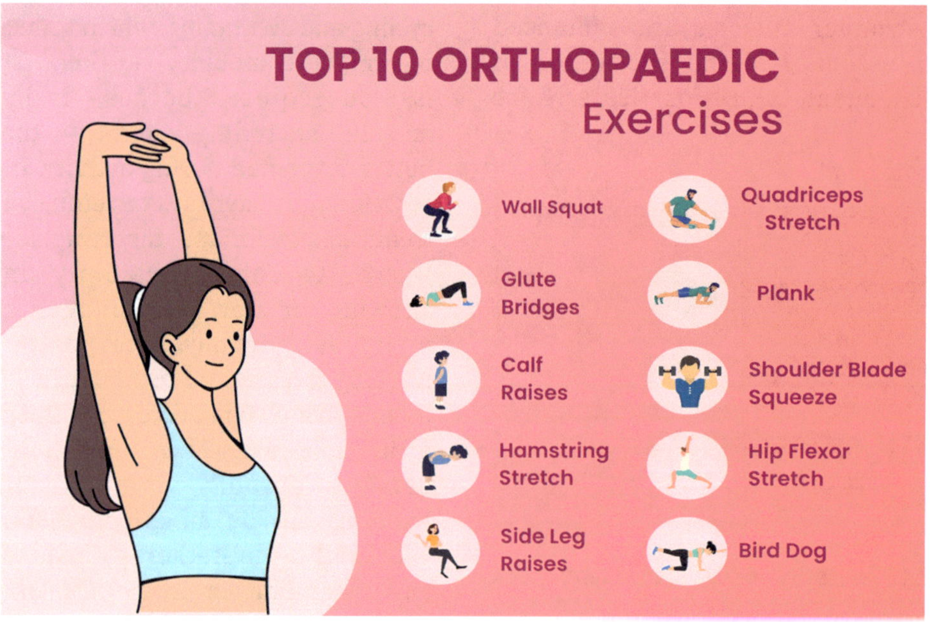

Figure 14.12. Top 10 orthopedic exercises.

Source: https://www.manipalhospitals.com/uploads/image_gallery/top-10-orthopedic-exercises.png.

14.4.3. Guidelines for Safe Exercise Practices

In orthopedic physiotherapy, safe exercise cannot be overstressed. A well-planned exercise program, besides giving relief from pain, encourages mobility and functional independence in musculoskeletal disorder patients. Some of the most important guidelines are to seek a full assessment by a qualified physiotherapist, who can devise programs based on people's needs and circumstances. This individualized strategy ensures that exercises are appropriate for the patient's current abilities as well as progress toward further advancement. In addition, patients must be instructed by physiotherapists regarding modifications so they understand how to effectively and safely execute each exercise. By establishing an empathic and constructive environment, health professionals can empower patients to fully engage in their rehabilitation and minimize the risk of injury or symptom exacerbation. Another major guideline addresses the application of warm-up and cool-down activities. Prior to any exercise, patients have to perform a dynamic warm-up to prepare the body for physical activity. This can include slow range-of-motion exercises and slow aerobic exercises, which induce high blood flow in the muscles and enhance flexibility. A cool-down with the inclusion of static stretching after exercise helps to sustain flexibility and reduce muscle stiffness.

Besides, patients need to be directed to listen to their bodies and notice any kind of pain or discomfort when performing exercise activities. Awareness plays an important role in preventing injuries and ensuring safe participation in rehabilitation exercises. Khachane et al. (2019) reaffirm that adherence to these guidelines not only facilitates a safe exercising environment but also lays the groundwork for effective long-term pain management and recovery. Paying attention to cross-training and variation in exercise is also important. Training in multiple modes of exercise may prevent overuse injuries and result in an even fitness program. On the orthopedic rehabilitation front, incorporating low-impact exercises such as swimming, cycling, or yoga into a program for a patient with arthritic pain or restrictions can be highly beneficial. This approach allows for muscle strengthening and improved cardiovascular conditioning without undue stress on the sites of injury. Regular monitoring with physiotherapists to adjust programs based on patient response is essential in maintaining attendance and adherence to programs. With the implementation of these diverse, risk-free exercise techniques, patients are able to enhance their rehabilitation process as well as reduce pain associated with orthopedic ailments, ending up with healthier lives and improved quality of life.

14.5. Patient Education and Self-Management

Effective patient education and self-management are central to pain management in orthopedic physiotherapy. Patient education with precise information about their condition and accompanying pain management techniques empowers them to become invested in the recovery process. By learning about their diagnosis, potential treatment, and the necessity of adherence to recommended exercise regimens, patients can minimize pain and improve functional status. Teachers need to tailor information to learning styles, presenting it in plain language and creating a questioning learning environment. Such collaboration not only generates trust but also strengthens the therapeutic partnership between practitioner and patient, which is key to maximum rehabilitation success. Self-management abilities, like the execution of ordered exercises and the use of pain coping tools, are important in patient recovery. There is evidence that noncompliance with home exercise programs is a major determinant of failure of rehabilitation, with approximately 50% of patients being noncompliant. The most frequent barriers to compliance are related to a lack of knowledge or motivation on the part of the patient to do exercises independently. Increased utilization of networked health technologies, such as mobile apps and wearable technology, can promote compliance by providing users with significant feedback, reminders, and monitoring of progress. By including such technology in their curriculum, practitioners can help patients overcome participation barriers, staying committed to their rehabilitation objectives and pain management strategies (Argent et al., 2018). Moreover, the interface between education and technology enhances not just compliance but more knowledge of pain management principles. Enhanced practices, such as the use of surface electromyography for quantitative assessments, will be able to enable clinicians to better document the efficacy of individually prescribed exercises (Campanini et al., 2020). The technology serves as a linking concept between theoretical comprehension and practical application and provides information guiding practice-based decision making and fostering patient confidence in treatment approaches. Bridging education tools into practice prepares patients to cope with their pain more effectively and empowers them with the skills necessary for long-term wellness beyond the clinic. Ultimately, there needs to be an emphasis on creating a culture of education and self-management in orthopedic physiotherapy to optimize patient outcomes and ensure long-term independence.

14.5.1. Importance of Educating Patients About Pain

Effective management of pain in orthopedic physiotherapy is, to a large extent, dependent on patient education about their pain. Understanding the nature of their condition allows patients to have realistic expectations of their treatment and recovery process. Education is a potent tool in eradicating myths about pain, which are predisposed to perpetuate catastrophizing and poor coping strategies. For instance, when patients are misinformed, they may confuse their pain with irreversible damage, such as in a case study where a patient who had been misdiagnosed with osteochondrosis of the spine went on to develop chronic misconceptions, which hampered proper planning for treatment. Therefore, comprehensive education processes involving the removal of these misconceptions and phobias are key to the rehabilitation process, which ultimately results in improved outcomes and increased participation in one's care. Besides, education on pain management practices enhances autonomy and self-efficacy. If educated on effective strategies, including therapeutic exercises and the appropriate use of ergonomics, patients will be more disposed to be actively involved in their rehabilitation and everyday functioning.

This information can alleviate helplessness and encourage adherence to recommended therapies. For example, by means of educative counseling supported by kinesiotherapy, patients can learn how to constructively manage their pain experience, reducing the impact of psychosocial determinants like anxiety and catastrophizing, documented in clinical observation. Active patients like these are more likely to be content with their care, as they perceive themselves to be part of the process rather than mere receivers of care. Lastly, educational intervention is able to bridge gaps between research and clinical practice, eliminating learned barriers in professional training. Rehabilitation clinicians are too frequently inadequate in basic knowledge to properly interpret quantitative pain measurements or to best utilize new technologies, as concluded in controversies for explanations of discrepancies between the large scientific literature and practice. Improving pain management education not only equips clinicians to care for their patients better but also promotes interdisciplinary collaborative communication in healthcare environments. As emphasized, the absence of equipment that is easy for users and the absence of standard measures are factors that lead to unfavorable patient outcomes. Therefore, integrating evidence-based educational models into pain management can revolutionize clinician practices and patients' experiences and lead, ultimately, to more encompassing and effective rehabilitation in orthopedic physiotherapy (Figure 14.13).

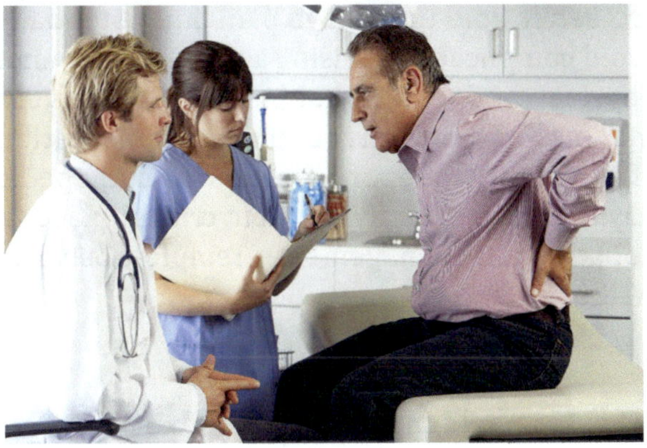

Figure 14.13. Educating patients about pain.

Source: https://www.gebauer.com/hubfs/pain_management.jpg.

14.5.2. Strategies for Self-Management of Pain

Effective self-management of pain is a vital element of orthopedic physiotherapy to empower patients to take charge of their pain management and facilitate their recovery. Mindfulness techniques, cognitive behavior therapy, and self-hypnosis have all proven effective in modifying the pain experience. Patient focus on the present moment characterizes mindfulness, encouraging acceptance of pain, and thereby reducing its emotional impact. Cognitive behavioral therapy assists patients in identifying and combating pain-related negative thoughts, promoting more adaptive coping. Self-hypnosis, also highlighted in literature, assists patients in going into a trance state, whereby they can detach from pain sensations, thus promoting physical therapy involvement and rehabilitation (Khachane et al., 2019). Not only do these techniques have the pain-reducing effect, but also a more general psychological impact on the patient, reinforcing their sense of control over their health. Physical self-management techniques are also a significant contribution to orthopedic physiotherapy, in addition to cognitive techniques. Systematic exercise programs tailored to the individual's needs can significantly alleviate pain and optimize function for the patient. Therapeutic procedures such as strengthening and stretching also aid in joint stabilization and stress reduction in the affected regions. Furthermore, teaching interventions on posture correction and ergonomic re-adjustment can assist in preventing the aggravation of pain through proper daily movements. Adherence to such protocols has been discovered to enhance outcomes, as ongoing participation in assigned exercises fosters both physical change but also self-efficacy in controlling one's state (Négrini et al., 2018). This multi-component protocol empowers the patient, more heavily equipping them with the means to take back control of their rehabilitation process. Lastly, a critical component of pain self-management addresses the role of social support and community resources. Communication with peers who share similar challenges can provide emotional support and motivation, which is essential for patients undergoing chronic pain. Physical or online support groups provide platforms for experience and planning exchange, enhancing motivation to adhere to self-managed regimes. Furthermore, collaboration with healthcare professionals, e.g., physiotherapists and psychologists, can ensure that patients are provided with tailored approaches that fit individual pain profiles. With the formation of an efficient support system, patients are better positioned to handle their rehabilitation process, hence increasing the quality of life as well as engagement in self-management strategies (Khachane et al., 2019). Lastly, the application of these strategies in orthopedic physiotherapy can lead to long-term pain management interventions and patient autonomy.

14.5.3. Role of Support Systems in Pain Management

Amongst the systems that have been hypothesized to play a role in the successful management of pain in orthopedic physiotherapy is the support system. Support systems denote a broad array of help, whether emotional, social, or medical, which helps create an atmosphere for healing. Emotional support from members of one's family and friends has a very significant impact on a patient's perception of pain and coping. Such individuals are likely to adhere to therapies that are prescribed to them and remain engaged in their rehabilitation process, hence reducing their overall experience of pain. This concept is in agreement with the biobehavioral model, which states the relationship between psychological well-being and physiological responses to pain and emphasizes that an overall support system should be incorporated in programs of pain management. The integration of support systems extends to healthcare providers and institutional facilities as well. A multidisciplinary service, combining orthopedic physiotherapy and psychological counseling with pain management specialists, will greatly enhance patient outcomes. Such teamwork encourages a broad assessment of pain, considering physical as well as psychological factors. Clinical evidence indicates that patients who are involved in schemes that apply alternate support systems report reduced pain and improved functional outcomes. This reinforces the necessity for orthopedic physiotherapists to organize and enhance contacts between patients and other support systems in order to foster collaboration in the participation of pain management intervention programs for complex pain phenomena (Négrini et al., 2018). Moreover, the dynamic character of evidence-based practices has recognized the importance of sustained support systems in the post-operative environment. Enhanced recovery strategies, as described in more contemporary research, encourage early mobilization and establish nutrition guidelines that highlight the role of support systems during recovery. For instance, immediate emotional and logistic support has been found to decrease anxiety and facilitate compliance with postoperative care procedures. By maximizing recovery through an effectively coordinated support system, patients are better able to manage pain and potentially avoid complications arising as a result of unmet physical and emotional needs. Collectively, the findings encourage the implementation of systematic support systems in orthopedic physiotherapy, justifying their critical place in holistic pain management (Temple-Oberle et al., 2017).

14.6. Challenges in Pain Management

Pain management is quite difficult in orthopedic physiotherapy, particularly due to the multifactorial basis of pain perception and individual variability in response to intervention. Psychological state, cultural background, and previous history of pain can strongly influence patients' perception and report of pain. This complexity complicates the implementation of universal pain management programs, as what may be effective for one patient may not be so for another. Therefore, orthopedic physiotherapists need to approach each case with a tailored combination of assessment and intervention specific to every individual's condition and needs. Understanding of these subtleties is necessary to the creation of comprehensive treatment plans that, in addition to pain relief, allow patients to become active participants in their recovery process, promote adherence to rehabilitation courses, and enhance the outcome as a whole in orthopedic practice. Additionally, the application of pharmacological approaches brings other difficulties to pain control. Although drugs, and particularly opioids, have been used for many years in postoperative pain management, their associated risks, including addiction and side effects, warrant reassessment of their role in orthopedic physiotherapy. Multimodal methods of pain management are becoming an attractive alternative by employing a group of non-opioid analgesics and regional anesthetics to target pain through various modes of action, minimizing opioid dependency. However, health inequities, unequal availability of advanced pain management techniques, and the need for extensive training in multimodal application restrict the application of these practices among professionals. The urgency for state-of-the-art solutions also highlights the need for ongoing research and education to equip orthopedic physiotherapists with effective application of these practices in different clinical environments (Machado et al., 2025). In addition, the multidisciplinary nature of pain management creates unique challenges, like unifying various healthcare providers into coordinated care. Effective pain management can sometimes require orthopedic surgeons, physiotherapists, pain physicians, and mental health professionals to conform to a collective pain management strategy. However, noncommunication, differences in philosophy of treatment, and resource constraints could prevent that. An instance of a case is observed in primary malignant giant cell tumor management, wherein multimodal treatment enhanced patient outcomes significantly. By incorporating surgical treatment along with postoperative physiotherapy, medical teams were able to demonstrate that there was scope for increased mobility and function (Prasad et al., 2025). Hence, establishing a spirit of teamwork and communication among the healthcare providers is crucial in an effort to optimize pain management in orthopedic physiotherapy, ultimately leading to enhanced patient outcomes and satisfaction.

14.6.1. Barriers to Effective Pain Management in Physiotherapy

Effective pain management in physiotherapy is riddled with numerous challenges that impede optimal patient outcomes. These challenges include cultural, educational, and technical barriers, among others. Cultural barriers include generic compliance with quantifiable pain management procedures, whereby some practitioners are opposed to abandoning traditional protocols for more objective assessments. This is compounded by training and educational differences between areas, which lead to variation in clinicians' ability to utilize advances in technology, such as surface electromyography (sEMG). Clinicians' reluctance to embrace evidence-based practice may significantly influence patient care to the extent of underutilization of potentially valuable methods to enhance recovery in orthopedic settings (Campanini et al., 2020). Therefore, breaking these cultural beliefs and creating a culture of innovation and knowledge transfer becomes a priority in assisting in advancing pain management practice in physiotherapy. Another highly significant barrier to effective pain management is compliance issues with home exercise programs (HEPs) prescribed by physiotherapists. Studies indicate that adherence levels range from 50%, significantly affecting the treatment outcome and patients' overall recovery (Argent et al., 2018). All of these are contributing factors towards nonadherence, including the unawareness of the patient about the importance of exercise, poor motivation, and the inability to integrate such exercises into activities of daily living. Also affecting compliance are individual patient factors, including pain severity and mental disorders. To counteract these difficulties, physiotherapists must deploy connected health technologies that enable patient empowerment. By embracing mobile applications and evidence-based practice, physiotherapists are able to provide guidance and support and hence improve patient compliance with exercise regimens and eventually pain management strategies. Also, technical inefficacies of pain management technologies are the culprits of inefficiency in the use of physiotherapy intervention. Despite advances in sensor technology and measurement tools, issues related to the cost, ease of use, and lack of standardized protocols for the equipment remain (Campanini et al., 2020). The cost and scarce training in the interpretation of such technology pose limitations to widespread clinical use. Additionally, the lack of a common vocabulary for rehabilitation clinicians and engineers could hinder synergistic efforts, preventing translation of research into practice. With the growing demand for contemporary pain management practices, the priority in expenditure on user-friendly equipment, uniform training, and improved communication between specialties is essential. By surmounting these technical barriers, physiotherapy can become a more effective discipline in pain management in orthopedic clinics with lasting implications on patient care.

14.6.2. Ethical Considerations in Pain Treatment

Ethics in pain management and orthopedic physiotherapy, in particular, are vital components influencing clinical practice and patient outcomes. Perhaps the foremost principle is informed consent, wherein practitioners need to clearly educate patients regarding treatment options, benefits, and risks of interventions aimed at managing pain. They need to be made aware of the choices, including the use of technology, which will have ramifications for facilitating self-management but may pose ethical issues in relation to data protection and security. These touch on the need for professionals to be responsive to, but not oblivious to, patients' autonomy so they become active agents, rather than passive consumers, of care, resulting in an ethically sound therapeutic bond. Further, inclusion of innovative technological interventions, such as mobile apps for pain management, presents a wonderful ethical challenge and opportunity. One of the significant cases is using health apps for self-management of conditions like low back pain. As indicated by research surrounding the Kaia App, the technology has proved effective in improving pain and physical functioning when compared to standard physiotherapy alone (Toelle et al., 2019). Ethical concerns do arise concerning the question of fair access to technology, as socioeconomic determinants might potentially disqualify some communities from accessing benefits. It becomes essential that healthcare systems strive to balance innovation and equity such that all patients can gain advantage from these effective interventions for pain relief, strengthening the ethical commitment to justice in healthcare delivery.

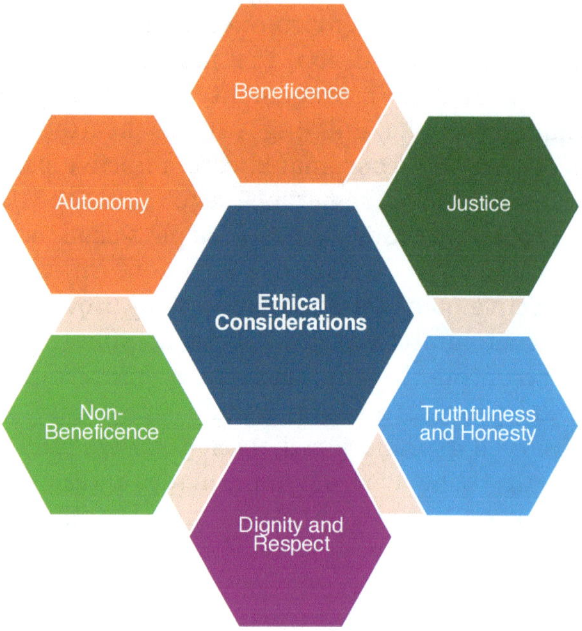

Figure 14.14. Ethical considerations.

Source: https://www.researchgate.net/profile/I-Made-Dwi-Adnyana/publication/377655909/figure/fig2/AS:11431281219610881@1706107451467/Ethical-considerations.png.

Furthermore, the ethics of pain treatment require care to consider the potential biases in clinical practice. For instance, evidence shows that if patients are actively involved in recovery, equipped with personalized educational information, they can have better results in pain management after surgical interventions, e.g., total knee replacement (Timmers et al., 2019). This also needs to be balanced against the individual variations within patient background that encompass cultural, psychological, and social intricacies that may affect treatment success and adherence. Ethical practice in orthopedic physiotherapy thus calls for practitioners to adopt a holistic approach, considering the individual circumstance and requirements of each patient, and what they are capable of doing for themselves in terms of pain management. In this manner, physiotherapists can maximize the ethical integrity of their interventions and an individualized model of care (Figure 14.14).

14.6.3. Future Directions for Improving Pain Management

The future of pain management in orthopedic physiotherapy necessitates global, individualized models of care going beyond traditional drug-based interventions. Utilization of high technology such as telehealth facilitates making things more accessible and allows for continued monitoring of patient progress. Using digital media, physiotherapists are able to offer individualized rehabilitation protocols, adjust treatment in real-time, and offer patients education materials that promote independence in self care for pain. Moreover, future directions could involve the utilization of data analytics to identify trends and results of pain management, further enhancing treatment procedures with collective outcomes and experiences of patients. The data-driven method has the potential to establish a proactive and individualized experience for patients, resulting in enhanced overall satisfaction and efficacy in pain control. The other direction is to integrate multidisciplinary approaches to deal with the complexity of pain management. As quoted by the recent hip fracture rehabilitation guidelines, successful recovery calls for a combined strategy of physical therapy, occupational therapy, and medical ecomanagement of related ailments (Min et al., 2021). Orthopedic physiotherapists should work in liaison with an interprofessional team of healthcare providers to create cohesive pain management plans attuned to patient-specific requirements. This blending can make not only pain management but also the enhancement of physical function and quality of life possible. Facilitation of this multidisciplinary collaboration will enable practitioners to share understanding and techniques and ultimately lead to enhanced outcomes in care and reduced overall burden of chronic pain syndromes. Apart from this, ongoing research and education in pain mechanisms and treatment strategies should persist as the foundation for future pain management. Research into non-invasive techniques such as neuromodulation and psychotherapy has promising future potential for pain reduction (Lagier et al., 2021). By understanding the physiological and psychological dimensions of pain, physiotherapists can develop more powerful, targeted interventions that address not just the symptoms but also the origin of pain. Furthermore, patient education in treatment programs encourages increased awareness and engagement in self-management strategies. With advancements in healthcare, being up-to-date on the latest evidence-based practice will keep orthopedic physiotherapists in a good position to tackle the unique issues of pain management within their specific patient populations.

SUMMARY

The effective orthopedic physiotherapy pain management has a pivotal position towards the optimization of patient results and maximizing optimal recovery. The interaction among therapeutic exercises, manual therapy, and application of modalities has been most beneficial in reducing pain and improving functional movement. Also, the increasing number of clinical trials of evidence supports the application of methodical treatment protocols, for example, those presented in the conservative treatment guidelines, which could significantly reduce the pain burden of such conditions as idiopathic scoliosis. The integration of these methods into one holistic system not only responds to the physical aspects of pain but also targets psychological features, which are crucial in developing an inclusive rehabilitation process for patients (Négrini et al., 2018). Further, the emphasis on evidence-based interventions highlights ongoing progress within orthopedic physiotherapy. The ERAS protocols, for instance, are the perfect example of a perioperative multi-modal management that rightfully enhances recovery with minimal pain following surgery. Such interdisciplinary approaches facilitate seamless transition from surgery to rehabilitation, hence rightfully addressing the issue of pain management along the care continuum. Collectively, these behaviors speak to the need for clinicians to be current with new guidelines and evidence to ensure optimal quality care for patients undergoing orthopedic rehabilitation (Ljungqvist et al., 2017). In conclusion, the role of orthopedic physiotherapists is more than the alleviation of pain; it involves empowering and informing patients and encouraging self-management. By equipping patients with the knowledge and skills required to manage their pain and become active participants in recommended therapies, physiotherapists enhance independence and general well-being. Ongoing communication with other healthcare professionals also maximizes the pain management process, providing patients with coordinated and integrated care best suited to their individual needs. As the profession evolves, it will continue to be imperative to utilize innovation and evidence-based practices in transcending adversity related to pain management in orthopedic physiotherapy, leading to enhanced patient function and satisfaction.

Orthopedic pain management in physiotherapy is comprehensive, with an emphasis on the integration of clinical evidence and individually tailored care methods. A central component of this approach is insight into complex pain syndromes, i.e., CRPS, which are multifactorial in nature and therefore require individually tailored treatment approaches. Recent advances highlight the importance of carrying out systematic reviews of available literature, with results showing a landscape of largely low to medium quality evidence. This discrepancy points to a necessity to combine current evidence in spite of the constraints of small sample size and rarity of such conditions. Practitioners are therefore required to modify treatment protocols where there is insufficient research evidence, being cautious about the unique presentation of every patient and how to appropriately combine several therapeutic strategies to optimize outcomes of pain reduction and functioning (Harden et al., 2022). In addition, the contribution of multidisciplinary collaboration cannot be undermined when it comes to orthopedic physiotherapy. Involving multiple healthcare workers encourages better comprehensiveness of pain management modalities, especially in dealing with conditions incurred with complicated genetic disorders like Neurofibromatosis Type 1 (NF1). NF1 patients tend to have multi-problematic orthopedic conditions that cause high morbidity. Therefore, the adoptive patient-centered longitudinal care strategy necessitates long-term observation and proper intervention of complications. The use of protocols, like France's Protocole national de diagnostic et de soins (PNDS), illustrates efforts towards the development of standardized care and maximizing therapeutic outcomes in different healthcare settings, thereby maximizing the efficacy of orthopedic pain management treatments (Bergqvist et al., 2020). Ultimately, continued research and development of therapeutic practice are key to furthering the evolution of pain management in orthopedic physiotherapy. Emerging evidence shows that incorporating new treatment modalities, such as neuromodulation techniques and targeted physical rehabilitation, can make significant contributions to altering outcomes for patients with chronic pain. While professionals remain dedicated to responding to individual patient needs, there is value in noting the importance of new information and integrating it into practice. This evidence-based practice pledge will facilitate enhanced symptom control in addition to the facilitation of recovery-supportive environments and enhanced quality of life for those with chronic pain conditions in orthopedic practice. Through the interweaving of clinical information with evolving research, orthopedic physiotherapists are better able to adapt practice to challenge the complex pain experiences of patients (Golovacheva et al., 2024).

CLOSER LOOK

PAIN MANAGEMENT

Pain management is a multidisciplinary approach aimed at reducing pain, improving comfort, and enhancing the quality of life for individuals suffering from acute or chronic pain. Pain can result from injury, surgery, illness, nerve damage, or long-term conditions such as arthritis, cancer, and musculoskeletal disorders. Effective pain management focuses not only on symptom relief but also on addressing the underlying causes of pain. Treatment strategies include pharmacological methods such as analgesics, anti-inflammatory drugs, muscle relaxants, and, in some cases, opioid medications under careful supervision. Non-pharmacological approaches play an equally important role and include physical therapy, exercise, heat and cold therapy, acupuncture, massage, relaxation techniques, and cognitive-behavioral therapy. Interventional procedures, such as nerve blocks, epidural injections, and minimally invasive surgeries, may be used for persistent or severe pain. A comprehensive pain management plan is personalized, considering the patient's medical history, pain intensity, lifestyle, and emotional well-being. Patient education and self-management strategies help individuals cope with pain and prevent recurrence. Psychological support is also essential, as chronic pain often affects mood, sleep, and daily functioning. Overall, effective pain management promotes physical recovery, emotional balance, and functional independence, enabling individuals to lead active, productive, and fulfilling lives.

REFERENCES

1. Argent, R., Daly, A., & Caulfield, B. (2018). Patient involvement with home-based exercise programs: Can connected health interventions influence adherence? *JMIR mHealth and uHealth, 6*, e47. https://doi.org/10.2196/mhealth.8518 (accessed on 26th June 2025).
2. Bergqvist, C., Servy, A., Valeyrie-Allanore, L., Ferkal, S., Combemale, P., & Wolkenstein, P. (2020). Neurofibromatosis 1 French national guidelines based on an extensive literature review since 1966. *Orphanet Journal of Rare Diseases, 15*. https://doi.org/10.1186/s13023-020-1310-3 (accessed on 26th June 2025).
3. Campanini, I., Disselhorst-Klug, C., Rymer, W. Z., & Merletti, R. (2020). Surface EMG in clinical assessment and neurorehabilitation: Barriers limiting its use. *Frontiers in Neurology, 11*. https://doi.org/10.3389/fneur.2020.00934 (accessed on 26th June 2025).
4. Castillo-González, W. (2023). Tratamiento kinésico sobre la rigidez, la calidad de vida y la independencia funcional en pacientes con artritis reumatoide. *AG Salud*. https://www.semanticscholar.org/paper/c7b2cff2597724429218496a2aa8bd0a2f7b45b4 (accessed on 26th June 2025).
5. Cho, C. H., Bae, K. C., & Kim, D. H. (2019). Treatment strategy for frozen shoulder. *Clinics in Orthopedic Surgery, 11*, 249. https://doi.org/10.4055/cios.2019.11.3.249 (accessed on 26th June 2025).
6. Cobb, E., Hurst, J., & Konshuk, E. (2016). Use of a mobile application to increase patient compliance to a prescribed home exercise program and improve outcomes. https://digitalscholarship.unlv.edu/cgi/viewcontent.cgi?article=4542&context=thesesdissertations (accessed on 26th June 2025).
7. Faletra, A., Bellin, G., Dunning, J., Fernández-de-las-Peñas, C., Pellicciari, L., Brindisino, F., Galeno, E., et al. (2022). Assessing cardiovascular parameters and risk factors in physical therapy practice: Findings from a cross-sectional national survey and implication for clinical practice. *BMC Musculoskeletal Disorders, 23*. https://doi.org/10.1186/s12891-022-05696-w (accessed on 26th June 2025).
8. Fan, H., Hooper, L., Horton, S., Wilsher, H., et al. (2016). Systematic overview of economic evaluations of health-related rehabilitation. https://core.ac.uk/download/41991060.pdf (accessed on 26th June 2025).
9. Geng, R., Li, J., Yu, C., Zhang, C., Chen, F., Chen, J., Ni, H., et al. (2023). Knee osteoarthritis: Current status and research progress in treatment (Review). *Experimental and Therapeutic Medicine, 26*. https://doi.org/10.3892/etm.2023.12180 (accessed on 26th June 2025).
10. Geroin, C., Artusi, C. A., Nonnekes, J., Aquino, C. C., Garg, D., Dale, M. L., Schlosser, D., et al. (2023). Axial postural abnormalities in parkinsonism: Gaps in predictors, pathophysiology, and management. *Movement Disorders, 38*, 732–739. https://doi.org/10.1002/mds.29377 (accessed on 26th June 2025).
11. Gualtierotti, R., Tafuri, F., Arcudi, S., Solimeno, P. L., Acquati, J., Landi, L., & Peyvandi, F. (2022). Current and emerging approaches for pain management in hemophilic arthropathy. *Pain and Therapy, 11*, 1–15. https://doi.org/10.1007/s40122-021-00345-x (accessed on 26th June 2025).

12. Haffner, D., Emma, F., Eastwood, D. M., Biosse Duplan, M., Bacchetta, J., Schnabel, D., Wicart, P., et al. (2019). Clinical practice recommendations for the diagnosis and management of X-linked hypophosphatemia. *Nature Reviews Nephrology, 15*, 435–455. https://doi.org/10.1038/s41581-019-0152-5 (accessed on 26th June 2025).

13. Harden, R. N., McCabe, C., Göebel, A., Massey, M., Suvar, T., Grieve, S., & Bruehl, S. (2022). Complex regional pain syndrome: Practical diagnostic and treatment guidelines, 5th edition. *Pain Medicine, 23*, S1–S53. https://doi.org/10.1093/pm/pnac046 (accessed on 26th June 2025).

14. Khachane, Y., Kozlowska, K., Savage, B., McClure, G., Butler, G., Gray, N., Worth, A., et al. (2019). Twisted in pain: The multidisciplinary treatment approach to functional dystonia. *Harvard Review of Psychiatry, 27*, 359–381. https://doi.org/10.1097/hrp.0000000000000237 (accessed on 26th June 2025).

15. Lagier, D., Zeng, C., Fernandez-Bustamante, A., & Vidal Melo, M. F. (2021). Perioperative pulmonary atelectasis: Part II. Clinical implications. *Anesthesiology, 136*, 206–236. https://doi.org/10.1097/aln.0000000000004009 (accessed on 26th June 2025).

16. Le, H., Lee, S., Nazarian, A., & Rodriguez, E. K. (2016). Adhesive capsulitis of the shoulder: Review of pathophysiology and current clinical treatments. *Shoulder & Elbow, 9*, 75–84. https://doi.org/10.1177/1758573216676786 (accessed on 26th June 2025).

17. Ljungqvist, O., Scott, M. J., & Fearon, K. C. H. (2017). Enhanced recovery after surgery. *JAMA Surgery, 152*, 292. https://doi.org/10.1001/jamasurg.2016.4952 (accessed on 26th June 2025).

18. Machado, V. G., de Figueiredo Azevedo, A. C., Dutra Alves, B. P. S., Valadares, J. F. M., Dias, M. T. H., Souza, L. D. Q., Tiveron, E., et al. (2025). Anesthesiology in multimodal pain management for orthopedic patients. *Journal of Medical Science and Evidences*. https://www.semanticscholar.org/paper/9e60e7ee3b0d370d0bda26992541dc0677837045 (accessed on 26th June 2025).

19. Maher, C. G., O'Keeffe, M., Buchbinder, R., & Harris, I. A. (2019). Musculoskeletal healthcare: Have we over-egged the pudding? *International Journal of Rheumatic Diseases, 22*, 1957–1960. https://doi.org/10.1111/1756-185x.13710 (accessed on 26th June 2025).

20. Min, K., Beom, J., Kim, B. R., Lee, S. Y., Lee, G. J., Lee, J. H., Lee, S. Y., et al. (2021). Clinical practice guideline for postoperative rehabilitation in older patients with hip fractures. *Annals of Rehabilitation Medicine, 45*, 225–259. https://doi.org/10.5535/arm.21110 (accessed on 26th June 2025).

21. Mishra, R., Narayanan, M., Umana, G. E., Montemurro, N., Chaurasia, B., & Deora, H. (2022). Virtual reality in neurosurgery: Beyond neurosurgical planning. *International Journal of Environmental Research and Public Health, 19*, 1719. https://doi.org/10.3390/ijerph19031719 (accessed on 26th June 2025).

22. Négrini, S., Donzelli, S., Aulisa, A. G., Czaprowski, D., Schreiber, S., de Mauroy, J. C., Diers, H., et al. (2018). 2016 SOSORT guidelines: Orthopedic and rehabilitation treatment of idiopathic scoliosis during growth. *Scoliosis and Spinal Disorders, 13*. https://doi.org/10.1186/s13013-017-0145-8 (accessed on 26th June 2025).

23. Patel, D. R., Neelakantan, M., Pandher, K., & Merrick, J. (2020). Cerebral palsy in children: A clinical overview. *Translational Pediatrics, 9*, S125–S135. https://doi.org/10.21037/tp.2020.01.01 (accessed on 26th June 2025).

24. Paul, S., Nahar, A., Bhagawati, M., & Kunwar, A. J. (2022). A review on recent advances of cerebral palsy. *Oxidative Medicine and Cellular Longevity, 2022*, 1–20. https://doi.org/10.1155/2022/2622310 (accessed on 26th June 2025).

25. Prasad, R., Shukla, S., Acharya, S., Mittal, G., & Wanjari, M. (2025). Primary malignant giant cell tumor (PMGCT): Diagnosis and management challenges in low resource settings. *Narra J, 5.* https://www.semanticscholar.org/paper/eabfc46f0d59739f47ebbd0ef9387ff2f252dfe4 (accessed on 26th June 2025).

26. Sivhugwana, Innocentia (2022). Factors related with the functional outcome of patients who sustained tibial plateau fractures. Dissertation (MSc (Physiotherapy))--University of Pretoria, 2022. https://core.ac.uk/download/565849089.pdf

27. Temple-Oberle, C., Shea-Budgell, M., Tan, M., Semple, J. L., Schrag, C., Barreto, M. P., Blondeel, P., et al. (2017). Consensus review of optimal perioperative care in breast reconstruction: Enhanced Recovery after Surgery (ERAS) Society recommendations. *Plastic & Reconstructive Surgery, 139*, 1056e–1071e. https://doi.org/10.1097/prs.0000000000003242 (accessed on 26th June 2025).

28. Timmers, T., Janssen, L., van der Weegen, W., Das, D., Marijnissen, W. J. C. M., Hannink, G., van der Zwaard, B. C., et al. (2019). The effect of an app for day-to-day postoperative care education on patients with total knee replacement: Randomized controlled trial. *JMIR mHealth and uHealth, 7*, e15323. https://doi.org/10.2196/15323 (accessed on 26th June 2025).

29. Toelle, T., Utpadel-Fischler, D., Haas, K. K., & Priebe, J. A. (2019). App-based multidisciplinary back pain treatment versus combined physiotherapy plus online education: A randomized controlled trial. *npj Digital Medicine, 2.* https://doi.org/10.1038/s41746-019-0109-x (accessed on 26th June 2025).

30. Wu, P. H., Kim, H. S., & Jang, I. T. (2020). Intervertebral disc diseases PART 2: A review of the current diagnostic and treatment strategies for intervertebral disc disease. *International Journal of Molecular Sciences, 21*, 2135. https://doi.org/10.3390/ijms21062135 (accessed on 26th Junc 2025).

31. Zhang, X., Yang, Y., Shen, Y., Zhang, K. R., Ma, L., Ding, C., Wang, B., et al. (2022). Quality of online video resources concerning patient education for neck pain: A YouTube-based quality-control study. *Frontiers in Public Health, 10.* https://doi.org/10.3389/fpubh.2022.972348 (accessed on 26th June 2025).

32. Golovacheva VA, Golovacheva AA, Tarshilova AR. Chronic musculoskeletal low back pain: mistakes in patient management and optimization issues. *Nevrologiya, neiropsikhiatriya, psikhosomatika = Neurology, Neuropsychiatry, Psychosomatics.* 2024;16(3):103-109. (In Russ.) https://doi.org/10.14412/2074-2711-2024-3-103-109 (accessed on 26th June 2025).

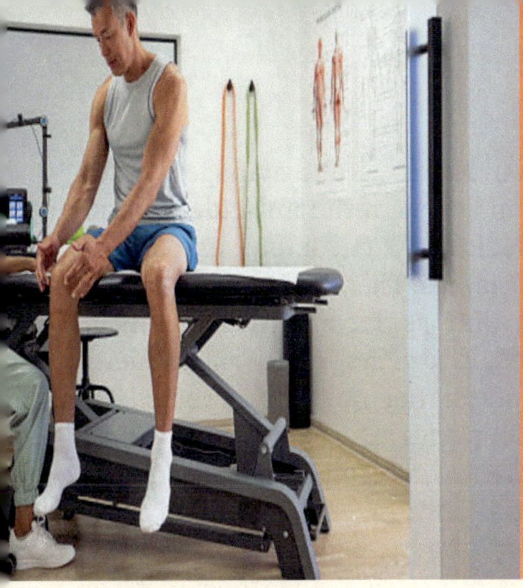

Chapter 15

RECENT ADVANCES IN ORTHOPEDICS AND PHYSIOTHERAPY

Contents

Introduction....481
15.1. Technological Innovations in Orthopedics....485
15.2. Advances in Physiotherapy Techniques....488
15.3. Regenerative Medicine in Orthopedics....492
15.4. Pain Management Strategies....496
15.5. Evidence-Based Research and Clinical Trials....500
15.6. Interdisciplinary Collaboration....503
Summary....508
References....511

Introduction

The field of orthopedics and physiotherapy has undergone remarkable progress driven by the advancements in diagnostic techniques and therapeutic modalities. With increasing awareness and perception given to musculoskeletal disorders, the medical community is increasingly realizing the intricacies of conditions such as cervical radiculopathy and subacromial impingement syndrome. Such conditions prevalent in most populations need accurate diagnosis and effective management strategies. Recent studies indicate the importance of a proper assessment, which combines patient history and clinical exams to enhance diagnostic specificity. For instance, some interview items and physical examination tests have been identified as critical in cervical radiculopathy diagnosis, as described in recent literature (Sleijser-Koehorst et al., 2020). Such increases not only enable accurate diagnoses but also help to develop tailored treatment plans that can greatly boost patient outcomes. Of shoulder conditions, the subacromial impingement syndrome is a significant issue, particularly in working overhead populations. Impingement syndrome is defined by specific biomechanical changes of the glenohumeral joint, influencing treatment plans and exercise programs. Imaging technology and best practice based on evidence have allowed clinicians to identify differential humeral head translations, especially with symptoms of impingement in overhead workers. By educating on therapeutic treatment with a better understanding of the mechanics at play, practitioners are better able to individualize rehabilitation programs. The literature highlights that abnormal translations are prevalent in this population, so it is clear evidence-based, specific treatment in physiotherapy is important (Shinde et al., 2023). These results accentuate the interconnectedness of clinical practice and research in shoulder pain and outcomes management. With the hue of orthopedics and physiotherapy continuously evolving, practitioners are required to be compliant in integrating new knowledge into practice. Advances in technology and enhanced research methodologies have opened up the channels of both diagnosis and therapy, rendering care approaches patient-centered and evidence-based. The collaborative effort between orthopedic surgeons and physiotherapists aids in developing holistic treatment models that address the complete needs of patients. Through the incorporation of surgical interventions combined with rehabilitation techniques, practitioners can more than double recovery rates and quality of life. Ongoing research into therapeutic techniques and the potential for these techniques to have outcomes will undoubtedly shape orthopedic and physiotherapy practice in the future, allowing practitioners to deliver the best possible care.

Definition of Orthopedics

The term orthopedics has evolved dramatically since its humble origins, reflecting the growing complexity and breadth of musculoskeletal medicine. Once a specialty of medicine devoted to the prevention, diagnosis, and management of diseases and conditions of the musculoskeletal system, orthopedics now encompasses a broad range of subspecialties. These encompass sports medicine and joint replacement, as well as geriatric and pediatric orthopedics. The modern orthopedic professional not only specializes in surgery, one performs rehabilitation and physiotherapy treatment. Modern advancements of orthopedics uphold the need for an interdisciplinary practice model, whereby a mutual relationship with physiotherapists is crucial towards patient care and rehabilitation, embracing medical and rehabilitative measures in managing the multifaceted nature of musculoskeletal disorders. With continued research in the area, orthopedics continues to advance as it adapts new innovations that enhance both surgery and post-surgical care. The advent of minimally invasive surgery, for instance, has revolutionized the way joint repair as well as replacement has been carried out. Techniques such as arthroscopy enable precise intervention with a shorter recovery period, thus significantly improving the patient's quality of life. Similarly, imaging advances have brought diagnostic accuracy closer to enabling the orthopedist to plan more effectively. Perhaps most notably, the confluence of rehabilitation techniques has grown, which has led to a more comprehensive approach to addressing problems such as cerebral palsy. The partnership between orthopedics and physiotherapy has grown, with greater focus on a model of partnership in care as necessary in developing pragmatic rehabilitation programs, as emphasized in current studies (Morris, 2002). In addition to a greater acknowledgment of the multi-factorial basis of musculoskeletal well-being is a greater requirement to redefine the scope of orthopedics. The influence of technology, and particularly that of virtual health technologies and telemedicine, is framing the future of orthopedic medicine. Telemedicine and virtual consultations can enhance compliance and participation of patients with treatments, ultimately generating adaptive recovery pathways. Population health research also indicates preventive care and early intervention strategies in orthopedics. For instance, the interrelatedness of exercise, injury prevention, and the role of physiotherapy points to a preventive approach towards musculoskeletal health. Combined, these advances underscore the value of a broad orthopedic expertise, advancing its position as an evolving field that responds to the overall health environment but maintains distinct lines of vision on patient care and interprofessional collaboration (Reynolds & Tansey, 2009) (Figure 15.1).

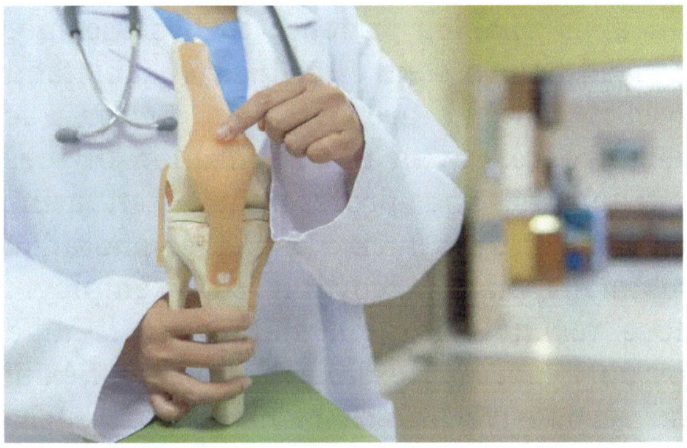

Figure 15.1. The definition of orthopedics has evolved significantly from its inception.

Source: https://drmrinalsharma.com/wp-content/uploads/2023/10/female-doctor-holds-knee-model-with-copy-space-text_747x467.webp.

Definition of Physiotherapy

Physiotherapy, a therapeutic branch of medicine, is truly scientifically defined as the art and science of movement, dealing with the testing, diagnosis, treatment, and prevention of physical dysfunction. The subject encompasses a large number of practices aimed at the rehabilitation of movement and function in patients afflicted by injury, illness, or disability. Central to physiotherapy is evidence-based practice intended to meet the needs of individual patients, and these can be comprised of manual therapy, exercise programs, and modalities such as electrotherapy. Furthermore, physiotherapists also play a key role in educating patients about their condition, enabling them to self-manage, and optimizing quality of life. This multi-dimensional approach is not only concerned with rehabilitation but also emphasizes the necessity of preventing further complications, particularly in orthopedic ailments that tend to necessitate physiotherapeutic intervention. Advances made in orthopedics in recent times have emphasized the interdependence of surgical intervention and physiotherapy. With enhanced techniques in surgery, such as minimally invasive procedures, the subsequent process of rehabilitation has itself been tuned to incorporate enhanced physiotherapeutic intervention. Physiotherapy is no longer merely a post-surgical intervention, but rather an integral part of the preoperative planning phase, maximizing physical status and preparing patients for the demands of recovery. Modern orthopedic physiotherapy often utilizes evidence from consensus conferences, where healthcare professionals critically appraise multiple treatment modalities. For instance, successful treatment of conditions such as cerebral palsy can be contingent on the recommendation for occupational and physical therapy interventions, based on in-depth analysis of these interventions (Morris et al., 2011). Incorporation of such evidence-based practices is hence essential to patient-focused care. The application of physiotherapy has broadened its definitional domain, encroaching on the domains of sport medicine and prevention, thereby reflecting ongoing advancement in the field. As defined in historical overviews, the roles of physiotherapists have dramatically shifted since their establishment as an accepted branch of medicine in 2005 and their concentration on not only rehabilitation but injury prevention and performance enhancement among athletes (Reynolds & Tansey, 2009). This evolving definition is symptomatic of a broader trend toward an integrated notion of health that prioritizes proactive care rather than reactive intervention. With increasing focus on lifestyle-related diseases and long-term conditions, physiotherapy stands at the threshold, offering innovative solutions that address the changing healthcare environment. Such an adaptability identifies the crucial role of physiotherapy in maximizing patient outcomes and building a wider understanding of health and mobility (Figure 15.2).

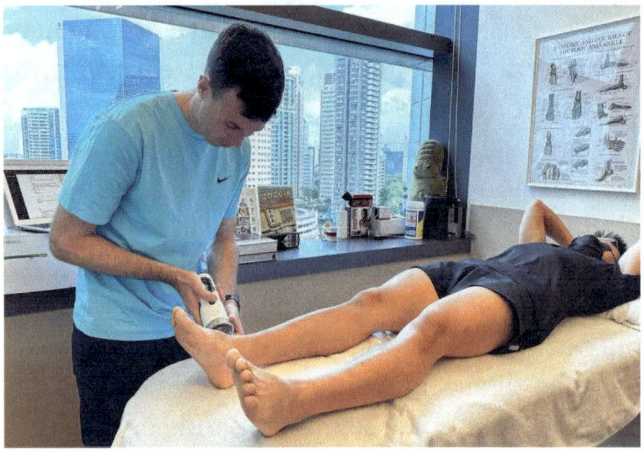

Figure 15.2. Physiotherapy.

Source: https://www.hellophysio.sg/wp-content/uploads/who-is-a-physiotherapist-1024x683.jpg.webp

Importance of Recent Advances in These Fields

Orthopedic and physiotherapeutic developments over the last few years are key to enhanced patient outcomes and more effective treatment protocols. Development in minimally invasive surgery, for instance, has greatly reduced recovery time as well as postoperative morbidity. Such developments in surgery allow quicker rehabilitation and easier return to normal activities with less compromise to the quality of a person's life due to injuries. In addition, advances in imaging technology enable orthopedic surgeons to make more informed decisions regarding diagnoses and treatment. Such technologies bring orthopedics into the forefront of patient-centered care by leading the way to meet the need for more personalized management of musculoskeletal disorders. As technology evolves, the integration of surgical interventions with new rehabilitation techniques forms an interdisciplinary methodology that is critical in responding to the demands of contemporary healthcare (Baldacchino et al., 2014). The integration of digital health technologies into physiotherapy has also enhanced the efficiency of the discipline. Telehealth offerings are becoming more prevalent, and practitioners can consult remotely while also personalizing rehabilitation programs for individual patients and expanding healthcare access to remote groups. The application of digital treatments like websites and apps enables patients to become more engaged and in control of their rehabilitation process. Patients are helped to better track their progress with the application of these instruments, and professionals can utilize data analytics to track compliance and adjust treatment plans accordingly. By employing these technologies, physiotherapy is made not only more accessible but also a flexible and responsive branch of healthcare. Such a development is indicative of the importance afforded to maintaining a forward-thinking approach to patient care that is increasingly answering the complex challenges of modern society (Baldacchino et al., 2014). Also, professionalization of practice in orthopedics and physiotherapy is an indicator of broader societal trends toward the value placed on multispecialty collaboration and evidence-based practice. The coming together of specialisms, as in the treatment of wounded soldiers during and after the First World War, illustrates the benefits of interdisciplinary rehabilitation. The development of physiotherapy as an established profession, distinct but increasingly combined with orthopedics, indicates a crucial turning point in healthcare. It emphasizes the role of massage and rehabilitation techniques as part of holistic care that has evolved to become scholarly and clinically legitimate through the decades. This background stresses the fact that current developments are a result of a foundation of interdisciplinary collaboration towards the formulation of a better composite image of patient care, ultimately resulting in improved health outcomes in these areas.

15.1. Technological Innovations in Orthopedics

The integration of technological innovation in orthopedics has profoundly transformed the setting of surgical procedures and rehabilitation protocols. One of the most important achievements is the development of wearable tracking technology that is able to monitor patient recovery in real time. This is particularly brought to attention with elbow rehabilitation, which depends on less accurate and less adaptable traditional techniques. With the help of sophisticated sensors integrated in wearable devices, doctors can gather rich information about joint movement, including rotation, position, and flexion. Such accuracy not only enhances diagnosis but also allows for tailored rehabilitation programs that closely align with individual patient needs. This shift towards a more data-centric pattern in orthopedics is a giant leap forward, streamlining the recovery times and improving overall compliance of the patient with the prescribed rehabilitation procedures, evident from the significant improvements in accuracy and performance associated with such technologies (Alonso-Rollán et al., 2024). Tele-rehabilitation is also one of the giant leaps in the area of orthopedics, greatly enhancing patient engagement and access to therapy. Blending virtual platforms with traditional therapeutic procedures, tele-rehabilitation allows physiotherapists to monitor and guide patients from afar, thus reducing geographical barriers to quality treatment. With telecommunication technologies, patients can take advantage of customized rehabilitation sessions tailored to address their specific illnesses without physically going to a clinic. This is particularly convenient for patients with mobility problems or who live in remote locations. Research has now begun to demonstrate that such a new approach not only maximizes patient compliance but also optimizes outcomes by allowing timely adjustments in the rehabilitation protocols based on real-time feedback. With the evolving landscape of healthcare, tele-rehabilitation is an important component in controlling orthopedic disorders, bridging the gap between technology and patient care (Nkhata & Mweshi, 2024). Moreover, the introduction of robotic-assisted surgical operations has revolutionized orthopedic operations into procedures of unprecedented accuracy and efficacy.

The technologies allow surgeons to perform intricate operations with increased precision, thereby limiting complications as well as enhancing the recovery rate of the patients. Robotic systems integrate advanced imaging and navigation features that allow for accurate planning as well as accurate implementation of the surgical treatments, particularly in joint replacement operations. The capacity to execute complex maneuvers with millimeter accuracy significantly reduces postoperative morbidity and enhances overall outcomes of surgery. With additional evidence being accrued on the effectiveness of robot-assisted surgery, its application can be anticipated to expand, enabling continued refinement of orthopedic intervention. In addition, ongoing studies on the relationship between robotic technology and patient outcomes further emphasize the groundbreaking possibilities of this innovation among the orthopedic world, with a new era of surgery norms that prioritize safety and effectiveness (Alonso-Rollán et al., 2024) (Figure 15.3).

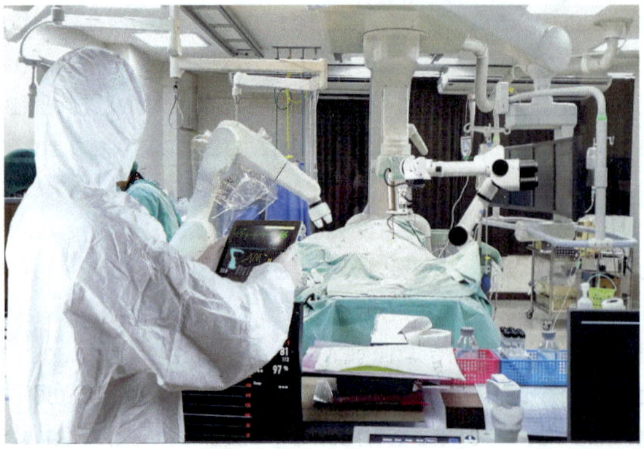

Figure 15.3. The integration of technological innovations in orthopedics.

Source: https://wp02-media.cdn.ihealthspot.com/wp-content/uploads/sites/476/2023/12/iStock-1219176880-1.jpg.

15.1.1. Robotics in Surgical Procedures

Robotics advancements in recent years have transformed surgical procedures, particularly in orthopedics and physiotherapy. Robotic surgery guarantees higher precision and control, less invasive procedures, and improved outcomes for patients. One of the major benefits of using robotic systems in surgical procedures is that they can perform intricate procedures with minimal cutting. This results in reduced postoperative pain, shorter recovery times, and smaller scars relative to traditional operations. Moreover, the real-time imaging and enhanced imaging capabilities of robotic systems enhance the surgeon's ability to manage challenging anatomical relationships, thereby making intervention more exact. This technology significantly contributes to the development of orthopedic practice and enables medical professionals to offer patient-centered care that enhances treatment pathway effectiveness as a whole. As orthopedic surgery continues to adapt to technological advancements, the role of robotics is increasingly intertwined with artificial intelligence (AI) and evidence-based tools. Since the introduction of AI and telemedicine to preoperative planning, robots apply big data sets to aid in evaluating patient needs and tailoring surgery approaches. The ability to process and interpret medical images through sophisticated algorithms allows for more extensive planning of surgical paths, which can significantly influence surgical outcomes. With the implementation of these digital platforms (Youssef et al., 2024), clinicians can perform interventions entirely optimized to patient profiles, thus optimizing recovery pathways. In addition, robotic systems in surgery promote interdisciplinary teams, which welcome input from disciplines like radiology and pathology, and thus provide a comprehensive means of surgical care. Along with enhancing surgical procedures, robotics has a key role in postoperative rehabilitation and care in orthopedics.

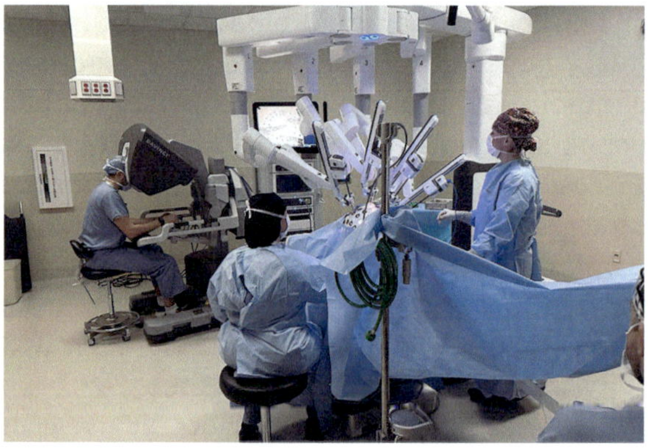

Figure 15.4. Robotics in surgical procedures.

Source: https://www.uofmhealthsparrow.org/sites/default/files/styles/scale_to_max_width_1920/public/2024-01/surgery-levy.png?itok=zwj7ka5c.

Robotic-assisted rehabilitation technology is coming forward as an integral element in physiotherapy, which allows patients to participate in monitored and guided exercises in the course of recovery. These systems can control the level of resistance and intensity of movements so that practitioners can tailor rehabilitation programs to specific patients. Such a personalized approach not only improves patient engagement but also promotes a healthier healing process by allowing mobility and strength reconstruction. Further, the ongoing development of immersion technologies such as virtual and augmented reality, as well as robotics, remains to redefine rehabilitation strategies to be more efficient and interactive (Sivhugwana, 2021). Robotics thus paves the way to new-generation solutions that can greatly improve patient care through the entire surgical process from preoperative planning to rehabilitation (Figure 15.4).

15.1.2. 3D Printing for Custom Implants

The advent of 3D printing technology has transformed the specialty of orthopedics, particularly through the development of patient-specific implants based on the unique anatomy of a patient. Unlike the traditional method of production leading to one-size-fits-all products, 3D printing allows the creation of implants that precisely fit the patient's unique biometrics. Implant personalization enhances the fit, leading to improved functional outcomes and reduced postoperative complications. Recent studies emphasize how implants produced via 3D printing can result in enhanced positioning and stability, ultimately shortening healing time and patient satisfaction. In the more complex cases of limb fracture, the ability to include 3D imaging data during the design process enables more efficient surgical planning and procedure. Therefore, this emerging technology promises to pave the way for even more innovation in personalized orthopedic medicine, redefining the parameters for recovery and treatment effectiveness. Furthermore, the sophisticated capability of 3D printing transcends mere customization; it makes it possible to produce biocompatible materials that can integrate seamlessly with human tissue. These implants are intended to mimic the structure of natural cartilage and bone, which is an important factor for enhancing the implant compatibility within the body. As highlighted in most clinical investigations, 3D-printed implant application has proven to improve the integration process with a remarkable increase in quicker healing and restoration of functions. The ability to customize not only the shape but also the design of implants allows for more strategic patient management. Based on recent literature, the use of 3D printing has transformed surgical outcomes, with pelvic and limb surgery experiencing significant advancement in accuracy and times of operation, indicating the extensive implications of such technology in modern surgery (Vera et al., 2024).

The contribution of 3D printing to orthopedic surgery extends to the improvement of the rehabilitation process. With improved fit and increased functionality of the implants, patients can more comfortably go through physical therapy, which helps in their recovery. Additionally, personalized implants reduce the occurrence of such incidents as infection and implant failure, which are some of the most common issues arising during the process of rehabilitation. More patient satisfaction and engagement have the prospect of leading to more successful rehabilitation outcomes, as the psychological aspect of seeing one's recovery made easier by personalized solutions cannot be discounted. Technologies like Percutaneous Endo Prosthetic Osseointegration for Limbs (PEPOL), underpinned by 3D technologies, are a direct indicator of the potential for drastic improvement in the quality of life of amputees. With ongoing research in developing the technologies of implant design and integration, the future offers the potential for even more patient-centered care in orthopedics and physiotherapy (Al Muderis, 2021) (Figure 15.5).

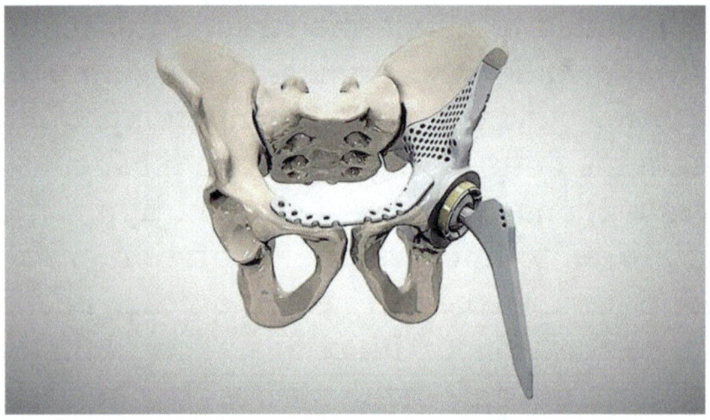

Figure 15.5. The advent of 3D printing technology has significantly transformed the landscape of orthopedics.

Source: https://wevolver-project-images.s3.us-west-1.amazonaws.com/0.d62tvezbzyimage16.jpg.

15.1.3. Telemedicine for Pre- and Post-Operative Care

Application of telemedicine in post-operative and pre-operative care is a leap in orthopedics and physiotherapy. Telemedicine employs digital communication technologies to remotely deliver healthcare services to patients, reducing the necessity of direct face-to-face consultation. Telemedicine facilitates it to be simple to carry out various steps in the course of surgical care, ranging from pre-operative assessment to post-operative checking. Patients can have virtual consultations whereby medical experts assess their conditions, prescribe treatment options, and map out surgical procedures, thereby simplifying the pre-operative process. This combined method not only increases accessibility for patients in remote locations but also enables them to access care in a timely manner without risking delays due to having to navigate conventional healthcare facilities. Post-operative care, a similarly crucial element of the patient care continuum, is also transformed by telemedicine. Post-operative patients, such as those who have undergone hip replacement, no longer need to go for repetitive clinic visits for follow-up treatment and rehabilitation guidance. Now they can simply use telerehabilitation devices to engage in telerehabilitation, which unlocks therapeutic exercises and recovery protocols as interactive online modules. The ability to monitor progress remotely enables healthcare practitioners to tailor rehabilitation programs along the individualized recovery pathway of each patient, further enhancing individualization in postoperative care. In addition to reducing healthcare costs and physical facility loads, these digital technologies also empower patients to take greater ownership of their recovery, fostering greater self-management and adherence to treatment regimens. The COVID-19 pandemic has catalyzed to usher in the acceleration of telemedicine adoption, with the latter unearthing the imperative of digital solutions for healthcare. Surgeons and physiotherapists have increasingly incorporated telehealth into their practice during the enforced social distancing, representing a seismic shift in the provision of orthopedic care. The swift growth of telemedicine applications over this time has underscored the capability of digital platforms to drive patient outcomes. New technologies, including remote monitoring with wearables and artificial intelligence, also enhanced clinical decision-making. These technologies, in literature, result in more data-driven, individualized patient care, thus improving treatment quality and efficiency in general (Esparza et al., 2019; Back et al., 2024). The continued use of these technologies can further revolutionize the pre- and post-operative care field in orthopedics and physiotherapy.

15.2. Advances in Physiotherapy Techniques

In recent years, physiotherapy has made tremendous progress that maximizes rehabilitation processes, particularly after surgical interventions. Of note is the arthroscopic suture-bridge method of rotator cuff tear repair. The new technique, as reported in studies, has improved contact between the tendon and footprint with improved functional outcome in patients. With the application of early rehabilitation protocols to patients undergoing such repairs, studies produce findings of a significant range of motion improvement immediately post-surgery. However, there is a very thin line between promoting movement and avoiding re-tears, an aspect that renders competent and well-organized physiotherapy regimens post-surgery essential to enable patients to enjoy optimal recovery without compromising structural integrity in the shoulder joint (Dias & Sera, 2020). Furthermore, the professional evolution of massage therapy has set a precedent for contemporary physiotherapeutic practices. Established in Britain in the late 19th century, massage transitioned from a lay treatment to a recognized component of medical rehabilitation, especially during and after the First World War. This evolution speaks to massage's increasing acceptance within medicine, contributing significantly to the development of physiotherapy as a formalized discipline. Understanding the history of how massage became involved in rehabilitative interventions gives clinicians the skill to grasp the socio-cultural orientations of patient care, valuing more the intricate relationship patterns between practitioner and patient. The historical context not only promotes current practice but also reveals the value of empathy and communication in successful practice rehabilitation (Nias, 2017). The integration of evidence-based practice has reformatted the character of physiotherapy to one of continued improvement and adaptation. Techniques such as myofascial release and neuromuscular reeducation illustrate how a better understanding of human anatomy and biomechanics can aid in more efficient ways of treating patients with chronic illnesses. The application of technology, including therapeutic ultrasound and electrical stimulation, adds to the effects of physiotherapy by acting to directly address pain relief and the healing of tissues. These developments accentuate the tremendous growth in the field, which strives to embrace scientifically validated approaches for the delivery of holistic treatment. As physiotherapists embrace these developments, the overall efficacy and quality of patient rehabilitation in orthopedics and physiotherapy are further enhanced, providing a platform where recovery is more effective and efficient (Nias, 2017; Dias & Sera, 2020) (Figure 15.6).

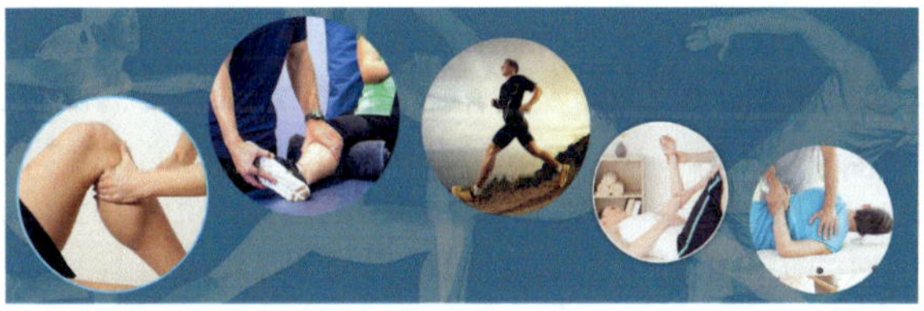

Figure 15.6. Advances in physiotherapy techniques.

Source: https://advancephysiotherapyclinic.co.in/assets/img/page-banner-bg.jpg.

15.2.1. Use of Virtual Reality in Rehabilitation

The application of virtual reality (VR) technology to the rehabilitation environment has been revolutionizing the setting of orthopedics and physiotherapy. Through the mimicry of real environments, VR establishes a setting where patients are able to feel a sense of immersion to perform therapy that enhances cognitive ability and motor function recovery. For those recuperating from surgery or injury, traditional rehabilitation is monotonous and challenging. On the other hand, VR introduces game-like elements to rehabilitation, not only making rehab fun but also increasing patient motivation and adherence to prescribed therapeutic routines. Research suggests that incorporating VR within rehabilitation can lead to improved physical outcomes, including increased range of motion and strength, by enabling patients to practice movements in a controlled and stimulating environment (Youssef et al., 2024). Moreover, VR's adaptability makes it a handy tool in rehabilitation. It can be tailored to meet the specific needs of patients, such as stroke or cerebral palsy. Unlike conventional methods that are not customizable, VR rehabilitation can also change the degree of difficulty in exercises based on real-time feedback, ensuring that each patient's improvement is optimized. Individualized rehabilitation allows for a better healing environment and the option of customized exercises to deal with the most overlooked regions. Emphasized in many studies, systematic use of VR has also been shown to have possible advantages in functional recovery for a variety of patient populations, suggesting a paradigm shift regarding how rehabilitation is managed in orthopedics and physiotherapy (Morris, 2002).

Additionally, the use of VR is not limited to individual patient care but promotes better interdisciplinary interaction between healthcare professionals. Through the application of VR systems, therapists are able to monitor patient interactions and body movements in the virtual environment, enabling the gathering of important information to be used in making treatment decisions. Not only does this data-driven method simplify the process of rehabilitation, but it also allows practitioners to better communicate with patients regarding their prognosis and expectations. With the continued advancement of the healthcare landscape, the application of VR in rehabilitation is a commitment to leveraging technology to the best effect for improved patient outcomes. With an emphasis on accessibility and customization, VR is a critical advancement in orthopedics and physiotherapy that affirms general movements in healthcare to optimize the efficacy and efficiency of treatment methods (Youssef et al., 2024).

15.2.2. Evidence-Based Practice in Treatment Protocols

The evolution of evidence-based practice (EBP) in treatment protocols has revolutionized orthopedics and physiotherapy to a large extent. EBP emphasizes the integration of clinical expertise, patient values, and best available external clinical research evidence to guide decision-making in patient care. This system serves to ensure that treatment recommendations are not only derived from well-conducted scientific research but also tailored according to individual patient needs. The application of EBP has facilitated the shift away from traditional, occasionally anecdotal therapies toward statistical, evidence-based results and methodical processes, enhancing the quality of care. In orthopedics, for instance, the incorporation of evidence from new clinical trials has led to more efficient surgical practices and rehabilitation protocols based on patients' restoration and satisfaction, a significant step forward in the effectiveness and safety of treatments. Recent studies provide an enlightening illustration of the use of evidence-based practices in orthopedic treatment protocols. The examination of Actovegin, a biologic drug with a storied clinical history, is an illustration of the nuanced insight required in the choice of treatments utilizing EBP. Reports are that Actovegin does not enhance performance for athletics, but it has anti-inflammatory and anti apoptotic properties beneficial for the treatment of injury, stroke, and diabetes. The drug is discussed in relation to the need to interpret the drug's effects with caution due to the heterogenelty of study designs and outcomes. As EBP encourages critical appraisal of such evidence, orthopedic clinicians are encouraged to make informed decisions from a fair analysis of the benefits and risks by using systematic reviews and randomized controlled trials, thus ensuring optimal patient outcomes in practice (Lee et al., 2016). In rotator cuff repair, evidence-based practice has played a crucial role in the choice of postoperative rehabilitation regimes. Evidence on the comparison of functional outcomes of patients who underwent an arthroscopic suture-bridge procedure with an early exercise regimen provides evidence of the contribution of research evidence to practice.

The results indicated a tremendous improvement in patient outcomes, where the majority reported having satisfactory levels of satisfaction and no re-tears were reported post-surgery. The evidence supporting it is that early ROM exercises work by helping the patient recover without compromising the integrity of the surgical repair. These advancements illustrate the manner in which EBP not only guides surgical procedures but also extends to rehabilitative measures, promoting methodologies that reflect the state of the art in clinical research (Dias & Sera, 2020). All these comprehensive inclusions of EBP into treatment protocols continue to frame the boundaries of the fast-changing discipline of orthopedics and physiotherapy, thereby ensuring that treatment modalities are patient-centered and effective.

15.2.3. Integration of Manual Therapy and Exercise

Both exercise and manual therapy together constitute the hallmark progress in the field of orthopedics and physiotherapy, particularly in musculoskeletal disorders. Manual therapy, also known as mobilization and manipulation techniques, is employed to eradicate pain, improve joint mobility, and facilitate the healing of tissues. Used in combination with exercise, which increases strength, flexibility, and overall physical function, this interdisciplinary approach has been shown to result in higher success rates than when used individually. Current clinical guidelines encourage their simultaneous application, pointing out that the musculoskeletal system can be conditioned to exercise through manual therapy, making the patient more receptive to physical rehabilitation measures, and thereby improving long-term recovery and long-term health (Silumesii, 2025). Apart from this, the need to combine manual therapy and exercise is also based on their complementary effects on proprioception and neuromuscular control. As the individual performs therapeutic exercises after manual therapy, the increase in joint mobility and reduction of pain add to a facilitative setting for enhanced sensory input and motor learning. This is particularly relevant in fall-risk or functional decline groups, such as older adults. By mitigation of the loss of proprioception and balance that is typically associated with increasing age, such a two-pronged strategy can prevent the adverse consequences entailed in fall risk.

Thus, collaborative care plans incorporating these modalities can ensure not only that patients regain their health but that they also maintain functional autonomy (Barnard & Carpenter, 2024). Besides, emerging technologies and individualized rehabilitation programs have emerged to advance the processes of manual therapy and exercise integration. With innovations such as virtual reality and biofeedback systems, therapists can enhance the outcomes of therapeutic treatments. These technologies facilitate easier training of proprioceptive and balance functions, which are important for rehabilitation and recovery. Additionally, customized exercise programs according to the specific needs of the patient can optimize the outcomes of manual therapy. Professionals are instilled with the embracement of adopting a multi-professional model involving these innovations through inter-professional practice amongst experts in developing systematic treatment protocols beyond customary practices. These concerted efforts are required in managing changing orthopedic and physiotherapy conditions (Silumesii, 2025) (Figure 15.7).

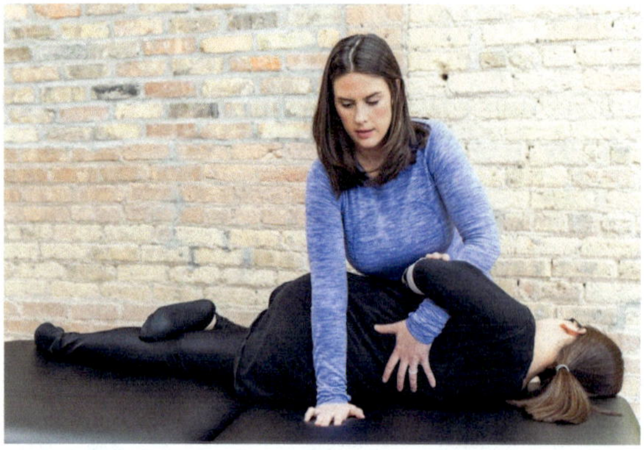

Figure 15.7. The integration of manual therapy and exercise.

Source: https://prepperformancecenter.com/wp-content/uploads/2022/03/prep_manultherapy.webp.

15.3. Regenerative Medicine in Orthopedics

Regenerative medicine has come a long way, particularly in orthopedics, where the limitations of traditional healing processes are being addressed using new technologies. Regenerative medicine tries to restore or replace damaged tissue and organs by using the body's own healing capabilities. This is especially pertinent in orthopedics, where trauma results in chronic pain and reduced functionality. Traditional repairs are usually only partially successful, and therefore inclusion of concepts of regeneration is essential. Employing methods that induce biological regeneration, such as stem cell therapy and novel biocompatible scaffolds, clinicians now achieve improved outcomes in tendon and joint repair. The enhanced healing potential afforded by these methods is resulting in more effective treatment protocols in orthopedic medicine. The latest advances in the use of bio-scaffolds provide the best evidence yet of the revolutionary influence that regenerative medicine is having on orthopedic practice. Scaffolds are three-dimensional structures that provide cell attachment and growth support, allowing functional tendon tissues to be regenerated. They are designed to be broken down naturally as the tissue repairs, providing a smooth integration with the host tissue. The current literature has identified the therapeutic potential of bio-scaffolds, demonstrating the ability to create an adequate environment for tendon regeneration. Despite the promising evidence, limitations remain, e.g., the necessity of wide-ranging studies to ascertain the best scaffold design and functional longevity. The knowledge of various biodegradable materials and their integration with cellular structures is the key to maximizing such scaffolding systems for application in clinical settings (Hafeez et al., 2021).

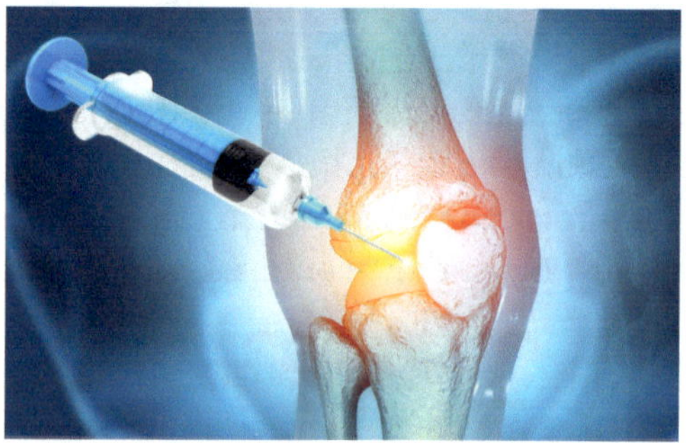

Figure 15.8. The field of regenerative medicine has made significant strides.

Source: https://www.caryortho.com/wp-content/uploads/2024/07/illustration-of-regenerative-orthopedics-knee-injection.png.

Moreover, the nanomedicine-tissue engineering interface is of enormous potential in regenerative medicine for orthopedic patients. With the incorporation of nanoparticles in therapeutic treatment, it is feasible to directly target the delivery of bioactive agents locally to the injured site, leading to faster healing and reduced inflammation. Using nanoparticles, local cellular response and scaffold integration can be enhanced and thus enable more efficient repair. The material sciences advancements are also coming up with innovations that improve the biocompatibility and functionality of such regenerative options. With ongoing growth in the demand for regenerative medicine, further research will be pivotal to addressing the complexities of tendon healing and joint rehabilitation. Multidisciplinary strategies combined will only increase the efficacy of treatment, which can be delivered to orthopedic patients (Richardson et al., 2018) (Figure 15.8).

15.3.1. Stem Cell Therapy for Joint Repair

Of late, orthopedic advances have turned to stem cell therapy as a promising procedure for joint reconstruction. Stem cells' ability to differentiate into several cell types, including chondrocytes and osteoblasts, makes them a significant tool in the healing of damaged joint tissues. Research indicates that mesenchymal stem cells (MSCs) can enable recovery of conditions like cartilage loss and rotator cuff injury that were previously untreatable.

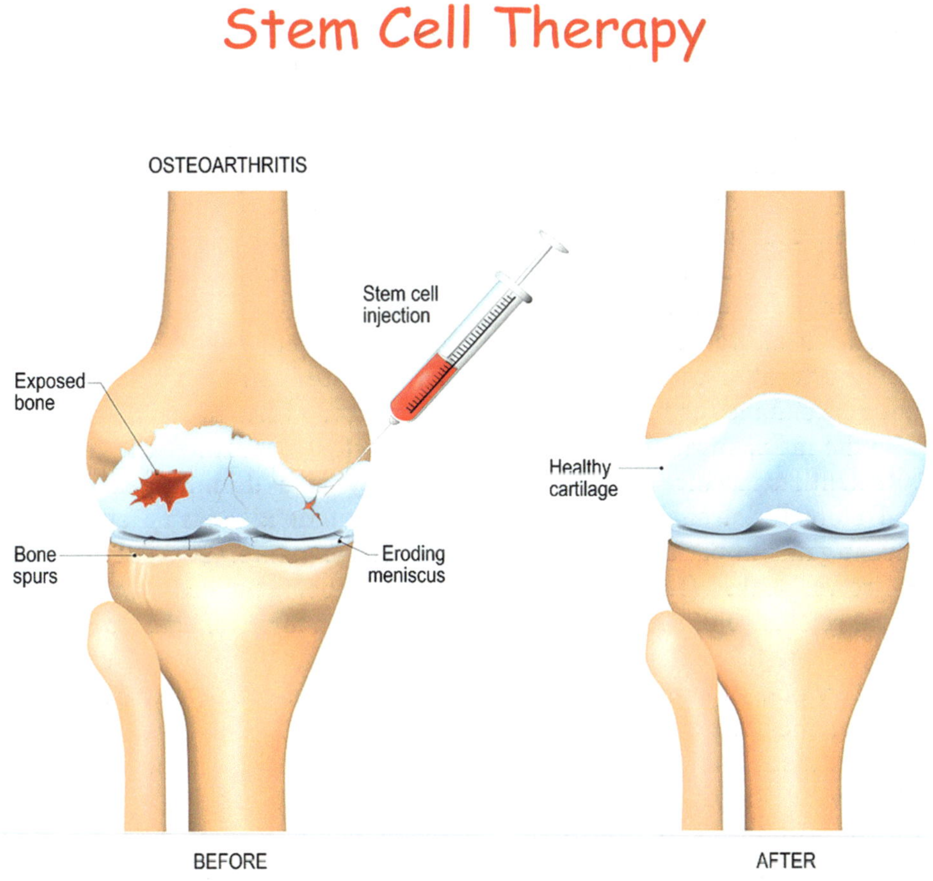

Figure 15.9. Stem cell therapy for joint repair.

Source: https://images.squarespace-cdn.com/content/v1/5b58b1cef8370aa14856d69c/1620239685176-HTRH043FSZWZY3QKPVW5/bigstock-Stem-Cell-Therapy-For-Pain-In-327218539.jpg.

The use of MSCs, especially in the scenario of rotator cuff reconstruction, holds promise to improve chronic pain and functional restoration by addressing the root cellular deficiencies pertaining to joint injuries. As discussed, increased understanding of joint pathophysiology and healing mechanisms is advancing the creation of personalized regenerative therapies, which will potentially supplant conventional surgical methods, creating better outcomes for patients and quality of life (Abdulwahab et al., 2017). Furthermore, the synergy between tissue engineering and stem cell therapy provides fertile soil for innovation in joint repair strategies. The development of scaffolds to allow cells to attach and grow is critical to enhance the therapeutic effects of stem cells in damaged tissues such as the meniscus and intervertebral discs. Fibrocartilaginous tissues of this type are likely damaged by accidents that cannot be treated effectively by conventional approaches. The use of stem cell therapy with advanced biomaterials has led to the creation of hybrid approaches that combine biological components with either synthetic or natural scaffolds for the reconstruction and restoration of joint integrity. The methods not only enhance cellular function but also replicate the mechanical properties of native tissue. As scientists advance methods for cell therapy and biomaterial engineering, the hope for significant gains in patient treatment in orthopedics grows clearer (Roberts et al., 2016). The clinical relevance of adopting stem cell therapy for joint repair extends beyond the transient restoration of function to the potential of altering the long-term trajectory of degenerative joint diseases. Current studies suggest that intervention early with MSCs may prevent progression of the arthritic joint degeneration and decrease the need for more invasive procedures such as joint fusion or replacement. Using minimally invasive techniques to deliver stem cells to the area of injury, doctors can treat specific damage without long downtime and accompanying complications of traditional surgeries. The promise unveiled by initial research has stimulated interest in standard protocols for the application of stem cell therapies to the treatment of a variety of joint conditions. As additional clinical trials continue to assess safety and effectiveness, the integration of stem cell therapy into conventional orthopedic intervention could transform therapeutic fashion, offering a regenerative and more holistic treatment of musculoskeletal well-being (Roberts et al., 2016; Abdulwahab et al., 2017) (Figure 15.9).

15.3.2. Platelet-Rich Plasma (PRP) Injections

Current advances in the application of Platelet-rich plasma (PRP) injections have drawn significant attention in orthopedics and physiotherapy. PRP is synthesized from a patient's own blood and contains a greater concentration of platelets, growth factors, and cytokines, which are critical to the healing and regeneration of tissues. Its application has been shown to be useful in the management of several musculoskeletal conditions, particularly chronic tendon injuries and osteoarthritis. As doctors turn to new, less invasive means to accelerate healing, the application of PRP therapy is a defining example of the shift towards individualized therapeutic approaches. The surge in interest is not unsubstantiated but rather is being fueled by an increasing empirical foundation for its efficacy to optimize functional recovery with fewer side effects compared to standard treatments. Comparative effectiveness of PRP injections with respect to corticosteroid injections has also been challenged to a great extent, particularly for disorders like lateral epicondylitis, or better known as tennis elbow. In randomized controlled trials, administration of PRP has proved more frequently superior in long-term benefits for pain improvement and functional gain compared to traditional corticosteroid therapy. For instance, in a particular study, it was found that while both corticosteroids and PRP effectively decrease symptoms in the short term, PRP significantly achieved greater improvements in patient-reported outcomes, such as the Visual Analog Scale (VAS) and Disabilities of the Arm, Shoulder, and Hand (DASH) scores. These findings underscore the therapeutic promise of PRP injections in chronic elbow pain and demand more research into protocols that could maximize its therapeutic promise (Ramanan, 2014). Despite the promising results, controversy regarding PRP therapy is not devoid of setbacks and disadvantages. Heterogeneity in preparation methods, platelet numbers, and injection techniques has a tendency to resist standardization of PRP treatment protocols. Moreover, considerations of cost-effectiveness and accessibility may affect its adoption in wide groups of clinical use. As more research is still discovering the optimal uses and enduring consequences of PRP injections, researchers and clinicians must remain critical in its adoption and use. Last, repeated clinical trials and systematic reviews are required to supply strict guidelines, thereby ensuring that patients receive effective evidence-based care in their recovery pathways, thereby solidifying PRPs place in present orthopedic and physiotherapeutic interventions (Singh & Gangwar, 2013) (Figure 15.10).

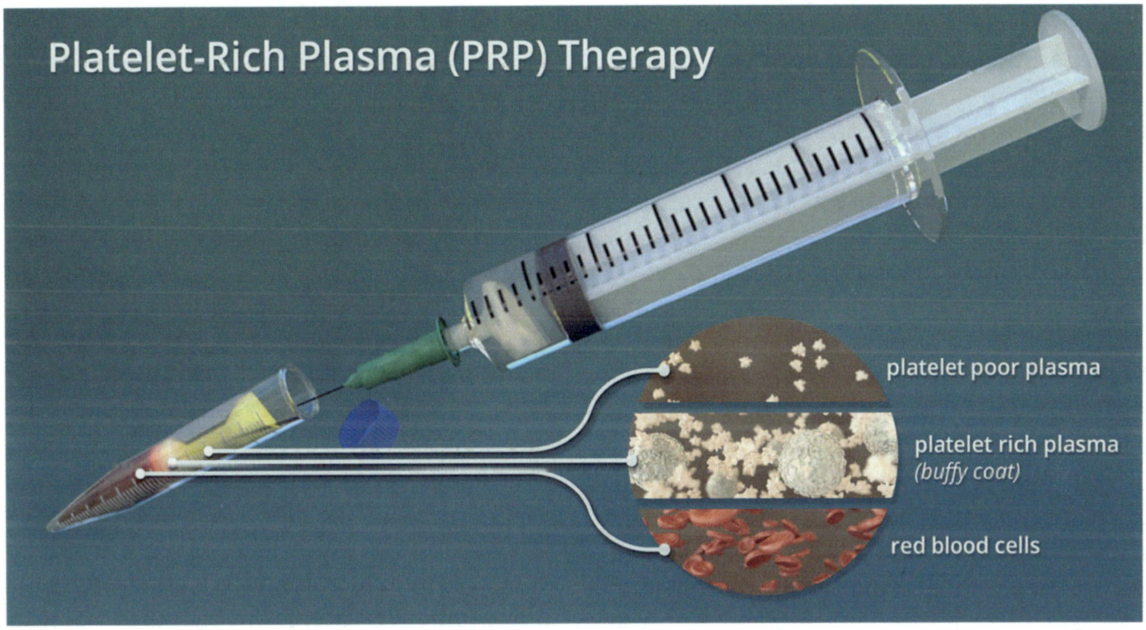

Figure 15.10. Platelet-rich plasma (PRP) injections.

Source: https://gopt.co/wp-content/uploads/2022/01/PRP-front-page.jpg.

15.3.3. Tissue Engineering for Cartilage Regeneration

Over the last decade or two, tissue engineering has come a long way, particularly in cartilage regeneration. Cartilage injury, especially within joints such as the knee and spine, poses enormous clinical challenges, leading to joint pain, swelling, and dysfunction. Conservative therapy and surgery are generally ineffective due to the cartilage's inherent avascular condition and lack of scope for self-repair. This has prompted researchers to search in new directions, and tissue engineering is offering possibilities for stimulating cartilage regeneration. By using cell therapy, growth factors, and biomaterials, a cartilage-promoting environment can be provided. Understanding the complex structure and biology of cartilage is crucial since it dictates how well engineering solutions will perform in terms of mimicking the composition and function of the native tissue. Among all the cartilages, the articular cartilage is unique because it has a role in keeping the joints healthy. Damage to the articular cartilage can lead to osteoarthritis, an inflammatory and degenerative joint disease with reduced joint function. Because of the cartilage's poor regenerative capability, the mesenchymal stem cells (MSCs) are a hot research topic for the field of tissue engineering. Recent studies indicate that MSCs possess the capability to differentiate into chondrocytes, the primary cartilage cells, and thereby modulate the repair and regeneration of damaged tissue. Advances in technology applied to the use of MSCs have broadened the reach of treatment, and refining cell delivery methods and scaffold architectures is of utmost significance. By using scaffolds with structural support in combination with appropriate biofunctional cues, scientists aim to direct cell behavior and enable proper cartilage regeneration to overcome the limitations of conventional treatment approaches (Fuentes-Mera et al., 2017). Furthermore, the use of new biomaterials and growth factors combined with MSCs represents a primary change in the cartilage tissue engineering paradigm. Scaffold materials, ranging from natural polymers to synthetic, play an important role in mimicking the extracellular matrix of cartilage for the attachment and function of cells. Techniques such as 3D bioprinting are now revolutionizing the design of scaffolds with the capability to manipulate the spatial distribution of cells and biomaterials to mimic the native cartilage architecture. Additionally, the incorporation of bioactive factors has also shown promise in promoting chondrogenesis and cartilage repair. Novel strategies that incorporate these elements promise not only functional repair but also long-term host integration of engineered tissue. Combined, these technologies are the new face of cartilage tissue engineering and its potential to revolutionize the clinical outcomes of physiotherapy and orthopedics (Roberts et al., 2016).

15.4. Pain Management Strategies

Incorporation of new strategies for pain management has been the thrust area in recent advances in orthopedics and physiotherapy. Effective management of pain, particularly in patients with chronic illnesses like hemophilia, where joint pain contributes significantly to the impact on quality of life. There is evidence to show that behavioral and psychological factors play an essential part in the control of joint pain associated with hemophilia. Interventions for enhancing self-management of pain might include the strengthening of pain evaluation, the construction of pain drug knowledge, and enacting pain acceptance. This multi-dimensional approach is not just targeted at reducing pain severity but also at maximizing physical and mental quality of life, suggesting that the integration of psychological and behavioral processes plays a central role in chronic pain management (Fuentes-Mera et al., 2017). Therefore, the use of evidence-based interventions for other chronic pain conditions could potentially lead to effective self-management strategies in haemophilia. Besides psychological management, pain measurement following some shoulder conditions, such as subacromial impingement syndrome (SAIS), emphasizes the importance of pain outcome measures for pain management interventions. The application of validated instruments—such as the McGill Pain Questionnaire and the Oxford Shoulder Score—provides a general template for measuring pain experience, functional capacity, and psychological function in patients. These tests reveal significant differences in pain experience and quality of life when contrasted with healthy controls. The inclusion of generic as well as shoulder-specific instruments provides a more sensitive understanding of a patient's condition and response to therapy. This approach emphasizes the need for customized management protocols that address the unique needs of SAIS patients in order to enhance an active collaboration between patients and healthcare professionals (Fuentes-Mera et al., 2016). Emerging technologies and techniques further add to the tale of pain management in orthopedics and physiotherapy. Virtual reality and biofeedback, for instance, have just started to demonstrate promising results in pain modulation, offering patients active, non-invasive options for pain relief.

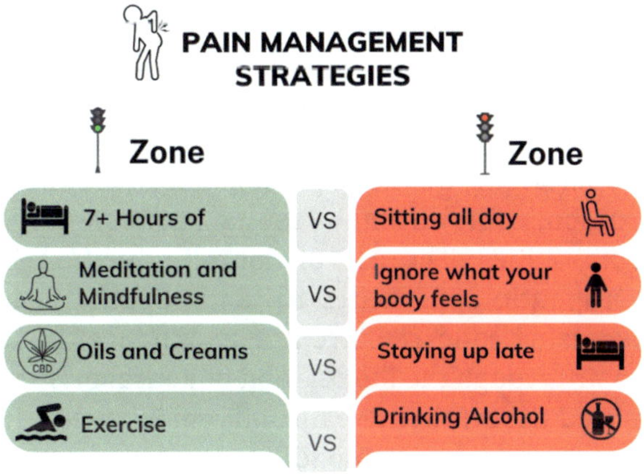

Figure 15.11. The integration of innovative pain management strategies.

Source: https://www.biaww.org/uploads/1/2/5/7/12574140/sessions-1-5-infographics1_orig.png.

Further, integrative treatment approaches such as functional exercise training and mindfulness-based interventions are gaining popularity for their capacity to facilitate greater acceptance and coping with pain. In designing such programs, clinicians attempt to develop patient-tailored pain management plans that address not just physical pain but also incorporate mental health services. Such integrated approaches can help augment enhanced self-efficacy and coping ability, empowering patients to handle pain better. Ultimately, these innovations not only contribute to the alleviation of pain but also enhance the general health and well-being of individuals who endure chronic conditions (Figure 15.11).

15.4.1. Multimodal Analgesia Approaches

Orthopedic and physiotherapy advancements have raised the focus on multimodal analgesia methods as a method of optimizing pain therapy. This multi-modal plan integrates a number of pharmacologic and non-pharmacologic methods individually discussed to cater to the requirements of each individual, to address pain from various directions. Traditional analgesics such as NSAIDs and acetaminophen can be supplemented effectively with adjuvant therapies that consist of regional anesthetic techniques and local anesthetic administration. These new approaches yield better pain control, prevent undesirable side effects, and improve postoperative recovery trajectories. The application of multimodal analgesia also promotes the use of tailored treatment in orthopedic centers. By considering patient-specific factors, including medical history, pain history, and surgery type, clinicians can design tailored analgesic plans to optimize outcomes. For instance, in total hip replacement surgery, the use of nerve block modalities together with systemic medications not only decreases postoperative pain severity but also enables earlier mobilization and rehabilitation interventions consistent with patient-centered care principles (Ferguson et al., 2018). This strategic overlap of functional restoration and pain management is a perfect example of how contemporary orthopedics is trending toward broader models of patient care. Beyond that, more recent studies have validated the efficacy of multimodal analgesia procedures in enhancing patient satisfaction and outcomes of recovery. With a multi-modal approach to pain management, patients exhibit significant reductions in pain scores, minimizing opioid dependence and hospital stay duration. Innovations such as the enhanced recovery after surgery (ERAS) protocols also point to the revolutionary nature of medical practices, as they seek to optimize the entire perioperative continuum (Pardeshi, 2023). The concerted effort on the part of medical professionals towards adopting the same points towards the paradigm shift in managing postoperative care. With ongoing research, the data for multimodal analgesia as the norm in orthopedic and physiotherapy treatment will change the face of pain management, bringing about improved patient outcomes and experiences (Figure 15.12).

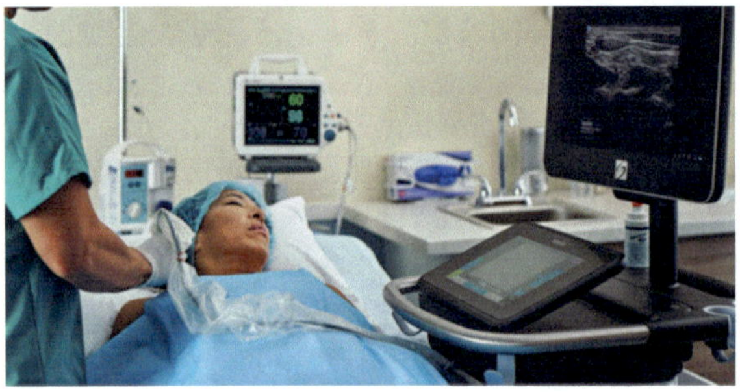

Figure 15.12. Multimodal analgesia approaches.

Source: https://www.sonosite.com/sites/default/files/styles/media_gallery_large/public/OpiodReduction_0.jpg?itok=N4yOK1Oy.

15.4.2. Neuromodulation Techniques

The evolving landscape of physiotherapy and orthopedics continues to validate the significance of using neuromodulation techniques in pain alleviation and rehabilitation outcomes. These techniques, by modulating nerve function with targeted intervention, are now pivotal in addressing chronic pain syndromes and musculoskeletal diseases. Several modalities of neuromodulation, like transcutaneous electrical nerve stimulation (TENS) and spinal cord stimulation, have become increasingly popular due to their non-invasive nature and the potential to improve the quality of life of patients. As healthcare professionals turn to alternative treatments rather than conventional pharmacological intervention, neuromodulation has become an acceptable alternative, with the additional benefit of twin effects on pain management as well as the ability to ease the rehabilitative processes involved for patients suffering musculoskeletal injury. Recent studies have revealed the relationship between the use of neuromodulation techniques and the severity of pathologies of the tendons, particularly in tendinopathy pathogenesis, a condition that affects a high percentage of the population. Tendons play a critical role in transmitting forces from muscles to bones and have maladaptive responses to mechanical loading, resulting in pain and disability. Therapies of tendinopathy range from conservative therapeutic approaches to operations, but need personalized treatment protocols for optimal results (Canosa-Carro et al., 2022). The use of neuromodulation in therapeutic approaches to tendinopathy is of increasing concern since it may enhance tissue repair through the modulation of neural drive to injured tissues, hence pain and rehabilitation. In cerebral palsy and complications, the application of neuromodulation has also shown promising outcomes. The conventional management normally entails orthopedic care, for example, braces and orthoses, to improve functional mobility among the affected individuals. Recent advancements have brought to the fore the role of neuromodulation procedures in supplementing the conventional modes by targeting certain neural pathways to facilitate improved coordination of muscles and reduced spasticity (Morris, 2002). The synergistic action of a combination of neuromodulation with physiotherapeutic training has the potential to optimize rehabilitation protocols, providing an integrated approach to management. With ongoing research in this field, future investigations will play a vital role in establishing the efficacy of neuromodulation techniques for orthopedic disorders, subsequently leading to more individualized and effective treatment strategies (Figure 15.13).

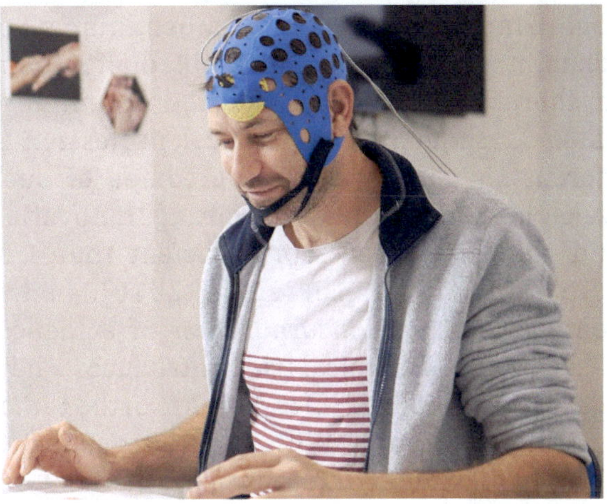

Figure 15.13. Neuromodulation techniques.

Source: https://ionclinics.com/wp-content/uploads/2024/02/1.jpg.

15.4.3. Role of Physiotherapy in Pain Management

Physiotherapy is a significant component of pain management in patients with musculoskeletal disorders and other musculoskeletal disorders. Current advancements in physiotherapeutic interventions aim at the combination of manual therapy, therapeutic exercises, and patient education, which collectively contribute to pain reduction and functional improvement. Through individualized rehabilitation plans, the physiotherapist assesses the unique characteristics of each patient and selects interventions to promote active engagement in the rehabilitation process. For instance, interventions such as dry needling and myofascial release can be directly targeted at areas of pain, minimizing pain and maximizing mobility. As evidence-based physiotherapy increases, the utilization of digital measurement tools to track patient progress is important in maximizing therapeutic input and outcomes. Such integration of therapy with patient response underscores the value of physiotherapy in creating a comprehensive pain management program that supports patient autonomy and overall well-being. With the development of orthobiologics, the use of physiotherapy in managing pain has found greater application, particularly in joint degeneration and injury. Condron et al. (2021) highlight how platelet-rich plasma and hyaluronic acid injections, among regenerative therapies, can be combined with physiotherapy to enhance tissue repair and minimize inflammation. This multi-modal therapy not only diminishes pain but also provides a more conducive platform for the body's own repair processes. Through cooperation with orthopedic specialists, physiotherapists formulate multidisciplinary treatment plans that integrate such biological therapy with rehabilitation exercises. Such cooperation between physiotherapy and orthobiologics has proven to be a powerful tool, maximizing patient outcomes while at the same time offering multifaceted pain management solutions. Interpreting the interaction of biological therapy and physiotherapeutic intervention is essential in formulating customized treatment regimens that optimize effectiveness and foster long-term recuperation. Moreover, since the incorporation of digital phenotyping, pain management has been handled differently by physiotherapy, as real-time data supplies information regarding the behavior of the patient as well as responses to interventions. Jayakumar et al. (2020) elaborate on the possibility of wearable device data being used to quantify activity level and track pain occurrence, such that one understands an individual patient's condition. With this technology, it is possible for physiotherapists to tailor treatment protocols according to objective measures, thus individualizing care to the unique needs of each individual. This not only assists in identifying patterns of contributing to chronic pain but also aids in patient engagement through self-tracking and feedback loops. As the practice develops with the advances of digital health technologies, physiotherapy continues to play a central role in pain management through the delivery of evidence-based interventions based on patient-centered care to bring about both instant pain relief and sustainable health gains.

15.5. Evidence-Based Research and Clinical Trials

The orthopedic and physiotherapy environment is significantly shaped by advances in evidence-based research and clinical trials that provide rigorous models for improving outcomes for patients. Evidence-based practice involves the integration of clinical judgment with the best available external clinical evidence from systematic research. Specifically, in orthopedic rehabilitation, this means using outcomes of randomized controlled trials and observation studies to inform treatment protocols and interventions. The evidence-based character of iterative research allows clinicians to adapt their techniques in accordance with the latest scientific discoveries so that interventions are not just effective, but also individually tailored to each patient's requirements. For instance, recent studies have underlined the importance of sets of outcome measures, as demonstrated with studies on balance interventions, which function to further solidify the connection between good research design and everyday clinical practice in orthopedics and physiotherapy (Sibley et al., 2015). In the context of clinical trials, the role of randomized controlled trials (RCTs) has been priceless to the confirmation of the efficacy of new therapies and interventions in orthopedics. The RCTs enable robust treatment comparison with variables controlled to isolate their effect to see the impact of specific interventions. RCTs also identify best practices by reducing biases that might mislead clinical judgment. The advent of modern technologies, including telemedicine and wearable technology, is also advancing the possibility of such trials. Trials involving such technologies have yielded information regarding postoperative mechanisms of rehabilitation, which has prompted alterations in therapy protocols supported by massive data. Consequently, the clinical profession is increasingly informed by outcomes of such well-planned studies, promoting innovation and providing safer, more efficient routes to cure for patients (Lee et al., 2016). In the coming years, the incorporation of evidence-based science in clinical trials introduces a new age of personalized medicine in orthopedics and physiotherapy. With regard to patient-centered outcomes, future research activity will increasingly put equal weight on both the safety and the acceptability of interventions from the patient's perspective and also their efficacy. This is being prompted by large databases and international collaborations that will strive to establish consensus about core outcome measures that are relevant to patients and practitioners alike.

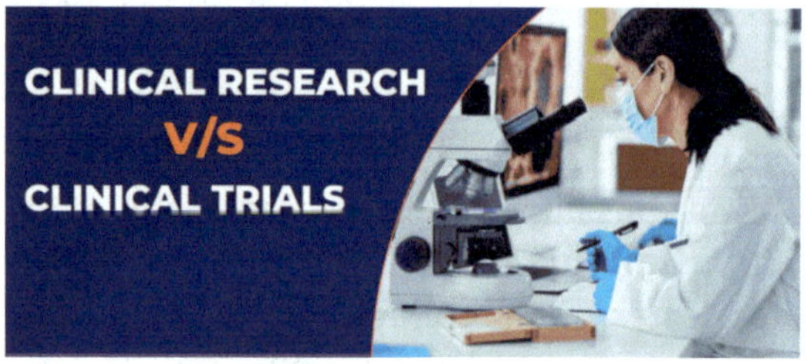

Figure 15.14. The landscape of orthopedics and physiotherapy.

Source: https://careerinpharma.com/wp-content/uploads/2025/04/Difference-between-Clinical-Research-and-Clinical-Trials-1-768x403-1.png.

Applying systematic approaches of identifying and validating these measures, as demonstrated in recent scoping reviews, can also result in effective knowledge translation to clinical practice. As there is more evidence, there is a greater ability on the part of practitioners to overcome rehabilitation challenges, ultimately resulting in improved functional recovery and quality of life for patients receiving treatment in the field (Sibley et al., 2015) (Figure 15.14).

15.5.1. Importance of Clinical Trials in Orthopedics

Clinical trials are an integral part of the development of orthopedic medicine, primarily through rational evaluation of new treatments, surgical methods, and rehabilitation protocols. Clinical trials allow for the comparison of new interventions against old standard practices, providing important information about efficacy and safety. In orthopedics, this is essential as it not only promotes innovation but also ensures that patients are being offered evidence-based interventions. Through hypothesis testing rigorously and analysis of findings, clinical trials play a crucial role in establishing best practice guidelines that contribute to effectively shortening recovery periods as well as patient satisfaction. Further, involvement of large populations in clinical trials leads to the identification of any treatment effect difference, allowing medical research to become inclusive and ensuring that findings are generally applicable across different groups. In recent years, the significance of evidence derived from clinical trials has been underscored by the emerging trend of personalized medicine in orthopedics. Personalized medicine personalizes interventions according to the distinct features of the patient, optimizing the impact of care. Clinical trials play a critical role in defining parameters that describe such personalized strategies, including maximum dose, timing of intervention, and target populations. With more orthopedic clinics adopting techniques like biophysical interventions and advanced surgery, it is increasingly necessary to look for robust clinical evidence. For instance, emerging evidence on pain management and psychological factors' impact on rehabilitation—comparable to that with illnesses like hemophilia—is reflective of an evolving perspective of patient need, seeking more coordinated treatment strategies (Elander, 2014). Through these multi-layered analyses, clinical trials pave the path to enhancing and validating effective treatments that enhance patient outcomes.

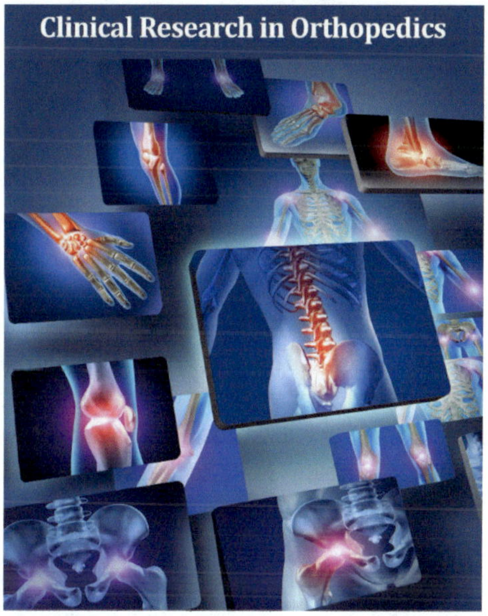

Figure 15.15. Importance of clinical trials in orthopedics.

Source: https://www.scitechnol.com/assets/img/flyer-images/Clinical-Research-in-Orthopedics-flyer.jpg.

Additionally, clinical trials seek to standardize measurement tools, which can be useful not only in research but also in the clinical setting of orthopedics. For example, developing a core outcome set (COS) for assessing standing balance stresses the importance of standardized measurement criteria for both intervention and outcome assessment. As has been recognized in recent research, the absence of standard instruments has hindered the synthesis of study data across studies, thereby limiting clinical practice development (Sibley et al., 2015). In an effort to offer more consistent assessment and comparison of treatments, trials seek consensus on effective measurement tools. Standardization not only assists in meeting the requirements of regulations but also in enhancing clinicians' faith in adopting new treatments. Lastly, clinical trials can also bridge the gap between implementation and development, advancing the front of orthopedics and physiotherapy (Figure 15.15).

15.5.2. Recent Studies on Physiotherapy Outcomes

Recent studies in physiotherapy outcomes have demonstrated profound enhancements in treatment efficiency, particularly in the rehabilitation of musculoskeletal trauma and postoperative recovery. Evidence-based practice has allowed physiotherapists to tailor their interventions more specifically to the patient, leading to improved functional outcomes and patient satisfaction. Research has established that individualized exercise programs and manual therapy techniques, when used systematically, can enhance mobility, reduce pain, and reduce healing time. Interestingly, with advances in primary healthcare systems, there is more focus on prevention and rehabilitation standards that ultimately further strengthen the role of physiotherapy as an integral part of the overall healthcare model. The incorporation of recent technology advancements also speaks for itself in terms of supporting these therapeutic activities, with technologies like telehealth and mobile apps being used to provide continuous support and monitoring of patient recovery (Baldacchino et al., 2014). Furthermore, meta-analyses and systematic reviews have also clarified the efficacy of some physiotherapy treatments, particularly in chronic disease management. For instance, studies on the rehabilitation of cerebral palsy have shown the importance of early intervention through targeted physiotherapy interventions. Some evidence supports that ankle-foot orthoses (AFOs) and other orthotics are effective in improving gait efficiency in children in Gross Motor Function Classification System (GMFCS) levels I through III, but the quality of evidence is low since most of the studies lack reporting strength and transparency in methodology. As such, the recent convention debates underscore the necessity of strictness in subsequent research, demanding standardized protocols and longer periods of follow-up to determine long-term results associated with such interventions (Morris et al., 2011). In addition to the standard physiotherapy parameters, recent studies are also examining the broader impact of these interventions on patients' quality of life and emotional well-being. Emerging literature highlights the interplay between physical rehabilitation, psychological health, and social rehabilitation, particularly for surgery or chronic pain patients. Physiotherapy is not limited to the physical recovery process; it encompasses patient teaching, self-management strategies, and psychosocial rehabilitation. Addressing such multifaceted variables makes physiotherapists key players in integrated patient care, ensuring optimal physical health as well as psychological resilience. This integrated approach is increasingly becoming clearer as an important element in helping patients manage the complexities of recovery in accordance with an emerging trend in the practice of physiotherapy towards integrative health approaches that target function and general welfare (Baldacchino et al., 2014).

15.5.3. Impact of Research on Treatment Guidelines

Research plays a crucial role in the development of treatment plans for orthopedics and physiotherapy. Clinical practice is dynamic, and evidence-based studies provide the foundation upon which practitioners develop more effective interventions. Evidence from such studies allows patient needs to be comprehensively understood, and tailored treatment methods are developed to enhance recovery rates. For instance, new evidence in multimorbidity and the application of advanced technologies in primary care have remarkably influenced the therapeutic approach. As discussed in Baldacchino et al. (2014), these innovations, in addition to improving the management of patients, interface with health equity and the measurement of outcomes. With these guidelines being updated based on new evidence coming to light, the improved care of patients is evidence that the provision of health services is dynamic and consistently aimed at improving the effectiveness of treatment. The conformity between interprofessional panels regarding treatment approaches is significant in guiding best practice for the treatment of complex diseases. For example, there has been a global consensus in the management of cerebral palsy that has presented several different interventions from physical and occupational therapy to orthotic and surgical interventions. While the majority of this evidence is robust, challenges are still encountered in enhancing the quality and transparency of evidence as presented in Morris et al. (2011). Particularly, the prohibitions against patient specificity and intervention design require continuous refinement of the research procedures used. This underscores the need for robust studies not just to confirm existing treatments but also to explore new treatments that can be tailored to meet the diverse requirements of patients, ultimately maximizing treatment guidelines. Translation of evidence into treatment guidelines is required to advance therapeutic protocols in physiotherapy and orthopedics. Research findings have revealed the utility of certain interventions—for instance, ankle-foot orthoses have been proven to enhance gait efficiency, and thus their application is advocated among targeted patient populations. However, that more research needs to be conducted cannot be overemphasized, as existing guidelines must maintain pace with emerging evidence. The present gap between high-level evidence of long-term efficacy of orthotic devices, as identified in Morris et al. (2011) provides an imperative need to pursue further research. Accordingly, the integration of new evidence into practice not only explains the treatment advice but also reinforces an environment of evidence-based medicine and ensures that patient care is at the forefront of physiotherapy and orthopedics clinical developments.

15.6. Interdisciplinary Collaboration

The collaboration of interdisciplinary teams is a more and more essential concept within the fields of orthopedics and physiotherapy due to the complexity of patient care that requires collective different expertise. The involvement is not only between physicians and physical therapists, but also that of health information professionals whose contribution is essential in the management of patient data and evidence-based practice advocacy. Through integrating these disciplines, medical practitioners can formulate more holistic treatment programs that consider the physical, psychological, and social needs of patients. For example, the evolving nature of healthcare technology enhances communications between specialists, which facilitates quicker decisions on patient interventions as well as methods of rehabilitation. Such cooperative systems are driven by shared emphasis on producing improved patient outcomes, thus constituting an engaged model of care that responds to the complexity of issues in modern healthcare. Interdisciplinary collaboration is not only critical in clinical practice but also for education and research within orthopedics and physiotherapy. University structures are currently embracing multidisciplinary training models in preparation to equip future practitioners to work together across various branches of medicine. This holistic education system imparts to learners the competence needed to engage in inter-professional communication with colleagues from other specialty backgrounds for a smooth transition from theory to practice. Along with this, inter-professional research attempts have also been initiated, welcoming teams of researchers to collaborate and exchange their knowledge and resources to solve advanced clinical questions. Interdisciplinary research attempts to aid in advancing the specialty as collective research findings may lead to more effective therapeutic methods and rehabilitation methodologies. Research has demonstrated that these combined approaches are more likely to generate more innovation and improved patient treatment outcomes, which are central to the ongoing progression of healthcare services. With further change within healthcare, the place of interdisciplinary practice will become increasingly prominent in orthopedics and physiotherapy. Patient-centered approaches underscore the importance of uninterrupted collaboration among healthcare professionals in addressing patients' entire needs.

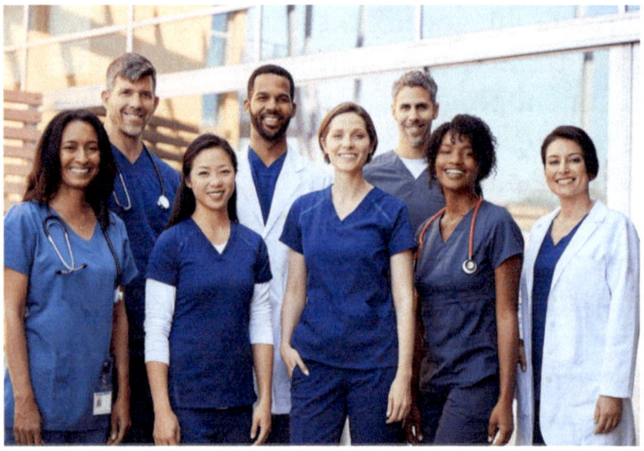

Figure 15.16. The concept of interdisciplinary collaboration.

Source: https://media.licdn.com/dms/image/v2/D4D12AQE6E4LN_3iuHw/article-cover_image-shrink_720_1280/article-cover_image-shrink_720_1280/0/1692194104118?e=2147483647&v=beta&t=hjJC9Q4XDQ4mFrtS3MDEt948qhM0LpD-6hmdeSPOeGI.

This shift in focus captures a broad definition of health that encompasses physical, emotional, and social well-being. Additionally, as technology continues to transform the way healthcare is delivered, the capacity of interdisciplinary teams to adapt becomes increasingly critical. Emphasizing shared knowledge and strategies, these collaborations foster an environment conducive to innovation, allowing for more personalized care solutions. Therefore, the convergence of diverse professionals along lines of treatment not only enhances the quality of care but also reflects the necessity for integration as a continuous process in driving the discipline towards better health outcomes for all, hence articulating an enormous call for thematic consistency in modern developments in healthcare (Kelly, 2009; Schmitt, 2022) (Figure 15.16).

15.6.1. Role of Orthopedic Surgeons and Physiotherapists

The role of orthopedic surgeons and physiotherapists in managing musculoskeletal disorders has become a new paradigm with the existing advancements in orthopedics and physiotherapy. The orthopedic surgeons have a primary function in diagnosing and surgically correcting structural deformities, including fractures, joint dysplasia, and spinal deformities. This empowerment empowers them with the practice of advanced surgical techniques that enhance recovery times and reduce complications, such as minimal intervention procedures or arthroscopic surgeries. With the evolution of the practice, surgeons increasingly rely on multimodal treatment approaches that integrate the services of physiotherapists to ensure effective patient results after surgery. Such collaboration ensures that professional integrity between both branches is necessary for the sustenance of a continuum of care that focuses on the surgical intervention and the rehabilitation process that follows. Physiotherapists are at the forefront of the rehabilitation aspect of orthopedic practice, with the aim of restoring function and quality of life for the patient. Recent developments in physiotherapy have seen the development of evidence-based treatment plans that are patient-centered, particularly post-surgery. For instance, physiotherapists utilize high-tech modalities such as dry needling, ultrasound therapy, and exercise prescription to manage pain and facilitate recovery. They are also vital in educating patients about their conditions and facilitating their ability to contribute to their own rehabilitation. Additionally, with the emphasis on functional recovery and early mobilization, physiotherapists collaborate closely with orthopedic surgeons so that rehabilitation protocols are aligned with operative objectives, thereby optimizing the overall efficiency of treatment protocols. Furthermore, the application of technology to both spheres highlights the dynamic nature of patient care. Innovations such as telehealth and wearable devices enhance the ability of physiotherapists to monitor progress and adapt interventions in real-time, particularly in emergency situations or where remote access to healthcare professionals exists. Similarly, the use of advanced imaging modalities in orthopedics helps surgeons to receive more accurate diagnoses and make proper treatment plans. For example, the combination of 3D printing technology helps in patient-specific implants. As well, more recent findings highlight the importance of developing referral guidelines, for example, in cases of rotator cuff damage, to enhance the effectiveness and appropriateness of surgery, acknowledging the interdependent role of orthopedic surgeons and physiotherapists with an integrated treatment approach (Griffiths, 2013; Haug, 2014).

15.6.2. Benefits of a Team Approach in Patient Care

The implementation of team practice in patients has revolutionized the clinical processes, particularly physiotherapy and orthopedics. Interdisciplinary care is characterized by the collective experience of the different healthcare providers, like surgeons, physiotherapists, occupational therapists, and nurses. Interdisciplinary practice yields integrative treatment plans reflecting the multifaceted needs of rehabilitation patients. These general approaches have the result of addressing every phase of a patient's recovery, from pain management to improvement in mobility, all at once. Patient outcome is enhanced according to evidence, suggesting that when multiple health professionals coordinate their work together, they shorten patients' recovery times and enhance patients' satisfaction and participation in their care processes. Technology and modern advancements further supplement the benefits of a team-based approach. For instance, the development of wearable technology and sensor-powered devices has provided healthcare teams with valuable tools for closely tracking patient recuperation. With the help of these technologies, medical practitioners and other healthcare providers can collaborate to track a patient's rehabilitative milestones, thereby facilitating real-time adjustment of treatment protocols when such is needed. As noted in current literature, their use in rehabilitation also allows for the ability of practitioners to witness in real-time the reaction of a patient, leading to more responsive and individualized care methods. Responsiveness is crucial in orthopedics and physiotherapy, where individualized treatment is critical in gaining optimal outcomes (Szabo et al., 2023). Additionally, the COVID-19 pandemic has recognized the value of new models of care, including telerehabilitation, encouraging greater collaboration in patient care. Remote therapy techniques have facilitated new ways of patient engagement without risking safety during health emergencies. Through the application of digital tools and online collaboration systems, multidisciplinary teams are able to provide remote support, fostering continuity of care in even restrictive environments. As has been highlighted by recent studies, the convergence of technological advancements, such as the use of digital twins for rehabilitation robots, emphasizes a paradigm shift in therapy delivery that is not only efficient but also customized to the individual needs and situation of each patient (Falkowski et al., 2023). Such a breakthrough in team approaches foretells a rosy future for the outcomes of patients in the fields of orthopedics and physiotherapy (Figure 15.17).

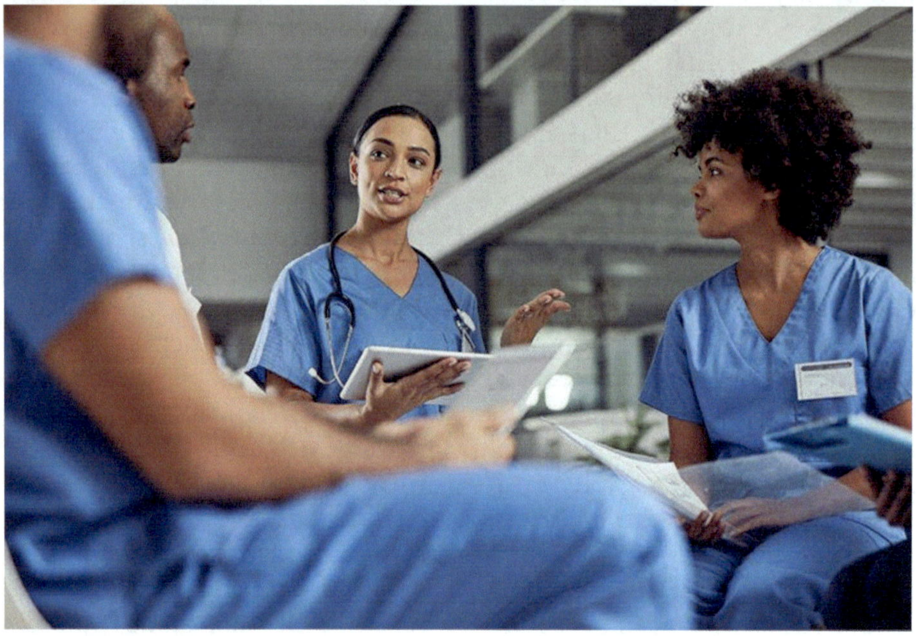

Figure 15.17. The implementation of a team approach in patient care.

Source: https://nursing.maryville.edu/blog/media_1b818676e4a45e1997114f6df03016af73c5872d5.jpeg?width=750&format=jpeg&optimize=medium.

15.6.3. Case Studies Showcasing Successful Collaboration

The culture of collaboration among physiotherapists and orthopedic practitioners has had a tremendous influence on the quality of treatment outcomes, as shown in a number of case studies. For instance, an international consensus conference hosted by the International Society for Prosthetics and Orthotics was employed to bring together a multidisciplinary panel of specialists who reviewed cerebral palsy care. The exercise of collaboration highlighted the importance of multidisciplinary research, revealing that successful interventions such as ankle-foot orthoses (AFOs) can significantly contribute to enhancing gait efficiency in children with mobility impairments. The discussion also stressed the importance of transparency and openness in study reporting, which ultimately contributes to improving clinical practice and guidelines. By bringing together knowledge from many professionals, the conference yielded practical recommendations for enhancing the effectiveness of orthotic treatment and identified areas of relevance to future research, thus showing productive collaboration in optimizing treatment methods (Morris et al., 2011).

Another celebrity instance of productive collaboration appears in a research study on Western Australian orthopedic surgeons' management of rotator cuff disease. The study enlightened how surgeons varied in surgical decision-making, reflecting a deficit in consensus concerning indications for operation and the utility of physical examination tests. Through sending a comprehensive anonymous questionnaire to regional surgeons, the researchers aimed to acquire knowledge about their attitudes, operative outcomes, and prognostic variables. The cooperative research emphasis drew attention to the shared goal of enhancing clinical practice by finding successful outcomes like pain relief and increased functional ability. This case also illustrates the need for collaborative expertise, coupled with the necessity of developing standard practices grounded in empirical proof, eventually creating consistency and better patient care in orthopedic surgery (Thorpe et al., 2017). Combining evidence from collaborative case studies in the treatment of cerebral palsy and rotator cuff surgery is proof of a broader shift throughout the orthopedics and physiotherapy professions toward interprofessional collaboration. By engaging experts from multiple specialties, these initiatives can create a comprehensive knowledge base that informs best practices and enhances patient outcomes. Sharing divergent perspectives encourages innovation and critical thinking, enabling practitioners to resolve complex clinical challenges with greater coherence. As seen through the collaborative work of the case studies presented, productive collaboration ultimately leads to bridging knowledge and practice divides and improving standards of care. This model of co-learning not only improves treatment modalities in patients but also contributes to the professional development of orthopedics and physiotherapy as professions (Morris et al., 2011; Thorpe et al., 2017).

SUMMARY

The exploration of recent advances in orthopedics and physiotherapy is characterized by both innovation and evidence gaps. The application of external fixation devices, though ubiquitous in management, entails a discrepancy in rehabilitation protocols across various clinical settings. A systematic review revealed that there existed a wide shortage of high-quality evidence to inform rehabilitation protocols in patients who employed these devices, and therefore, intense research is needed to establish effective strategies. This inconsistency can impact not just patient outcomes but also the validity of practice throughout the field. With the aim of optimizing recovery, it is imperative to close these gaps and establish a consistent approach on firm evidence (Pawson et al., 2024). The development of cryotherapy also reflects the need to evaluate new methods in orthopedic practice. Despite the emergence of devices with the aim of delivering sustained, stable temperatures for pain management following total knee arthroplasty (TKA), recent evidence shows that such technology may not possess significant benefits over conventional procedures. The systematic review did not find any obvious differences in the severity of pain or recovery from function when comparing continuous cryotherapy to conventional ice packs. Such evidence persuades healthcare practitioners to reassess the effectiveness and economic viability of new technologies to guarantee effective and cost-effective patient care (Liu et al., 2023). In conclusion, the contemporary body of orthopedics and physiotherapy literature emphasizes a critical necessity for continuous research and multidisciplinary collaboration between health practitioners. By prioritizing well-designed studies and encouraging innovative rehabilitation techniques, the science can pave the way for improved outcomes in recovery and increased patient satisfaction. Inconsistent findings on rehabilitation following external fixation and the efficacy of cryotherapy remind us that not all that moves is progressive. To successfully promote the field, combined efforts must ensure that the gap between innovation and practice is closed and clinical practice is guided by sound, empirical evidence (Liu et al., 2023; Pawson et al., 2024).

The history of orthopedics and physiotherapy has been marked by a series of milestone developments that have significantly advanced patient outcomes. The most sophisticated progress in orthopedics is the development of state-of-the-art surgical techniques, particularly minimally invasive treatments. The methods reduce recovery times, diminish scarring, and lower the risk of complications compared to traditional open surgery. These techniques have changed the management of such complicated musculoskeletal conditions, allowing the achievement of earlier rehabilitation and greater mobility. Thus, patients have a faster return to daily activities, particularly for patients with high lifestyle demands. Furthermore, advances in technology, such as MRI and CT scanning, have greatly improved diagnostic accuracy, helping practitioners develop tailored treatment plans that are individually aimed, leading to better management of orthopedic conditions. In parallel, physiotherapy has also dramatically improved, most notably with the introduction of evidence-based practices and advancing rehabilitation methods. The incorporation of technology, such as virtual reality and telehealth, has changed the way physiotherapy is delivered, making it accessible to patients in remote or underserved areas. Not only do they enhance communication, but they also enable practitioners to monitor progress in real-time. Professionalization of massage therapy, as discussed in the background, has further influenced the practice of physiotherapy significantly. As massage found its way into the medical practice in the late 19th century, it opened doors to contemporary rehabilitation procedures. The practice has developed an interdisciplinary procedure in which other therapies are incorporated to formulate complete rehabilitation plans to ensure that patients receive holistic care while undergoing the recovery process. Another field that is of utmost improvement is merging patient-centered care, which espouses the principles of inter-professional practice among patients and healthcare providers. This model has been one of really involving patients in decision-making regarding treatment plans. By developing a partnership model, practitioners foster patient compliance and satisfaction with rehabilitation programs. Moreover, the recognition of psychological aspects of recovery has facilitated interventions that address both the physical and emotional sides of healing. This combined strategy will aim to empower patients so that they are no longer mere passive receivers of treatment but active participants in their recovery. With advances continuing to be developed in orthopedics and physiotherapy, patient-centered care is set to inform future practice, involving more effective and compassionate treatment approaches that consider the individual's needs and circumstances (Pawson et al., 2024).

CLOSER LOOK

RECENT ADVANCES IN ORTHOPEDICS AND PHYSIOTHERAPY

Orthopedic medicine focuses on the diagnosis, treatment, and prevention of disorders of the musculoskeletal system, including bones, joints, muscles, ligaments, tendons, and nerves. It plays a vital role in restoring mobility, reducing pain, and improving the quality of life for patients of all ages. Advances in medical science have significantly transformed orthopedic care, making treatments more precise, effective, and patient-centered. Modern orthopedic medicine combines clinical examination, advanced imaging techniques such as X-rays, MRI, and CT scans, and laboratory investigations to accurately diagnose conditions. Common orthopedic problems include fractures, arthritis, osteoporosis, sports injuries, spinal disorders, and congenital deformities. Treatment approaches range from conservative methods, such as medication, physiotherapy, and lifestyle modifications, to surgical interventions like joint replacement, arthroscopy, and spinal surgery. Pharmacological management is an essential component of orthopedic care. Pain relievers, anti-inflammatory drugs, muscle relaxants, and supplements like calcium and vitamin D help manage symptoms and promote healing. In conditions such as rheumatoid arthritis, disease-modifying antirheumatic drugs (DMARDs) and biologic agents are used to control inflammation and prevent joint damage. Advances in regenerative medicine, including platelet-rich plasma (PRP) therapy and stem cell treatments, offer promising options for tissue repair and faster recovery. Rehabilitation and physiotherapy are equally important, focusing on restoring strength, flexibility, and function after injury or surgery. Personalized rehabilitation programs help patients regain independence and prevent future complications. Preventive strategies, such as ergonomic education, proper posture, and injury prevention programs, further enhance long-term musculoskeletal health.

REFERENCES

1. Abdulwahab, T. A., Bhangra, N., Jain, N. B., et al. (2017). Complete rotator cuff tear: An evidence-based conservative management approach. https://core.ac.uk/download/322432491.pdf (accessed on 26th June 2025).
2. Canosa-Carro, L., Bravo-Aguilar, M., Abuín-Porras, V., Almazán-Polo, J., García-Pérez-de-Sevilla, G., Rodríguez-Costa, I., López-López, D., Navarro-Flores, E., & Romero-Morales, C. (2022). Current understanding of the diagnosis and management of the tendinopathy: An update from the lab to the clinical practice. *Disease-a-month : DM*, *68*(10), 101314. https://doi.org/10.1016/j.disamonth.2021.101314(accessed on 26th June 2025).
3. Elander J. (2014). A review of evidence about behavioural and psychological aspects of chronic joint pain among people with haemophilia. *Haemophilia : the official journal of the World Federation of Hemophilia*, *20*(2), 168–175. https://doi.org/10.1111/hae.12291(accessed on 26th June 2025).
4. Thorpe, A., Hurworth, M., O'Sullivan, P., Mitchell, T., & Smith, A. (2017). Rotator cuff disease: opinion regarding surgical criteria and likely outcome. *ANZ journal of surgery*, *87*(4), 291–295. https://doi.org/10.1111/ans.13862(accessed on 26th June 2025).
5. Al Muderis, M. (2021). Osseointegration for amputees: Past, present and future: Basic science, innovations in surgical technique, implant design and rehabilitation strategies. https://core.ac.uk/download/534373910.pdf (accessed on 26th June 2025).
6. Esparza, W., Ramón Aladro-Gonzalvo, A., Baldeon, J., & Ortiz, S. (2019). Toward a Design of a Telerehabilitation Program for the Functional Recovery in Post-Hip Arthroplasty Patients. IntechOpen. doi: 10.5772/intechopen.85768(accessed on 26th June 2025).
7. Alizadehkhaiyat, O., Roebuck, M. M., Makki, A. T., & Frostick, S. P. (2017). Pain, functional disability, psychological status, and health-related quality of life in patients with subacromial impingement syndrome. *Cogent Medicine*, *4*(1). https://doi.org/10.1080/2331205X.2017.1406631(accessed on 26th June 2025).
8. Roberts et al. (2016). Tissue Engineering of Fibrocartilaginous Tissues: The Intervertebral Disc and the Meniscus. Reference Module in Biomedical Sciences, 321-329. https://doi.org/10.1016/B978-0-12-801238-3.99809-X. https://core.ac.uk/download/76978447.pdf (accessed on 26th June 2025).
9. Alonso-Rollán, S., Márquez-Sánchez, S., Carrera, A., Froes, I. M. S., & Blanco, J. F. (2024). Evaluation and refinement of elbow recovery in sports medicine using smart tracking technologies. *adcaij: Advances in Distributed Computing and Artificial Intelligence Journal*, *13*, e31939–e31939. https://doi.org/10.14201/adcaij.31939 (accessed on 26th June 2025).
10. Baldacchino, M., Bezzina, G., Sammut, M. R., Scerri, C., et al. (2014). A review of certain recent advances in primary healthcare. https://core.ac.uk/download/46603060.pdf (accessed on 26th June 2025).
11. Hafeez MN, d'Avanzo N, Russo V, et al. Tendon Tissue Repair in Prospective of Drug Delivery, Regenerative Medicines, and Innovative Bioscaffolds. *Stem Cells Int.* 2021;2021:1488829. Published 2021 Nov 16. doi:10.1155/2021/1488829(accessed on 26th June 2025).
12. Barnard, C. C., & Carpenter, E. (2024). A classification for medical and veterinary libraries. https://doi.org/10.56920/lshtmp-1 (accessed on 26th June 2025).

13. Morris C. (2002). A review of the efficacy of lower-limb orthoses used for cerebral palsy. *Developmental medicine and child neurology*, *44*(3), 205–211. https://doi.org/10.1017/s0012162201001943(accessed on 26th June 2025).

14. Morris, C., Bowers, R., Ross, K., Stevens, P., & Phillips, D. (2011). Orthotic management of cerebral palsy: recommendations from a consensus conference. *NeuroRehabilitation*, *28*(1), 37–46. https://doi.org/10.3233/NRE-2011-0630.pdf (accessed on 26th June 2025).

15. Fuentes-Mera, L., Camacho, A., Moncada-Saucedo, N. K., & Peña-Martínez, V. (2017). Current Applications of Mesenchymal Stem Cells for Cartilage Tissue Engineering. InTech. doi: 10.5772/intechopen.68172 (accessed on 26th June 2025).

16. Vera, M. D. F., Dávila, D. A. D., Valdés, C. A. J., Zambrano, K. N. M., Chimbo, N. de J. P., & Montero, F. G. S. (2024). 3D imaging techniques for the diagnosis and surgical planning of complex limb fractures: a systematic review. *International Journal of Research in Orthopaedics*, *11*(1), 178–185. https://doi.org/10.18203/issn.2455-4510.IntJResOrthop20243418(accessed on 26th June 2025).

17. Condron, N. B., Kester, B. S., Tokish, J. M., Zumstein, M. A., Gobezie, R., Scheibel, M., & Cole, B. J. (2021). Nonoperative and operative soft-tissue, cartilage, and bony regeneration and orthopedic biologics of the shoulder: An Ortho regeneration Network (ON) Foundation review. *Arthroscopy: The Journal of Arthroscopic and Related Surgery, 37*, 3200–3218. https://doi.org/10.1016/j.arthro.2021.06.033 (accessed on 26th June 2025).

18. Sleijser-Koehorst, M. L. S., Coppieters, M. W., Epping, R., Rooker, S., Verhagen, A. P., & Scholten-Peeters, G. G. M. (2021). Diagnostic accuracy of patient interview items and clinical tests for cervical radiculopathy. *Physiotherapy*, *111*, 74–82. https://doi.org/10.1016/j.physio.2020.07.007(accessed on 26th June 2025).

19. Shinde, S. B., Dalvi, S. K., & Shinde, R. V. (2023). Glenohumeral Translations in Overhead Workers with Sub-Acromial Impingement Syndrome: A Review. *International Journal of Occupational Safety and Health*, *13*(4), 548–559. https://doi.org/10.3126/ijosh.v13i4.51630(accessed on 26th June 2025).

20. Dias, N. K., & Sera, R. (2020). An assessment of the functional outcomes of patients undergoing early exercise physiotherapy following arthroscopic rotator cuff repair using the double-row suture bridge technique. *International Journal of Research in Orthopaedics*, *7*(1), 66–72. https://doi.org/10.18203/issn.2455-4510.IntJResOrthop20205562(accessed on 26th June 2025).

21. Falkowski, P., Osiak, T., Wilk, J., Prokopiuk, N., Leczkowski, B., Pilat, Z., & Rzymkowski, C. (2023). Study on the applicability of digital twins for home remote motor rehabilitation. *Sensors, 23*, 911–911. https://doi.org/10.3390/s23020911 (accessed on 26th June 2025).

22. Ferguson, R. J., Palmer, A. J., Taylor, A., Porter, M. L., Malchau, H., & Glyn-Jones, S. (2018). Hip replacement. *Lancet (London, England)*, *392*(10158), 1662–1671. https://doi.org/10.1016/S0140-6736(18)31777-X(accessed on 26th June 2025).

23. Singh A, Gangwar DS, Shekhar. Autologous Blood versus Corticosteroid Local Injection for Treatment of Lateral Epicondylosis: A Randomized Clinical Trial. Online J Health Allied Scs. 2013;12(2):11. Available at URL:http://www.ojhas.org/issue46/2013-2- 11.html (accessed on 26th June 2025).

24. Griffiths, S. (2013). Evaluating referral appropriateness in primary care extended scope physiotherapists through the development of referral criteria for rotator cuff tears. https://core.ac.uk/download/161888715.pdf (accessed on 26th June 2025).

25. Haug, L. (2014). Bruddbehandling i Malawi: Pasienters og fagfolks erfaringer med strekkbehandling. "Pasientene er nesten som fengslet i sykehusavdelingen." https://core.ac.uk/download/630806088.pdf (accessed on 26th June 2025).

26. Richardson, S. M., Kalamegam, G., Pushparaj, P. N., Matta, C., Memic, A., Khademhosseini, A., Mobasheri, R., Poletti, F. L., Hoyland, J. A., & Mobasheri, A. (2016). Mesenchymal stem cells in regenerative medicine: Focus on articular cartilage and intervertebral disc regeneration. *Methods (San Diego, Calif.)*, *99*, 69–80. https://doi.org/10.1016/j.ymeth.2015.09.015(accessed on 26th June 2025).

27. Jayakumar, P., Lin, E., Galea, V. P., Mathew, A. J., Panda, N., Vetter, I., & Haynes, A. B. (2020). Digital phenotyping and patient-generated health data for outcome measurement in surgical care: A scoping review. *Journal of Personalized Medicine, 10*, 282–282. https://doi.org/10.3390/jpm10040282 (accessed on 26th June 2025).

28. Kelly, K. (2009). Health science libraries: Future trends. https://core.ac.uk/download/pdf/60772733.pdf (accessed on 26th June 2025).

29. Paul Lee., et al. "Should We Treat Soft Tissue Injuries with Actovegin?". EC Orthopaedics 4.4 (2016): 600-604(accessed on 26th June 2025).

30. Liu, M., Tian, M., Luo, C., Wang, S., & Shao, L. (2023). Continuous cryotherapy vs. traditional cryotherapy after total knee arthroplasty: A systematic review and meta-analysis of randomized controlled trials. *Frontiers in Surgery, 9*. https://doi.org/10.3389/fsurg.2022.1073288 (accessed on 26th June 2025).

31. Nias, K. (2017). Negotiating intimacies: Gender, rehabilitation and the professionalization of massage in Britain, c.1880–1920. https://core.ac.uk/download/158354636.pdf (accessed on 26th June 2025).

32. Nkhata, L. A., & Mweshi, M. M. (2024). A retrospective review of postgraduate physiotherapy research at the University of Zambia. *Rehabilitation Advances in Developing Health Systems, 1*. https://doi.org/10.4102/radhs.v1i1.13 (accessed on 26th June 2025).

33. Pardeshi, C. Z., et al. (2023). Perioperative care innovations: Optimizing recovery and reducing complications in general surgery. https://core.ac.uk/download/596247492.pdf (accessed on 26th June 2025).

34. Pawson, J., Church, D., Fletcher, J., Wood, R. A., Hilton, C., Lloyd, J., Brien, J., et al. (2024). Rehabilitation techniques for adults undergoing external fixation treatment for lower limb reconstruction: A systematic review. *Strategies in Trauma and Limb Reconstruction, 19*, 45–55. https://doi.org/10.5005/jp-journals-10080-1609 (accessed on 26th June 2025).

35. Ramanan, N. S. (2014). Treatment of lateral epicondylitis with platelet rich plasma or corticosteroid injection: A short-term comparative study. https://core.ac.uk/download/235658624.pdf (accessed on 26th June 2025).

36. Reynolds, L. A., & Tansey, E. M. (2009). The development of sports medicine in twentieth-century Britain. https://core.ac.uk/download/30696172.pdf (accessed on 26th June 2025).

37. Schmitt, J. (2022). Rehabilitation/recovery journals. https://core.ac.uk/download/588619943.pdf (accessed on 26th June 2025).

38. Sibley, K. M., Howe, T., Lamb, S. E., Lord, S. R., Maki, B. E., Rose, D. J., Scott, V., Stathokostas, L., Straus, S. E., & Jaglal, S. B. (2015). Recommendations for a core outcome set for measuring

standing balance in adult populations: a consensus-based approach. *PloS one*, *10*(3), e0120568. https://doi.org/10.1371/journal.pone.0120568 (accessed on 26th June 2025).

39. Silumesii, L. (2025). Peripheral and central contributions to age-related proprioceptive decline, clinical implications and management. *Galore International Journal of Health Sciences and Research, 9*, 27–54. https://doi.org/10.52403/gijhsr.20240403 (accessed on 26th June 2025).

40. Sivhugwana, Innocentia (2022). Factors related with the functional outcome of patients who sustained tibial plateau fractures. Dissertation (MSc (Physiotherapy))--University of Pretoria, 2022. https://core.ac.uk/download/565849089.pdf

41. Szabo, D. A., Neagu, N., Teodorescu, S., Apostu, M., Predescu, C., Pârvu, C., & Veres, C. (2023). The role and importance of using sensor-based devices in medical rehabilitation: A literature review on the new therapeutic approaches. *Sensors, 23*, 8950. https://doi.org/10.3390/s23218950 (accessed on 26th June 2025).

42. Youssef, Y., De Wet, D., Back, D. A., & Scherer, J. (2024). Digitalization in orthopedics: A narrative review. *Frontiers in Surgery, 10*. https://doi.org/10.3389/fsurg.2023.1325423 (accessed on 26th June 2025).

INDEX

A

Acetabulum 79, 280
Achilles tendonitis 153, 156
Achilles tendon rupture (ATR) 394
ACL Injury Risk Estimation Quiz (ACL-IQ) 207, 218, 219
Active exercise patients 464
Acute care protocols 38
Acute–chronic workload ratio (ACWR) 38
Acute injuries 38, 39, 202, 204, 234
Acute medical management 6
Acute pain 35, 38, 40, 51, 64, 71, 77, 78, 107, 391, 404, 428, 453
Acute trauma 8, 35, 36, 39, 121, 123, 140, 142, 146, 165, 179, 234
Adaptive designs 374
Adolescent Idiopathic Scoliosis (AIS) 240, 253, 254
Adult population failing 44
Advanced-level interventions 78
Adverse drug reactions (ADRs) 282
Aerobic exercises 145, 385, 467
Age-adjusted evaluation 247
Age-dependent orthopedic diseases 139
Aging population 139, 141, 271, 277, 291, 293, 399
Ambroise Paré 3
American Cancer Society 335, 349, 359
Anesthetic techniques 278, 497
Aneurysmal bone cyst (ABC) 348
Ankle-foot orthoses (AFOs) 502, 506
Ankle sprain 40, 50, 53, 68, 107, 215, 222
Ankle sprains 65, 210, 222, 230
Ankylosing spondylitis (AS) 173
Anterior cruciate ligament (ACL) 204, 205, 207, 217, 250
Anterior cruciate ligament avulsion 70
Anterior talofibular ligament (ATFL) 213, 215
Antibiotic therapy 304, 306, 308, 311, 317, 318, 319, 323, 324, 329
Anti-inflammatory drugs 21, 43, 46, 51, 150, 190, 285, 462
Antimicrobial therapy 308, 309, 310, 316, 319
Aquatic exercise 386
Area under the curve (AUC) 215
Arthritis 7, 144, 146, 274, 275, 279, 308
Arthritis and joint disorders 7, 8
Arthroscopy 31, 138, 482
Artificial intelligence (AI) 25, 138, 486
as Open Reduction and Internal Fixation (ORIF) 122
Athlete welfare 202
Autoimmune disorder 139
Auto-inflammatory 144
Autologous chondrocyte implantation (ACI) 370

B

Back pain 39, 45, 67, 122, 145, 170, 173, 174, 175, 179, 185, 187, 453, 463, 464, 472, 479
Bacterial infections 244, 305, 312, 315
Bacterial Pathogens 311
Berg Balance Scale 269
Biofilm formation 310, 318
Biofilm-related infections 318
Biological annular repair techniques 174
Biological behaviors 335, 357
Biomechanical examination 208
Biomechanics 37, 43, 106, 107, 139, 157, 160, 165, 172, 179, 194, 207, 208, 217, 244, 374, 489
Biopsy 339, 345, 347, 348, 361, 364, 366
Bio-psychosocial intervention 287
Bio-scaffolds 492
Blood vessels 50, 86, 111, 117, 344
Body labor 56
Body's immune system 144, 353
Body surgery 371
Bone density drops 276
Bone fragility 238
Bone infections 304
Bone mineralization loss 276
Bone sarcomas 254, 264, 350
Bone structure 75, 83, 239, 346
Bone tumors 18, 249, 316, 336, 338, 339, 340, 341, 346, 348, 349, 350, 353, 357, 359
Botulinum toxin type A (BoNT-A) 4
Bursitis pain 157

C

Calcaneofibular ligament (CFL) 215
Cancer treatment-related operations 370
Candid dialogue 370
Cardiac surgeries 372
Cardiopulmonary exercise testing (CPET) 214
Cardiovascular disease 270, 276, 278, 284, 285, 373, 409
Casting 89
Celebrity instance 506
Central nervous system (CNS) 412, 413, 414, 415, 418, 428
Cerebral Palsy (CP) 425
Childhood growth 238
Children heal faster 239
Children's musculoskeletal conditions 253
Child's growth potential 241
Child's quality 235
Chosen therapeutic exercises 376
Chronic contusions 112
Chronic injury 40
Chronic low back pain 65, 453
Chronic musculoskeletal pain 4, 14, 31, 61, 322
Chronic neck pain (CNP) 159
Chronic pain syndromes 456, 458, 473, 498
Chronic problems 241
Chronic process 40
Chronic rehabilitation programs 86
Chronic spinal patients 170
Chronic Traumatic Encephalopathy (CTE) 208, 222, 223
Clinical observations 14
Clinical prediction rules (CPRs) 8, 16, 222
Cognitive appraisal 454
Cognitive impairment 271, 273, 276, 284, 289, 290, 421, 423, 424, 439
Cognitive worsening 277
Community environment 271
Complex Regional Pain Syndrome (CRPS) 458
Comprehensive assessment 175
Computational simulation 245
Computed tomography (CT) 187, 214, 280, 314, 316, 431
Conducive environment 143, 383
Congenital deformities 1, 237, 241, 242, 260
Congenital deformity 242
Conservative management 118, 122, 146, 153, 176, 177
Conservative management fails 19
Constructing resilience 393
Constructive environment 467
Contemporary treatment 354
Conventional antibiotic 317, 318
Conventional antibiotic therapies 317
Copy number variants (CNVs) 351

Core outcome set (COS) 501
Coronary artery bypass grafting (CABG) 372
Corrigendum 311
Craft interventions 4, 246
Cumulative neurotrauma 208
Customized rehabilitation 7, 377, 388, 425, 441, 485
Cutting-edge developments 202
Cyclooxygenase-2 (COX-2) 462
Cyclooxygenase enzymes 51

D

Data protection 472
Deep infections 306
Degenerative cervical myelopathy (DCM) 182
Delayed onset muscle soreness (DOMS) 52
Devastating malignancy 338
Diabetes mellitus 313
Diabetic patients 276, 307, 314
Diagnostic imaging 85, 210, 316, 334, 340, 345
Diagnostic imaging modalities 316
Dietary restriction 278
Digital video fluoroscopy (DVF) 172
Disastrous injuries 109
Disc disease 170, 171, 172, 173, 174, 175, 180, 184, 187, 191, 453, 479
Diverse clinical environments 380
Drastic repercussions 128
Dry needling 384, 407, 499, 505

E

Early Wound Healing Score (EHS) 117
Effective communication 37, 211, 212, 216, 234, 327, 353, 389
Effective interventions 114, 271
Effective palliative interventions 340
Effective pediatric orthopedic 236
Effective prevention and management 43, 81
Effective prevention strategies 56, 83
Elbow dislocations 72, 101
Elbow trauma 81
Elderly patients 80, 149, 268, 270, 271, 276, 278, 279, 280, 281, 282, 283, 284, 286, 287, 288, 289, 290, 291, 293, 295, 296, 299, 300, 342, 404
Electrical stimulation 3, 9, 24, 143, 152, 180, 190, 384, 386, 425, 461, 489
Embryological development 237, 238
Emergency department (ED) 273
Emotional stability 147
Empirical antibiotics 317
Empirical evidence 221, 303, 402, 508
Endurance athletes 204
Enhanced recovery after surgery (ERAS) 498
Enhanced Recovery After Surgery (ERAS) 449
Environmental factors 42, 80, 154, 180, 210, 305, 326, 336
Epiphyseal plates 238
Etiological conditions 152
Etiological factors 303
Etiology 5, 6, 37, 38, 42, 46, 80, 109, 111, 112, 152, 157, 158, 174, 178, 179, 180, 184, 185, 187, 205, 207, 208, 210, 243, 256, 284, 299, 303, 305, 309, 311, 324, 328, 336, 427, 444, 458
European Society of Cardiology (ESC) 370
Evidence-based programs 286
Evidence-based treatment 3, 221, 260, 505
Ewing sarcomas 338
Exacerbate symptoms 175
Exercise prescription 1, 9, 11, 124, 159, 385, 386, 409, 465, 505
Exercise Prescription 385
Exertional heat illnesses (EHI) 59
External anal sphincter (EAS) 106
External fixation (EF) 122

F

Falls and injuries 82
Fecal incontinence (FI) 105
Fetal development 241, 425
Fine-tuning interventions 357
Finger dislocation 78, 79
Fixed-dose combinations (FDCs) 288
Fluorescence 342
Foreign bodies 318
Formal rehabilitation processes 151
Fracture-associated infection (FRI) 315
Fracture immobilization 94

Fracture management 88
Fracture-related infections (FRI) 306, 328
Fractures 6, 41, 69, 70, 72, 73, 74, 75, 76, 84, 85, 88, 89, 99, 104, 133, 137, 140, 145, 148, 149, 158, 206, 241, 242, 271, 273, 287, 298
Frozen shoulder 5, 6, 7, 8, 11, 12, 15, 18, 22, 27, 30, 451, 460, 464, 477
Functional assessment tools 353
Functional autonomy 10, 96, 148, 236, 268, 452, 491
Functional testing 213

G

Game-changer 336
Gamma-aminobutyric acid (GABA) 418
Gastrointestinal hemorrhage 462
Gender distribution 341
Geriatric fracture programs (GFP) 273
Geriatric nutritional assessment 278
Geriatric orthopedic management 283
Geriatric orthopedic procedures 285
Geriatric orthopedics 267, 268, 269, 270, 271, 273, 274, 275, 276, 277, 278, 279, 280, 281, 282, 283, 284, 285, 286, 288, 289, 290, 291, 292, 293, 295, 296
Geriatric patients 264, 268, 269, 270, 273, 275, 277, 278, 279, 280, 282, 283, 285, 286, 288, 291, 294, 295, 298, 300
Glasgow Coma Scale 189
Glial fibrillary acidic protein (GFAP) 207
Good assessment 203
Good communication 162
Gross Motor Function Classification System (GM-FCS) 502
Gustilo-Anderson classification system 306

H

Harsh management 73
Heal effectively 95, 287
Healing process 1, 14, 18, 38, 42, 49, 55, 89, 95, 117, 118, 120, 122, 125, 151, 207, 219, 239, 260, 293, 371, 377, 381, 389, 393, 395, 414, 425, 459, 461, 487
Healthcare professionals 4, 10, 15, 24, 42, 51, 56, 57, 67, 70, 92, 138, 139, 154, 191, 218, 251, 253, 268, 288, 305, 307, 316, 327, 370, 378, 379, 380, 382, 386, 388, 389, 390, 399, 402, 418, 425, 441, 450, 469, 474, 483, 490, 497, 498, 504, 505
Healthcare system 13, 16, 18, 43, 276, 287, 306, 315, 322, 398, 402
Healthcare systems 27, 48, 83, 146, 149, 162, 193, 255, 273, 276, 321, 382, 389, 399, 402, 472
Healthcare treatment 116
Health professionals 141
Heat therapy 461
Hematogenous infections 306
Hemiarthroplasty (HA) 93
Hereditary multiple exostosis (HME) 139
Herniated discs 171, 174, 175, 176, 179, 180, 182, 184, 186, 187
Heterogeneity 252, 261
High-entropy alloys (HEAs) 75
High-intensity narrow-spectrum (HINS) 311
Hip arthroplasty 31, 93, 100, 102, 270, 278, 299, 321, 332
Hip dislocation 79, 80
Hip fractures 79, 85, 140, 270, 271, 273, 274, 276, 278, 281, 284, 287, 289, 295, 299, 300, 478
Hip fracture surgery 269, 290, 298
Hip hemiarthroplasty (HHA) 79
Hip replacement 33, 95, 100, 333, 488, 497
Home exercise programs (HEPs) 471
Hospital Anxiety and Depression Scale (HADS) 392
Human sports 37
Hyperglycemia 313

I

Imaging modalities 17, 46, 187
Imaging technology 48, 87, 182, 184, 213, 258, 336, 339, 438, 439, 484
Immediate postoperative prostheses (IPOP) 374
Immunosuppressive diseases 313
Inefficient hospital resources 287
Infection control 305
Inflammatory cytokines 45, 174, 324, 354
Inguinal disruption (ID) 117, 401
Injury mechanism 122

Injury mechanisms 85, 96, 203, 207, 222
Innovative eye-movement 203
International Skeletal Society 70
Intervertebral discs 39, 172, 173, 174, 175, 179, 182, 188, 464, 494
Intra-articular hyaluronic acid (IAHA) 275
Invasive treatments 19, 508
Ionizing radiation 17, 121, 215, 243

J

Joint cartilage 145
Joint degeneration 267, 270, 494, 499
Joint diseases 3, 7, 8, 494
Joint fluid 309
Joint function 25, 46, 78, 145, 147, 154, 157, 158, 162, 236, 270, 309, 460, 464, 496
Joint mechanics function 46
Juvenile idiopathic arthritis (JIA) 236

K

Kinesio Taping (KT) 53
Kinesiotherapy 468
King-Devick (KD) 213, 215
Knee laxity 120, 134

L

Lacerations 108, 109
Lateral epicondylalgia 142, 143, 167
Ligament sprain 116, 147
Limb deformity 234, 240
Limb-salvage reconstruction 339
Liposarcoma 341, 344
Long-term infections 304
Lower motor neuron (LMN) 413, 415, 420, 422, 428, 431, 436, 437, 438
Lower motor neurons (LMNs) 418, 425
Low-level laser therapy (LLLT) 53
Low-load blood flow restriction training (LLB-FRT) 375
Lumbar 68, 172, 174, 176, 177, 197, 453, 464, 465

M

Magnetically-controlled growing rod (MCGR) 243
Magnetic resonance imaging (MRI) 16, 47, 87, 119, 178, 188, 214, 280, 314, 316, 347, 431
Malignancy 149, 339, 344, 345, 346, 347
Malignant bone neoplasms 340
Malta's specialist geriatric medicine 287
Manual skills therapists 385
Manual therapy 10, 143, 155, 384, 385, 491
Manual therapy treatments 384
Mechanical stressors 175
Medial Tibial Stress Syndrome (MTSS) 115, 117, 131, 208, 210, 219
Medical practitioners 2, 8, 27, 48, 49, 61, 70, 107, 187, 189, 206, 214, 217, 219, 247, 282, 288, 304, 326, 421, 503, 505
Medical staff 217
Medical technology 1, 137, 339, 401
Medical treatment 202, 271, 346, 428
Mental health interaction 271
Mesenchymal stem cells (MSCs) 493, 496
Metabolic pathways 45
Metastatic bone disease diagnosis 339
Metastatic disease 338, 342
Metastatic disease control 338
Microbial agents causing infection 316
Microwave diathermy 2
mild traumatic brain injury (mTBI) 221
Mind sound resonance technique (MSRT) 142, 159
Mini Balance Evaluation Systems Test 269
Minimally Invasive Plate Osteosynthesis (MIPO) 122
Minimally invasive spinal surgery (MISS) 191
Minimally invasive surgery (MIS) 256, 291
Mitigate risk 127
Modern healthcare systems 2
Modified-Delphi procedures 304
Modulate patient-specific treatment plans 281
Multiaxial loading 77
Multi-dimensional function 10
Multidisciplinary coordination 375
Multidisciplinary management strategy 4, 356
Multifaceted conditions 70

Multi-faceted interventions 111
Multifilament knee injuries (MLKIs) 221
Multimodal interventions 37
Multimodal strategy 270
Multiple sclerosis (MS) 415, 418, 431, 432, 434, 438, 439
Muscle loss 276
Muscles 2, 4, 17, 22, 24, 36, 41, 43, 44, 46, 54, 56, 57, 87, 105, 106, 107, 108, 109, 111, 113, 115, 116, 118, 119, 120, 124, 126, 127, 128, 129, 137, 138, 142, 152, 153, 154, 157, 170, 172, 173, 176, 181, 206, 215, 216, 240, 245, 246, 278, 336, 384, 411, 412, 413, 415, 430, 431, 461, 465, 467, 498
Muscle tearing 108
Muscular disorders 195
Musculoskeletal disorders 3, 4, 5, 15, 16, 18, 19, 42, 43, 48, 53, 55, 59, 60, 61, 64, 67, 100, 129, 138, 139, 142, 145, 167, 170, 234, 235, 237, 241, 244, 245, 252, 255, 256, 259, 260, 261, 277, 279, 285, 286, 334, 453, 481, 482, 484, 491, 499, 504
Musculoskeletal health 3, 4, 21, 40, 42, 43, 44, 45, 61, 111, 115, 155, 233, 236, 239, 441, 483
Musculoskeletal injury 10, 35, 36, 37, 38, 39, 41, 44, 45, 46, 49, 51, 52, 53, 55, 56, 57, 59, 61, 62, 64, 71, 216, 462, 498
Musculoskeletal trauma 21, 35, 36, 39, 46, 47, 48, 49, 52, 53, 54, 55, 61, 70, 215, 245, 314, 502
Musculoskeletal Tumor Society Score 353
Musculoskeletal ultrasound (MSKUS) 53

N

National productivity 139
Natural stability 74
Neoadjuvant treatment modalities 357
Nerve impingement 87, 176, 188
Nerve Roots 174
Nervous System 412, 413, 414
Neurological disorders 184, 411, 412, 413, 414, 415, 416, 417, 418, 420, 424, 425, 428, 429, 432, 433, 434, 435, 436, 437, 438, 439, 440, 441, 442, 444, 445
Neurological examinations 188
Neurological illness 411, 424, 428
Neurological signs 184
Neurologic deficits 177
Neuromuscular disorders 4, 184, 199
Neuromuscular electrical stimulation (NMES) 24
Neurotransmitters like dopamine 418
Non-athletic populations 107
Non-operative methods 250
Non-operative spinal disorder management 190
Non-operative spinal disorder treatment 190
Non-physician clinicians 280
non-steroidal anti-inflammatory agents (NSAIDs) 386
Nonsteroidal anti-inflammatory medications (NSAIDs) 283
Non-surgery 283
Non-surgical management 20, 49, 75, 285
Novel combinations 359
Numeric Rating Scale (NRS) 456

O

Occupational hazards 44
Occupational health and safety (OSH) 44
Occupational therapists 382
Omega-3 fatty acids 49, 181
Oncology discipline 335
Optimal communication 288
Optimal healing 74, 90, 109, 111, 125
Optimal management plan 41, 79
Oral and maxillofacial injuries 108, 130, 135
Orthopedic 1, 3, 4, 5, 13, 14, 16, 25, 64, 68, 99, 101, 102, 103, 137, 139, 146, 164, 167, 230, 240, 241, 254, 255, 258, 259, 263, 269, 271, 272, 276, 278, 283, 287, 303, 304, 305, 306, 307, 310, 313, 314, 315, 317, 321, 333, 334, 404, 411, 449, 450, 460, 464, 465, 473, 474, 477, 478, 484, 497, 504
Orthopedic conditions 5, 138, 139, 140, 142, 143, 146, 147, 150, 154, 155, 157, 158, 159, 161, 162, 164, 165, 233, 237, 240, 241, 245, 247, 249, 250, 253, 254, 255, 256, 260, 267, 271, 272, 280, 295, 324, 450, 463, 474, 508
Orthopedic disorders 26, 137, 139, 142, 144, 146, 147, 158, 160, 162, 163, 164, 240, 276, 293, 322, 450, 460, 461, 465, 485, 499
Orthopedic geriatrics 273, 280

Orthopedic infection management 304, 305, 316
Orthopedic infections 244, 303, 304, 305, 306, 311, 312, 313, 314, 315, 316, 317, 318, 319, 320, 321, 323, 324, 325, 326, 327, 328, 334
Orthopedic patients 151, 254, 284, 286, 288, 295, 324, 457, 478, 492, 493
Orthopedics 1, 2, 4, 16, 19, 29, 64, 67, 103, 138, 142, 145, 146, 148, 149, 153, 154, 156, 157, 159, 161, 163, 164, 233, 234, 235, 252, 267, 268, 279, 290, 332, 481, 482, 485, 492, 501, 510
Orthopedics management plans 142
Orthopedics services 146
Orthopedic surgery 10, 14, 23, 32, 91, 99, 250, 255, 258, 276, 277, 279, 284, 293, 304, 305, 311, 319, 321, 327, 331, 371, 396, 411, 486, 487, 507
Orthopedic Trauma Association-Open Fracture Classification (OTA-OFC) 306
Oslo Sports Trauma Research Center Overuse Injury Questionnaire (OSTRC-O2) 209
Osteoarthritis 6, 7, 19, 83, 91, 133, 137, 139, 141, 142, 143, 144, 145, 146, 147, 148, 154, 155, 157, 158, 160, 164, 167, 168, 175, 270, 271, 274, 275, 300, 309, 365, 453, 460, 464, 465, 477, 494, 496
Osteomyelitis 235, 236, 241, 243, 244, 264, 305, 306, 307, 308, 315, 316, 323, 328, 333, 347, 365
Osteoporosis 83, 99, 135, 270, 272, 298, 340
Osteosarcoma 338

P

Pain management 10, 11, 14, 38, 39, 43, 44, 51, 64, 118, 130, 137, 138, 147, 150, 159, 165, 174, 182, 183, 184, 186, 192, 251, 273, 277, 285, 290, 299, 339, 340, 369, 374, 384, 386, 387, 391, 449, 450, 451, 453, 454, 455, 456, 457, 458, 459, 460, 461, 462, 463, 464, 465, 466, 467, 468, 469, 470, 471, 472, 473, 474, 475, 477, 478, 496, 497, 498, 499, 500, 501, 505, 508
Pain perception 46, 454
Pain relief 11, 39, 40, 43, 46, 52, 53, 74, 89, 93, 108, 118, 123, 138, 140, 154, 159, 187, 206, 270, 273, 340, 384, 386, 459, 461, 462, 465, 470, 472, 489, 497, 500, 507
Pain symptoms 247, 451
Palpation Methods 212
Parkinson's disease 181, 199, 415, 418, 421, 436, 438
Partial restoration 429
Particularly pediatric orthopedics 235
Patellar tendinopathy (PT) 21
Patellofemoral pain (PFP) 21
Pathology 6, 19, 21, 46, 47, 49, 114, 117, 143, 173, 176, 185, 187, 191, 194, 203, 245, 247, 256, 277, 285, 287, 295, 309, 336, 337, 340, 345, 349, 401, 431, 454, 455, 486
Pathophysiological mechanisms 307, 421
Patient assessments 13, 282
Patient care continuity 148
Patient compliance 396
Patient-controlled analgesia (PCA) 340
Patient education 2, 11, 53, 122, 124, 125, 143, 156, 162, 184, 185, 242, 269, 325, 326, 327, 370, 387, 388, 389, 390, 393, 398, 451, 452, 462, 463, 467, 468, 473, 479, 499
Patient engagement and treatment 160, 293
Patient motivation 377, 383, 396, 489
Patient satisfaction 2, 8, 14, 15, 22, 36, 49, 80, 139, 150, 156, 187, 192, 291, 295, 324, 382, 386, 387, 402, 412, 487, 497, 501, 502, 508
Patient-specific needs 336, 441
Patient's recovery process 287, 450
Patient's symptoms 211
Patient tolerance 357
Pedal pulses 308, 323
Pediatric orthopedic program 241
Pediatric orthopedics 233, 234, 235, 241, 252, 260
Pediatric patients 234, 253, 260
Pediatric population 238, 243
pediatric Toronto Extremity Salvage Score (pTESS) 254
Perioperative management 284
Peripheral nervous system (PNS) 412, 413, 414, 415, 428
Photoacoustic imaging (PAI) 121
Physeal injury 238
Physical activity 6, 8, 12, 44, 45, 83, 111, 113, 127, 140, 179, 185, 192, 237, 272, 278, 463, 467
Physical examination 18, 47, 48, 117, 119, 120, 186,

187, 211, 214, 247, 280, 378, 430, 437, 481, 507
Physical limitation 180
Physical rehabilitation 2, 6, 10, 12, 36, 39, 40, 49, 54, 55, 95, 118, 145, 147, 151, 183, 203, 225, 231, 244, 254, 292, 296, 373, 374, 380, 381, 382, 384, 390, 394, 396, 449, 455, 475, 491, 502
Physical symptoms 56, 159, 183, 185, 441
Physical therapists 49, 54, 95, 125, 126, 138, 158, 187, 219, 220, 250, 251, 255, 295, 373, 374, 380, 381, 382, 383, 404, 408, 412, 461, 466, 503
Physical therapy 1, 3, 12, 19, 24, 25, 39, 42, 43, 46, 49, 50, 52, 53, 54, 55, 71, 74, 79, 95, 106, 107, 108, 111, 118, 122, 124, 125, 130, 138, 145, 147, 150, 153, 154, 164, 171, 172, 176, 179, 183, 185, 189, 190, 193, 194, 237, 249, 250, 255, 270, 275, 283, 285, 286, 290, 370, 372, 375, 381, 383, 384, 386, 412, 441, 459, 461, 469, 473, 477, 483, 487
Physiological function 194, 287
Physiological mechanisms 453
Physiotherapeutic developments 484
Physiotherapeutic scoliosis-specific exercise (PSSE) 21
Physiotherapists 2, 4, 8, 9, 10, 11, 13, 14, 15, 16, 20, 22, 23, 25, 27, 30, 80, 91, 95, 139, 140, 141, 143, 147, 148, 151, 152, 153, 157, 158, 159, 162, 164, 165, 189, 205, 225, 235, 251, 256, 271, 386, 389, 400, 412, 414, 415, 416, 418, 420, 421, 424, 425, 438, 449, 450, 451, 453, 455, 456, 458, 459, 462, 467, 469, 470, 471, 473, 474, 475, 482, 483, 485, 488, 489, 499, 502, 504, 505, 506, 512
Physiotherapy 1, 2, 3, 4, 5, 6, 7, 8, 9, 10, 11, 12, 13, 14, 15, 16, 17, 18, 19, 20, 21, 22, 23, 24, 25, 27, 29, 31, 32, 33, 39, 49, 53, 81, 89, 91, 117, 140, 141, 142, 143, 144, 145, 146, 147, 148, 149, 150, 151, 152, 154, 155, 156, 157, 158, 159, 160, 161, 162, 163, 164, 168, 175, 177, 191, 192, 193, 199, 203, 207, 225, 230, 236, 265, 268, 283, 284, 301, 375, 383, 390, 395, 396, 398, 401, 402, 405, 409, 412, 413, 415, 416, 417, 418, 419, 423, 424, 425, 430, 431, 432, 434, 439, 441, 442, 447, 449, 450, 451, 452, 453, 454, 455, 456, 457, 458, 459, 460, 461, 462, 463, 464, 465, 466, 467, 468, 469, 470, 471, 472, 473, 474, 475, 479, 481, 482, 483, 484, 486, 487, 488, 489, 490, 491, 494, 496, 497, 498, 499, 500, 502, 503, 504, 505, 506, 507, 508, 509, 510, 512, 513, 514
Physiotherapy interventions 6, 143, 145, 147, 152, 164, 430, 502
Plain radiography 316
Plantar fasciitis 8, 15
Platelet-rich plasma (PRP) 25, 106, 118, 191, 494, 495
Point-of-care ultrasound (POCUS) 216
Polyvinyl alcohol (PVA) 40
Positron emission tomography (PET) 347
Post-burn patients 393
Posterior spinal fusion (PSF) 170, 177
Post-intensive care syndrome (PICS) 381
Postmenopausal women 83, 99
Postoperative care 325, 326
Postoperative discomfort 256, 283
Postoperative experiences 290
Postoperative management 326
Post-operative pain 386, 391
Post-operative phase 325, 373, 374
Postoperative rehabilitation 191, 251, 370, 371, 377, 378, 380, 383, 384, 385, 386, 387, 391, 397, 398, 399, 401, 478, 486, 491
Post-reduction therapy 93
Post-surgical infections 318
Potential disinfection 311
Preoperative assessments 90, 216, 277, 325, 350
Preoperative measures 325
Preoperative planning 138, 185, 257, 258, 290, 353, 483, 486, 487
Pre-rehabilitation assessment 377, 378
Preventing recurrence 116, 312
Primary management 88
Primitive neuroectodermal cells 338
Procalcitonin (PCT) 324
Professional education and training 12
Prognosis 356, 357
Prognostic scenario 358
Prompt intervention 8
Prophylactic interventions 311
Propionibacterium acnes 310, 317, 331
Prosthetic joint infection 319
Prosthetic joint replacement surgery 310

Prosthetic Osseointegration for Limbs (PEPOL) 487
Psychological and emotional support 236
Psychological assistance 275
Psychological dimensions 55
Psychosocial healing 269

R

Radiation therapy 339, 348, 350, 351, 352, 354, 355, 359
Radiographic assessment 280
Randomized controlled trials (RCTs) 500
Range of motion (ROM) 118
Real-time feedback 19, 216, 290, 379, 393, 397, 459, 485, 490
Reduce waiting times 146
Regenerative medicine 4, 25, 39, 190, 191, 256, 258, 492, 493, 513
Rehabilitation 11, 31, 38, 41, 49, 52, 64, 68, 71, 89, 91, 93, 95, 96, 106, 124, 138, 148, 150, 162, 165, 192, 198, 203, 222, 229, 244, 251, 270, 286, 300, 364, 369, 371, 372, 373, 374, 375, 376, 377, 379, 383, 390, 392, 393, 395, 397, 399, 401, 404, 408, 409, 414, 418, 421, 422, 429, 435, 460, 464, 468, 478, 489, 513
Rehabilitation standards compliance 370
Rehabilitative function 147
Repetitive motion injury 115
Repetitive movements 42, 46, 113, 115, 209
Repetitive stress 6, 38, 43, 69, 73, 172, 202, 206, 210
Repetitive tendon stress 39
Responsive management approach 247
Responsive physiotherapy 2
Retrospective examination 72
Return-to-play (RTP) 218, 224
Reverse shoulder arthroplasty (RSA) 78
Revolutionary transformation 399
Rhabdomyosarcoma 344, 351, 356, 366
Rheumatoid arthritis 7, 137, 139, 145, 146, 158, 159, 164
Rheumatoid arthritis (RA) 144
Robust knowledge 314
Rotator cuff related shoulder pain (RCRSP) 13
Routine evaluation techniques 378

S

Sarcoma patients 335, 355, 357, 364
Self-confidence 370
Self-esteem 254, 286
Semi-automated systems 9, 27
Septic arthritis 305, 306, 308, 309, 315, 332
Short Bowel Syndrome (SBS) 372
Shoulder dislocation 77, 78
Shoulder joint 5, 101, 118, 489
Slip under stress 76
Social care 276
Social contact 278
Social participation 278
Soft tissue injury 75, 87, 105, 106, 107, 108, 109, 111, 113, 114, 115, 116, 117, 118, 119, 121, 123, 124, 125, 126, 127, 128, 129, 130, 131, 133, 148, 215, 321
Soft tissue manipulation 143, 162
Soft tissue repair 52
Soft tissue sarcomas 349, 350, 354, 355, 357, 358, 359, 366
Soft tissue trauma 70, 110, 113, 119, 120, 121, 125
Spatial quantitative systems pharmacology (spQSP) 355
Specific imaging biomarkers 341
Specific patient populations 286, 473
Spinal anatomy 172, 173
Spinal canal 175, 177, 182, 187
Spinal cord injury (SCI) 415, 418, 422, 432, 434, 438, 440
Spinal deformities 17, 21, 178, 194, 243, 504
Spinal disease 171, 173, 174, 179, 181, 184, 185, 194
Spinal disorders 169, 170, 171, 172, 173, 174, 175, 176, 178, 179, 180, 181, 182, 183, 184, 185, 186, 187, 188, 189, 190, 191, 192, 193, 194, 195
Spinal elements 453
Spinal flexibility 173
Spinal fusion procedures 310
Spinal musculature 249
Spinal stenosis 170, 171, 174, 177, 178, 179, 180, 182, 184, 185, 186, 188, 190, 191, 194
Spiral fractures 6, 73, 75
Sport injury 43
Sports activities 110, 111, 113, 402

Sports and exercise medicine (SEM) 160
Sports injury management 160, 214, 219, 221
Sport-specific movements 38
Sports physicians 218
Sports-Related Injuries 43, 81
Staphylococcus aureus 331
Strains 108, 111, 206
Stress fractures 6, 38, 70, 73, 81, 115, 148, 161, 202, 206, 207
Subacromial impingement syndrome (SAIS) 496
Sufficient nutrition 277
superior labral anterior-posterior (SLAP) 47
surface electromyography (sEMG) 450, 453, 460, 471
Surgical excision 345, 353, 354
Surgical intervention 17, 21, 39, 41, 48, 49, 52, 73, 77, 89, 96, 109, 125, 126, 138, 146, 179, 182, 221, 247, 250, 268, 278, 280, 283, 285, 308, 309, 319, 323, 329, 347, 381, 401, 407, 464, 483, 504
Surgical interventions 21, 88, 90, 91, 125, 126, 174, 191, 192, 285, 349, 350, 395
Surgical patients 95, 138, 305, 307, 374, 375, 401, 406
Surgical site infections (SSIs) 304, 310, 319, 321, 324
Surgical therapy 348
Surgical trauma 78, 255, 312, 314
Surgical treatment 20, 52, 85, 90, 99, 186, 189, 191, 221, 251, 261, 274, 283, 312, 313, 317, 319, 349, 376, 380, 391, 471
Surgical treatment materials 85
Symptomatic adult spinal deformity (SASD) 178, 194
Synovial sarcoma 344
Systematic method 126
Systemic inflammatory response syndrome (SIRS) 324

T

Tackling 158, 299, 394
Target-oriented interventions 375
Tearing ligaments 38
Telehealth facilitates 282
Tendon healing capacity 39
Therapeutic choice 289
Therapeutic decision-making 211
Therapeutic interventions 19, 22, 38, 49, 106, 157, 158, 175, 192, 221, 225, 244, 284, 315, 324, 328, 341, 344, 347, 370, 374, 378, 386, 415, 418, 425, 426, 439, 453, 458
Titanium elastic nailing (TENS) 249
Total hip arthroplasty (THA) 93
Totalistic recovery process 390
Total knee replacement (TKR) 162, 300
Traditional infection-management techniques 311
Traditional rehabilitation 384, 397, 489
Transcutaneous electrical nerve stimulation 2, 11, 498
Transtibial amputation (TTA) 380
Traumatic injury 77, 81, 83, 312, 414
Treat existing infections 310
Tumor biology 336, 337, 344, 347, 349, 350
Tumor diagnosis 336, 339, 348, 361
Tumor malignancy 342
Tumor pathophysiology 336
Tumor's biological profile 339

U

Ulnar Collateral Ligament Reconstruction (UCLR) 372, 376
Ultrasound imaging (USI) 16
Upper motor neuron (UMN) 413, 415, 420, 422, 425, 428, 431, 436, 437, 438

V

Vacuum-assisted closure (VAC) 320
Vascular response 117
Vertebrae anatomy 173
Video-assisted thoracoscopic surgery 291
Virtual health technologies 482
Virtual reality (VR) 24, 151, 160, 400, 489
Visual Analog Scale (VAS) 456, 495
Visual Analogue Scale (VAS) 216, 292
Visual examination 212
Vital significance 107

Volumetric muscle loss (VML) 40
Vulnerable population 234, 252, 274, 284

W

Weight-bearing joints 139, 140, 145, 271
Western Ontario and McMaster Universities Osteoarthritis Index (WOMAC) 216
Whiplash Associated Disorders (WAD) 205
World Health Organization 272, 294
Wrist extension movements 142

X

X-linked hypophosphatemia (XLH) 4, 450
X-ray imaging 215, 220
X-rays 3, 17, 46, 47, 71, 85, 87, 120, 121, 186, 187, 215, 246, 339, 345

Y

Yasunori Suematsu demonstrates 385
Yellow discharge 315
Younger patients 7, 149, 234, 258